SENSATION AND MEASUREMENT

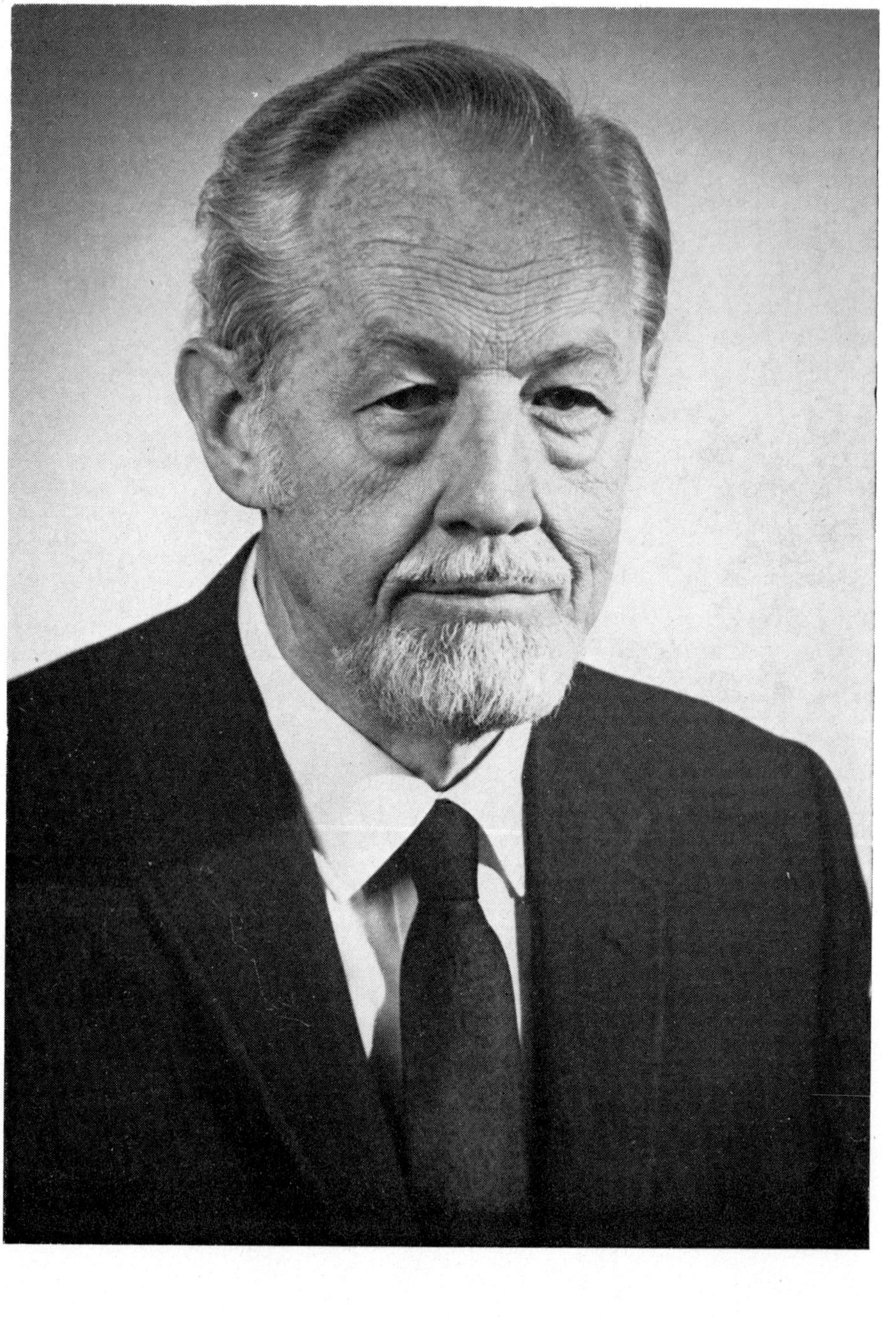

S S Stevens

SENSATION AND MEASUREMENT

Papers in Honor of S. S. Stevens

Edited by

HOWARD R. MOSKOWITZ

U.S. Army Natick Laboratories, Natick, Mass., U.S.A.

and

BERTRAM SCHARF

Northeastern University, Boston, Mass., U.S.A.

and

JOSEPH C. STEVENS

John B. Pierce Foundation Laboratory and Yale University, New Haven, Conn., U.S.A.

D. REIDEL PUBLISHING COMPANY

DORDRECHT-HOLLAND / BOSTON-U.S.A.

Library of Congress Catalog Card Number 74–77966

ISBN 90 277 0474 0

Published by D. Reidel Publishing Company,
P.O. Box 17, Dordrecht, Holland

Sold and distributed in the U.S.A., Canada, and Mexico
by D. Reidel Publishing Company, Inc.
306 Dartmouth Street, Boston,
Mass. 02116, U.S.A.

Printed in The Netherlands by D. Reidel, Dordrecht

TABLE OF CONTENTS

PART III / VISION, TASTE, WARMTH

PART IV / A BRIEF AUTOBIOGRAPHY

PREFACE

We planned this book as a Festschrift for Smitty Stevens because we thought he might be retiring around 1974, although we knew very well that only death or deep illness would stop Smitty from doing science. Death came suddenly, unexpectedly – after a full day of skiing at Vail, Colorado on the annual trip with wife Didi to the Winter Conference on Brain Research. Smitty liked winter conferences near ski resorts and often tried to get us other psychophysicists to organize one.

Every person is unique. Smitty would have said it's mainly because each of us has so many genes that two combinations just alike would be well-nigh impossible. But most of us strive in many ways to be like others, and to abide by the norms (some smaller number try even harder to be unlike other people); as a result many persons seem to lose their uniqueness, their individuality. Not Smitty. He tried neither to be like others nor to be different. He took himself as he found himself, and ascribed peculiarities, strengths, and weaknesses to his pioneering Utah forebears, in whom he took much pride. His was the true and right nonconformity. He approached each task, each problem, ready to grapple with the facts and set them into meaningful order. And if the answer he came up with was different from everyone else's, well that was too bad. Smitty was responsible only to what the facts told him, and he labored long and hard to get straight what the data were trying to tell him – whether data on the loudness function or brightness adaptation or scales of measurement or the neural quantum or somatotypes or the ups and downs of the stock market or the optimal length of skis.

In his last years, Smitty took to riding a bike from his home on Francis Avenue the half mile or so to the Laboratory of Psychophysics in Harvard's William James Hall. He rode a woman's bike, no horizontal bar, because it was easier getting on and off, and because he had ascertained that he didn't need the support provided by that extra bar with the high-carbon steel of today's bike frames. And so no wonder that when Smitty made psychophysics his field, he challenged the superfluous and the obvious, the traditional and the accepted, and went on to carve out a whole new branch of science involving the scaling of sensation magnitude, and so became the father of modern psychophysics.

Under Smitty's guidance, psychophysics became a broad-based, far-reaching discipline that reflected his own wide range of interests. Those interests appear in the nature of this volume's contributions, even though the forty papers are arbitrarily squeezed into only three categories: scaling and sensory physiology, hearing and speech, and vision and other senses. But the categories hardly do justice to the scope of their contents, for there are articles about evoked potentials, single-unit recordings, the scaling of opinions and attitudes, as well as about loudness and brightness, the neural quantum, and the sweetness of sugars. Thus closely intertwined with the man it memorializes, this collection of papers speaks to a variety of readers. To students and professors, specialists and generalists. To sensory psychologists and physiologists, to workers in psychological scaling and measurement, and to those scientists of an historical bent who will see the volume as a culmination of a forty-year period in the history of psychology during which Smitty Stevens revived psychophysics, gave it a new aspect and rigor, and made it once again a vital part of the study of man.

Having opened this book, you are likely already to know something about Smitty Stevens. His autobiographical Notes for a Life Story and his bibliography, which come at the end of the book, will tell you more. So, we think, will the papers here printed in his honor, for they are the products of some of the students and colleagues whom Smitty taught and worked with during his forty years at Harvard.

Boston and New Haven,
February 1974

HOWARD R. MOSKOWITZ,
BERTRAM SCHARF,
JOSEPH C. STEVENS

ACKNOWLEDGMENTS

The editors thank Geraldine Stevens for her valuable advice and assistance in connection with many aspects of this volume dedicated to the memory of her husband. We also wish to acknowledge the unusually close cooperation accorded us by all the contributors.

For permission to use previously published materials we thank the American Psychological Association for the papers by Georg von Békésy and Wendell Garner; Audiology for the paper by James P. Egan; the British Psychological Society for the paper by Robert J. Irwin and A. William Mills; John Wiley and Sons, Inc. for the chapter by William J. McGill; and the Clinical Psychology Publishing Company for the contribution by William H. Sheldon. We are also grateful to Geraldine Stevens and Prentice-Hall, Inc. for permission to include 'Notes for a Life Story' by S. S. Stevens.

H.R.M.
B.S.
J.C.S.

LIST OF CONTRIBUTORS

(The dates in parentheses indicate when the contributor was student, colleague, or long-term visitor at Harvard, working closely with S. S. Stevens during part or all of that period.)

Georg von Békésy (deceased), Professor of Sensory Sciences, Laboratory of Sensory Sciences, University of Hawaii (1947–1966)

David V. Cross, Professor of Psychology, State University of New York, Stony Brook, New York 11790 (1965–1972)

Hallowell Davis, Director of Research Emeritus, Central Institute for the Deaf, 818 South Euclid, St. Louis, Missouri 63110 (1934–1946)

William E. Dawson, Assistant Professor of Psychology, University of Notre Dame, Notre Dame, Indiana 46556 (1963–1969)

A. Leonard Diamond, Professor of Psychology, Simon Fraser University, Burnaby 2, British Columbia, Canada (1963–1964)

James P. Egan, Professor of Psychology, Mezes Hall 211, The University of Texas at Austin, Austin, Texas 78712 (1940–1947)

Hannes Eisler, Senior Research Fellow, Psychological Laboratory, University of Stockholm, Box 6706, S-113 85 Stockholm, Sweden (1960–1961)

Gordon Flottorp, Physicist, The Institute of Audiology, University of Oslo, Oslo, Norway (1950–1952; 1956)

Robert Galambos, Professor of Neurosciences, University of California, San Diego, La Jolla, California 92037 (1947–1951)

Eugene Galanter, Professor of Psychology, Columbia University, New York, New York 10027 (1955–1956)

Wendell R. Garner, James Rowland Angell Professor of Psychology, Yale University, New Haven, Connecticut 06510 (1942–1945)

Julius Goldstein, Professor of Electrical Engineering, Tel-Aviv University, Ramat-Aviv, Tel-Aviv 69978, Israel (1966–1968)

David M. Green, Professor of Psychophysics, Harvard University, Cambridge, Massachusetts 02138 (Coauthor of the article contributed by R. Duncan Luce.)

Donald D. Greenwood, Associate Professor, Division of Audiology and Speech Sciences, University of British Columbia, Vancouver, British Columbia, Canada (1956–1960)

Roland Harper, Leverhulme Senior Fellow, Department of Food Science, University of Reading, Reading, RG1 5AQ, England (1962)

Rhona P. Hellman, Senior Research Assistant, Laboratory of Psychophysics, William James Hall, Harvard University, Cambridge, Massachusetts 02138 (1967–1973)

Ira J. Hirsh, Professor of Psychology, Washington University and Director of Research, Central Institute for the Deaf, St. Louis, Missouri 63110 (1946–1951)

Davis H. Howes, Research Professor of Neurology (Neuropsychology), Boston University School of Medicine and Boston Veterans Administration Hospital, 150 South Huntington Avenue, Boston, Massachusetts 02130 (1946–1951)

Tarow Indow, Professor of Psychology, Keio University, Mita, Minato-ku, Tokyo, Japan 108 (1963–1966; 1972)

R. J. Irwin, Professor of Psychology, University of Auckland, Auckland, New Zealand (Coauthor of the article contributed by A. William Mills.)

Karl D. Kryter, Director, Sensory Sciences Research Council, Stanford Research Institute, Menlo Park, California 94025 (1943–1946)

Edwin H. Land, President and Director of Research, Polaroid Corporation, Cambridge, Massachusetts 02139 (1966–1973)

Harlan Lane, Professor and Chairman, Department of Psychology, Northeastern University, Boston, Massachusetts 02115 (1958–1960)

R. Duncan Luce, Professor of Social Science, School of Social Science, University of California, Irvine, Irvine, California 92664 (1957–1959)

Richard J. W. Mansfield, Assistant Professor of Psychology, Harvard University, Cambridge, Massachusetts 02138 (1966–1970; 1972–1973)

Lawrence E. Marks, Associate Fellow, John B. Pierce Foundation Laboratory, and Assistant Professor of Environmental Physiology and Research Associate in Psychology, Yale University, New Haven, Connecticut 06519 (1962–1965)

William J. McGill, President, Columbia University, Room 202 Low Library, Columbia University, New York, New York 10027 (1949–1953)

George A. Miller, Professor, The Rockefeller University, New York, New York 10021 (1942–1951; 1955–1968)

A. William Mills, Associate Professor of Psychology, Tufts University, Medford, Massachusetts 02155 (1952–1955; 1957–1959)

Howard R. Moskowitz, Research Psychologist, U.S. Army Natick Laboratories, Natick, Massachusetts 01760 (1965–1969)

Edwin B. Newman, Professor of Psychology, Harvard University, Cambridge, Massachusetts 02138 (1932–1937; 1943–1973)

Irwin Pollack, Professor of Psychology, Mental Health Research Institute, University of Michigan, Ann Arbor, Michigan 48103 (1945–1949)

Patricia Pliner, Erindale College, University of Toronto, Toronto, Canada (Coauthor of the article contributed by Eugene Galanter.)

Bertram Scharf, Professor of Psychology, Northeastern University, Boston, Massachusetts 02115 (1955–1958)

William H. Sheldon, Clinical Professor of Medicine Emeritus, University of Oregon Medical School, Portland, Oregon 97201 (1938–1943)

Esther M. Smith, University of Hawaii, Honolulu, Hawaii (Coauthor of the article contributed by A. Leonard Diamond)

Joseph C. Stevens, Fellow, John B. Pierce Foundation Laboratory, and Research Associate and Lecturer in Psychology, Yale University, New Haven, Connecticut 06519 (1953–1966)

Charles F. Stromeyer, Postdoctoral Fellow, Department of Psychology, Stanford University, Stanford, California 94305 (1964–1969)

Martha Teghtsoonian, Research Associate, Department of Psychology, Smith College, Northampton, Massachusetts 01060 (1955–1957; 1969)

Robert Teghtsoonian, Professor of Psychology, Smith College, Northampton, Massachusetts 01060 (1955–1957; 1969)

A. P. van Teslaar, Associate Professor of French, New York University, and Director, New York University in France, 9, Avenue Franklin-Roosevelt, 75008 Paris, France (Coauthor of the article contributed by Harlan Lane.)

John Volkmann, Professor of Psychology Emeritus, Mount Holyoke College, South Hadley, Massachusetts 01075 (1931–1937; 1942–1945)

W. Dixon Ward, Director, Hearing Research Laboratory, University of Minnesota, Minneapolis, Minnesota 55455 (1949–1953)

Eberhard Zwicker, Professor and Director, Institut für Elektroakustik, Technische Universität München, Arcisstr. 21, 8 München 2, Germany (1956)

Jozef J. Zwislocki, Professor and Director, Institute for Sensory Research, Syracuse University, Syracuse, New York 13210 (1951–1957)

PART I

PSYCHOPHYSICS, MEASUREMENT, SENSORY PHYSIOLOGY

SIMILARITIES OF INHIBITION IN THE DIFFERENT SENSE ORGANS[1,2]

GEORG VON BÉKÉSY[3]

University of Hawaii

I would like to show in the following text the scientific framework of observations that made me interested in inhibition. Since I worked for many years in telephone engineering, the input and output system as represented in Figure 1 was, at that time, the basis of all my thinking. It is almost an electrical model of the causality principle. Unfortunately, the simple input-output model does not hold for many situations. For instance, the sound of a speaker is reflected from all the walls of a room and the listener hears two types of sounds, first the direct sounds representing the simple input-output system, and then the reflections from the walls. To localize the speaker correctly, all the reflected sounds coming from the walls have to be suppressed. I would like to call this suppression inhibition.

Inhibition is not new. By looking at Greek statues, it is obvious that sculptors realized that it is impossible to contract all the muscles simultaneously. During movement, when one muscle is contracted its opponent is always relaxed. The relaxed muscle is the one that is inhibited by the nervous system. If we stimulate electrically both muscles simultaneously, we do not move, but have a cramp. If we look at Roman copies of Greek statues, we may feel that something is wrong and misunderstood. My impression was that the Roman copies did not understand the principle of in-

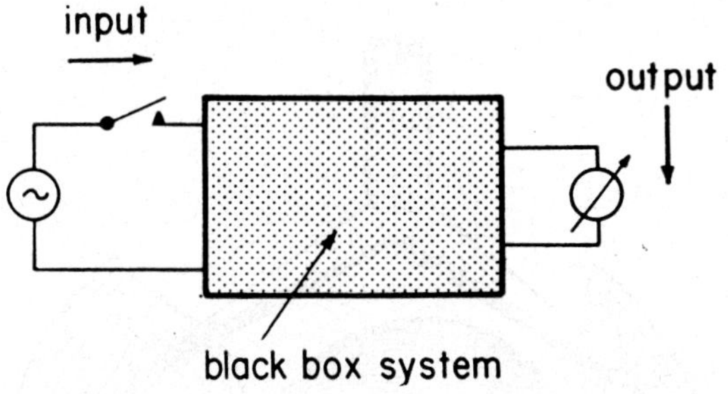

Fig. 1. The input-output system. (The electrical analogy of the causality principle.)

[1] Invited lecture presented at the meeting of the American Psychological Association, September 1, 1968, in San Francisco. The research was supported in part by the American Otological Society Grant M-14, the National Science Foundation Grant GB-5768, and the National Institute of Health Grant NB-06890.

[2] Reprinted from *American Psychologist* Vol. 24, No. 8, August 1969, pp. 707–719.

[3] Prior to his death in June 1972, Professor von Békésy dedicated this paper to S. S. Stevens for the Festschrift then being planned. The original article contained no abstract; the editors decided not to attempt to write one, since the article's title and Professor von Békésy's reputation provide adequate notice to the reader of the article's contents.

H. R. Moskowitz et al. (eds.), Sensation and Measurement. 3–21.

hibition so they represented in action large groups of muscles, contracted, which is physiologically not possible. Therefore, some muscles seem to stand out as bulges on the wrong place. It is this misunderstanding of the inhibitory process during movements that makes the Roman statues somehow unreal.

In the early Renaissance, there was no interest in the human figure. Leonardo da Vinci was the first to study anatomy, but he was so involved in anatomy that he represented most of the muscles in a completely relaxed status. There is no stimulation, and there is no inhibition whatsoever. Therefore, most of his drawings and most of his paintings look flat and really represent half-dead people. The famous Mona Lisa painting shows the fascinating smile of a cadaver. This is one of the reasons why, during the Renaissance, most of the pictures showed no dynamics. In the later period, the muscles were put in action. But again, there was no discrimination between inhibited muscles and excited muscles. Many of the statues, especially the very much admired Hercules, looked, according to Cellini (the most famous goldsmith), like sacks of potatoes.

However, Eustachius, who lived from 1515 until 1574, had a new theory. His theory was that at any place that there is a joint, there has to be a muscle. I had the impression that in his later years, he found that to every joint, two muscles were attached. It was his pupil Varolius (1543–1575) who discovered in this way the stapedius muscle of the middle ear, because there was a joint between the incus and the stapes. In my opinion, the discovery of the stapedius muscle, which is the smallest muscle in the human body, is an important discovery predicted by a theory.

I would like to call the law, that every joint is connected with a muscle, the Law of Eustachius. It is the first law in anatomy. We need many other laws of exactly that type that are able to integrate our views on anatomy and that lead to new discoveries.

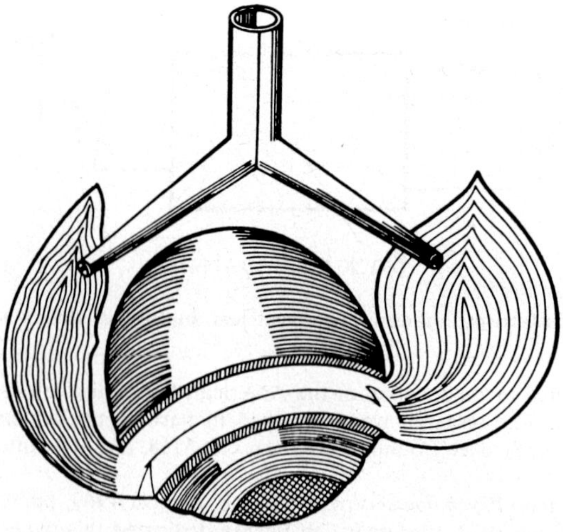

Fig. 2. Eyeball with the two muscles to rotate them. The muscle on the right side is contracted, the muscle on the left side relaxed. In this situation, the eyeball is rotated counterclockwise. The upper part in the drawing represents the nerve supply. (After Descartes.)

The first scientist who clearly described muscle activity was Descartes (1677). As can be seen from Figure 2, he shows for the rotation of the eyeball two muscles, one of them is excited and the other one is inhibited and flat. It was evident to him that the only way to produce a rotation of the eyeball is to have this interaction between the two muscles, so that when one muscle is excited and contracted, at the same time his companion is inhibited and relaxed. This holds for every degree of freedom. There is a little too much seventeenth-century hydraulics in Figure 2. The muscles do not change their volume that much during contraction and the nerve tracks are not like pipe lines.

In the nineteenth and twentieth centuries, inhibition was well known. I would like to quote here Hering's (1878) theory of color vision, which is based on the assumption that there are groups of colors, which mutually inhibit each other. The work of Sherrington (1947) and Eccles (1957) is very well known, and lateral inhibition in vision was mainly described by Hartline (1949) and Ratliff (1965). Central inhibition was discovered early by the Russian scientist Sechenov (1935).

It is the discrimination between central inhibition and lateral inhibition that clarified many facts we know today. The difference can be best illustrated by some examples. It is a well-known fact that a miller hears the noise of the grinding with a very much reduced loudness. The loudness reduction is the same for all frequencies and any small event can make the loudness jump back to its original value. We think this type of inhibition is produced on the higher level of the nervous system and we would like to call it central inhibition. To say that there is a central inhibition is equivalent to the statement that the sensation magnitude is reduced. In some cases it is even difficult for the subject to say if the sensation was reduced by central inhibition or a reduction of the stimulus.

Lateral inhibition, on the other hand, is the interaction between two similar stimuli on a sense organ, particularly with a large surface area. It can produce a reduction or an increase of the local sensation magnitude. It produces a sharpening of the edges of a stimulus pattern and it may change the localization of a stimulus considerably.

The general concept in sensory sciences has been that inhibition is a relatively small effect that only modifies slightly the input-output system seen in Figure 1. Of course, the system had to be modified to the type shown in Figure 3 to fulfill the more complicated requests of today where one input controls several outputs. But in general the input-output system remained and it was successful even in investigations of the brain. The reason for this is easy to understand if we look at Figure 4, a drawing made by Aerospace Medical Research Laboratory. It shows the interconnections of different parts of the nervous system in the brain. It can be seen that there are many interconnections that are very similar to the input-output system. They are connections from one central part to other parts. It is in this type of nervous connections where electrophysiology is successful, because it has all the possibilities of investigating an input and an output.

But we do not have to look around too much to be aware of the fact that this type of input-output system can be used to explain only some aspects of our sensation. Some of the problems of modern rocketry illustrate the limits of the input-output

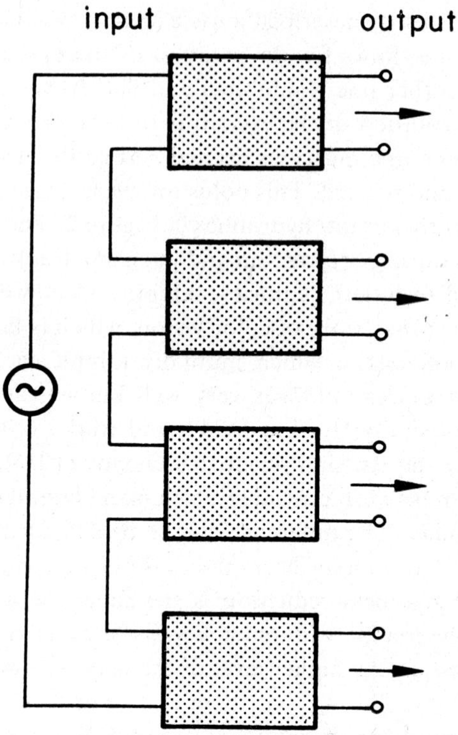

Fig. 3. Improved input-output system with many outputs.

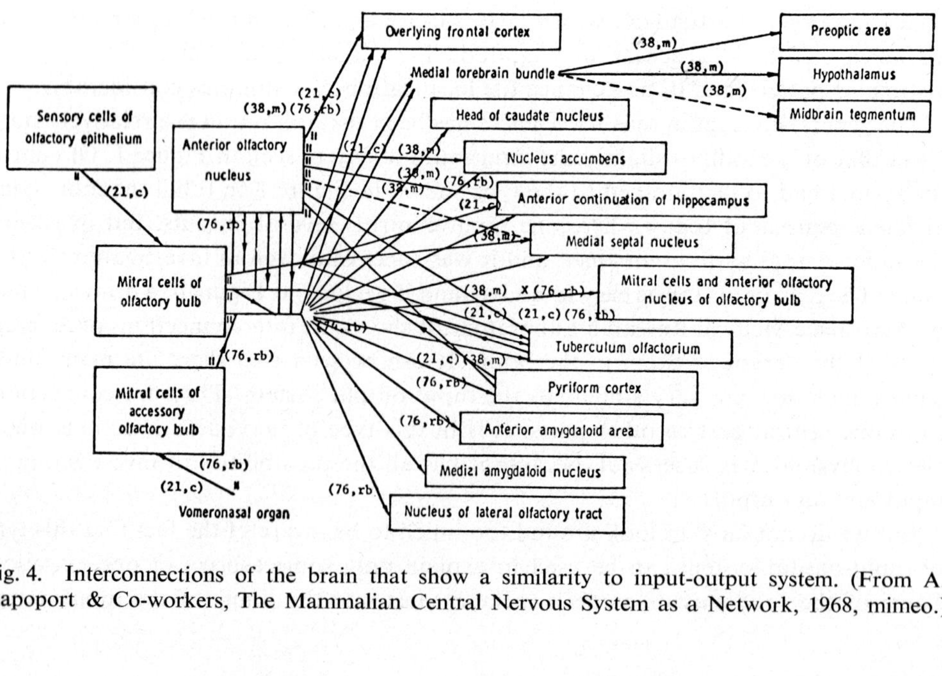

Fig. 4. Interconnections of the brain that show a similarity to input-output system. (From A. Rapoport & Co-workers, The Mammalian Central Nervous System as a Network, 1968, mimeo.)

system as an explanatory model. When we aim a missile at Mars, for example, in addition to the initial aiming, after it is already on its way, we constantly correct its position and direction, using the data we get fed back as the rocket approaches the planet. The important progress of the past years in technology is that we are able to correct our aim continuously by the process of feedback. Similarly, it is quite obvious that if we want to move our finger with a high speed to a certain point, we do not use an input-output system with one single adjustment. On the contrary, we try to get a continuous feedback from our arm and from the finger, and compare the hand position with the position of the object we want to touch.

It is exactly the same procedure that is used today in modern aiming techniques. Naturally, if we have a very simple process, we would always prefer an input-output method. But, if we have to achieve something complicated, then it is obvious that the system with the feedback is much more effective and much more precise. There was a time when in mass production all the adjusting was done once. In situations where the amount of material used was not important, this method is still used. But today, for the more complicated productions, we have to use a feedback system that will readjust the manufacturing process if anything is wrong with the end product.

In spite of the fact that in manufacturing more and more feedback systems are used, there are some very important fields where the resistance against the introduction of feedback considerations is very high. For instance, economists still insist on a five-year plan, a strict application of an input-output concept. It is a good system for the start but during later development it becomes questionable. The education program of a university with 20000 students handled as a five-year plan without feedback can be quite a risk. Maybe the worst applications of the input-output concept are some military war projects that are maintained until there is no more input left.

If we use however a feedback system, immediately the question comes up, what should we feed back? Any electronic device will put up a great deal of information that we might not want to feed back, if it is unimportant for our purpose. Therefore, we need a selective feedback. This can be done by filter action, etc., and this filter action is the sort of inhibition that I would like to describe. We can see already from this simple description that feedback and inhibition have to be applied together.

Figure 5 shows again a drawing made by the Aerospace Medical Research Laboratory. It shows another part of the nervous system with many feedback lines. This is the part in the brain in which corrections are produced, and I think it is the more important one. It is this type of network that is found mainly also in the microstructures of the nervous system. We immediately realize that in this type of interconnection, simple input-output measurements are difficult to make. But, if we want to go ahead with electrophysiology in the way we are doing it now, the only possibility is the use of simultaneous multi-electrode recording.

About two or three decades ago, there were very few known interconnections in the brain between the left side and the right side of the auditory tract. I almost had the feeling that some of the connections were missing and therefore I decided to wait. In the meantime, the whole picture changed completely. Today, we have so many

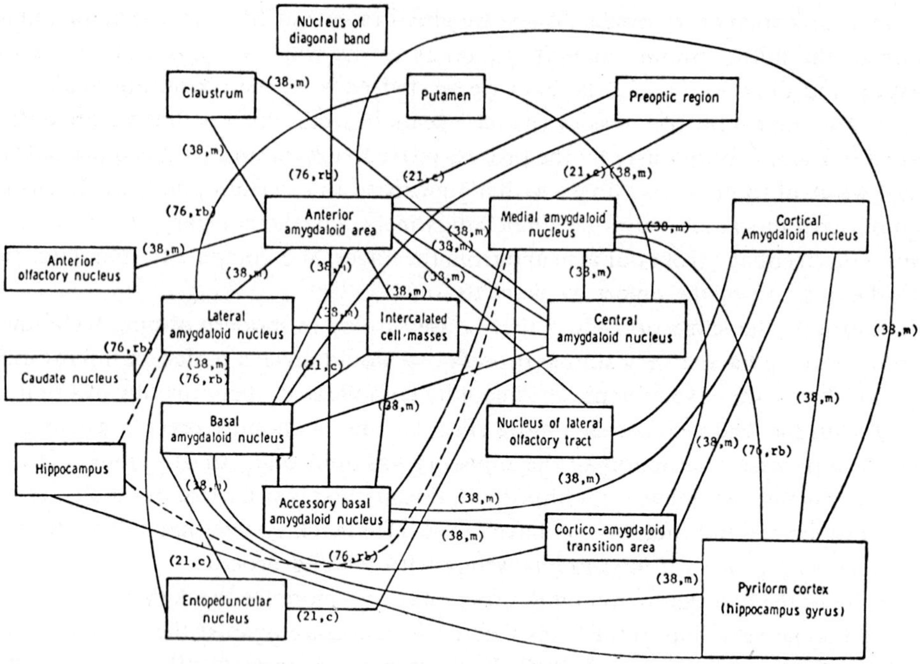

Fig. 5. Interconnections of the brain that show mainly a feedback system. (From A. Rapoport & Co-workers, The Mammalian Central Nervous System as a Network, 1968, mimeo.)

interconnections, as you can see from Figure 5, that it is impossible to decide which one will play the role in direction hearing, to mention one example. It is almost so that every point of the brain seems to be interconnected with every other point. Unfortunately, neuroanatomy is at the moment still mainly descriptive rather than functional.

Similarities between the Different Sense Organs

If we look at any handbook of physiology or psychology, it is surprising how neatly the different sense organs are separated into different chapters and each one is treated, in general, by a different author. Unfortunately, I find this disturbing because it creates an artificial separation barrier between different parts of physiology where we would expect some cross-correlations. After all, we know that all the sense organs develop from the skin. They are surely modified during evolution, but there must be some remaining similarities. From the point of view of experimental work, any similarity is of outstanding importance since there are many experiments we cannot do on one sense organ, which can be done easily on another one. For instance, it is difficult to do experiments on the basilar membrane of the cochlea, which could be done very easily on the surface of the human skin. Therefore, it is useful at least to do the preliminary experiments on the human skin, then to extrapolate what we may expect in the cochlea. There are other experiments that are simple on the retina but are almost impossible to repeat on the basilar membrane.

If we look at Figure 5, the interconnections are so complicated that the question arises as to how can we start to do any experiments or any research in a field that is so difficult. As a beginning, we always can do one thing: we can investigate to see if this complication is about the same for all the sense organs. If the pattern is completely different for every sense organ, I definitely would give up research in sensory sciences. But, as it turns out, the patterns are similar, and there is a certain hope that by combining the different sense organs, we might make some progress. Furthermore, I think the investigation of the similarities between the sense organs is a new avenue.

From the engineering point of view, it would be most convenient to consider the whole sensory system as simply consisting of different receptors, adapted to the different stimuli in nature. The difference between the sense organs would then be in the end organs, which would then be the transformers of the physical stimuli. And after this is done we would prefer that all subsequent neural messages and their interactions should be similar. This assumption, to put all the differences between the sense organs into the periphery and make the rest of the higher nervous level similar, actually seems to be quite fruitful. It immediately points to the fact that similarities should be expected mainly in the processing of the nervous information.

On the basis of some preliminary experiments, this conclusion seems to be correct. The so-called Mach band may be used as an illustration. As shown in the top drawing

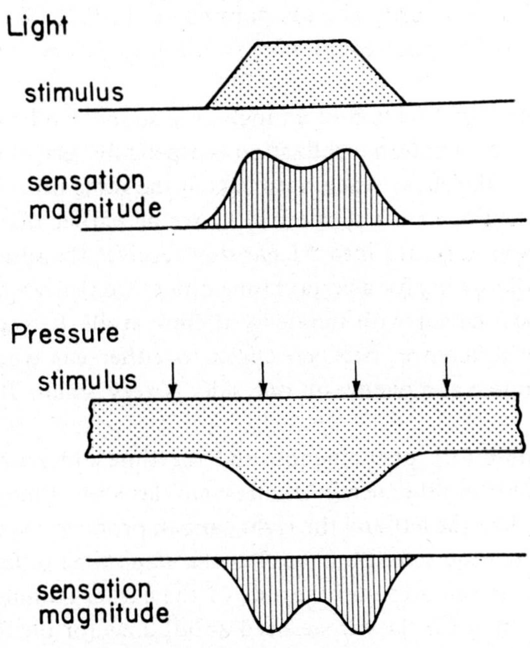

Fig. 6. Luminance distribution along the surface of the retina that has a trapesoidal form, as shown in the top drawing, produces a brightness distribution that shows two maxima. The two lower drawings indicate that a cardboard with a trapesoidal cut pressed against the surface of the skin will produce a pressure sensation similar to that of the brightness distribution with two maxima in spite of the fact that the original pressure stimulus has only one maximum.

of Figure 6, we can produce on the retina a light distribution that increases from zero up to a certain constant value, then drops continuously down to zero. This luminance (physical) distribution represents in this case a trapezoid. We will expect that the brightness (psychological) distribution would be very similar to a trapezoid also, which should show only one maximum with a flat top. But, as illustrated in the drawing below, this does not occur. We have two maxima. These two maxima are called white Mach bands. They were discovered 100 years ago by Mach (1865–1868) and they indicate that the distribution of the sensation magnitude does not completely correspond to the stimulus distribution, rather the sensation emphasizes discontinuities in the stimulus distribution. As we can see from the second drawing, the corners particularly are emphasized. This phenomenon is not small and it is very easy to demonstrate with simple equipment.

It is not difficult to conduct the analog experiment for the pressure sensation on the skin of the arm. To produce a certain pressure distribution we can cut out from a cardboard the shape seen in the third drawing. Again, the pressure distribution will be in the form of a trapezoid. We can test the magnitude of the pressure distribution by measuring under a microscope the indentations of the skin, and it turns out that it follows exactly the pattern of the trapezoid. Any observer will immediately say he feels practically only the corners as it is shown in the lowest drawing of Figure 6. We have the Mach bands not only in the retina, therefore, but we have them also on the surface of the skin, a similarity already pointed out in 1928. Since that time, I have been interested in discovering more and more similarities between the different sensory perceptions.

It is well known that the direction of an incoming sound can be well determined by the use of both ears. The direction localization is especially very sharp for clicks. If the sound is in front of us, the clicks reach both ears at the same time. But, if the sound is a little on the side, then one ear will receive the sound earlier than the other. In this case we localize the sound source into the ear that receives the sound first. The localization phenomena is so strong for a certain time difference that we have the impression that no sound reaches the ear with the delayed click at all. It is an almost complete inhibition. The time difference, between clicks to either ear which is necessary to localize the sound source completely on one side, is very small. It is of the order of one millisecond.

Since this is an inhibitory phenomenon and the time difference is so short, it is interesting to find out if in other sense organs a similar short time delay between two points of stimulation like the left and the right ear can produce a similar phenomenon. If we then explore the taste sensation, we find the same time difference of one millisecond produces a taste sensation on the side of the earlier stimulus. We know from previous experiments that for the ear we need about 0.2 s for the full development of the loudness sensation. But the development of the taste sensation takes more than a second. Therefore, it was surprising to find that even for a sense organ with such a slow-acting receptor, the time difference of one millisecond between a two-point stimulation could be recognized.

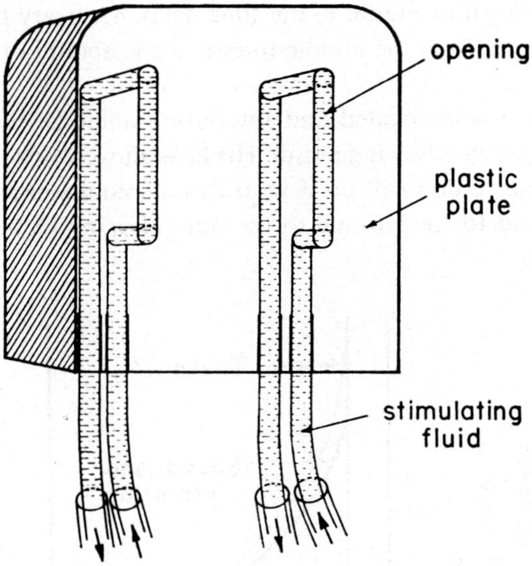

Fig. 7. A plastic block showing the tubes through which, for taste stimuli, a fluid can be conducted. (The surface of the plastic tube is open so that the plastic tube placed in the surface of the tongue will bring it in contact with the fluid stimuli, one on the left side and the other on the right side.)

The measurements for the taste experiments were extremely difficult and required a complicated equipment because we had to exchange the fluid on the surface of the tongue in a very short time interval. We used a plastic plate as is shown in Figure 7. In this plastic plate, two openings were drilled that were slit open on the surface of the plate. The plate placed in the middle of the tongue permitted a contact between the fluid and the surface of the tongue. There were two slits, one on the left and the other on the right side of the tongue. All connections to these slits have to be made extremely short and a special equipment was made to exchange the constantly streaming tap water or the physiological solution with the taste solution we wanted to investigate. The experiments indicated that the better the equipment, the shorter was the time delay necessary to change the localization of the taste sensation from the middle of the tongue to the left or to the right side. After the exchange of the water with the test solution was made as soon as possible and checked with special recording devices placed on the surface of the tongue, the necessary time difference to shift the taste sensation from the middle to the side was about the same as it was for sound. (See Figure 8.)

Next we explored the sensation of smell. For this experiment we introduced a tube in one nostril and a second tube in the nostril of the other side. If in the constant airflow of the two tubes an odorous substance was injected exactly at the same time, the observer located the smell in the middle plane of his nose, but if it had a time delay on one side, then he located the smell either into the left or the right nostril. This phenomenon is very pronounced and it is very similar to the general features of direction hearing. As is shown in Figure 8, the time delay necessary to displace the locus of an odorous substance from the middle to one side is about of the order of one-half millisecond.

There are even more complicated and interesting analogies between hearing and smelling if we watch a dog following a trail. His head movements during the maneuver are exactly the same as a dog will do if he traces a sound source. It is a continuous movement of the head to the left and to the right after which he tries to center into the correct direction.

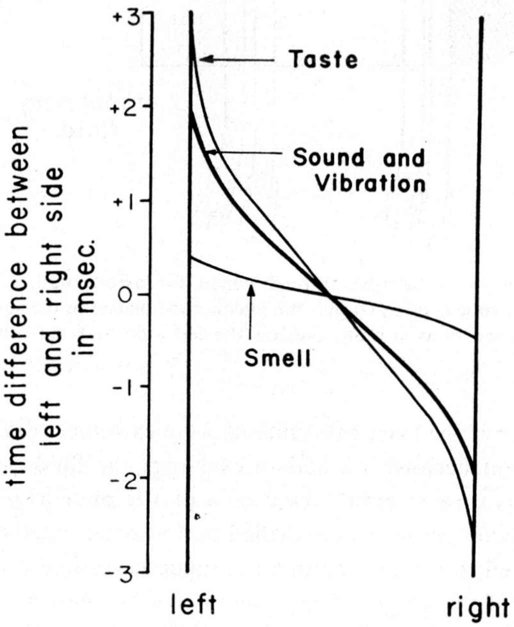

Fig. 8. If two stimuli are presented, and if there is no time delay, the sensation is localized into the middle between the two stimuli. (If the time delay is introduced, the sensation moves laterally. For vibrations, taste, and smell, the time delay necessary is about of the same order of magnitude.)

From Figure 8 we can see that if the sensation magnitude on both sides of the head are the same and if they stimulate the sense organs exactly at the same time, we will localize the sensation in the median plane. But, if the time delay of about one millisecond is introduced on one side, the sensation will shift to the side that received the stimulus first. For all different sensations like sound, taste, smell, and vibration, we found about the same time delay. This seems to indicate that the localization phenomenon involves a nervous process of inhibition that is very similar for all these different sensations.

This analogy holds even though different sense organs are innervated by different numbers of nerve fibers. For vibratory sensations, we may use about 1000 nerve fibers, but for hearing 30000. Olfaction has about one million nerve fibers.

In localizing a sensation, the apparent spatial size of the sensation plays an important role. It is well known in direction hearing that the apparent size of a click is small. Furthermore, the sharper the click is, the smaller the apparent size. On the other hand, a soft low-frequency tone appears much larger. We would expect then, on the basis of this difference in apparent size, that a low-frequency tone would be less precisely localized than a click. This is in fact what our experiments showed.

It is easy to observe further, that in audition, there is very little change of the apparent size of a sound image during its movement from the midline to the side. This is illustrated in Figure 9. However, it is not so for vibration sensations produced on

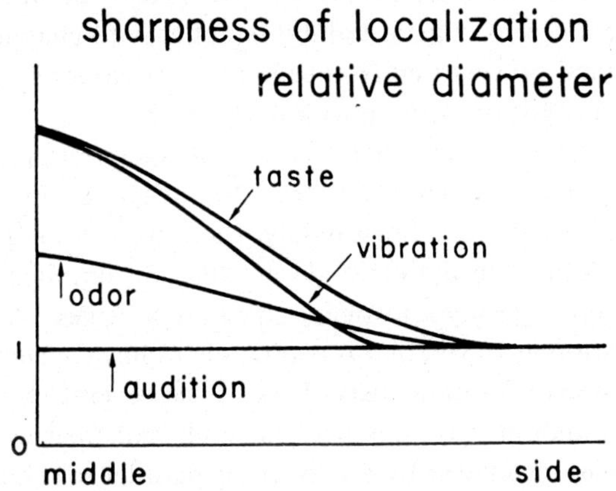

Fig. 9. For audition, the apparent magnitude of the sound image does not change if the localized sound is moved from the middle to the side by introducing a time delay. (Other sense organs do not show this constancy.)

the skin. If the two vibrators that are interacting are far away on the arm, the vibratory sensation in the middle between them is diffused. If the vibratory image is on one side, then we have a very well-defined image of the vibratory sensation that is not much larger than the vibrating surface that touches the skin. It is interesting to notice that if the two vibrators are placed close to each other, then the uncertainty becomes less pronounced. If we bring them very close together, we have practically no change in the extension of the vibratory sensation during its movement from the middle to the side. The situation for the taste sensation and olfaction is also shown in Figure 9. Here again, the closer the two stimuli are, the less is the change in the extension of the sensation area during movement. We may assume that if the two stimuli are closer together, then there is more neural interaction between the two points. We can conclude from the experiments that the more interaction is present, the less is the change of the sensation area during the movement from the middle to the side.

Summing up, it seems that the localization phenomena produced by time differences in the different senses are surprisingly similar. Localization in all the senses is produced by short time delays below one millisecond, despite the well-known fact that the time necessary to fully develop a sensation magnitude always takes more than 200 msec.

Oscillation of the Sensation Magnitude

An effective way to show that sensations are not produced by a simple input-output system is that in many sensations, oscillations can be observed. If we switch on a continuous stimulus, this will start a set of oscillations that decay under normal conditions of the nervous system. This phenomenon is known for vision. Especially, it can happen under certain conditions on the periphery of the visual field, that we see a continuous fluctuation of brightness. It is a yellow flicker around the whole periphery. The frequency of the flicker is constant and it is not easy to change anything about it. The flicker is an internal process that is not modified by external stimuli, for instance, by looking at a bright light or going into a dark room.

It is obvious that in any system that has a feedback, we expect oscillation. Most people of the older generation remember that the biggest problem of amplifiers was to make them free of oscillation. Fortunately, there were some rules that permitted the damping of oscillations in a simple system like an amplifier. But in a complex system as seen in Figure 5, to my knowledge there are no rules available. I was always interested in the question as to whether it is possible to have in such a complex system two different oscillations simultaneously. I had once several hundreds of telephone relays switched in a random way together. They all had their energy supply and in some cases a time delay produced by a condenser parallel to the relay coil. If one of the relays was switched on, then in general a large part of the relays also switched to a different position. But in most cases no oscillations were observed. Only by introducing long feedback lines was it possible to produce oscillation. These oscillations all had the same frequency. There was one type of oscillation that seemed interesting since it represented a sort of sweeping of the relay positions from one side of the whole set of relays to the other side in a periodic way. To produce this type of behavior, it is necessary to have very large number of relays with definite phase difference between one side of the set and the other one. If the traveling time is too short, no such sweeping will occur. I was never able to find the conditions under which such a sweeping oscillation was produced.

The last time I had the opportunity to see such a sweeping oscillation was at Cambridge in William James Hall. William James Hall consists of 15 floors and had three, more or less, automatic elevators. I was always surprised how long I had to wait for an elevator. For weekdays the explanation was that the elevators were busy. But, when I went to William James Hall on a Sunday, 7:30 A.M., it was obvious that nobody was in the building and still it took seven and more minutes until one elevator arrived. By listening to the doors, it was possible to hear the elevators running up and down, all three of them, and then suddenly like magic, all three doors opened simultaneously. After having waited so long, I was always afraid to step in any of those elevators. This type of elevator behavior is called, in elevator language, "hunting."

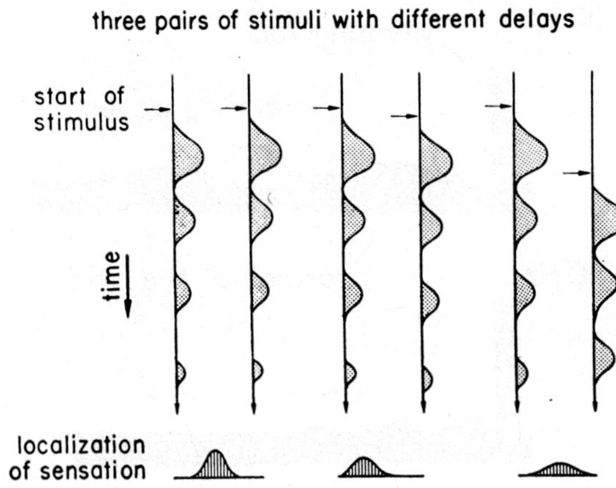

Fig. 10. Sensation localization can be used to determine if a constant stimulus may produce fluctuations in the sensation magnitude. (From G. v. Békésy, 1967.)

It is a very similar type of sweeping movement like we found in many systems. Unfortunately, again it was not possible to find out what the real conditions for this situation were. Naturally, by changing the resting location of the elevator, etc., the phenomenon could be eliminated.

To test experimentally if the switching on of a constant stimulus can produce oscillations in the sensation magnitude, the method illustrated in Figure 10 of two separate stimuli of equal sensation magnitude can be used. If both stimuli start exactly at the same moment, we may get sensation magnitude changes with time as illustrated in the drawings. Since both sensations are exactly the same, we will locate the sensation in the middle between the two stimulators, as indicated for the stimulus pair on the left side. In this case again, the sensation will be localized in the middle position. Naturally, the sensation magnitude will not be exactly the same for the second and third maximum. Therefore, the position in the middle is not as precise as it was when both stimuli were presented without any time delay.

We did this experiment on the surface of the tongue by using two concentric electrodes on both sides of the tongue. The current through these electrodes was adjusted so that a taste sensation was produced in the middle of the tongue if no time difference was present. If a continuously increasing time delay is introduced, the localization of the taste moves repeatedly from one side to the other. This indicates that for the taste sensation, stimulated electrically, there is an oscillation of sensation magnitude present. The frequency of the oscillation can be determined from the time delay necessary to produce a repetition. We could repeat the same observations for stimulations with a salt solution, and find about the same period as found for the electrical stimulation.

Inhibition is not Small

In general, it has been assumed that inhibition plays a very unimportant role in daily

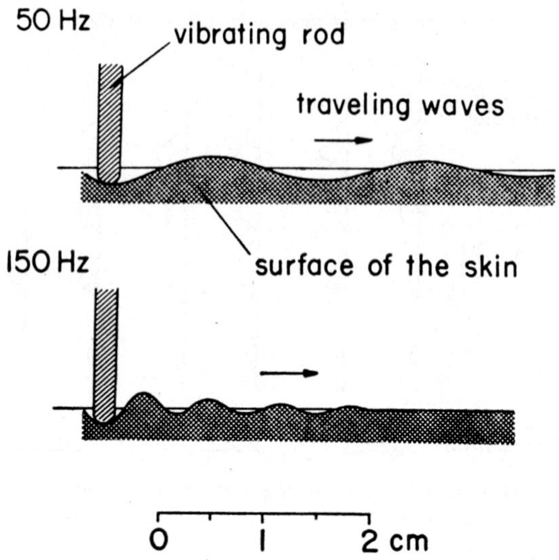

Fig. 11. A vibrating rod produces traveling waves along the surface of the skin.

life and in experiments with sense organs. Some forty years ago, I started to point out that between a stimulus distribution on a sense organ with a large surface and the observed sensation distribution, there is a very large difference under some conditions.

In Figure 11, you can see a vibrator vibrating with a frequency of 50 Hz. It is touching the surface of the skin on the lower arm. With stroboscopic illumination, we can see a traveling wave along the arm, and we can measure its wavelength and decay in amplitude and, therefore, we would expect to feel vibrations along the whole arm. But if we ask an observer, he reports that the vibratory sensation extends about one centimeter around the vibrator. The more remote sections of the traveling wave are completely inhibited. The inhibition is produced partially by the time delays of the successive sections of the traveling wave. This situation does not change even when we show to the observer his whole arm vibrating. The phenomenon is even more dramatic if the observer stands on a vibrating table. His whole body is seen vibrating and he still insists that he feels only vibration on his feet.

In the field of hearing, it is especially easy to devise experiments that show a large amount of inhibition. When we listen to a speaker in a room, we localize all the sounds reflected from the walls as coming from the place of the speaker. This process of inhibition is a very important phenomenon. If we place one microphone about one foot away from the speaker, and a second microphone about five feet away, the sound pattern of these two microphones is completely different, as can be seen in Figure 12. In the lower recording the reflections from the wall distort the original sound pressure pattern close to the speaker. In spite of the large difference between the sound pressures, a listener does not hear a difference when he moves his head from one microphone to the other, since in binaural hearing the reflections from the walls are inhibited.

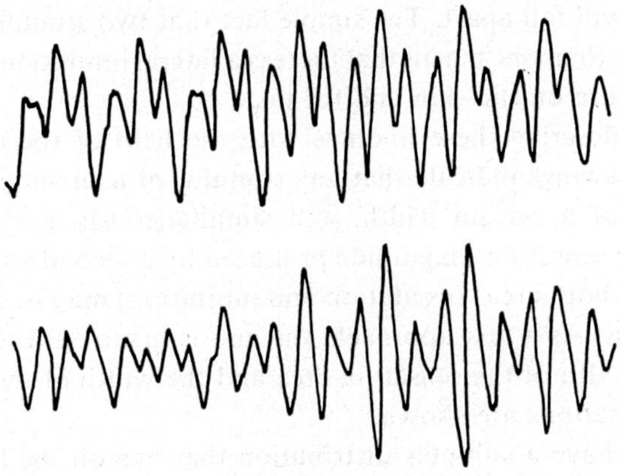

Fig. 12. The sound pressure can be very different on two places and still the ear will not recognize any difference.

The knowledge of these wall reflections and the inhibitory processes concerning localization is of utmost importance for the acoustics in concert halls and theaters. It can make the difference between a good or a bad concert hall.

The Neural Unit

There are many stimulus patterns by which a sense organ with a large surface area can be excited. It is of interest to find a general approach to such stimulation.

Mach, almost 100 years ago, developed a formula for transforming a stimulus distribution along the retina into the sensation magnitude distribution, that is, for transforming the luminance pattern on the retina into the brightness pattern in sensation. His formula contains, as a main distorting factor, the second derivative of the luminance function. Mach's formula describes very well the appearance of the white and the dark bands. It is in agreement with the observations that the smaller the curvature of the luminance distribution, the larger the brightness of the dark or white band. If the curvature is positive, we have a white Mach band, and if the curvature is negative, we have a black band. I became interested in finding some physiological background for this phenomena, in addition to the purely mathematical description. To test this question, the simplest approach seemed the investigation of how two stimuli interact with each other if presented to a sense organ with a large surface. The sensation produced by one single point stimulus has a certain spread, but it is not large. If we have two stimuli that are close together, the magnitude of the sensation increases, and the width of the spread also. We can go farther and farther apart with the two stimuli, and there is a certain distance when the sensation becomes as wide as the distance of the two stimuli. We have only then to increase the distance just a little more and, at that moment, we have the peculiar result that the magnitude of the combined sensation suddenly drops (Békésy, 1960). The more precise the two sensation magnitudes are adjusted to be equal, the larger is the drop. If we increase the distance, the two sensations will fall apart. The simple fact that two stimuli can give a smaller sensation magnitude than one means that there is a lateral inhibition. This phenomenon was tested for pressure on the skin and for taste.

It is possible to describe these findings with the help of the drawings shown in Figure 13. These drawings indicate that any stimulus of a small area will produce an area of excitation of a certain width, and simultaneously a surrounding area of inhibition where the sensation magnitude produced by a second stimulus is decreased. The combination of both areas (excitation and inhibition) may be called an inhibitory unit for one stimulus. As a first approach, the unit is made out of rectangles, and the dimensions of the width of the sensation area and the width of the inhibited area for vision and skin sensations are shown.

In Figure 14, we have a stimulus distribution that has on the left side a constant stimulus and then going to the right side increases linearly to a certain value that remains constant again. In order to analyze this distribution in terms of the above inhibitory unit, we use the following procedure. The stimulus distribution is cut in

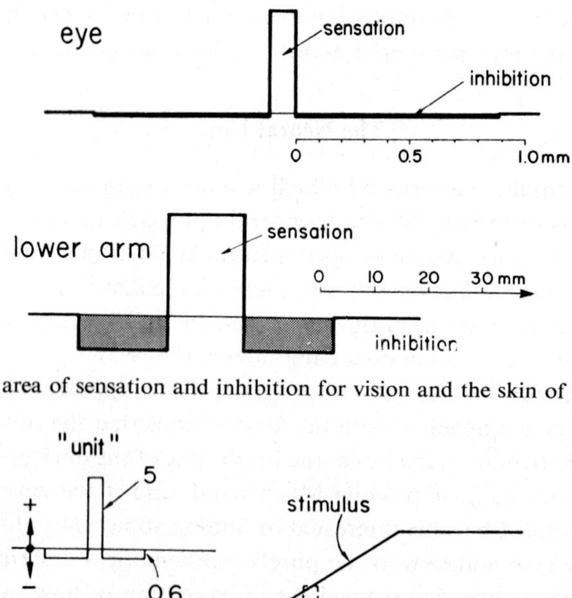

Fig. 13. The area of sensation and inhibition for vision and the skin of the lower arm.

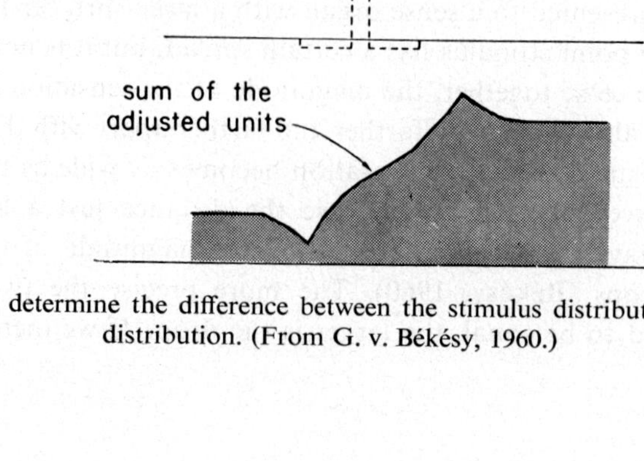

Fig. 14. Method to determine the difference between the stimulus distribution and the sensation distribution. (From G. v. Békésy, 1960.)

small vertical segments of the width of the excitation. The stimulus magnitude is multiplied by the excitation magnitude of the unit and they are plotted all along the stimulus distribution curve. The same thing is done for the inhibitory areas, and after the two curves are drawn, we subtract from the excitation magnitude distribution on the inhibitory magnitude distribution. As can be seen in the lower drawing of Figure 14, the resulting sensation magnitude curve shows a well-developed overshoot and undershoot. The width of this overshoot and undershoot is given by the width of the inhibitory area of the unit. It was found that for many stimulus distributions, this type of geometrical procedure is successful. The geometrical addition is different than the pure mathematical formula of Mach. For instance, for a very sharp corner, the curvature becomes infinite and therefore the mathematical overshoot and undershoot should be extremely high also. In the geometrical analysis, the overshoot has always a certain width but not an infinite height.

Displacement of the Sensation Maximum

Lateral inhibition can produce a difference between stimulus distribution and sensation distribution that is quite surprising. We cut out from a black sheet an opening as shown on the left side of Figure 15. This opening has at the top, and on the lower edge, a constant curvature. It can be rotated around the center of the curvature (marked by a cross). A rotation of the opening around its center will not change the stimulus magnitude or its second derivative.

We can plot the height of the opening in a curve as it is shown in the upper drawing of Figure 16 (Békésy, 1968). In the represented situation, the opening is symmetrical to the vertical line. From the stimulus distribution, we can calculate the sensation magnitude distribution by using the inhibitory unit. In this symmetrical situation, the stimulus has a maximum that falls together with the maximum of the sensation. We cannot see any reason why this should change if we rotate the opening in Figure 15 around the center point, because neither the stimulus magnitude nor the second derivative near the point of the maximum will change. But using again our geometrical

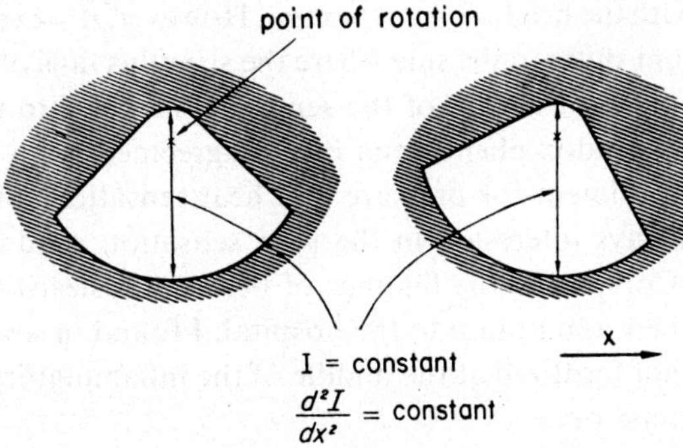

Fig. 15. Masks to produce a luminance distribution along the surface of the retina for which in a certain region the luminance and its second derivative are constant.

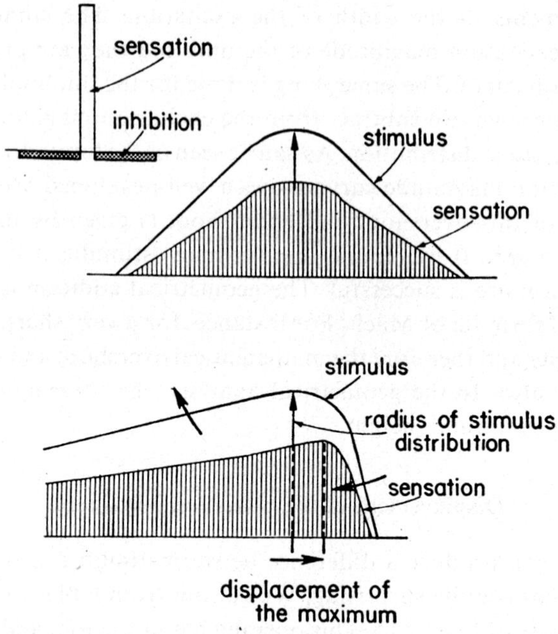

Fig. 16. A stimulus distribution that keeps its maximum and second derivative constant can still produce a displacement of the sensation maximum if the slopes on the side change. (From G. v. Békésy, 1968.)

method, we find that for the sensation distribution, the maximum is quite away from the maximum of the stimulus distribution, as shown by the shaded area in the lower drawing of Figure 16.

The question is, do we find the similar type of the shift of the sensation magnitude relative to the stimulus maximum in actual observations? To test this in vision we use an equipment that transforms the light of the openings in Figure 15 linearly into a luminance distribution (Békésy, 1968).

Experiments showed that for the symmetrical position of the opening the stimulus maximum coincided with the brightness maximum. However, if we rotated the opening, the brightness maximum shifts to the side where the stimulus falls off. During rotation, we have a feeling that the maximum of the sensation moves into the area where the stimulus is reduced, a paradox phenomena but in agreement with Figure 16.

We repeated this experiment for pressure and heat sensations of the skin with the same results. I was always interested in the pain sensation produced by certain inflammatory diseases. Comparing the findings of their autopsies with the descriptions patients gave during their admittance to the hospital, I found in several cases, that the pain localization was not localized at the middle of the inflammatory process, but near the edge of the inflammation.

After the war, it was quite common that the roots of the teeth on the lower jaw were inflamed. In general, the middle part of the teeth had the maximum inflammation and it dropped on different sides with a different slope. This could be demonstrated easily by X-ray pictures. But the patients, in general, did not localize the pain at the maximum of the inflammatory process, determined by the X-ray pictures, but more toward the edge, when the distribution of the inflammation did not drop equally on both sides. In this case, there was a danger to have the wrong tooth pulled.

References

Békésy, G. v. Neural inhibitory units of the eye and skin: Quantitative description of contrast phenomena. *Journal of the Optical Society of America*, 1960, **50**, 1060–1070.

Békésy, G. v. *Sensory inhibition*. Princeton: Princeton University Press, 1967.

Békésy, G. v. Location of maxima and minima in sensation patterns influenced by lateral inhibition. *Journal of Applied Physiology*, 1968, **25**, 200–206.

Descartes, R. *L'Homme*. (2nd ed.) Paris: Charles Angot, 1677. Esp. pp. 15–18.

Eccles, J. C. *The physiology of nerve cells*. Baltimore: John Hopkins Press. 1957.

Hartline, H. K. Inhibition of activity of visual receptors by illuminating nearby retinal areas in the Limulus eye. *Federal Proceedings*, 1949, **8**, 69.

Hartline, H. K., Ratliff, F., & Miller, W. H. Neural interaction in the eye and the integration of receptor activity. *Annals of the New York Academy of Sciences*, 1958, **74**, 210–222.

Hartline, H. K., Ratliff, F., & Miller, W. H. Inhibitory interaction in the retina and its significance in vision. In E. Florey (Ed.), *Nervous inhibition*. London: Pergamon, 1961.

Hartline, H. K., Wagner, H. G., & Ratliff, F. Inhibition in the eye of limulus. *Journal of General Physiology*, 1956, **39**, 651–673.

Hering, E. *Zur Lehre vom Lichtsinne* (Vienna: Gerolds Sohn, 1878). (Trans. by Leo M. Hurvich & Dorothea Jameson.) Cambridge: Harvard University Press, 1964.

Mach, E. Über die Wirkung der räumlichen Verteilung des Lichtreizes auf die Netzhaut, I. *Akademie der Wissenschaften in Wien, Sitzungsberichte, math.-nat. Cl.*, 1865, **52**, Abt. 2, 303–322. Über die physiologische Wirkung räumlich vertheilter Lichtreize. *Ibid.*, 1866, **54**, Abt. 2, 393–408, and 1868, **57**, Abt. 2, 11–19.

Ratliff, F. *Mach bands: Quantitative studies on neural networks in the retina*. San Francisco: Holden-Day, 1965.

Sechenov, I. *Selected works*. Moscow-Leningrad: State Publishing House for Biological and Medical Literature, 1935.

Sherrington, C. *The integrative action of the nervous system*. New Haven: Yale University Press, 1947.

SOME TECHNICAL NOTES ON PSYCHOPHYSICAL SCALING

DAVID V. CROSS

SUNY at Stony Brook, New York

Abstract. A simple theory of psychophysical scaling is presented. It is based on the power law and a multiplicative error model that treats magnitude judgments as lognormal variates. Conventional techniques for estimating power-law exponents are reviewed along with a solution to the problem of estimating parameters of psychophysical relationships when both variables in the relationship are measured with error. This problem arises when validating ratio scales of opinion by matching sensory magnitudes to social stimuli and thereby producing psychophysical cross-modality matching functions. The regression problem is reconsidered in this context and a method for dealing with it is proposed.

Much is said in this volume of the importance of S. S. Stevens' contributions to psychophysical measurement. The past two decades have indeed produced a proliferation of experimental findings based on the method of cross-modality matching that he popularized (Stevens, 1966). Although studies focused initially on the psychophysics of sensory function, with a major result being the revision of the psychophysical law, the new paradigms have also found fruitful application to the scaling of non-sensory variables such as seriousness of offenses, prestige of occupations, perceptions of national power and strength of opinion (Stevens, 1972). As applications have increased so have the methodological problems and issues (Stevens, 1971a). More than ever we are aware of the need for standard treatment of such matters as parameter estimation, measurement error or judgment variability, the identification of sources of bias, and the measurement of bias.

This paper outlines a simple theory of psychophysical scaling based on the power law and a multiplicative error model. Standard techniques for treating psychophysical data are reviewed. Most of them are familiar to psychophysicists but some of the results are derived from the proposed theory and are original solutions to some long standing problems in psychophysical scaling. Emphasis is placed on paradigms applicable to the scaling of social stimuli. The regression problem is reconsidered in this context and a method of dealing with it is proposed.

Basic Psychophysical Theory

It is assumed the presentation of a physical stimulus, Φ, produces a perceptual response of variable magnitude, Ψ_i, which is related to Φ by the following psychophysical law:

$$\Psi_i = \Phi^{\beta}\varepsilon_i. \tag{1}$$

The subscript i indexes the order of presentation of Φ. It also indicates that the symbol subscripted is interpreted as a random variate. It is suppressed when denoting an average value, or parameter, as in $\Psi = \prod \Psi_i^{1/n}$.

H. R. Moskowitz et al. (eds.), Sensation and Measurement. 23–36.

The exponent, β, is a characteristic of the continuum under investigation; it depends both on the transduction characteristics of the sensory system involved and on the mode of expression for Φ as, for example, whether Φ is measured in units of power or force.

The multiplicative error term ε_i is a random variate to which, for a fixed Φ, we attribute all variability in Ψ_i. The multiplicative average (geometric mean) of the ε_i is defined as $\varepsilon = \prod \varepsilon_i^{1/n}$. Alternative assumptions can be made concerning the interpretation or evaluation of ε; for example, the absence of systematic bias in the psychophysical relation implies that ε is constant, independent of Φ. This may be taken as $\varepsilon = 1$, for sufficiently large n, or more generally as $\varepsilon = \kappa$, $\kappa > 0$, thus incorporating in the average error term the usually arbitrary modulus or scale unit contained in the standard version of the power law: $\Psi = \kappa\Phi^{\beta}$. On the other hand, systematic departures from the power law, such as curvature near threshold, or systematic biases in empirical representations of the law may, in some cases, be suitably represented by a functional dependence between ε and Φ. One case in point is the occurrence of assimilative order effects in sequential magnitude estimations; this dependence of ε on both focal and preceding stimulus levels is expressible as a power function $\varepsilon = (\Phi_{i-1}/\Phi_i)^b$ (Cross, 1973).

The probability density function for ε_i is assumed to be lognormal; this means that the logarithm of ε_i is normally distributed with $E(\ln \varepsilon_i) = \mu$ (i.e., μ is related to ε by $\varepsilon = e^{\mu}$) and $\mathrm{Var}(\ln \varepsilon_i) = \sigma^2$. This notion has the equivalent representations

$$\varepsilon_i = \Lambda(\mu, \sigma^2) \quad \text{or} \quad \ln \varepsilon_i = N(\mu, \sigma^2).$$

A basic theorem concerning lognormal variates states that if X is $\Lambda(\mu, \sigma^2)$ and $Y = cX^b$ (for $c > 0$, say $c = e^a$) then $Y = \Lambda(a + b\mu, b^2\sigma^2)$ (Aitchison & Brown, 1963). This important result figures significantly in several places in the following exposition. It says simply that a power-function relationship between two lognormal variates implies a linear relation between their distribution parameters.

From the above definitions and the definition $\Psi = e^{\xi}$ it follows that the distribution of Ψ_i is lognormal with parameters $\xi = \beta \ln \Phi$ and σ^2; this is represented by $\Psi_i = \Lambda(\beta \ln \Phi, \sigma^2)$.

Magnitude Estimation

In a magnitude estimation experiment numbers are matched directly to a given Φ and they are assumed to be proportional to Ψ_i: thus

$$N_i = \kappa \Psi_i = \kappa \Phi^{\beta} \varepsilon_i .$$

An unbiased estimate of $\kappa\Phi^{\beta}$ is given by the geometric mean of the n independently produced N_i:

$$N = \prod_{i=1}^{n} N_i^{1/n} = \kappa\Phi^{\beta} \prod \varepsilon_i^{1/n} = \kappa\Phi^{\beta} \tag{2}$$

since, for sufficiently large n, $\varepsilon = 1$.

The arithmetic mean is not an appropriate average for lognormal variates since if $X = \Lambda(\xi, \sigma^2)$ then $E(X) = e^{\xi + \sigma^2/2}$ which is biased upwards in estimating e^{ξ}. The median is unbiased and it is occasionally used in place of the geometric mean but it is less efficient.

In a typical experiment Φ is presented at various predetermined levels of $\Phi_j (j = 1, \ldots, m)$. Levels are often selected that comprise a geometric progression in which each successive term is a constant multiple, a, of its predecessor in the progression: $\Phi_j = a\Phi_{j-1} = a^{j-1}\Phi_1$. The power-law maxim "equal stimulus ratios produce equal sensory ratios" entails that the geometric mean response corresponding to Φ_j will also enter a geometric progression, $N_j = bN_{j-1} = b^{j-1}N_1$, with a constant of progression, b, that is related to the a in the stimulus progression by $b = a^{\beta}$ where β is the exponent of the power-function relation given in (2). Any stimulus pair can define a ratio, a, which in turn determines a response ratio, b, and when both are known then so is β by the relationship $\beta = \ln b / \ln a$. However, an exponent is seldom obtained by such a simple calculation because the response ratios are fallible estimates of b and measurement error is likely to prevent a perfect geometric progression of response values. Consequently, with fallible data, statistical methods must be used to estimate function parameters. The most popular method invokes the criterion of least squares which minimizes the residual variance of deviations from the best fitting curve.

A Graphical Least-Squares Fitting Procedure

If logarithmically transformed, (2) can be made linear in the parameters to be estimated; hence

$$\ln N = \beta \ln \Phi + \ln \kappa . \tag{3}$$

If we let $Y = \ln N$, $X = \ln \Phi$ and $\alpha = \ln \kappa$, our data might form a plot in linear coordinates as in Figure 1. The data points are equally spaced on the X-axis (equal log intervals) in correspondence to a geometric progression of the Φ_j. A simple pencil-and-ruler construction is available (Askovitz, 1957) that allows us to locate the straight line about which the sum of squared vertical deviations of the points is minimum. Starting from point number 1 (Figure 1) we move toward point number 2 (in a straight line connecting the two points) until we have moved two-thirds of the horizontal spacing between them, placing us at the first p in Figure 1. We then move directly toward point number 3 until another two-thirds of this uniform step size, Δ, is traversed. This places us at the second p. We continue in this manner, moving to the right in steps of two-thirds of the horizontal spacing between stimuli and always heading toward the next data point, until we finally arrive at point P which is, by construction, two-thirds of the horizontal distance between or first and last data points. This entire procedure is repeated from the other end leading us from right to left to a point P' which is again two-thirds the distance between the last and first points. The points P and P' necessarily trisect the stimulus range defined by our extreme data points. The least-squares line passes through P and P'; it has a slope equal to β and a Y intercept equal to α.

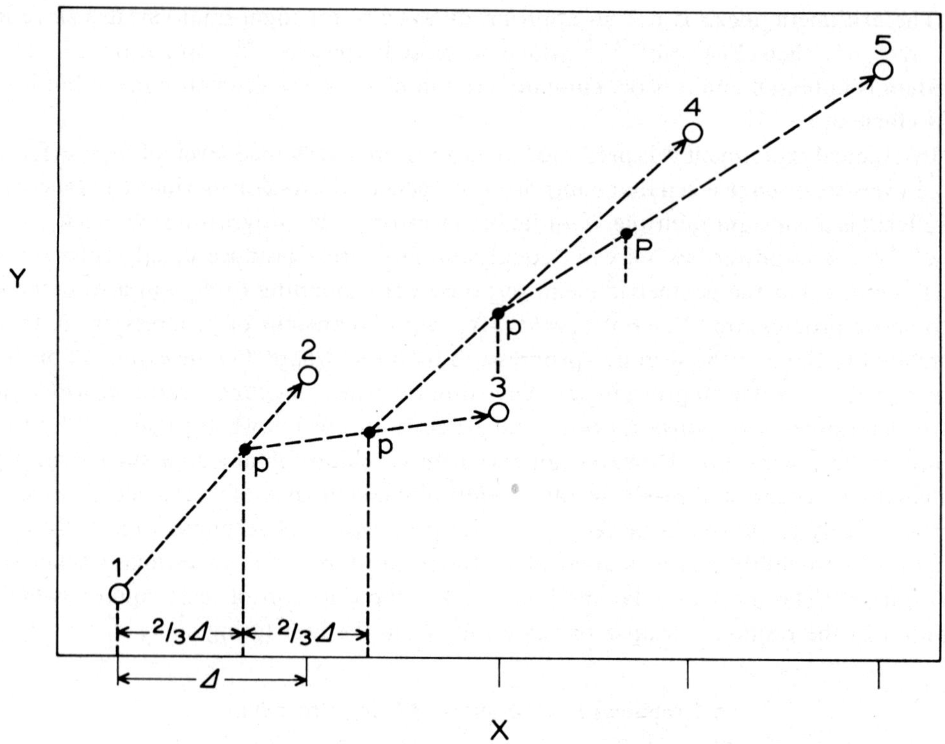

Fig. 1. A graphical least-squares fitting procedure.

This procedure, though simple and quick (it takes more time to describe than to actually do), lacks a measure of the residual variance about the line. Without this it is impossible to statistically evaluate the goodness of fit of the line or to establish confidence limits for the regression parameters.

Conventional Curve Fitting with Error only in the Dependent Variable

Given the linear functional relation $Y=\beta X+\alpha$ where, as in (3), $Y=\ln N$, $X=\ln \Phi$, and $\alpha=\ln \kappa$, the obtained Y is an unbiased estimate of a point on the functional relationship. But by definition it is also an estimate of a point on the regression line for predicted Y given X. Therefore, the regression of Y upon X is also an estimate of the functional relationship.

The method of least squares yields the following estimate of β:

$$b = S_{xy}/S_{xx}, \tag{4}$$

where

$$S_{xy} = \sum XY - \sum X \sum Y/n$$
$$S_{xx} = \sum X^2 - (\sum X)^2/n.$$

The n in these equations refers to the number of levels of X. The intercept α is estimated by $a = \bar{Y} - b\bar{X}$ from which the constant of proportionality in the power function is obtained by $\kappa = e^a$.

The sum of squares of deviations of Y about the regression line can be shown to be equal to the sum of squared deviations of Y about the mean $\bar{Y}$ less the sum of squares due to regression. These sums of squares can be conveniently presented in the form of an analysis of variance table as shown in Table 1.

TABLE 1

Analysis of variance for regression

Source of variation	Sum of squares	Degrees of freedom	Expected mean square
Due to regression	S^2_{xy}/S_{xx}	1	$\sigma^2 + \beta^2\Sigma(X-\bar{X})^2$
About regression	$S_{yy} - S^2_{xy}/S_{xx}$	$n-2$	σ^2
Total	S_{yy}	$n-1$	

Standard error of the regression coefficient, b, and confidence limits for β

The greater the residual dispersion about the regression line the less precisely will the slope, β, be known. The standard error of the estimate, b, is given by

$$\text{S.E.}(b) = \sigma/(S_{xx})^{1/2}. \tag{5}$$

We have to substitute for σ its estimated value, s, the square of which is the sum of squares about regression divided by its degrees of freedom, $n-2$ (the second variance line in the ANOVA table). Assuming the variation about the line is normal, the $100(1-2\alpha)\%$ confidence limits for β are

$$b \pm t_\alpha s/(S_{xx})^{1/2}, \tag{6}$$

where t_α is the value of t corresponding to probability α for $n-2$ degrees of freedom.

Functional Relationships when both Variables are Subject to Error

The situation discussed above applies when the stimulus levels are fixed and presumed measured with no (or negligible) error. Departures from a strict functional relationship are assumed due to errors in the dependent variable and the criterion for estimating the functional relationship is the minimization of squared vertical deviations from the estimated regression line. This procedure is not appropriate when the independent variable is uncontrolled and when measures of the independent variable are fallible. When this is true the conventional least squares estimation is biased and the line that results from it has a slope that is smaller than that of the true line. Error in the horizontal direction as well as in the vertical direction must be taken into account in estimating the true line. The literature on this problem is extensive (see references in: Madansky, 1959; Cochran, 1968). It turns out there are no generally simple solutions if nothing is known about the nature or magnitude of these errors.

Let us assume that a linear functional relationship exists between Y and X and that the only reason the data depart from this is the existence of random, independent errors in the sampling or measurement of both Y and X. Let the error variance of Y be σ_y^2 and that of X be σ_x^2. If these variances are known or, at least, the ratio $\lambda = \sigma_y^2/\sigma_x^2$ is known, then an unbiased estimate of β is obtained from

$$b = \frac{(S_{yy} - \lambda S_{xx}) + \{(S_{yy} - \lambda S_{xx})^2 + 4\lambda S_{xy}^2\}^{1/2}}{2S_{xy}}. \tag{7}$$

When $\lambda \to \infty$, corresponding to $\sigma_x^2 \to 0$, (7) tends to S_{xy}/S_{xx}, the regression coefficient of Y upon X. On the other hand, when $\lambda \to 0$ (7) reduces to S_{yy}/S_{xy} which is the slope $1/b'$ of the regression line of X upon Y. The linear functional relationship always lies between these two regression lines. When $\lambda = 1$, the case of equal error variances, (7) yields the line about which the sum of the squared *perpendicular* deviations is minimum.

The formula for determining confidence limits β_1 and β_2 for the true slope β is rather complex:

$$\lambda^{1/2} \tan\left(\tan^{-1}\{b\lambda^{-1/2}\} \pm \tfrac{1}{2}\sin^{-1}\left\{2t\left[\frac{\lambda(S_{xx}S_{yy} - S_{xy}^2)}{(n-2)\{(S_{yy} - \lambda S_{xx})^2 + 4\lambda S_{xy}^2\}}\right]^{1/2}\right\}\right), \tag{8}$$

where the value of t is that corresponding to $n-2$ degrees of freedom at the chosen confidence percentage. If 95% confidence limits are calculated, $(\beta_2 - \beta_1)^2/16$ provides a rough estimate of the variance for the slope b.

Cross-Modality Matching

Magnitude estimation is a special case of the cross-modality matching (CMM) paradigm, a case in which numbers are matched to stimulus presentations. The model, represented by (1) and (2), assumes that number is directly proportional to Ψ_i, a lognormal variate corresponding to the product of Φ^β and a lognormal error term, ε_i. In magnitude production, number plays the role of the stimulus. The presentation of a number produces a perceptual response of variable magnitude according to

$$N \to \Psi_i = \Lambda(\ln N, \sigma^2).$$

This expression asserts that a given number presentation produces a response that behaves as a lognormal variate with parameters $\xi = \ln N$ and σ^2. Two assumptions are made here in order to simplify exposition: it is assumed that apparent magnitude is a power function of number with unit exponent and that there is no regression effect ... i.e., the same functional relationship is established in both magnitude estimation and magnitude production. Neither of these assumptions are necessary as subsequent generalizations of the model will show when we attempt to accommodate the empirical relations that most often in fact obtain.

Of course, the Ψ_i produced in response to N is unobservable. It is measured by S's behavior in matching another physical stimulus to Ψ on the assumption that $\Phi = \kappa\Psi^{1/\beta}$. The physical stimulus is now adjusted by the subject so it produces an apparent magnitude that matches $\Psi(N)$. Since Ψ_i is a variate its stochastic properties are propagated to Φ_i:

$$\begin{aligned}\Psi_i \rightarrow \Phi_i &= \Lambda(1/\beta \ln \Psi,\ 1/\beta^2\sigma^2)\\ &= \Lambda(1/\beta \ln N,\ \sigma^2_\Phi).\end{aligned}$$

This expression asserts that the observed dependent variable Φ_i obtained in response to fixed N will be lognormally distributed with parameters $\xi = 1/\beta \ln N$ and $\sigma^2_\Phi = \mathrm{Var}\,(\ln \Phi) = 1/\beta^2\sigma^2$. β is the true exponent relating Ψ and Φ as in (1) and σ^2 is the variance associated with random fluctuations in Ψ_i $(\sigma^2 = \mathrm{Var}(\ln \varepsilon_i))$.

The magnitude estimation and production paradigms are distinctive only in that number serves as one of the matching variables. In principle, any pair of modalities or stimulus domains can be brought into a matching relationship. A sound, for example, may be adjusted so its loudness matches in magnitude the brightness of a light, or the light may be adjusted to match the sound.

This general paradigm is called cross-modality matching (CMM). It is illustrated graphically in Figure 2. Given any two stimulus domains, A and B, and the psychophysical relations $\Psi = A^\alpha$ and $\Psi = B^\beta$, Figure 2 represents the linear mappings between $\ln A$, $\ln \Psi$, and $\ln B$. For experimentally controlled and presented levels of A the lognormal perceptual responses Ψ_i in turn give rise to adjusted levels of B_i in which are propagated the errors inherent in Ψ_i: the mappings are in the order $A \rightarrow \Psi_i \rightarrow B_i$. The mapping from A to Ψ_i is represented as

$$A \rightarrow \Psi_i = \Lambda(\alpha \ln A,\ \sigma^2)$$

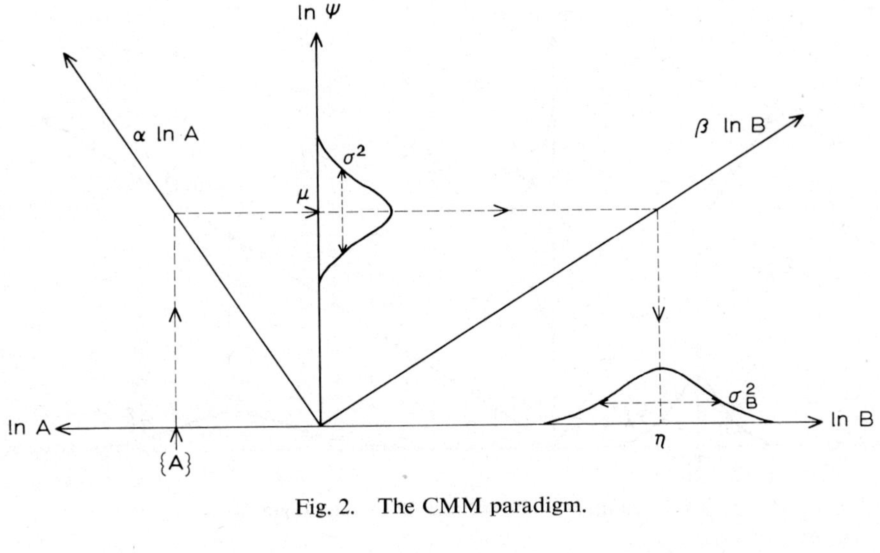

Fig. 2. The CMM paradigm.

and from Ψ_i to B_i we have

$$\begin{aligned}\Psi_i \to B_i &= \Lambda(1/\beta \ln \Psi,\ 1/\beta^2\sigma^2)\\ &= \Lambda(\alpha/\beta \ln A,\ \sigma_B^2).\end{aligned}$$

This last result asserts that the geometric mean, B, will enter a power-function relationship with A with an exponent equal to the ratio of the two exponents α and β as determined separately by magnitude estimation: $B = A^{\alpha/\beta}$.

The conventional curve-fitting techniques described above with (4) and the substitutions $X = \ln A$ and $Y = \ln B$ give an unbiased estimate of this exponent, α/β.

Indirect CMM and Scaling Strength of Opinion

The CMM paradigm and established psychophysical relations can be used to scale nonmetric variables such as seriousness of offenses or importance of public office. The item to be scaled is presented and a subject adjusts or produces a A_i and a B_i, stimuli from two different domains such as sounds and lights, or numbers and squeezes of a hand-dynamometer, so that both the loudness and brightness of the two dependent variables match the magnitude of the item on the dimension of interest. These modalities are matched on different occasions so that errors are likely to be independent. The item is assumed to produce an internal representation of variable magnitude Ψ_i which in turn induces a representation in both A and B. The following diagram illustrates these mappings (the stimulus item is denoted by Ω):

$$\Omega \to \Psi \begin{cases} \nearrow & A_i = \Lambda(1/\alpha \ln \Psi,\ 1/\alpha^2\sigma^2) \\ & = \Lambda(\ln \Psi,\ \sigma^2) \\ \searrow & B_i = \Lambda(1/\beta \ln \Psi,\ 1/\beta^2\sigma^2) \end{cases}$$

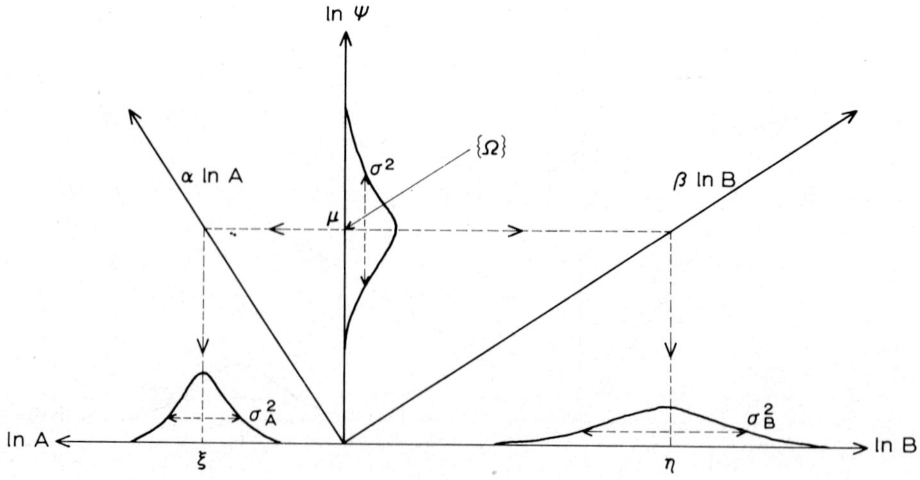

Fig. 3. The indirect CMM paradigm.

The linear mappings implied by the relationships expressed above are illustrated in Figure 3. As shown, the relationships among the parameters of the three distributions are functionally interdependent. The relations among the variances imply $\sigma_B^2/\sigma_A^2 = \alpha^2/\beta^2$ ... this result is an important relationship for the estimation of the CMM exponent, α/β, as will be seen below.

In constructing a ratio scale of strength of opinion for social stimuli, using indirect CMM, several items covering as extreme a range as practical are presented as criterion stimuli to which are matched stimulus levels from both A and B. Essentially, two ratio scales are constructed ... if it is presumed that the true psychophysical relations are known and faithfully rendered in the scaling task. One scale obtains by applying the transformation $\Psi = A^\alpha$ to the geometric mean of the levels of A produced in response to an item; the other is obtained from B and the assumed relation $\Psi = B^\beta$. These two scales should be in fairly close agreement although they are fallible and a perfect correlation would not be expected. However, the first step in validating the scales should involve evaluation of whether the data are in accord with the expected psychophysical relations. This is done by examining the linearity of regression of $\ln B$ upon $\ln A$ and comparing the empirical regression coefficient with the theoretical value of α/β.

A plot of $\ln B$ vs $\ln A$ is a plot of the logarithms of the geometric mean responses produced to each stimulus item; that is, each data point corresponds to one of the scaled items and the coordinates for each point are the logarithms of the A and B matched, on the (log) average, to that item.

Both variables are fallible in this type of regression because of variability in magnitude productions on both continua. Accordingly, the regression coefficient should be estimated by (7) rather than (4). A great simplification is possible, however, because of what we can assume about the relationship between the two error variances. As shown above, $\sigma_B^2/\sigma_A^2 = \alpha^2/\beta^2$ which is the square of the expected slope parameter of the linear functional relationship between $Y = \ln B$ and $X = \ln A$. If this value is substituted for λ in (7) it reduces to the simple expression

$$b = (S_{yy}/S_{xx})^{1/2}, \qquad (9)$$

where

$$S_{yy} = \sum Y^2 - (\sum Y)^2/n,$$
$$S_{xx} = \sum X^2 - (\sum X)^2/n.$$

This result is equal to the geometric mean of the two slopes $b = S_{xy}/S_{xx}$ and $1/b' = S_{yy}/S_{xy}$, the latter being the slope of the regression line of X upon Y.

Confidence limits for the true regression coefficient are given by (8). If this confidence interval does not contain the expected value α/β then the validity of one or both scales is contradicted. The utility of the indirect CMM paradigm lies in the vulnerability of the procedures to violations of the underlying scaling assumptions. If *S*s are not producing matches consistent, on the average, with the psychophysical relations presumed to be true for the experimental variables the scale based on their matches will be biased.

Assuming that our two psychophysical scales pass the acid test of log-linearity with a theoretically accordant slope, the computation of a single scale value for each Ω is based on the two magnitude productions A and B and the known exponents α and β:

$$\Psi(\Omega) = (A^{\alpha} B^{\beta})^{1/2}. \tag{10}$$

This estimate may still be wrong even though the above criterion is satisfied, for reasons made clear in the next section, but it has an interesting geometric interpretation which remains valid when (10) is replaced by (12) in order to accommodate the regression bias. In the X–Y plot relating $\alpha \ln A$ and $\beta \ln B$, data points representing the stimulus items will be scattered about a regression line with unit slope. The deviations from the regression line reflect the variability inherent in magnitude productions and less than perfect correlation between the dependent variables. Each (X, Y) data point is sampled from a bivariate distribution of potential observations with expected values for the true coordinates of the stimulus item being the distribution parameters $\xi = \alpha \ln A$ and $\eta = \beta \ln B$. The point (ξ, η) corresponding to (X, Y) is the perpendicular projection of (X, Y) onto the regression line. The logarithm of the estimate given by (10) corresponds to this projection.

The Regression Paradigm

Stevens and Greenbaum (1966) review the results of several experiments and show that CMM functions are often biased because of a tendency for *S*s to shorten the range of their adjustments of the variable under their control. Depending on which variable *S* controls, the matching procedures may yield two different regression lines (in log-log coordinates) and thus two different exponents for the power function presumed to hold between the variables. This so-called "regression effect" appears to be ubiquitous in psychophysical scaling and probably accounts for more variability in experimental determinations of exponents than any other factor. Hence, one reason the indirect CMM paradigm used in social scaling might fail the validation test is that the regression biases are likely to occur unequally on the two variables. This can result in an empirical relation between the two matching variables with an exponent different from that expected. This should and probably would result in rejection of the scales. But a hazard is presented when regression effects operate in a symmetric fashion. The simple validation criterion presented above would be satisfied but the ratio scale of opinion constructed by (10) would be seriously attenuated. The problem can be seen graphically in Figure 4. The equivalence between $\ln \Psi$ and $\alpha \ln A$ is depicted by the 45° diagonal line. An item having a magnitude $\Psi(\Omega)$ should be matched by A_t the theoretical (true) value corresponding to $A_t = \Psi^{1/\alpha}$. When a regression bias operates *S* produces a value A_e consistent with the empirical relation represented by the solid line drawn with a slope angle of $(45° + \theta)$. The parameter θ is called the angle of regression. The greater the regression toward mean levels the larger the regression angle. The exponent for the biased function is

$$a = \tan(45° + \theta) = X_t / X_e, \tag{11}$$

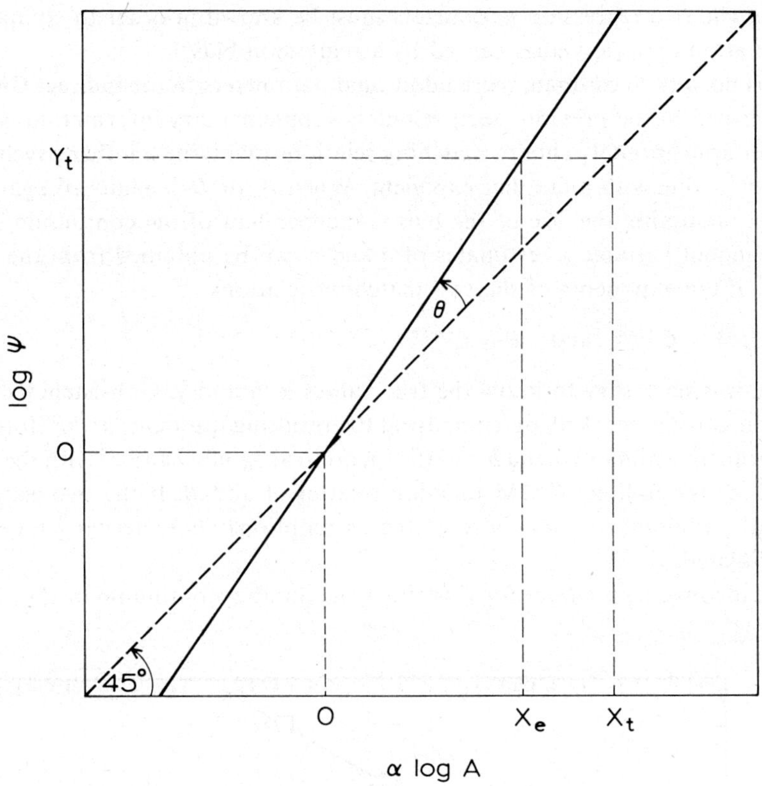

Fig. 4. The regression effect.

where $X_t = \alpha \ln A_t = \ln \Psi(\Omega)$ and $X_e = \alpha \ln A_e$ and where, for simplicity, levels of A are presumed measured relative to the abscissa of the point of intersection of the two curves.

From (11) it is easy to see that the relation between the value A_e actually produced by S and the value A_t that S should have produced in response to $\Psi(\Omega)$ is

$$A_t = A_e^a.$$

An equivalent relationship holds between the unbiased and biased productions on the other modality, B, although a different regression may be operating with an exponent equal to b, thus

$$B_t = B_e^b.$$

When these values are substituted in (10) the correct estimate of $\Psi(\Omega)$ based on the two obtained psychophysical matches is

$$\Psi(\Omega) = (A_e^{a\alpha} B_e^{b\beta})^{1/2}. \qquad (12)$$

Not only must the true exponents of the psychophysical relations be known but also the size of the two regression parameters must be known in order to compensate for the attenuation in scale values caused by a regression bias.

There is no way to estimate these additional parameters in the indirect CMM paradigm described in the previous section unless supplementary information is obtained from other appropriately chosen matching relations involving another psychophysical continuum ... one with a familiar exponent. When A, or B, is matched against C, for example ... assuming the size of the bias is independent of the continuum serving as the independent variable ... estimates of a and b can be obtained from the empirical estimates of the exponents of the two matching relations

$$A = C^{\gamma/\alpha a} \quad \text{and} \quad B = C^{\gamma/\beta b}.$$

Of course it is necessary to know the true values α, β and γ. Consistency of the representation can be checked by comparing the resulting quotient, $a\alpha/b\beta$ (formed from the independent estimates a and b and the theoretical values α and β) with the empirical exponent for the indirect CMM function relating A and B. If the two estimates are significantly different, one or more of the assumptions characterizing the paradigm may be violated.

The most convenient choice for C is either the number continuum or the continuum

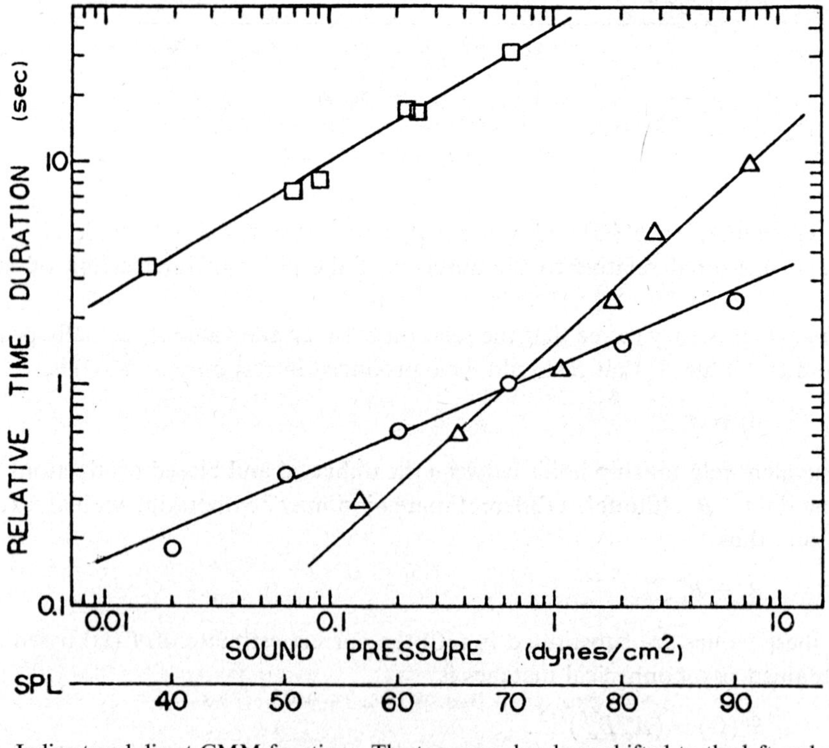

Fig. 5. Indirect and direct CMM functions. The top curve has been shifted to the left and upward by one log unit (Dawson & Brinker, 1971).

of line length ... both of which are easy to present and both have a theoretical exponent equal to one.

An alternative procedure that does not require the introduction of a third continuum is a combination of the direct and indirect CMM procedures. Only two psychophysical continua are involved, A and B, and the set of social stimuli to be scaled $\{\Omega\}$. Both A and B are matched to Ω as before and, in addition, A and B are matched to each other in a direct CMM procedure. This paradigm was first used, to my knowledge, by Dawson & Brinker (1971). They used two physical continua; sound pressure (A) and time duration (B). The nonmetric stimuli were trigrams differing in pronounceability. Loudness was matched to duration, duration was matched to loudness, and both loudness and duration were matched to pronounceability. The results are shown in Figure 5. The reported slopes for the direct CMM functions are 0.44 for the circles (duration adjusted), and 0.91 for the triangles (sound pressure adjusted). This shows a relatively large regression effect. The top line represents the indirect CMM curve obtained by plotting duration as a function of sound pressure for each trigram. This line has a reported slope of 0.60 (a value that is probably slightly underestimated because the method of fitting the line did not take into account errors in the horizontal direction). Either of these three different matching functions might be represented as the 'equal-sensation' functions relating apparent duration and loudness. They differ because the bias parameters figure differently in each exponent. In the first function duration is adjusted with a regression bias resulting in

$$(B^b)^\beta = A^\alpha \quad \rightarrow \quad B = A^{(\alpha/\beta)(1/b)} = A^{n_1}.$$

In the second function, the bias is in the adjusted variable; sound pressure

$$B^\beta = (A^a)^\alpha \quad \rightarrow \quad B = A^{(\alpha/\beta)a} = A^{n_2}.$$

In the third function both variables are separately adjusted, each with its regression bias, and in their mutual relationship with the trigrams they are indirectly brought into the following functional relation

$$(B^b)^\beta = (A^a)^\alpha \quad \rightarrow \quad B = A^{(\alpha/\beta)(a/b)} = A^{n_3}.$$

The theoretical exponents of the three power functions appearing on the right in each case are estimated by the empirical regression coefficients $n_1 = 0.44$, $n_2 = 0.91$, and $n_3 = 0.60$. Equating each n_i with its theoretical counterpart we get three equations in three unknowns. Their solution gives the following estimates of α/β, a, and b.

$$\begin{aligned} \alpha/\beta &= n_1 n_2/n_3 = (0.44)\,(0.91)/(0.60) = 0.67 \\ a &= n_3/n_1 = (0.60)/(0.44) = 1.36 \\ b &= n_2/n_3 = (0.91)/(0.60) = 1.52 \end{aligned} \tag{13}$$

The value of two thirds for the exponent relating duration and sound pressure is consistent with the loudness exponent which is assumed to be two thirds (Stevens, 1971b), and a unit exponent for apparent duration which is consistent with the value reported by Stevens and Greenbaum (1966).

If the estimate of α/β obtained by formula (13) is consistent with the assumed values for the true exponents of the psychophysical relations involved then computation of the bias free estimates of $\Psi(\Omega)$, comparable to those obtained in (12) is provided by

$$\Psi(\Omega) = (A^{\beta n_2} B^{\alpha/n_1})^{1/2}, \tag{14}$$

where n_1 and n_2 are exponents of the empirical relations given above in which B and then A is the variable adjusted to match Ω, and α and β are the theoretical exponents that transform unbiased values of A and B into perceived magnitude, Ψ.

References

Aitchison, J. & Brown, J. A. C. *The lognormal distribution.* Cambridge: The University Press, 1963.

Askovitz, S. I. A short-cut method for fitting the best straight line to a series of points according to the criterion of least squares. *Journal of the American Statistical Association*, 1957, **52**, 13–17.

Cochran, W. G. Errors of measurement in statistics. Technometrics, 1968, **10**, 637–666.

Cross, D. V. Sequential dependencies and regression in psychophysical judgments. *Perception and Psychophysics*, 1973, **14**, 547–552.

Dawson, W. E. & Brinker, R. P. Validation of ratio scales of opinion by multimodality matching. *Perception and Psychophysics*, 1971, **9**, 413–417.

Madansky, A. The fitting of straight lines when both variables are subject to error. *Journal of the American Statistical Association*, 1959, **54**, 173–205.

Stevens, S. S. On the operation known as judgment. *American Scientist*, 1966, **54**, 385–401.

Stevens, S. S. Issues in psychophysical measurement. *Psychological Review*, 1971a, **78**, 426–450.

Stevens, S. S. Perceived level of noise by Mark VII and decibels (E). *Journal of the Acoustical Society of America*, 1971b, **51**, 575–601.

Stevens, S. S. *Psychophysics and social scaling*. General Learning, 1972.

Stevens, S. S. and Greenbaum, H. Regression effect in psychophysical judgment. *Perception and Psychophysics*, 1966, **4**, 439–446.

RELATIONS OF PERIPHERAL ACTION POTENTIALS AND CORTICAL EVOKED POTENTIALS TO THE MAGNITUDE OF SENSATION[1]

HALLOWELL DAVIS

Central Institute for the Deaf, St. Louis, Mo.

Abstract. The magnitude of sensation is related to the stimulus according to Stevens' psychophysical "power" law $\Psi = k(\phi - \phi_0)^n$. Peripheral action potentials and central electric responses have both been examined for a possible parallelism. According to Mountcastle, somatosensory receptors impose the power law on the number or the frequency of impulses in the primary sensory neurons and higher-order neurons respond linearly to this input. Davis, however, found poor correspondence in auditory nerve of guinea pig, using number of active fibers as the measure.

The slow cortical *V*-potential response increases too slowly with increasing stimulus magnitude to determine whether the relation is linear, power law or more complex, and other properties of the *V* potential differ widely from sensation. A new experiment with constant stimuli, relates ratings of sensation magnitude to amplitude of individual *V* potentials. The correlation is about +0.20, very low but significant. The *V* potential does not seem to arise close to the physiological substrate of sensation.

A major interest of S. Smith (Smitty) Stevens was his "power law" of psychophysics (Stevens, 1961). This law states, in its simplest form, that "equal stimulus ratios produce equal sensation ratios." Smitty devoted many years of work to establishing its generality. The simplified mathematical form[2] of the law is $\Psi = k \cdot \phi^n$. Each sensory modality has a characteristic exponent.

A major interest of my own has been the slow cortical evoked potential as recorded from the human scalp at the vertex (referred to ears or mastoid). These potentials, evoked in the waking state by sound, light or electric shock, were first described by my wife, Pauline A. Davis (1939). They have come to be known as the *V* (or vertex) potentials. They are broadly similar across the three major modalities mentioned above and apparently they are generated in the primary cortical projection area of the modality in question (Vaughan & Ritter, 1970). Using the technique of averaged responses, I and my associates have explored many of the properties of this response, particularly in the auditory modality.

One obvious question has been whether the amplitude of the *V* potential follows the Stevens power law. A broader question is whether the *V* potential, as an output of the central nervous system, CNS, constitutes a useful "window" to the uncharted psychophysiological processes of sensation. The broad question has been the explicit

1 This research was supported in full by a U.S. Public Health Service, Department of Health, Education and Welfare research grant NSO3856 from the National Institute of Neurological Diseases and Stroke.

The author acknowledges with thanks the assistance of Mr Arnold Heidbreder in this experiment.

2 More fully the Stevens power law is $\Psi = K(\phi - \phi_0)^n$, where Ψ = magnitude of sensation, k = constant, ϕ = stimulus, ϕ_0 = stimulus at threshold.

H. R. Moskowitz et al. (eds.), Sensation and Measurement. 37–47.

hypothesis of many recent investigators, but in my own opinion it is not tenable. We shall see that the relation of the V potentials to sensation is very remote at best.

Auditory AP in Guinea Pig

Smitty and I discussed several times the possible congruence between neurophysiological and psychophysical processes and measurements, particularly about 1960 when the power law was new and when I had just measured the whole-nerve action potential of the auditory nerve in guinea pig to various intensities of sound (Davis, 1961). Here, under special conditions of stimulation by high-frequency tone-pips (to obtain an adequately synchronized volley of impulses) and intra-cochlear electrodes [to eliminate the receptor potential (the cochlear microphonic)], the amplitude of the action potential became a measure of the *number of fibers* excited by the tone-pip. Unfortunately for the hypothesis of congruence, the input-output curve showed a rapid rise of AP amplitude, a partial plateau and then a second larger and steeper rise. Apparently there were two populations of fibers: a smaller low-threshold group and a larger high-threshold group. This did not disprove congruence, however, as we did not know how the magnitude of sensation increased in guinea pig. Smitty and I were disappointed but remained hopeful, because central nervous-system activity is not entirely a direct linear reiteration of the input from the peripheral sensory units.

Cutaneous AP in Monkey

The CNS has proved to be more linear than we thought, however. Mountcastle and his associates (1966, 1967a, b; 1969.) have measured the input from cutaneous sensory units in glabrous skin of monkey and have compared it with the psychophysical responses of man to identical tactile stimulation of the hand. The measure of input to the CNS in this case was not the *number of fibers* responding but the *frequency of impulses* set up in a single sensory fiber by stimuli of various intensities. The result was a surprisingly accurate linear relation between stimulus and number of impulses. This corresponded to a power law with an exponent of 1.0. In the companion psychophysical experiment on man, magnitude estimations done according to Stevens' method yielded a power-law straight line (in double-logarithmic coordinates) with a slope corresponding to an exponent of 1.0. Very similar experiments in Stevens' laboratory had given an exponent of 1.1. This is probably the best congruence on record between a neurophysiological measure and the psychophysical power law. This correspondence is valid for a particular type of slowly-adapting receptor in a situation where the intensity of stimulation is coded by frequency of neural discharge, not by number of fibers. There are also other cutaneous receptors, however, such as the fast-adapting elements (probably Pacinean corpuscles) in hairy skin that mediate the sense of vibration or flutter. For this form of stimulation the exponent of the power law is about 0.5, both for the neurons of monkey and for psychophysical estimations by man (Werner & Mountcastle, 1965, 1968).

Linear Processing by the CNS

The experiments cited so far have all dealt with the input to the CNS at the level of the peripheral sensory nerve. This is a very strategic location and feasible for experimentation as well. Some measurements have also been made on single neural units in unanaesthetized monkeys in intermediate nuclei of brain stem or thalamus (Mountcastle, 1967), and, in the auditory system, on gross (large electrode) responses of superior olive, inferior colliculus, and cortical auditory area *I* in anaesthetized cats (Desmedt, 1962). Excellent correspondence was reported in each case between responses at the higher levels and the input in primary sensory units. Mountcastle (1967) cites similar results for the visual system (Poggio and Baker) and for taste (Zotterman). Evidently in some pathways in each sensory system there is a one-to-one correspondence of nerve impulses from level to level, although it is also well known that very different relations between input and output obtain for other pathways and transfer stations.

From these and related experiments on the cutaneous sensory system Mountcastle (1967) draws two conclusions. First:

> The CNS deals linearly with the input from primary sensory units. The exponent of the power law is thus determined by the properties of the receptors.

Second:

> For one and the same afferent system, and dealing with the same attribute of the same sensory quality, quite different relations obtain between stimulus and response (both neural and behavioral) depending upon whether glabrous or hairy skin is stimulated and these differences are uniquely set by the transforming properties of the two sets of receptors concerned. The brain operates upon either in a linear manner.

Parsimony forbade any more complicated hypotheses of compensating non-linearities in the particular system studied. It will be interesting to see how far the principle of linearity extends in other sensory systems such as auditory and visual.

It is obviously not feasible to study single neurons in humans with implanted electrodes, and even the summed activity of many neurons gives very small potentials with external electrodes. Mid-brain responses and early cortical activation can be recorded from the human head, it is true, but even with the averaged response techniques no one has yet reported satisfactory input-output curves.

The *V* Potentials

The slow *V* potentials have special strategic value. The responses are usually of the order of 10 μV and are readily separated from the EEG background by simple response-averaging (Donchin & Lindsley, 1969). Being cortical in origin, they are much closer to the site of the processes underlying sensation than the peripheral sensory units. They are slow enough to integrate the cortical input over several milliseconds, so that the input need not be exactly synchronous in all of the participating neurons. Finally the entire complex of slow *V* potential waves, between 50 and 250 ms, has seemed to reflect activity evoked by the fast lemniscal pathways associated with sensation and fine discrimination, as opposed to possible slower and more diffuse activation by way of the reticular formation. These *V* potentials are apparently a *second-order* cortical response of the primary projection area. They are at a high enough level in the CNS to be strongly influenced by the state of the subject (awake vs asleep). There is a clear but slow fatigue effect although no habituation in the strict sense of the term. Heightened alertness and focussing attention on the stimulus, as in making a difficult discrimination, significantly increase the amplitude of the response. The slow *V*

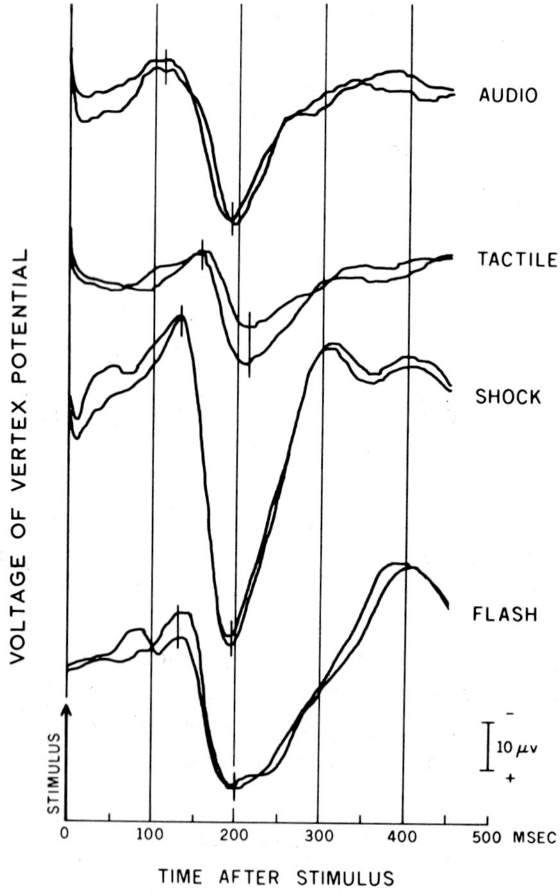

Fig. 1. Superimposed tracings of averaged vertex potentials, reference mastoid, evoked by stimuli ($n = 32$) in four modalities. The general form and properties are the same although the latencies of the major peaks (N_1 and P_2) differ slightly. This subject yielded unusually large responses, particularly to shocks (to his left median nerve). Subjects differ with respect to the voltages of their *V* potentials at a given interstimulus interval and sensation level. Here ISI was 5.5 s, and the stimuli were adjusted for equal sensation magnitudes, matched to shock at the threshold for muscle twitch as standard. (From Davis *et al.*, 1972, by permission from *Electroencephalography and Clinical Neurophysiology*.)

potentials do indeed offer a fine promise of psychophysiological congruence of some sort.

Thresholds

One requirement of congruence is met. The threshold of detection of the *V* potential corresponds very closely to the psychoacoustic (auditory) threshold. This is true both in the quiet and in the presence of a noise background. The *V* potentials are used as endpoints in electric response audiometry (Davis, *et al.*, 1967) and laboratory experiments confirm the correspondence between the two types of threshold (Hillyard *et al.*, 1971; Tanis, 1971). A necessary condition for the correspondence seems to be a high level of alertness or attention, but the range of uncertainty seems to be nearly as great for the behavioral as for the electrical threshold (Hirsh & Wier, 1973).

In favor of a possible relation of the slow *V* potential to sensation is the general similarity of the response in the visual, auditory, and tactile modalities (Figure 1). This invites comparison with some general psychophysical process such as sensation; and the latency is of the right order of magnitude.

The Power Law

On the other hand the input-output relation (intensity function) of the auditory *V* potential does not show a convincing power-law form with the proper exponent. An early claim of a power-law function (Keidel & Spreng, 1965) was based on scanty data, the important parameter of interstimulus interval was not controlled, and satisfactory confirmation is lacking. One of our own experiments (Davis *et al.*, 1968) yielded data that could be "fitted" by a straight-line function in double logarithmic coordinates, but in semi-logarithmic coordinates they fitted just as well. The increase in amplitude of the *V* potential over the entire dynamic range was small and the variability of the data was large. The only clear conclusion was that if the power law applied to the data the exponent was certainly smaller than that yielded by auditory magnitude estimations. Further study of unpublished data of the intensity function of the auditory *V* potential has convinced us that, like the total AP of the auditory nerve, the amplitude increases rapidly over a range of 20 dB above threshold, then very slowly up to about 70 dB. Above this level individuals differ. Some show large increases at high stimulus levels, others seem to "saturate" and yield rather small responses of nearly constant amplitude. There is little support here for congruence with respect to the power law.

Other Properties of *V* Potentials

Several other properties of the slow *V* potentials make it difficult to find a clear relation to *any* aspects of sensation. The *V* potential is a transient response, or more probably a sequence of responses, evoked by a transient stimulus such as a click or the onset (or the offset) of a steady tone or noise. The response depends on a *change* in the stimulus, on or off, or the sudden addition of an increment of intensity (ΔI) or a change in frequency (Δf) (McCandless and Rose, 1970; Nichols and Tanenholtz, 1970).

Another time-related property of the *V* potential is its extraordinarily long recovery period. If the voltage of the response is to be independent of the interstimulus interval (ISI) the interval must be no shorter than approximately 10 s. At ISI of 1 s the voltage is reduced to about one quarter of its maximum (Davis *et al.*, 1966). Another curious property is the interaction across modalities (Davis *et al.*, 1972). Flashes of light or electric shocks interposed between clicks reduce the voltage of the auditory evoked potentials, although the effect is not as great as if additional clicks are interposed with the same interstimulus intervals. The dependence of amplitude on interval and the cross-modality depression have no counterparts in the magnitude of sensation. In fact it is difficult to find any psychological function except perhaps short-term memory that has a half-time of the order of two seconds.

The obvious inference from this collection of facts is that the voltage of the slow *V* potential does not parallel sensation. This inference holds whether we measure N_{100} (the negative peak 100 msec after stimulus onset) alone or P_{170} (the positive peak 170 msec after stimulus onset) alone or more conveniently $N_{100}-P_{170}$. The *V* potential apparently lies on another processing pathway or else somewhere beyond the neural level at which the magnitude of sensation is determined. The voltage is influenced by several factors that do not affect the magnitude of sensation. The *V* potential is a good sign, as at threshold, but a poor measure.

An Experimental Demonstration of a Correlation

The question remains whether, among the variety of relevant factors, there is *any* correlation between the voltage of the slow *V* potential and the magnitude of sensation beyond the fact that both are rising functions of the intensity of the stimulus. With stimulus constant or nearly so is there any relation? An experimental answer to this question was made possible by our finding a cooperative subject whose *V* potentials, evoked by percutaneous electric shocks to a peripheral nerve, were unusually large. In his EEG tracing, filtered to pass 1 to 15 Hz, it was easy to measure the amplitude of *individual* responses, which were often more than 100 μV in amplitude at long interstimulus intervals. He was able to relax his muscles effectively and while sitting with eyes open, reading a magazine or making psychophysical judgments, his EEG background was relatively quiet. Rectangular pulses of current to his left median nerve at the wrist were adjusted to or just below the threshold for muscle twitch in the hand. (Large Beckman electrodes were employed, and the interelectrode resistance and the twitch threshold were very stable.) Two scalp electrodes were placed near C_3 and C_4, over the somatosensory projection area of each hand. Our usual interstimulus interval was 5 s. A longer interval would have yielded somewhat larger responses but it was important to collect, within an hour or so, enough responses for statistical evaluation before their amplitude became significantly reduced by fatigue or, as we called it, the "chair effect." The changes of state were monitored by the usual computer-averaged response for each series. The individual responses were measured by hand from the EEG tape, which moved at 60 mm s^{-1}. At this speed the responses could be clearly identified by their latencies.

Under these experimental conditions the shock-evoked V potentials varied considerably in amplitude from one response to the next, as shown in Figure 2. Some of

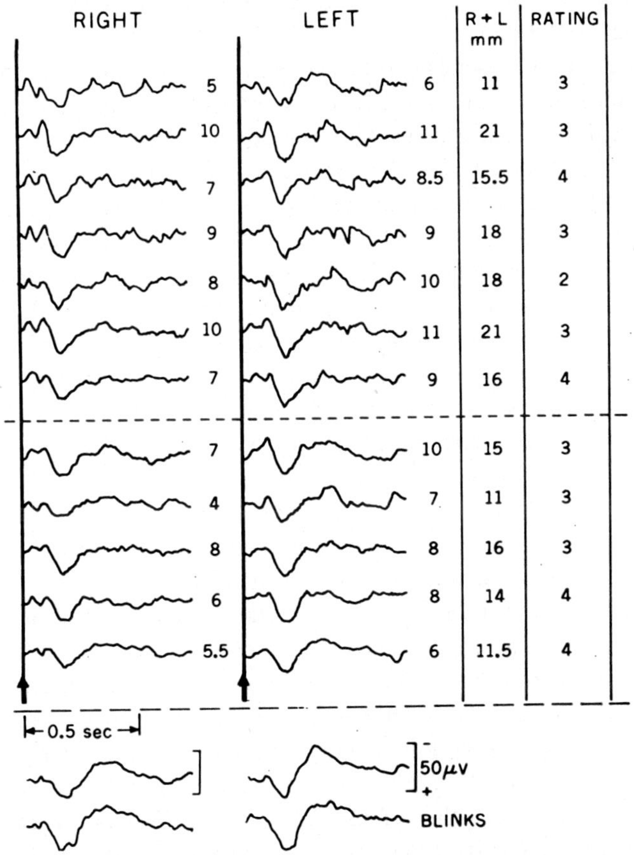

Fig. 2. Individual V potentials evoked by shocks to the left median nerve. Scalp electrodes were over the right and left hemispheres, approximately C_3 and C_4, each referred to its homolateral mastoid process (M_1 and M_2). Same subject as for Figure 1. ISI = 5 s. Speed of tape = 60 mm s^{-1}. Passband of Grass Polygraph (7P5A) = 1–15 Hz. Responses have been retraced by hand, aligned with respect to their stimulus signals at the vertical lines. Stimuli were constant, just at the threshold for muscle twitch. The subject gave orally his rating, on a five point scale (1 = weakest), of the magnitude of his sensation. The numbers adjacent to each tracing are the millimeters of the $N_1 - P_2$ wave as measured on the original tape. Two blink artifacts, R and L, are shown at the bottom. Note that the calibrations of the two channels were not exactly equal. This accounts for the slight systematic differences in amplitude. Note also the small negative wave (N_0) that regularly preceeds N_1 in the contralateral (right) but not in the homolateral response. The 7 top and the 5 bottom responses are consecutive at the beginning and the end of a block of 32.

this variability is due to the EEG background, but most of it is not.[3] The subject was not aware of any such variations in the magnitude of sensation of the shocks as occurred in the amplitudes of the responses. The responses from right and left hemispheres (each referred to the homolateral mastoid process) varied almost exactly in parallel ($r=0.84$); so closely that simultaneous right and left responses were summed for subsequent statistical treatment, in order to reduce the contribution from EEG to the variability. Furthermore the latencies of the (averaged) responses from the two hemispheres were identical within the uncertainty of measurement (contralateral, 138.4±3.9, homolateral 135.8±2.5 ms).

On the basis of earlier studies (Stohr & Goldring, 1969, and unpublished observations) of patients from whom one cortical somatosensory projection area had been excised (by Dr Sidney Goldring) we had anticipated *earlier* activation of the contralateral (right) cortex followed by secondary transcallosal activation on the left, with additional variability of amplitude introduced in the second cortical response. Our present observations suggest instead a *single sub-cortical source* of the variability of amplitude and simultaneous activation of the two hemispheres from this source. This suggests in turn activation of the *V* potential by way of the diffuse reticular formation rather than by the more discrete lemniscal pathway as we had supposed. The findings are in accord, however, with the inference made above that the *V* potential response is on a sensory pathway different from the one that determines the magnitude of the sensation. (It is not appropriate to try here to reconcile this model with the observations on Dr Goldring's patients. The task is not simple. It will be important to determine, when it becomes technically feasible, whether the fast components of the *V* potential share the variability of the slow components and whether they differ in latency between homolateral and contralateral hemispheres.)

The fluctuations in amplitude of the *V* potential were examined in our subject over several sessions in which he engaged in various activities such as reading, counting the stimuli, making discriminations, rating the magnitude of his sensations, or simply suffering fatigue in a very prolonged session. The correlations between successive individual responses were very low, averaging about +0.16, but most of them were positive. We have not as yet been able to identify any firm relation between the variations in amplitude and any other factor. We have an impression of nearly random variation (cf. Zerlin & Davis, 1967) but with periods of higher or lower average amplitude with durations of the order of half a minute. On the other hand the average responses ($n=32$), summed by the computer over periods of about 2.5 min, remained

[3] The variability due to the EEG background (including muscle) was assessed by comparing the blink artifacts recorded from right and left hemispheres respectively (see Figure 2). There is no alpha rhythm in the EEG under our experimental conditions and the right and left background EEGs are nearly independent of one another. In one experiment the subject was instructed to blink deliberately between the stimuli. The artifacts were of the same order of magnitude and varied in amplitude like the *V* potentials. The correlation between *R* and *L* blinks was +0.85 and between the *R* and *L V* potentials in the same trial it was +0.86. On the other hand the correlation between successive *V* potentials (sum of right and left) varied widely but averaged only about +0.16.

very stable and reflected the familiar influences of attention, difficult discrimination, fatigue, etc.

We (C. S. Watson, S. K. Hirsh, C. C. Wier and the present writer) next undertook to determine whether, as the amplitude of the *V* potential varied spontaneously, any relation between magnitude of sensation and the amplitude could be established. This is really the key question. In one series of trials the shocks were actually varied slightly in duration, adjusted so that the subject could just distinguish among three durations. After 5 or 6 shocks of medium duration to enable him to establish a criterion, the three durations were presented in random sequence, but always with 10 or 11 of each duration in the series of 32 stimuli. During the 5-s interval between shocks the subject rated the magnitude of his sensation on a five-point scale. In another series of trials he was told simply that his discrimination task would be more difficult, and the duration of the shocks was held constant. He nevertheless gave ratings that included some quite confident subjective differences, i.e., ratings of 1 or 5. This experiment was carried out first in March, 1972 (Watson *et al.* 1972), and was replicated in January, 1973 with almost identical results.

The correlation between the actual strength of the stimuli (when the strength was varied) and amplitude of *V* potential was only +0.07 (1972) and +0.08 (1973). On the other hand, between the actual strength and the magnitude rating it was +0.75 (1972) and +0.63 (1973). The critical correlation between the amplitude of response and the rating was +0.21 (1972) and +0.17 (1973). This correlation is low but it is positive and it is significant.

There is indeed a demonstrable correlation between amplitude of the slow *V* potential and subjective magnitude of sensation. On the other hand, as Dr Watson put it in conversation,

> If a cooperative person's state of consciousness is at issue, information out of his mouth is a lot better than that off the top of his head.

An Interpretive Comment

The power law, $\Psi = k \cdot \phi^n$, describes the relation between magnitude of sensation and the stimulus. The first step toward establishing this relation is the behavior of the receptors. Here the dynamic range of the system is established. The extent of the dynamic range is the chief factor that determines the characteristic exponent of each sensory system. Increments of neural activity related to increments of the stimulus are distributed over this range and a power-law relation is established, approximately, at this level. The coding of intensity among various sensory systems and even within a given system apparently differs, although in general it seems to involve some combination of number of fibers activated and frequency of discharge in individual fibers. A priori there may also be some weighting of the contribution of different fibers or else nonlinear addition of their effects. The experiments summarized or cited by Mountcastle seem to show that, to a rather surprising extent, the intermediate levels of the CNS deal in linear fashion with the neural input of the primary sensory fibers. Any smoothing or nonlinear adjustments (or integration in time or across neurons) that is needed to yield a straight-line power law in the hypothetical physiological process that underlies sensation is apparently carried out at a high level. This process is presumably a global activity of a group of neural elements. Somewhere, somehow a physiological measure may be found of such a global activity that corresponds to sensation in its latency, its time-course, and its relations to the various parameters of the stimulus, in addition to following the power law. This will be a "window" to the psychophysiology of sensation. But the slow *V* potential is not such a window. It is on a sensory pathway different from the one that determines magnitude of sensation and such relation between the two as is shown by our present experiments is probably quite indirect.

References

Davis, H. Peripheral coding of auditory information. In W. Rosenblith (Ed.), *Sensory Communication*, 1961, Ch. 7.

Davis, H., Mast, T., Yoshie, N., & Zerlin, S. The slow response of the human cortex to auditory stimuli: Recovery process. *Electroencephalography and Clinical Neurophysiology*, 1966, **21**, 105–113.

Davis, H., Hirsh, S. K., Shelnutt, J., & Bowers, C. Further validation of evoked response audiometry (ERA). *Journal of Speech and Hearing Research*, 1967, **10**, 717–732.

Davis, H., Bowers, C., & Hirsh, S. K. Relations of the human vertex potential to acoustic input: Loudness and masking. *Journal of Acoustical Society of America*, 1968, **43**, 431–438.

Davis, H., Osterhammel, P. A., Wier, C. C., & Gjerdingen, D. B. Slow vertex potentials: Interactions among auditory, tactile, electric and visual stimuli. *Electroencephalography and Clinical Neurophysiology*, 1972, **33**, 537–545.

Davis, P. A. Effects of acoustic stimuli on the waking human brain. *Journal of Neurophysiology*, 1939, **2**, 494–499.

Desmedt, J. E. Auditory-evoked potentials from cochlea to cortex as influenced by activation of the efferent olivo-cochlear bundle. *Journal of Acoustical Society of America*, 1962, **34**, 1478–1496.

Donchin, E., & Lindsley, D. B. (Eds.) Average evoked potentials: Methods, results and evaluations. *NASA (National Aeronautics and Space Administration SP-191*, 1969. Ch. 2, 4, and 6.

Hillyard, S. A., Squires, K. C., Bauer, J. W., & Lindsay, P. H. Evoked potential correlates of auditory signal detection. *Science*, 1971, **172**, 1357–1360.

Hirsh, S. K., & Wier, C. C. Personal communication based on unpublished experiments. 1973.

Keidel, W. D., & Spreng, M. Neurophysiological evidence for the Stevens power function in man. *Journal of the Acoustical Society of America*, 1965, **38**, 191–195.

McCandless, G. A., & Rose, D. E. Evoked cortical responses to stimulus change. *Journal of Speech and Hearing Research*, 1970.

Mountcastle, V. B. The problem of sensing and the neural coding of sensory events. In *The Neurosciences: A study program*, 1967, pp. 393–408. (a)

Mountcastle, V. B., Talbot, W. H., Darian-Smith, I. & Kornhuber, H. H. Neural basis of the sense of flutter-vibration. *Science*, 1967, **155**, 597–600. (b)

Mountcastle, V. B., Talbot, W. H., & Hornhuber, H. H. The neural transformation of mechanical stimuli delivered to the monkey's hand. In De Reuch & Knight (Eds.), *Touch, Heat and Pain*. A Ciba Foundation Symposium. London: J. & A. Churchill, 1966, pp. 325–351.

Mountcastle, V. B., Talbot, W. H., Sakata, H., & Hyvärinen, J. Cortical neuronal mechanisms in flutter-vibration studied in unanesthetized monkeys. Neuronal periodicity and frequency discrimination. *Journal of Neurophysiology*, 1969, **32**, 452–484.

Nichols, T. L., & Tanenholtz, S. D. Effect of increments in a sinusoidal pedestal on the vertex potential. *Journal of the Acoustical Society of America*, 1970, **47**, 97. (Abstract)

Stevens, S. S. The psychophysics of sensory function. In W. A. Rosenblith (Ed.), *Sensory Communication*, 1961, Ch. 1.

Stohr, P. E., & Goldring, S. Origin of somatosensory evoked scalp responses in man. *Journal of Neurosurgery*, 1969, **31**, 117–127.

Tanis, D. C. A signal-detection analysis of auditory evoked potentials in an intensity discrimination task. (Doctoral dissertation, Washington University) St. Louis, Mo., 1971.

Vaughan, H. G. Jr., & Ritter, W. The sources of auditory evoked responses recorded from the human scalp. *Electroencephalography and Clinical Neurophysiology*, 1970, **28**, 360–367.

Watson, C. S., Davis, H. & Hirsh, S. K. Relations between stimulus intensity, subjective magnitude and the cortical evoked response. Paper presented at the 13th meeting of the Psychonomic Society, St. Louis, November, 1972.

Werner, G., & Mountcastle, V. B. Neural activity in mechanoreceptive cutaneous afferents: Stimulus-response relations, Weber functions, and information transmission. *Journal of Neurophysiology*, 1965, **28**, 359–397.

Werner, G., & Mountcastle, V. B. Quantitative relations between mechanical stimuli to the skin and neural responses evoked by them. In D. R. Kenshalo (Ed.), *The Skin Senses*. Springfield, Ill.: Charles C. Thomas, 1965, pp. 112–137.

Zerlin, S., & Davis, H. The variability of single evoked vertex potentials in man. *Electroencephalography and Clinical Neurophysiology*, 1967, **23**, 468–472.

AN ASSESSMENT OF RATIO SCALES OF OPINION PRODUCED BY SENSORY-MODALITY MATCHING

WILLIAM E. DAWSON
University of Notre Dame

Abstract. The validity and potential usefulness of ratio scales of opinion are assessed by looking at some of the parallels that exist between these scales and those obtained by ratio scaling in psychophysics. Several experiments show that opinion scales can be validated by means of two or more sensory-modality matches. In addition, inverse opinion scales and scales for individual subjects are examined. The results show that ratio scales of opinion have many of the characteristics of sensory ratio scales. Preliminary efforts have been made to use sensory-modality scales in verbal learning, psycholinguistics, and with children.

As an outgrowth of efforts to measure loudness, Stevens found that a scale could be obtained by matching sensations from one intensive continuum to sensations from another. The earliest matching continuum he used was that of numbers in the method of magnitude estimation (ME). Later, cross-modality matching (CMM) entered the picture – here the sensory effects of stimuli from one physical continuum were matched to those from another.

In the 1960's, Ekman, Künnapas, and others of "the Stockholm group," showed that the ratio scaling methods of ratio estimation and magnitude estimation could be used to measure intensity of opinions. In a paper in 1966, Stevens summarized much of their activity in addition to work in the United States. In brief, he showed that many interscale relationships that hold in psychophysics between scales obtained using different methods (mainly ratio estimation, magnitude estimation, paired comparison, and category scaling) also are found when they are used to scale intensity of opinions. The invariance of these relations as one moves from impressions of physical stimuli to stimuli having no obvious physical metric led Stevens to assert that the newer direct scaling methods could supplant both the Thurstonian and the rating (or category) scale methods.

Another step was to move beyond matching just numbers to opinion intensity and it applied another psychophysical technique to the opinion domain. This entailed the use, as demonstrated by Dawson & Brinker (1971), of a procedure analogous to what is called cross-modality matching in psychophysics. It has been called *sensory-modality matching* (SMM) since it involves adjusting the sensory intensity to indicate ones intensity of opinion. For example, the loudness of a tone might be matched to each of several politicians in order to represent the degree of their political conservatism. It is no longer reasonable to call the method CMM here, since one modality is not being matched to a second sensory modality. In 1972, when Stevens reviewed the research on ratio scales of opinion for a second time, he added a discussion of these matches which employ continua other than just the number continuum. This paper will examine what is gained by use of the SMM method and will report the results of some ex-

H. R. Moskowitz et al. (eds.), Sensation and Measurement. 49–59.

periments that assess its potential usefulness in the scaling of attitudes, opinions, and the impressions of sets of stimuli in general.

Why Sensory-Modality Matching?

Many of the reasons for the use of SMM are the same as those for CMM. Neither requires the use of numbers and this can be an advantage in some situations. For example, Bond & Stevens (1969) showed that 5-year-old children could match the brightness of a light to the loudness of a 500-Hz tone. CMM was used because it was felt that such young children probably were numerically naive and would be unable to report their impressions in terms of numbers that indicate sensory ratios. Non-numerical matching continua should also be useful in cross-cultural studies where persons from different cultures have been exposed to different types of mathematical training. Their application would be perhaps most valuable with illiterate persons and cultures.

One reason CMM came into existence was the desire for a check on ME. As Stevens (1961) pointed out, many scientists were uneasy about a technique like ME in which subjects were asked to make sophisticated judgments in terms of the number system. CMM validated the method of ME by yielding a series of now familiar results which showed close agreement between empirical and predicted power-function exponents. The validation involved the prediction of CMM performance based on a pair of power functions obtained by ME: $\Psi_1 = \phi_1^{\alpha}$ and $\Psi_2 = \phi_2^{\beta}$. Here, Ψ_1 and Ψ_2 refer to the numerical judgments given to various stimulus intensities of the two physical continua ϕ_1 and ϕ_2, respectively. In a cross-modality match, sensations arising from ϕ_1 were matched to those from ϕ_2 and hence $\phi_1 = \phi_2^{\beta/\alpha}$ should and does describe the resulting match (Stevens, 1961). In logarithms, we have $\log\phi_1 = (\beta/\alpha)\,(\log\phi_2)$ which indicates that the equal-sensation power function is a straight line with a slope β/α when plotted in log-log coordinates. The method of SMM provides comparable advantages and it permits a somewhat similar validation in the realm of opinions regarding so-called nonmetric stimuli.

Some Tests of the Method

VALIDATION BY MULTIMODALITY MATCHING

With nonmetric stimuli, we cannot start out with two power functions involving two physical continua as the independent variables since there are no clear physical continua along which the stimuli can be arranged. Nevertheless, a comparable validation of opinion scales can be obtained if two different sensory-modality matches are made to the same set of nonmetric stimuli (see Dawson & Brinker for additional details). Since all of the stimulus items are matched twice, once for each matching continuum, we end up with a pair of SMM values for each item. Things matched as equal to a common item might in turn be expected to be equal. Therefore, the set of datum pairs are similar to a set of such pairs from a cross-modality match and they can be plotted

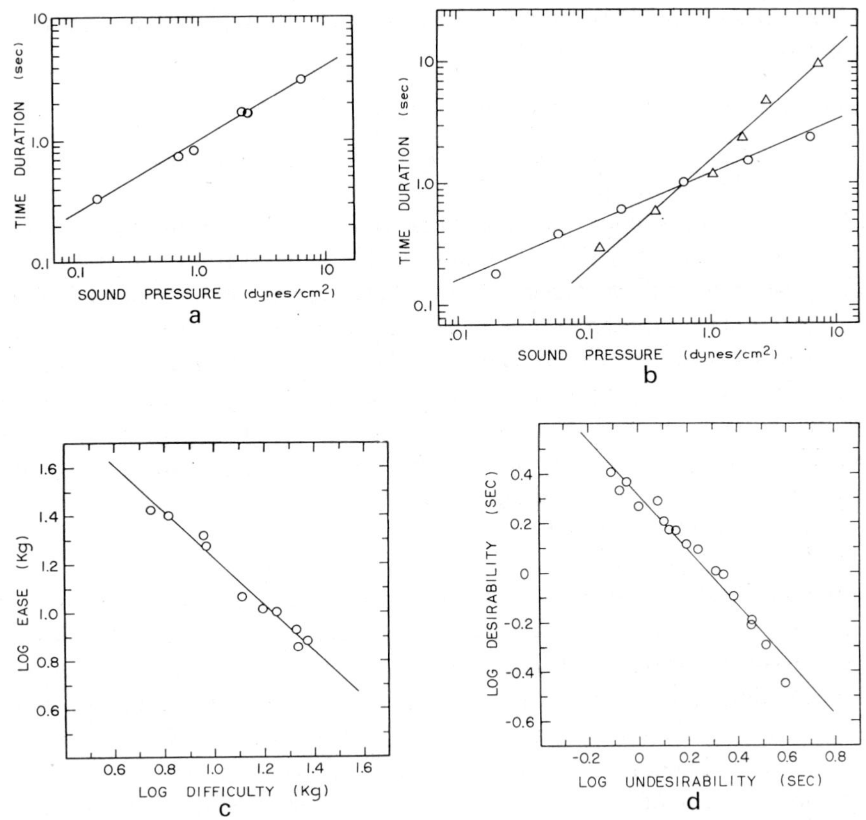

Fig. 1. Sensory-modality matches for (a) the multimodality matching of apparent time duration and loudness to trigram pronounceability, (b) the cross-modality matching of apparent duration to loudness (circles) and vice versa (triangles), (c) the inverse attributes of ease and difficulty of trigram pronounceability, and (d) the inverse attributes of desirability and undesirability of occupation.

graphically and compared with the results predicted for a direct cross-modality match. The results of one such plot are shown in Figure 1a. The time durations produced to indicate the pronounceability of each of six trigrams (YQG, RTI, TLF, IFO, VIZ, BAD) are plotted as a function of the corresponding sound pressures produced to represent their pronounceability. The straight line drawn through the six points in this log-log plot has a slope of 0.60. Since the latest reported exponent for apparent duration is 1.1 (Stevens, 1961) and that for loudness approximately 0.68 (Stevens, 1972), the predicted slope is 0.68/1.1, or 0.62, a value close to that obtained. The construction of two or more SMM scales, what we have called *multimodality matching* (MMM), is thus seen as one way of assessing whether ratio scales of opinion are consistent with findings in sensory psychophysics. Such a validation procedure permits the development of close quantitative ties between psychophysical and other scales of subjective impression. It means that scales for nonmetric variables can be assessed for consistency with the large set of psychophysical scales that are already known to be internally consistent.

COMPARISON WITH AN ACTUAL CROSS-MODALITY MATCH

The relation between the SMM results of a multimodality match can be predicted, as noted above, if the power function exponents are known for the two or more sensory modalities matched to the set of stimuli. These exponents, for the most part, have been obtained with the method of ME. Validation by MMM differs from validation by CMM in that it is a more indirect procedure. In CMM, one sensory modality is matched directly to another (and then vice versa if one wishes to balance for the "regression effect" discussed by Stevens & Greenbaum, 1966). The slope of a log-log plot of the two variables gives the empirical exponent. In MMM, each sensory modality is matched to a common intermediate set of stimuli and a pair of the resulting scales is examined in a log-log plot to determine the empirical exponent. Since construction of both of these scales involved the adjustment of a matching variable, the regression effect is already balanced out, much as it is in the CMM predictions discussed earlier where the predicted exponents are based on two ME scales.

The plotted results for a multimodality match agree with the results of a cross-modality match which has been balanced for the regression effect. The pair of curves in Figure 1b (from Dawson & Brinker, 1971) are for two cross-modality matches, one for apparent time duration matched to loudness and one for loudness matched to apparent duration. The former has a slope of 0.44 and the latter 0.91. Balancing for regression consists in taking their geometric mean (Indow & Stevens, 1966) and in this instance yields a value of 0.63 which agrees with the 0.60 cited above for MMM. The same *S*s took part in both the MMM and CMM tasks in an appropriately counterbalanced order.

INVERSE ATTRIBUTE SCALES

One of the first tests in psychophysics that aimed at validation of ratio scales was the construction and comparison of scales for inverse attributes of a fixed set of stimuli. Torgerson (1960, 1961) presented Munsell gray color chips and had *S*s give MEs of their lightnesses and also their darknesses. When he plotted average darkness judgments as a function of average lightness ones, he found, as would be expected if *S*s were judging ratios of attributes, that one scale was approximately the reciprocal of the other, i.e., $\Psi_1 = \Psi_2^{-1}$. Later studies (Stevens & Guirao, 1962, 1963) substantiated Torgerson's finding although there has been some debate about whether the relation is strictly reciprocal (Schneider & Lane, 1963).

If a pair of such inverse scales is plotted, in log-log coordinates, one as a function of the other, the expectation is a straight line with a slope of -1.0. Some of the psychophysical studies listed above have obtained close to such a result. The inverse attribute test can also be extended to SMM or ME opinion scales. Since our concern has been to assess the validity of SMM scales, we have made several such tests. Michael Mirando and I asked 24 *S*s to indicate both the ease and the difficulty of pronouncing each of ten trigrams by squeezing a hand dynamometer. An earlier experiment (Dawson & Mirando, 1973) had shown that these trigrams, ranging from BAD to YQG, covered a wide and fairly evenly spaced range of pronounceability. Figure 1c shows that the present results, although noisier than comparable psychophysical data, are fitted by a straight line in log-log coordinates and that the line of best fit has a slope of -0.98. Each datum point is based on the geometric means of the two sensory-modality matches for a trigram. The line was fitted to the data using a procedure described by Kenney (1939). This procedure fits a straight line to a set of datum pairs for the situation where both variables are subject to error. Since the ease and difficulty values both involve adjustment of the dynamometer by the *S*s, there is error present for both these variables. The figure shows that the two scales are very close to being reciprocals of one another.

In a second experiment, 38 *S*s evaluated 17 occupations both for their desirability and undesirability as a permanent, lifelong occupation. This time SMM was carried out by matching apparent time intervals in proportion to impressions. A key was depressed which held a small white light on for a period of time that *S* felt represented his impression. Figure 1d is a plot of the results and again the data suggest a reciprocal relationship with the best fitting line having -1.1 for its slope. The bottommost point lies below the line and there is a hint of concave-downward curvature, the type of departure from strict reciprocality noted in some of the studies cited earlier. By and large, however, the data are consistent with the theoretical prediction of reciprocality. Apparently, SMM scales of opinion are like strictly psychophysical scales in this regard.

SENSORY-MODALITY SCALES FOR INDIVIDUAL SUBJECTS

The same questions which have been asked regarding psychophysical scales can be asked of opinion scales. One of the first questions asked concerning Stevens' power law was whether it was an artifact of averaging across the data of individual subjects (Jones & Marcus, 1961). Actually two different questions have been asked – one about the mathematical form of the function and the other about the value of the exponent. First, do group results yield a power function while at the same time this function does not describe the data for any individual subject in the group? Second, are the exponents for individuals equal to that of the group? Although some studies have found that individual functions are not describable by power functions (Pradhan & Hoffman, 1963; Luce & Mo, 1965), most have found that individual data can be fit by such a function (Stevens & Guirao, 1964; Marks & Stevens, 1966). With regard to the second question, most studies have found that individual exponents vary widely across subjects – much more so than would be expected were only sensory factors involved.

Figure 2 presents individual results of a multimodality match for the difficulty of pronunciation of 12 trigrams. Eight *S*s were selected at random from a total of 16 *S*s who took part in an experiment conducted by Mirando and the author. The experiment was designed to answer questions about individual SMM scales. Although there is

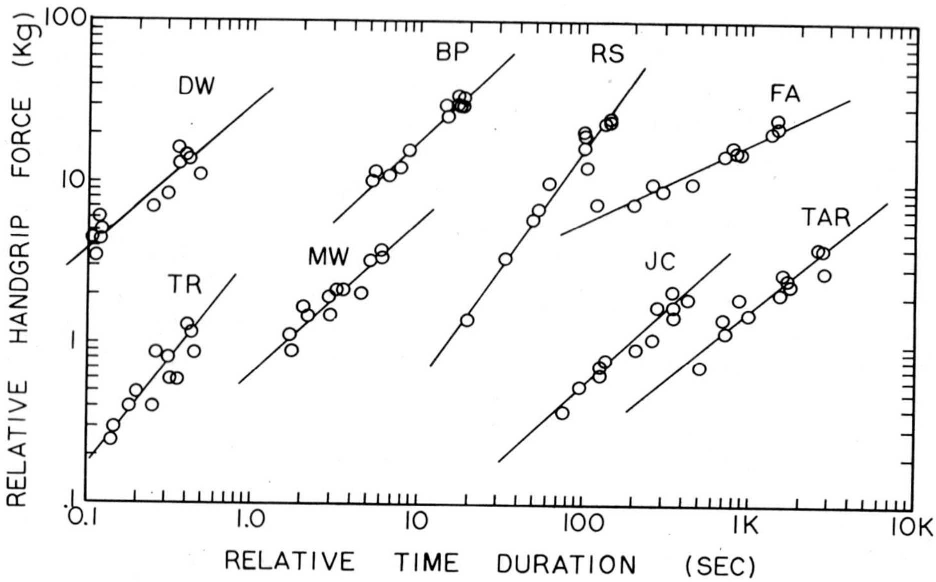

Fig. 2. Multimodality matches for eight subjects. Handgrip force and apparent time duration were both matched to pronunciation difficulty for each of 12 trigrams. The coordinates read properly for subject DW, but sets of data for the others in the top row have been successively displaced one log unit to the right. Data for subjects in the bottom row are presented similarly but have been displaced downward a log unit as well.

considerable scatter, the data appear to agree with the power function. The variability resembles that seen in the results of Stevens & Guirao (1964) and Marks & Stevens (1966). The present data are medians based on six adjustments per trigram, with three made in one session and the other three in a session that followed two to three weeks later. Lines of best fit were obtained in the manner mentioned earlier.

There is an important point to be made in connection with the multimodality plots for individuals in Figure 2 and for a group as in Figure 1a. Both sorts of findings could occur in a situation where there is little or no agreement among subjects about the attribute or characteristic being scaled. Plots of this sort could be obtained even if some subjects rated BAD as difficult and YQG as easy to pronounce, etc. As long as they did so consistently for both sensory-modality matches, such a judgment need not affect the linearity nor the slope of the power function recovered. In order to determine whether all persons agree in their opinions of the set of stimuli, some other check must be made. For the 16 *S*s in our experiment, the median matches were arranged in a Subjects *X* Trigrams matrix and Kendəll's coefficient of concordance (W) was calculated. These coefficients were highly significant and indicated strong agreement among *S*s about the stimuli for both the match by handgrip force ($W=0.88$, $p<0.001$) and that by duration ($W=0.90$, $p<0.001$).

The slopes of the best-fitting lines in Figure 2 vary considerably from person to person, a finding that parallels the results with individual psychophysical scales.

Although the latter tend to be power functions, their exponents, like those here, range widely for different persons. The factors which give rise to such individual differences are still in dispute. They have been attributed to individual differences in judgmental criteria (Marks & Stevens, 1966; Stevens & Guirao, 1964), response bias (Rule, 1966; Rule & Markley, 1971), perceptual sensitivity (Ekman *et al.*, 1968), reaction to the number of presentations per stimulus in a session (Teghtsoonian & Teghtsoonian, 1971), and in the regression effect (Stevens, 1971). Although their source is not clear yet, it is known that these effects persist over time when *S*s make repeated judgments (Teghtsoonian & Teghtsoonian, 1971). Generally, the effects are detected as a significant correlation between a group of *S*s' exponents for one session as compared to those for another session. Our SMM opinion scales provided no exception: the correlation between individuals' exponents from the first and second sessions was significant, $r=0.64$, $p<0.01$.

The exponents for the 16 *S*s ranged from 0.31 to 1.56 while the group data had 0.71 as its exponent. These results are reminiscent of the variation in exponents with psychophysical scales (e.g., Stevens & Guirao, 1964). They bear on Stevens' contention that most of the individual variability may be due to the regression effect. Stevens argues that when regression is compensated for, much of this variation will disappear. But it is in the nature of the MMM procedure to produce an exponent that is somewhat free of the regression influence. As Stevens (1971) himself has said, when two sensory continua *A* and *B* are matched against a common third sensory continuum *C*, "the two matching functions provide exponents whose ratio determines the exponent of the power function relating *A* to *B*," and this procedure may "cancel a major portion of the regression bias." But in spite of the analogous balance by MMM, the big range in individual exponents remains. In a related study, Wanschura & Dawson (1973) have shown that strong individual differences remain after a regression balance with scales obtained by CMM. Clearly, regression is neither the sole nor the main factor in the production of idiosyncratic exponents.

Some Applications of Sensory-Modality Matching

The existence of a scaling method, by itself, is not enough to warrant its widespread use. It will be used only if it allows construction of scales that are as good or better than those available. Some preliminary efforts toward application of SMM have been undertaken.

PRONOUNCEABILITY SCALE

In their 1960 book, Underwood & Schulz introduce a nine-point category or rating scale for the pronounceability (Pr) of three-letter sequences called trigrams. "One" stood for "easy to pronounce" while "nine" was for "hard to pronounce." Many of these trigrams have been used in the experiments discussed earlier in this paper. Their book was mainly concerned with problems and issues in verbal learning. Dawson & Mirando (1973) used SMM, matching with handgrip force, to scale the difficulty of pronouncing 18 trigrams and then compared their scale with that of Underwood and Schulz. The Pr category scale was roughly a concave downward function of the sensory-modality scale, the usual relation found between a category and a ratio scale for the same attribute (Stevens & Galanter, 1957). A product-moment-correlation of 0.96, $p<0.001$, was obtained between the values of the two scales for the 18 trigrams which indicated a high level of agreement between the two scales. When a new group of *S*s was given 12 trials to learn the trigrams, their recall performance correlated negatively with pronounceability for both SMM and category scales of pronounceability. The size of these correlations was the same for both types of scales. In addition, they were of the same magnitude as those reported for comparable experiments in Underwood and Schulz (1960). The sensory-modality scale, then, appears to be as good as its forerunner in addition to being relatable to a whole family of psychophysical scales. Since pronounceability has continued to be an important variable in verbal learning (cf. Heim, 1973), perhaps the new scale has a part to play.

ACCENTEDNESS SCALE

The manner in which a person speaks a language is known to affect the attitudes of others toward him (Lambert & Lambert, 1973). Those interested in such effects are students of what are called *language attitudes* (Shuy & Fasold, 1973). One problem in this area has been to find a measure of perceived accentedness for naive, non-linguistically trained listeners (Ryan, 1973). If a listener's behavior does indeed depend on how he perceives another's speech, then a measure of subjective accentedness should be helpful in exploration of these effects. In 1970, Eileen Muench[1], began a study of accentedness using both ME and SMM. Tape recordings of eight Mexican Americans, whose spoken English varied in degree of accentedness, were played to *S*s who in turn matched either numbers (ME) or handgrip force (SMM) to accentedness. The results, reported in Brennan *et al.* (1973), showed that observers agreed on the relative intensity of accentedness in the speech samples, that the two scales were highly correlated, and that the recovered MMM exponent, expressing ME as a function of handgrip force, was approximately 1.92. The latter finding is in agreement with Stevens and Mack (1959) who report that the exponent relating numbers and force lies between 1.6 and 2.0. Research in progress is attempting to relate accentedness to both language attitudes and to phonological variables.

SENSORY-MODALITY SCALING WITH CHILDREN

As mentioned earlier, direct scaling techniques have been used with young children. Children match brightness to loudness in much the same manner as adults (Bond & Stevens, 1969). But it is doubtful whether they make all such matches like adults. Siegel & McBurney (1970), for example, found that cross-modality matches of handgrip force to line lengths (and also to verbally-presented numbers) gave slopes that increased with age. Children from 6 to 13 years and adults both took part. It would

[1] Now Eileen Brennan.

appear that the stronger you are, the larger the range of force you may tend to use.

William Wozniak and I carried out a MMM study in which first graders were asked to indicate the "badness" of each of seven behaviors engaged in by a boy. A one-sentence description of a behavior was read to each *S* who indicated its badness by squeezing a hand dynamometer and by adjusting the loudness of a 1000 Hz tone. For example, one behavior was described as follows: The boy walked across the street when the stoplight was red. The 24 students were in agreement about the ordering of the behaviors with respect to badness as indicated by a significant Kendall's coefficient of concordance for each of the matches. And they were consistent across the two tasks as shown by a significant correlation. The exponent recovered, 0.73, was considerably larger than 0.40, the value predicted by the ratio of the loudness exponent (0.68) to the one for handgrip force (1.7). Since the same experimenter, using the same equipment and seven occupations in a pilot project, recovered a slope of 0.37 with six undergraduate students asked to judge occupational desirability, we concluded that the matching behavior of first graders is probably different than that of adults. More warmup familiarization with the adjustable stimuli might make a difference, however, since the children seemed very reluctant to use much of the range of loudnesses available to them. Further work is needed here much as it is with strictly psychophysical matches involving children.

Summary

At this point it appears that sensory-modality matching gives results that parallel those of cross-modality matching and magnitude estimation. Ratio scales of opinion seem to be very much like the magnitude scales of psychophysics. For the most part, however, we have avoided the problem areas in psychophysical scaling. Issues like the category vs ratio scale discrepancy, the range effect (Stevens, 1971), and the need for scale consistency (Cliff, 1973) have not been treated. Presumably the difficulties present with psychophysical scales will be found to occur for opinion scales as well.

The parallel between the sensory and opinion domains has some important implications. Although borne and fostered in sensory psychophysics, the scaling techniques allow the measurement and investigation of subjective impressions in general. Further, the parallel, as we have seen, provides a way of assessing the opinion scales we construct. The various scales will be characterized by a large number of quantitative interrelationships. As scales become available, the task of locating higher-order relations among psychological measures may become simpler (cf. Stevens *et al.*, 1965). In addition, as more and more scales are produced in the course of research of all kinds, they will provide an impetus to the search for relations between subjective impressions and other sorts of behavior.

References

Bond, B., & Stevens, S. S. Cross-modality matching of brightness to loudness by 5-year-olds. *Perception & Psychophysics*, 1969, **6**, 337–339.

Brennan, E. M., Ryan, E. B., and Dawson, W. E. Scaling of apparent accentedness by magnitude estimation and sensory modality matching. Submitted for publication.

Cliff, N. Scaling. *Annual Review of Psychology*, 1973, **24**, 473–506.

Dawson, W. E., & Brinker, R. P. Validation of ratio scales of opinion by multimodality matching. *Perception* and *Psychophysics*, 1971, **9**, 413–417.

Dawson, W. E., & Mirando, M. A. Sensory-modality scale for pronounceability of trigrams and its relation to free-recall learning. *Perceptual and Motor Skills*, 1973, **36**, 1219–1224.

Ekman, G., Hosman, B., Lindman, R., Ljungberg, L., & Akesson, C. Interindividual differences in scaling performance. *Perceptual and Motor Skills*, 1968, **26**, 815–823.

Heim, J. A comment on R. C. Johnson: "Reanalysis of 'Meaningfulness and verbal learning.'" *Psychological Review*, 1973, **80**, 235–236.

Indow, T., & Stevens, S. S. Scaling of saturation an dhue. *Perception* and *Psychophysics*, 1966, **1**, 253–271.

Jones, F. N., & Marcus, M. J. The subject effect in judgments of subjective magnitude. *Journal of Experimental Psychology*, 1961, **61**, 40–44.

Kenney, J. F. *Mathematics of statistics. Part One*. New York: Van Nostrand, 1939.

Lambert, W. W., & Lambert, W. E. *Social Psychology*. (2nd ed.) Englewood Cliffs, N. J.: Prentice-Hall, 1973.

Luce, R. D., & Mo, S. S. Magnitude estimation of heaviness and loudness by individual subjects: A test of a probabilistic response theory. *British Journal of Mathematical and Statistical Psychology*, 1965, **18**, 159–174.

Marks, L. E., & Stevens, J. C. Individual brightness functions. *Perception and Psychophysics*, 1966, **1**, 17–24.

Pradhan, P. L., & Hoffman, P. J. Effect of spacing and range of stimuli on magnitude estimation judgments. *Journal of Experimental Psychology*, 1963, **66**, 533–541.

Rule, S. Subject differences in exponents of psychophysical power functions. *Perceptual and Motor Skills*, 1966, **23**, 1125–1126.

Rule, S., & Markley, R. P. Subject differences in cross-modality matching. *Perception and Psychophysics*, 1971, **9**, 115–117.

Ryan, E. B. Subjective reactions toward accented speech. In R. Shuy & R. Fasold (Eds.), *Language attitudes: Current trends and prospects*. Washington, D.C.: Georgetown Univ. Press, 1973.

Schneider, B., & Lane, H. Ratio scales, category scales, and variability in the production of loudness and softness. *Journal of the Acoustical Society of America*, 1963, **35**, 1953–1961.

Shuy, R., & Fasold, R. (Eds.) *Language attitudes: Current trends and prospects*. Washington, D.C.: Georgetown Univ. Press, 1973.

Siegel, A. W., & McBurney, D. H. Estimation of line length and number: A developmental study. *Journal of Experimental Child Psychology*, 1970, **10**, 170–180.

Stevens, J. C., & Guirao, M. Individual loudness functions. *Journal of the Acoustical Society of America*, 1964, **36**, 210–213.

Stevens, J. C., & Mack, J. D. Scales of apparent force. *Journal of Experimental Psychology*, 1959, **58**, 405–413.

Stevens, S. S. The psychophysics of sensory function. In W. A. Rosenblith (Ed.), *Sensory communication*. New York: Wiley, 1961.

Stevens, S. S. A metric for the social consensus. *Science*, 1966, **151**, 530–541.

Stevens, S. S. Issues in psychophysical measurement. *Psychological Review*, 1971, **78**, 426–450.

Stevens, S. S. *Psychophysics and social scaling*. Morristown, N.J.: General Learning Press, 1972.

Stevens, S. S. Perceived level of noise by Mark VII and decibels (E). *Journal of the Acoustical Society of America*, 1972, **51**, 575–601.

Stevens, S. S., & Galanter, E. H. Ratio scales and category scales for a dozen perceptual continua. *Journal of Experimental Psychology*, 1957, **54**, 377–411.

Stevens, S. S., & Greenbaum, H. B. Regression effect in psychophysical judgments. *Perception and Psychophysics*, 1966, **1**, 439–446.

Stevens, S. S., & Guirao, M. Loudness, reciprocality, and partition scales. *Journal of the Acoustical Society of America*, 1962, **34**, 1466–1471.

Stevens, S. S., & Guirao, M. Subjective scaling of length and area and the matching of length to loudness and brightness. *Journal of Experimental Psychology*, 1963, **66**, 177–186.

Stevens, S. S., Guirao, M., & Slawson, A. W. Loudness, a product of volume times density. *Journal of Experimental Psychology*, 1965, **69**, 503–510.

Teghtsoonian, M., & Teghtsoonian, R. How repeatable are Stevens' power law exponents for individual subjects? *Perception and Psychophysics*, 1971, **10**, 147–149.

Torgerson, W. S. Distances and ratios in psychophysical scaling. MIT Lincoln Laboratory Report 58-G-0014, October, 1960.

Torgerson, W. S. Distances and ratios in psychophysical scaling. *Acta Psychologica*, 1961, **19**, 201–205.

Underwood, B. J., & Schulz, R. W. *Meaningfulness and verbal learning*. New York: Lippincott, 1960.

Wanschura, R. G., & Dawson, W. E. Regression effect and individual power functions over sessions. Submitted for publication. Also presented as paper at meeting of Midwestern Psychological Association, Chicago, Ill., May, 1973.

THE DERIVATION OF STEVENS' PSYCHOPHYSICAL POWER LAW[1]

HANNES EISLER

University of Stockholm, Sweden

Abstract. Stevens' psychophysical power law is derived from the empirical finding of linearity between variable and standard in ratio setting experiments. The uniqueness of the solution depends on an invariance assumption.

It is a common finding in ratio setting experiments (e.g. half-setting) that the adjusted ratios are a linear function of the standards. (Taves, 1941; Reese, 1943; Ross & Katchmar, 1951; Ekman & Frankenhaeuser, 1957; Ekman, 1958; Eisler & Ekman, 1959; Björkman & Holmkvist, 1960.) Denoting standards by x and variables (set ratios) by y, both in physical units, we have

$$y = ax + b. \tag{1}$$

Let us assume that there are two psychophysical functions, one for the standard (u) and one for the variable (v). (Note that we thus do not make the customary assumption that the psychophysical function is the same for the standard and the variable.) Thus

$$u = u(x), \tag{2}$$

and

$$v = v(y). \tag{3}$$

If the subject is required to set the ratio p (e.g. $p=0.5$ when the subject is to adjust the variable magnitude so that it is experienced as half the standard magnitude), then

$$v(y) = pu(x). \tag{4}$$

Equations 1–4 yield

$$pu(x) = v(ax + b), \quad p > 0. \tag{5}$$

In order to be able to solve Equation 5 uniquely we have to introduce some restrictions. Let us make the invariance assumption that both u and v are independent of p; in other words that the psychophysical functions are the same regardless of the ratio the subject is to set, and that different ratios are reflected only by different values of a and b.

We will investigate whether there are functions u and v such that

(i) u and v are independent of p, whereas

(ii) a and b may depend on p,

(iii) Equation 5 holds for all $p > 0$, and all x such that $u(x)$ and $v(ax+b)$ are defined.

[1] This work was supported by the Swedish Social Science Research Council. I am indebted to Dr Sören Holm for mathematical assistance.

H. R. Moskowitz et al. (eds.), Sensation and Measurement. 61–64. *All Rights Reserved.*

We also assume that u, v, a, and b are derivable with respect to their relevant arguments. Taking the derivative of Equation 5 first with respect to p, and then to x, yields respectively

$$u(x) = (a'x + b')\cdot v'(ax + b) \tag{6}$$

and

$$pu'(x) = a\cdot v'(ax + b). \tag{7}$$

Let $a'x+b' \neq 0$. The division of Equation 7 by Equation 6 yields

$$\frac{pu'(x)}{u(x)} = \frac{a}{a'x + b'}. \tag{8}$$

Consider Equation 8 as a function of x for a fixed p. Integration yields

$$p\cdot \ln u(x) = (a/a')\cdot \ln|a'x + b'| + C_1(p) \tag{9}$$

if $a' \neq 0$, i.e.

$$u(x) = |a'x + b'|^{a/a'p}\cdot C_2(p)^{1/p}, \quad C_2 = e^{C_1}. \tag{10}$$

If $a' = 0$ we obtain

$$p\cdot \ln u(x) = \frac{a}{b'}\, x + C_3(p), \tag{11}$$

i.e.

$$u(x) = e^{ax/pb'}\cdot C_4(p), \quad C_4 = e^{C_3}. \tag{12}$$

The case with $a' = 0$ is at variance with empirical findings, since it implies that the slope in Equation 1 does not depend on the ratio p. Therefore Equation 12 can be discarded.

For $a'x+b' \equiv 0$, Equation 6 yields $u(x) \equiv 0 \equiv v(x)$. Also this case is at variance with empirical findings and can likewise be discarded.

We have required that $u(x)$ be independent of p. If there exists an a and a b such that Equation 5 holds, $u(x)$ must become (using cancellation in Equation 10)

$$u(x) = \alpha(x - \gamma)^{\beta}, \quad x > \gamma. \tag{13}$$

Next we have to investigate whether there are an a, a b, and a v such that Equation 13 implies Equation 5.

Rewriting Equation 5

$$pu\left(\frac{x - b}{a}\right) = v(x),$$

i.e.

$$v(x) = p\alpha\left(\frac{x - b}{a} - \gamma\right)^{\beta} = \frac{p\alpha}{|a|^{\beta}}(x - b - a\gamma)^{\beta}. \tag{14}$$

For $v(x)$ to be independent of p

$$p/|a|^{\beta} = C_5, \quad b + a\gamma = C_6.$$

Setting $C_5\alpha = \alpha_1$, $C_6 = \gamma_1$ we obtain

$$v(x) = \alpha_1 (x - \gamma_1)^\beta, \quad x > \gamma_1 \tag{15}$$

i.e. the psychophysical function is Stevens' power law both for the standard (Formula 13) and the variable (Formula 15). The two functions 13 and 15 may or may not differ in the scale unit ($\alpha \neq \alpha_1$), the subjective zero ($\gamma \neq \gamma_1$), or both.

As can be shown by inserting, Equations 13 and 15 satisfy Equation 5.

Discussion

That Stevens' power law is compatible with a linear relation between variable and standard in ratio setting experiments was known earlier (Ekman, 1958; Eisler, 1958). Let us now scrutinize the premises from which the uniqueness of this psychophysical function is derived.

1. The existence of subjective counterparts to stimuli in the physical world, namely sensations. Considering these "sensations", denoted by u and v in this paper, as intervening variables should obviate possible objections regarding their "existence".

2. The ability of a subject to carry out the task required, i.e. to find a stimulus which evokes a sensation standing a given ratio to the sensation of the standard. This problem can be divided into two parts: (a) does the *S* follow the instructions so that Equation 4 holds, and (b) if he does, is the value of p in Equation 4 really the prescribed ratio, say 0.5 in half-setting. The latter problem has to do with the subject's number behavior and is of minor interest here. Provided that p is constant for a given prescribed ratio, Stevens' law must follow as shown above, though the exponent β obtained may be at fault. The rather good agreement between exponents obtained from series of experiments with different ratios on the same continua, supports the assumption of agreement between p in Equation 4 and the prescribed ratio. Point (a) may be questioned. However, as long as there is no other description of the subject's behavior that ties in better with known facts, there seems to be no reason to reject the premise described by Equation 4. (See also Eisler, 1965.)

3. Variable and standard in ratio setting experiments are linearly related. This is an empirical finding. It goes without saying that to the extent to which this linearity is an approximation, so is the power law.

4. The invariance assumption that neither the psychophysical function for the standard nor the one for the variable is affected by the particular ratio to be set by the subject. This assumption is required for any psychophysical theory of some generality – it should not be abandoned without compelling reasons.

References

Björkman, M., and Holmkvist, O. The time-order error in the construction of a subjective time scale. *Scandinavian Journal of Psychology*, 1960, **1**, 7–13.

Eisler, H. *A note on treatment of ratio setting data for constructing psychological scales.* Reports from the Psychological Laboratory, The University of Stockholm, 1958, No. 54.

Eisler, H. On psychophysics in general and the general psychophysical differential equation in particular. *Scandinavian Journal of Psychology*, 1965, **6**, 85–102.

Eisler, H., and Ekman, G. A mechanism of subjective similarity. *Acta Psychologica*, 1959, **16**, 1–10.

Ekman, G. Two generalized ratio scaling methods. *The Journal of Psychology*, 1958, **45**, 287–295.

Ekman, G., and Frankenhaeuser, M. *Subjective time scales*. Reports from the Psychological Laboratory, The University of Stockholm, 1957, No. 49.

Reese, T. W. The application of the theory of physical measurement to the measurement of psychological magnitudes with three experimental examples. *Psychological Monographs*, 1943, **55**, No. 251.

Ross, S., and Katchmar, L. The construction of a magnitude function for short time-intervals. *American Journal of Psychology*, 1951, **64**, 397–401.

Taves, E. H. Two mechanisms for the perception of visual numerousness. *Archives of Psychology*, 1941, **37**, No. 265.

CROSS-MODALITY MATCHING OF MONEY AGAINST OTHER CONTINUA[1]

EUGENE GALANTER
Columbia University

and

PATRICIA PLINER
Erindale College, Univ. of Toronto

Abstract. Cross-modality matching of hypothetical increments of money against loudness recover the previously proposed exponent of the utility function for money within a few percent. Similar cross-modality matching experiments for decrements give a disutility exponent of 0.59, larger than the utility exponent for increments. This disutility exponent was checked by an additional cross-modality matching experiment against the disutility of drinking various concentrations of a bitter solution. The parameter estimated in this fashion was 0.63.

The application of direct scaling techniques to the measurement of the utility of money is made difficult by the numerical nomenclature for money. Galanter (1962) bypassed this problem by having subjects judge the degree of happiness money would bring, and from these data concluded that the incremental utility function for monetary increases was a power function with an exponent of approximately 0.43. He also reported extreme difficulty in getting people to estimate the disutility of monetary decrements.

Further support of a power law as an appropriate form for the utility function was provided by Galanter & Holman in psychophysical detection experiments (1967). Here, pay-off matrices were changed to show that equal ratios of money lead to the same decision behaviors. This was taken to mean that equal ratios of money were interpreted by *S* as equal ratios of utility. Other studies of the empirical utility function have not significantly disconfirmed the power function nor the exponent (Galanter, 1974). But all of the data are sketchy, and the field is more populated with theory and derivations from a variety of models than it is with a wealth of empirical information (cf. Lee, 1971, Ch. 4). The experiments reported here are aimed at enlarging our data base in respect of ways in which people appreciate increments and decrements of money.

The experiments described below involve hypothetical increments and decrements. That is to say, the people never receive or lose actual amounts of money in these experiments. Therefore, one may reasonably argue that what is being observed is the utility function for hypothetical increments and decrements, and that the utility function for real money may be different both in form or parametric value. We shall remark briefly on this question later and touch upon the nature of experiments that could enlighten us.

[1] Partial support of Miss Pliner's efforts was provided by a grant from the General Electric Company. The research was supported in part by the Office of Naval Research.

H. R. Moskowitz et al. (eds.), Sensation and Measurement. 65–76. All Rights Reserved.

Experiment I

Cross-modality matching experiments, one of S. S. Stevens' most ingenious inventions, are indistinguishable from magnitude estimation experiments except that the comparison dimension is not a set of numerical responses that *S* makes, but rather the adjustment of some stimulus magnitude until it is subjectively equal to the magnitude of the stimulus being judged. Naturally, when conceptualized in this fashion, the exponents of the compared subjective scales only represent ratios. Their numerical values are determined by selecting some continuum as representative, and then using the slopes of other perceptual dimensions against that representative continuum as the preferred nomenclature. The importance of cross-modality scaling resides in its demonstration of the coherence of people's judgments about a variety of continua whose synaesthetic similarities are hardly expressible in common language. And yet, a wide literature supports the essential unity of this class of judgments.

The utility of cross-modality matching rests upon the assumption that the comparison of the two continua is made possible by subjective scales that have ratio properties. Furthermore, if the subjective scales are themselves power functions of objective dimensions, then cross-modality comparisons will also be power functions. In its simplest form, if one dimension is represented in the physical domain by the exponent a, and the other dimension is represented by the exponent b, then if the two dimensions are matched by a subject who follows these psychophysical laws, the first dimension can be represented by the second dimension to the b/a exponent. Consequently, if we know any two of the three exponents in a cross-modality matching experiment, then the third can be calculated directly. It is this operation that we perform in the following experiments. As a first step, we attempt to confirm the value of the exponent for money increments observed earlier by comparing the magnitude of monetary increments with the loudness of a tone that *S*s are free to adjust.

SUBJECTS

We chose names at random from the directory of Columbia College and obtained seven male college students as volunteers for the experiment.

APPARATUS

The apparatus consisted of a Hewlitt-Packard HP-200 AD audio oscillator calibrated to produce a 300-Hz tone. The tone was fed into a Dynaco amplifier whose output was led to a sone potentiometer and thence through a switching box to either a set of ear phones (PDR 8 in home-made Zwislocki semi-plastic ear muffs) or a Ballentine voltmeter. The earphones had been previously calibrated.

PROCEDURE

Although we could have used existing values of the magnitude estimation exponent for loudness, we chose instead first to conduct a magnitude estimation experiment to obtain a loudness scale for the group of *S*s we used. These loudnesses could then be compared with the cross-modality judgments for utility on the assumption that any bias in the loudness judgments would be transferred intact to the cross-modality judgments, and consequently we would obtain a more purified estimator of the utility function exponent.

*S*s gave five judgments of each of fifteen different amplitudes. Before making each judgment *S* was presented with a standard tone called 1000. (We were at that time experimenting with the use of a standard for every trial. We have since given up that procedure. However, the results obtained by this technique are not seriously distorted in comparison to the literature by the procedure itself.) *S*s were given the following specific instructions:

As I mentioned to you on the telephone, this experiment involves sound. Specifically what you will be doing is judging the loudness of tones. In order for you to communicate your judgments to me, I would like you to assign a number to each tone. You may use any numbers you wish, but I would like you to use smaller numbers if the tone is softer and larger numbers if the tone is louder. I would also like the numbers to be proportional to how loud you think the tone is. If one tone is twice as loud as another tone, you should give it a number twice as large (the subject then put on the earphones). Arbitrarily, let us call the loudness of this tone 1000. (The subject was presented with a tone arbitrarily assigned the value of 35 dB). This is the comparison tone. Now, if another tone is $\frac{1}{2}$ as loud as the comparison tone, what number would you assign to it? (Wait for answer). If another tone is three times as loud as the comparison tone, what number would you assign to it? (Wait for answer). On each trial, I will present you with two tones. The first will always be the comparison tone, and you are to judge the second in relation to it. Do you have any other questions?

After the *S*s had completed this segment of the experiment, they were then required to match the stimuli from the two modalities: the subjective loudness of the 300-Hz tone and the utility of money. To accomplish this task, the *S*s were given the following instructions:

This part of the experiment involves receiving money. Of course, you are not really going to receive money during the experiment, but I want you to imagine as realistically as you can that you have received as gifts the amounts of money that I will mention. Now, receiving money would probably make you happy to a certain extent, and what I want to do is to make an analogy between how happy you would be and the loudness of a tone. Specifically, here is what you will be doing. You will put the earphones on again and will hear a tone of a certain loudness. This will be the comparison tone. We will assume that receiving $90.00 is analogous to the loudness of this comparison tone. Then, I will mention other amounts of money and you will adjust the tone with this device (show sone potentiometer) so that its loudness is analogous to how happy you would feel in receiving those amounts of money.

For example, let us say that receiving $50.00 would make you $\frac{1}{2}$ as happy as receiving $90.00, then you would set the tone so that it would sound $\frac{1}{2}$ as loud as the comparison tone. Or, for example, if receiving $150.00 would make you three times as happy as receiving $90.00, you should set the tone so that it sounds three times as loud as the comparison tone. Are there any questions? (Answer all questions).

In order to eliminate visual and kinesthetic cues, the position of the sone potentiometer was randomized from trial-to-trial and its calibration dial was concealed from *S*s view. The various amounts of money were presented in an irregular order and the subjects made three more or less independent matches by adjusting the sone potentiometer for each of the monetary values told to him.

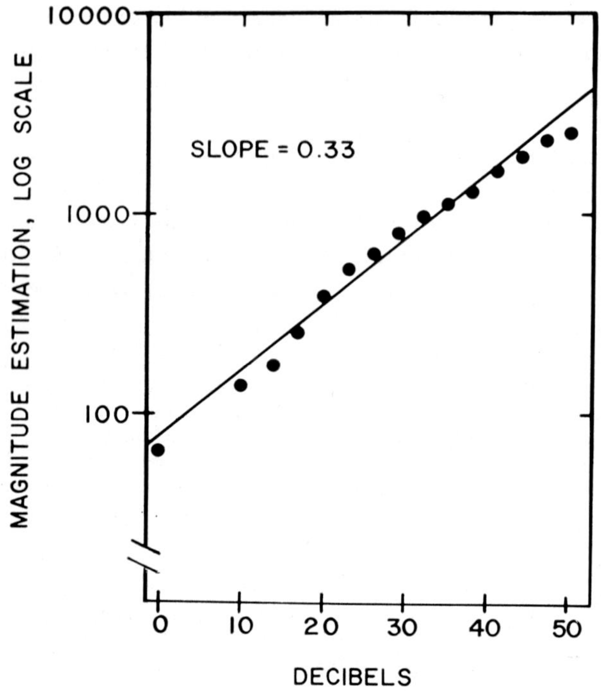

Fig. 1. Magnitude estimations of the loudness of a 300-Hz tone plotted against relative dB. Each data point represents 35 judgments from seven different subjects.

RESULTS

The geometric mean of each of the five loudness judgments that *S* made to the various amplitudes of the tones were computed. A regression analysis of these means was used to find the best fitting line for the data points. The slope against relative dB was 0.33, which is within 0.03 of the generally accepted value. Figure 1 shows the data points obtained in this magnitude estimation of loudness experiment.

The cross-modality matching procedure resulted in the data points shown in Figure 2. A regression analysis of these data yield a slope of 0.74. Using these values we calculate the exponent of the utility function for money by taking the ratios of these two slope functions. This value is 0.45. This obtained exponent is within 4% of the value reported earlier (1962).

Experiment II

The successful replication of the utility function by the method of cross-modality matching emboldened us to attempt to estimate the disutility of monetary losses by the same procedure.

SUBJECTS

Again, seven male Columbia students were used as *S*s based on their random selection

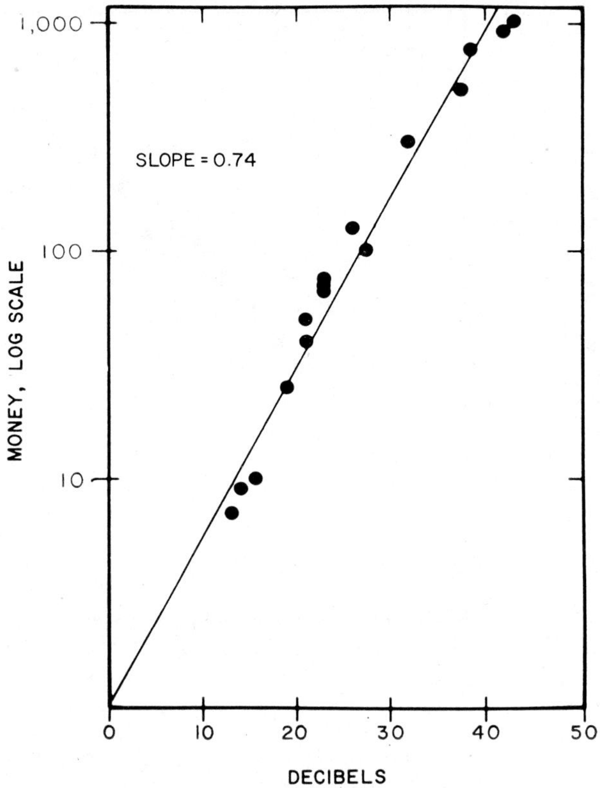

Fig. 2. A cross-modality matching function by the same subjects whose data are shown in Figure 1, between the amplitude of a sound judged equal in loudness to the value of varying amounts of monetary gain.

from the directory of students with the provision that the telephone recruiting succeeded in bringing them to the laboratory.

PROCEDURE

The apparatus, procedure, and instructions to the *S*s were exactly the same as in Experiment I except that the instructions were revised for the cross-modality matching part of the experiment so that their sense was that of comparisons of losses of money rather than of gains.

RESULTS

The magnitude estimation values of subjective loudness against relative dB yielded an exponent of 0.38. The graph of this function is shown in Figure 3. This number was larger than we would have anticipated. However, for seven subjects making five judgments each, it is certainly within the acceptable region. The exponent of the matching function for losses of money was 0.64. This function is plotted as Figure 4. Conse-

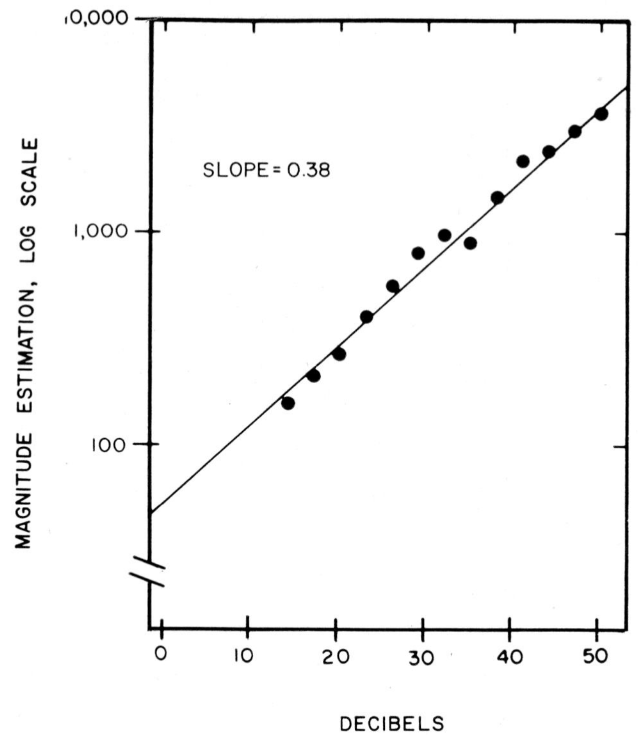

Fig. 3. Magnitude estimations of subjective loudness against relative dB. This is the analogue of Figure 1 for a new group of seven subjects.

quently, the derived exponent of the function relating monetary loss and disutility was 0.59. This value is considerably larger than the exponent for monetary gain.

This result creates a disharmony in our estimates of the value of the exponents of monetary increments and decrements. One would have expected that either the exponents would be of widely divergent values, or they would be symmetric. The fact that they are so close together, and yet so decidedly different, begs for a further examination of the disutility function to see if, in fact, its magnitude is consistently larger than the exponent for increments of utility. To that end, Experiment III was conducted.

Experiment III

One can operationalize the notion of "negative amounts of money" in at least two ways. First of all, one can couch the idea in terms of losses of money; this was the procedure that we used in the previous experiment. In that case, the dependent variable may be feelings of unhappiness at the loss, or some other consequential affective event whose magnitude is assessed by the subject. On the other hand, one may assume that the degree of unwillingness of a person to spend money is a measure of the disutility of negative sums of money. In that case, we may assume that a person would

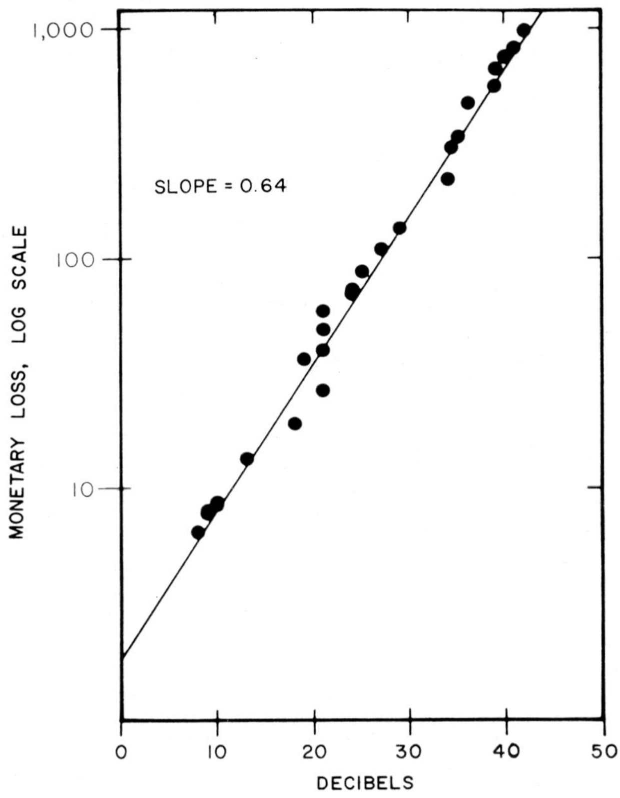

Fig. 4. The cross-modality matching function for monetary losses matched to the loudness of the amplitudes of a 300-Hz tone for the subjects who generated the data of Figure 3.

refuse to spend money for an item or service unless the utility of that item or service exceeded the disutility involved in spending the money. The maximum amount of money spent for an item or service should be that amount whose disutility is just exceeded by the utility of the item or service.

In the present experiment, we chose to have subjects make cross-modality matches in such a way that the second operational characterization of disutility could be represented. In order to do this in a fashion that avoids comparisons among a jumble of events, we would like to "sell" the subjects a product that varies along some reasonable scalable perceptual continuum. An additional constraint on our commodity is that the continuum should not be one for which there is a decreasing marginal utility. This immediately suggests some form of aversive continuum. Once we have established and scaled such a continuum, we may then extract from the subject his willingness to pay to avoid the degree of aversiveness particular values of the continuum generate.

This is the plan of the present experiment. First, we scale an aversive continuum, and then we obtain estimates of how much a subject would be willing to pay in order to avoid any value of that continuum. Beneath it all, of course, we assumed that the aversiveness of any event is some linear function of its subjective magnitude.

SUBJECTS

*S*s were nine undergraduate male students at Columbia University who were enrolled in an introductory psychology course. They were induced to participate in the experiment by a course requirement. In addition, they were compensated at the prevailing rate of $2.25 per hour.

APPARATUS

The aversive continuum in this experiment was represented by solutions of various concentrations of sucrose octaacetate manufactured by Matheson, Coleman and Bell of East Rutherford, New Jersey. Sucrose octaacetate is a synthetic, nontoxic compound, intensely bitter to man in dilute concentrations. The concentrations (by volume) we used in the present experiment were: 10^{-3}, 5×10^{-4}, 2×10^{-4}, 10^{-4}, 5×10^{-5}, and 2×10^{-5}. Corresponding log concentrations are: -3.000, -3.3010, -3.6990, -4.000, -4.3010, and -4.6990. The concentration of the solution named as the standard was 10^{-4}.

PROCEDURE

In this cross-modality matching experiment, it was necessary first that we obtain magnitude estimation values of the aversive continuum. The procedure for the construction of this scale was as follows. *S* was blindfolded and seated at a table. Three cubic centimeters of the standard solution or the solution to be judged were put in a 30 cc^3 shot glass by means of an eyedropper and presented to *S*. *S* sipped the contents of the glass and held it in his mouth until it reached a peak intensity. He then spit it out, and rinsed his mouth with tap water. On each trial, *S* first tasted the standard solution, rinsed his mouth out, then tasted the solution to be judged, rinsed and then made his judgment. Trials were separated by an interval of 30 s. *S*s made two judgments of each of the six stimuli. They were given the following instructions:

> This experiment involves taste. Specifically, I would like you to judge the bitterness of various solutions of a bitter substance. In order for you to communicate your judgments to me, I would like you to assign a number to the bitterness of each solution. You may use any numbers you wish, but I would like you to use smaller numbers if the solution tastes less bitter and larger numbers if the solution tastes more bitter. Also, I would like you to assign the numbers so that they are proportional to how bitter the solution tastes. So, for example, if one solution tastes twice as bitter as another, you should assign to it a number twice as large as you would to the other. Or, if a solution tastes two-thirds as bitter as another to which you have already assigned the number, "150," you should assign to it the number, "100." (*S* is presented with the standard solution). Arbitrarily, let's call the bitterness of this solution, "100," and you judge each other solution in relation to it. On each trial, I will present you with two solutions – first, the standard which has been assigned the number, "100," and then the solution to be judged in relation to the standard.

E assured himself that *S* understood the instructions.

After each *S* had completed the magnitude estimation portion of the experiment, he was given a five minute rest period followed by the cross-modality experiment. This new phase of the experiment was introduced to *S* with the following instructions:

Actually, this experiment is the pretest of an experiment I am going to be doing later on in the year. In the experiment proper, I am going to ask subjects to drink eight ounces of each of these bitter solutions instead of merely tasting them as you did. Obviously, that will be rather unpleasant, and since the subjects will be students from psychology courses just as you are, I don't feel that I can force them to drink these vile-tasting solutions. However, it is important to me that each subject drinks as many of the solutions as possible, so this is the procedure I am going to use to see that they do so. I am going to give each subject a certain amount of money and inform him that if he wants to avoid drinking a particular solution, he may, but in order to do so, he will have to return a specified amount of the money to me. In other words, he will have to pay to avoid drinking a solution, and the more unpleasant a solution tastes, the more he will have to pay to avoid drinking it. Subjects will be permitted to keep any money they have left over. That way, I hope subjects will have an incentive to drink the solutions.

What I would like you to do is to help me set a price for each of the solutions. You can't do this in an absolute sense since I am not sure yet how much money I will have at my disposal, but you can do it in a relative sense in the following manner. Just as before, on each trial, I will present you with the standard solution to be judged. This time, I would like you to tell me the maximum amount of money you would pay to avoid drinking the solution to be judged in relation to the standard. So, if you pay twice as much to avoid drinking a particular solution as you would to avoid drinking the standard, you should say "twice as much." If you would pay one-half as much, you should say "one-half as much". Please keep in mind that I am not asking you in different words to judge the bitterness of the solutions again. While one solution may taste exactly twice as bitter as the standard, it is possible that you would be willing to pay more than twice as much to avoid drinking it. It is also possible that you would be willing to pay less than twice as much to avoid drinking it. Your judgments should depend on how much you would be willing to pay to avoid drinking the solution.

Following these instructions, *S*s were interrogated to insure that they understood exactly what it was they were to do. They then made their judgments. The presentation of the stimulus materials were identical to those used previously. The same six concentrations of sucrose octaacetate were used and again, *S*s made two judgments to each of the six stimuli.

In part, the adequacy of *S*s judgments are contingent upon his acceptance of the rationale provided in the instructions above. Informal evidence of *S*s belief in this rationale is given by the fact that many of them volunteered to serve in the future when the alleged experiment was to be run.

RESULTS

Figure 5 shows the relation between log concentrations of sucrose octaacetate and the logarithms of the magnitude estimation judgments of bitterness. Each data point represents the geometric mean of 18 judgments. The slope of a straight line obtained by means of regression analysis of the logarithms of the magnitude estimation judgments is 0.44. Once again, the data for this continuum seem well approximated by a power function.

In Figure 6, we show the results of the cross-modality matching procedure. The line drawn in the figure has a slope of 0.70. By taking the appropriate ratio of exponents we are able to calculate that the disutility exponent associated with payments for drinking these bitter solutions is 0.63. This value is similar to that based on the

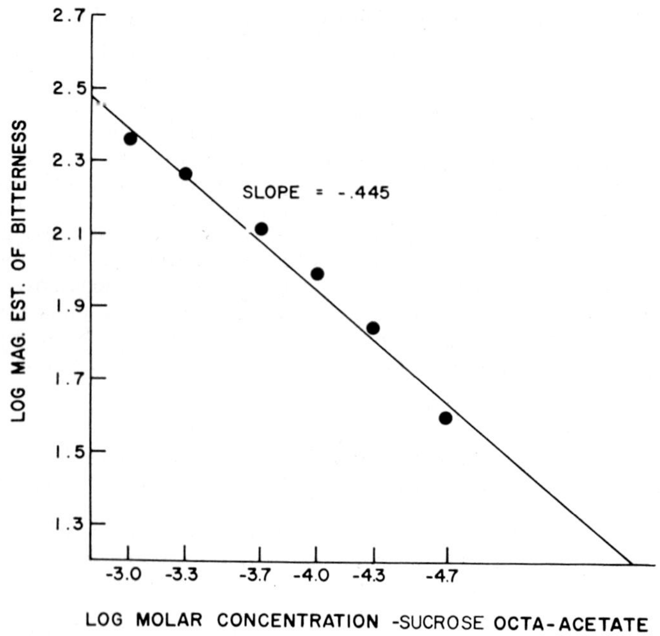

Fig. 5. The magnitude estimation function of judged bitterness vs log concentration of sucrose octaacetate.

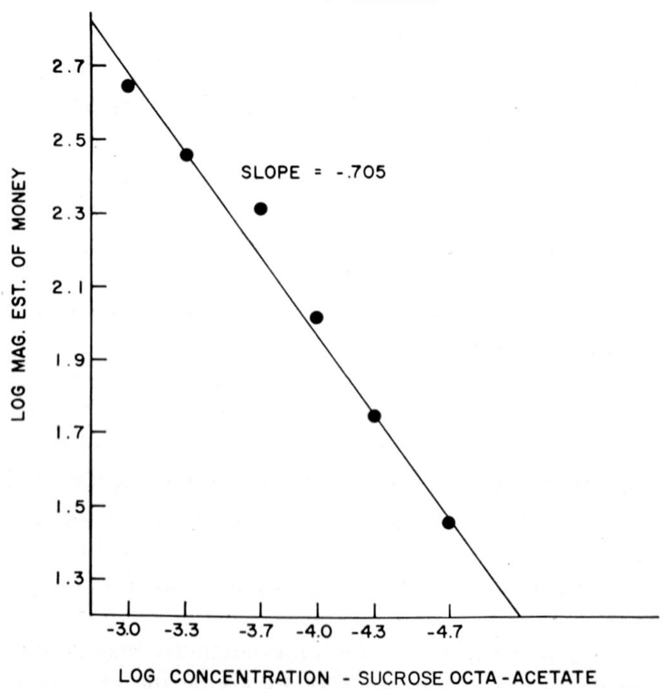

Fig. 6. A cross-modality matching function between the degree of bitterness of solutions of sodium octaacetate and the amount of money a subject would be willing to pay in order to avoid drinking that solution.

data of Experiment II. Even though these data are thin, in the sense that the number of observations entering into the calculations are small, they clearly represent a reasonable approximation to the previous observations.

Discussion

The remarkable consistency of the power function as a representation of data that show how people judge events that have a quantitative character is once again supported in these studies. Continuing criticism of cross-modality matching experiments (cf. Anderson, 1974) cannot vitiate the enormous descriptive simplification these methods provide. Regardless of the theoretical elegance of functional measurement, conjoint measurement, or other structural attacks on quantitative psychophysical judgments, the hard reality is that the judgments and behavior of people in situations of the kind described here fall nicely into place. Furthermore, these psychophysical descriptions represent an extensive generalization of a variety of behavior, not merely the organization of some simple verbal responses.

On the question of the hypothetical nature of these judgments, we would advance the argument that all monetary decisions, including expenditures and the acceptance of tasks for expected monetary returns, are intrinsically hypothetical. Of course, it is true that these hypothetical events have consequences, and one can justifiably compare the evaluation of the events subsequent to their occurrence relative to their evaluation prior to their returns. Indeed, this question is represented in an extensive theoretical and empirical literature (Festinger, 1957). Suffice it to say here that in other experiments in our laboratory in which the bias effects of monetary pay-offs are evaluated on the hypothesis that certain theories of the psychophysical judgments are appropriate, our preliminary results suggest that the consequential evaluations are not remarkably different from these hypothetical judgments.

We turn now to the question of the possible symmetry of the positive and negative limbs of the utility function. On the basis of intuition and anecdote, one would expect the negative limb of the utility function to decrease more sharply than the positive limb increases. Indeed, it has been conjectured that the positive limb is probably "truly" a square root function and the negative limb a square. This would go far toward explaining the apparently irrational behavior involved in the purchase of insurance and other such "risky" schemes. What we have observed, if anything, is an asymmetry of much less magnitude than would have been expected. In particular, the asymmetry is one only of the magnitude of the exponent on the same side of unity. That is to say, the curvature of the function does not change in going from positive to negative.

What is not immediately obvious is the profound effect that a change in exponent of this magnitude produces. In one informal experiment, we informed a group of *S*s that they were to participate in a ten-minute game in which they would use money to play for chances of winning and losing. We gave them $5.00. A prestigeful confederate (the professor) entered at this point and apologized for the inadequacy of his assistant, explaining to the group that their stake was to be only $2.00. They would have to return $3.00 of the $5.00 they had already received. Another group of *S*s were given $2.00 with similar instructions concerning the game that they were going to play. Although the actual experiment was never successfully accomplished, *S*s were interviewed after this stage in the procedure, and in particular, were questioned about their conception of the worth of their stake. The judgments of the group who had arrived at a $2.00 stake via plus $5.00 and minus $3.00 uniformly valued the $2.00 as "hardly adequate for anything these days." On the other hand, the group that had received the $2.00 directly, considered it an adequate if not enormous amount of cash to be used in a game that would take only ten minutes, and from which they might emerge richer or poorer.

A final comment is in order about the nature of the "unit" parameter or multiplicative constant in the utility power function. We nowhere attempted to estimate the magnitude of the multiplicative parameter, but one must recognize an important feature that that parameter constrains. Observe that with a power function having an exponent less than 1, the value of the ordinate or dependent variable, "utility," grows more slowly than the value of the abscissa, "money," but this is true only for values of money and of utility greater than unity. At the unit point, or below, utility grows more rapidly than money and consequently, for small increments, that is increments all remaining below the unit value, the value of an increment increases more rapidly as the magnitude of the increment increases. We have not examined systematically the psychological consequences of this feature of a power function utility scale, but remark here merely on its existence.

References

Anderson, N. Algebraic models in perception. In Carterette and Friedman (Eds.), *Handbook of Perception*. Vol. II. New York: Academic Press, Inc. In press.

Coombs, C., Dawes, R., & Tversky, A. *Mathematical Psychology:* An Elementary Introduction. Englewood Cliffs, N.J.: Prentice-Hall, Inc., 1970.

Festinger, L. *A Theory of Cognitive Dissonance*. Stanford, Calif.: Stanford University Press, 1957.

Friedman, M. & Savage, L. The utility analysis of choices involving risk. *Journal of Political Economics*, 1948, **56**, 279–304.

Galanter, E. The direct measurement of utility and subjective probability. *American Journal of Psychology*, 1962, **75**, 208–220.

Galanter, E. Psychological decision mechanisms and perception. In Carterette and Friedman (Eds.), *Handbook of Perception*. Vol. II. New York: Academic Press, Inc. In press.

Galanter, E. & Holman, G. Some invariances of the isosensitivity function and their implications for the utility function of money. *Journal of Experimental Psychology*, 1967, **73**, 333–339.

Lee, W. *Decision Theory and Human Behavior*. New York: John Wiley & Sons, 1971.

THE STIMULUS IN INFORMATION PROCESSING[1,2]

WENDELL R. GARNER
Yale University

Abstract. It is argued that the nature of the stimulus must be understood before we can ask meaningful questions about human information processing since it is the stimulus that determines the nature of the information to be processed. As one example, it is shown that redundant stimulus dimensions provide an improvement in information processing only if the dimensions combine to produce in effect a new dimension; and such dimensions are termed integral. And as a second example, inadequate performance may occur because stimuli are process-limited in that inadequate differentiation of stimuli occurs, or they may be state-limited in that inadequate energy is available for the stimulus to be represented in the organism.

My thesis today is simply that too many of the experiments, interpretations, and concepts that have been used in studies of information processing have emphasized the processing part of the problem to the neglect of the information part of it. Too often has the nature of the input been ignored, with the consequence of incorrect assessment of the nature of information processing at worst, or an inadequate picture at best. Today I want to argue and demonstrate that more attention to the nature of the stimulus, the input without which no processing can take place, will be generously rewarding to those of us trying to understand how the organism processes information.

STIMULUS AS AN EXPERIMENTAL VARIABLE

The nature of the stimulus must become an important and frequent experimental variable. In preparing this talk, I reread, with the usual pleasure, James Gibson's (1960) presidential address to the Eastern Psychological Association on the concept of the stimulus in psychology. My original hope had been that I might be able to make use of some of the distinctions he made to outline how the stimulus should be considered in information processing. But I found myself unable to do that, and realized that this inability is the very reason why we must keep the nature of the stimulus as part of the experimental problem. For example, Gibson asks: When does a sequence constitute a single stimulus? That is not a question to be answered a priori. Rather, it is truly an experimental question. Or, Gibson asks: When is a relation to be considered a single stimulus and when a number of separate stimuli? Once again, this is properly an experimental question, not one to be answered before we undertake an experiment.

[1] Reprinted from *American Psychologist*, vol. 25, No. 4, April 1970.
[2] This article is the text of an invited address delivered to the Division of Experimental Psychology at the meeting of the American Psychological Association, Washington, D. C., September 1969. The research was supported by Grant MH 14229 from the National Institute of Mental Health to Yale University. Robert Crowder and Richard Gottwald made valuable comments about an earlier version of the paper.

H. R. Moskowitz et al. (eds.), Sensation and Measurement. 77–90.

In other words, we need experimental questions that concern the very nature of the input. Understanding the nature of the stimulus is exactly what I am arguing is necessary in the study of information processing, and we need experiments and concepts pertinent to the input just as we need them pertinent to the processing. Certainly at the very least our experiments should contain more than one type of stimulus – stimuli that are perhaps logically equivalent but could conceivably function quite differently for the organism.

We would never consider drawing conclusions from an experiment based on a single subject, because we know that a different subject might give us a different answer. And we have even learned to be cautious about drawing general conclusions based on the use of a single task. Continuous and discrete reaction-time tasks, for example, might just lead to different results. Why, then, are we apparently so happy drawing sweeping conclusions about how information is processed when we have used only one kind of stimulus? I am not about to argue that we forgot what we have learned about subject and task variations in our studies; I do want to argue that we become equally concerned about the nature of the information input.

MULTIPROCESS ORGANISM

Another point that has not been given sufficient consideration in our studies of information processing is that the organism is truly capable of many different types of information processing. Yet psychologists have often assumed that only a single information process operates for the organism. How many papers have been published in the past two years in which the question being asked was whether the organism processes information in serial or in parallel? Why must the organism do just one or the other? Very probably it can do either, depending on the task and the stimuli. And even as likely is that the organism frequently does both, not in the sense of doing first one and then the other, but in the sense of doing both simultaneously.

Now the particular pertinence of arguing for a multiprocess organism when I want to emphasize the role of stimulus concepts in information processing is this: One of the most important variables in determining how the organism will process information is the nature of the input itself, the very thing that has received so little attention in our research. If we want to understand how the organism processes information, we must be prepared to ask under what circumstances a particular form of processing is used. And one of the most important of these circumstances has to do with the nature of the stimulus input, the information to be processed.

Multidimensional Stimuli

In recent years there has been a heavy experimental use of stimuli defined by multiple dimensions, and such stimuli have been used with a variety of experimental tasks. Before discussing some of my own research, let me briefly outline three of these experimental tasks. These are tasks whose experimental results and the concepts derived from them should be, and as we shall see are, related.

MULTIDIMENSIONAL STIMULUS SCALING

One experimental task has been direct stimulus scaling of multidimensional stimuli. With this task our goal is to discover the psychological dimensional structure that is pertinent to the stimulus dimensional structure. These experiments are directly in the perceptual tradition, and it is therefore not surprising that from them have come stimulus concepts, in particular one that I will be using today.

The usual scaling question has been whether psychological distances correspond more nearly to a Euclidean structure or to a city-block structure. With the Euclidean structure, the distance between two stimuli differing on two dimensions is the familiar hypotenuse relation, which becomes the square root of two if the two distances for the two dimensions separately are equal; with the city-block structure, the multidimensional distance is the sum of the unidimensional distances. The experimental result has been that the type of dimensional structure obtained depends on the nature of the stimulus dimensions.

Torgerson (1958) suggested that the city-block metric would hold when the stimulus dimensions were "obvious and compelling [p. 292]," and that otherwise some metric closer to the Euclidean model would hold. Shepard (1964) referred to perceptually distinct dimensions as those that give a city-block metric. Still later, Hyman & Well (1968) made a direct experimental comparison of scaling of Munsell colors, using the dimensions of value and chroma. In one case they varied value and chroma within a single color patch, and they refer to unanalyzable dimensions in this case. In another case they varied value on one patch and chroma on another patch, and they refer to analyzable dimensions in this case. These authors found that the city-block metric was appropriate for their analyzable stimuli, but that the Euclidean metric was appropriate for their unanalyzable stimuli. (See also Attneave, 1962; Handel, 1967.)

So from this research we have a clear stimulus concept. I will use the term integrality for this concept, following the use of Lockhead (1966a), and the term separability seems an appropriate antonym.

ABSOLUTE JUDGMENTS

A second task frequently used with multidimensional stimuli is absolute judgment. With this task several different levels are used per stimulus dimension; and accuracy is the dependent variable, measured either with percentage of correct identifications or with information transmissions. The primary experimental problem studied with this technique has been to ask whether information transmission is increased when new stimulus dimensions are added to an existing one. The experimental literature, reviewed by Garner (1962), shows that when dimensions are added orthogonally, and judgment of all dimensions is required, performance improves, but not as much as would be expected if the subject were able to deal with each dimension independently. On the other hand, if a new dimension is added redundantly by being correlated with an existing dimension, there sometimes is a gain in performance, but in other cases there is little or no gain.

Very little of this research, unlike the case with direct multidimensional scaling, has been concerned with the nature of the stimulus dimensions. Lockhead (1966a) first used a stimulus concept in suggesting that a gain in absolute judgment accuracy with redundant stimulus dimensions would occur only if the dimensions were integral, and in another study (1966b) justified his suggestion by showing that if the dimensions of hue and value were made redundant but with separate stimulus patches, no gain in judgmental accuracy occurred.

TABLE 1

Experimental design and possible experimental outcomes in the Garner-Felfoldy experiments

Dimension sorted	Stimulus set Single dimension	Correlated dimensions	Orthogonal dimensions
A or *B*	Base speed	Equal or faster	Equal or slower

SPEEDED CLASSIFICATION

A third task commonly used with multidimensional stimuli is speeded classification. With this task the subject is required to classify stimuli by one of the two or more dimensions represented in a set of stimuli, and speed of classification is measured. The usual experimental question has been whether the addition of irrelevant stimulus dimensions interferes with classification on the basis of the relevant dimension; that is, can subjects selectively attend to a stimulus dimension? Egeth (1967), in a review of this literature, argued that interference occurs only when there is response competition. Thus at that time there was no evidence that properties of the stimuli were pertinent to the presence or absence of interference in the classification task.

So here we have three lines of research all using multidimensional stimuli, all asking apparently unrelated questions, and naturally getting unrelated answers. With the scaling approach we are concerned with how the stimuli are related to each other. With absolute judgments we are concerned with whether performance is improved by the addition of stimulus dimensions. With speeded classification we are concerned with whether performance becomes poorer with the addition of stimulus dimensions.

The number of experiments that have crossed these boundaries of task and experimental question is small indeed. In fact, what is truly remarkable is that there is practically no cross-referencing of the literature between these three areas defined jointly by task and problem. But surely there must be some sensible relations between those conditions that produce interference in speeded classification and those that produce improved discrimination in absolute judgment tasks, and even further between each of these and those conditions in which the city-block metric holds rather than the Euclidean metric. There are indeed, and what makes sense out of some of these relations is this stimulus concept of dimensional integrality, first derived from experiments on multidimensional scaling.

A STUDY OF CLASSIFICATION SPEED

Now I will describe some research I have been doing at Yale, with the collaboration of Gary Felfoldy (Garner & Felfoldy, 1970, in press). Four different experiments are involved in this research, but these four are identical in all respects except one – and that is the particular stimulus dimensions used. So I can describe a single experiment, and then discuss the results with four different pairs of stimulus dimensions.

We used speeded classification as our experimental task, in which subjects were required to sort a deck of 32 stimulus cards into two piles as rapidly as they could. Sorting time was our measure. Errors are, of course, low in this type of experiment, and I shall not discuss the few that occurred.

Each experiment involved two stimulus dimensions, with two levels or values per dimension. Thus four different stimulus values could exist. We used three different types of stimulus set, and with each type of stimulus set we required the subjects to sort by each of the two dimensions. Thus for each experiment there were six different experimental conditions. These six conditions, plus some possible outcome expectations, are schematized in Table 1.

One type of stimulus set had only two stimuli differing on a single dimension, and in these cases the subject simply sorted by that dimension. A second type of stimulus set had the two dimensions occurring in a perfectly correlated or redundant manner. In this case there were still only two different stimuli. Nevertheless, we required the subjects to sort by each of the two different dimensions separately. The third type of stimulus set was the orthogonal set, in which each value of each of the dimensions occurred with both values of the other dimension, with a resultant four different stimuli. And, as with the correlated stimulus set, we required the subjects to classify or sort the stimuli separately by each dimension.

Now the comments within the table concern the possible experimental outcomes. The sorting time obtained with each single dimensional deck is, of course, the base time for that particular dimension. This is the control condition. But now when we require sorting by that same dimension with correlated stimulus dimensions, we expect either that there will be no change in discrimination speed, or that there will be faster sorting if use is made of the additional dimension. We could logically get slower speeds with the correlated stimulus dimensions, but such a result would be most unlikely. At least it would be most unexpected since we do not ordinarily entertain the possibility of interference in such a task. And last, when we require sorting by just one dimension from the orthogonal stimulus set, we expect either no change in speed or a slower speed, indicating interference from what is now an irrelevant dimension. Once again, notice that we could logically get facilitation, but such a result would be most unlikely and unexpected.

The question we are concerned about, of course, is the relation between results with these latter two cases: Should stimulus dimensions that give facilitation with the correlated stimulus set give interference with the orthogonal set; or should facilitation occur only with dimensions that produce no interference; or is there no meaningful relation?

Integral Colors

One pair of dimensions we used were value (or brightness) and chroma (or saturation) of single Munsell color chips. These are the same stimulus dimensions that Hyman & Well (1968) used in their experiment on direct multidimensional scaling, and that were found to produce the Euclidean metric indicative of integral dimensions.

The result in our experiment is very straightforward. When we required sorting of the correlated stimulus sets, sorting speeds were faster than either base rate for each dimension, indicating facilitation. When we required sorting of the orthogonal stimulus sets, sorting speeds were slower in each case, indicating interference. Thus for these stimulus dimensions, the result is clear and simple: Both facilitation and interference occur: facilitation with redundant dimensions, and interference with orthogonal dimensions.

Separated Colors

As Hyman and Well had also done, we used these two dimensions in a way that makes them clearly separable, by literally having one color chip varying in value and another color chip on the same card varying in chroma. Hyman and Well had, in this case, obtained the city-block metric indicative of separable dimensions. Furthermore, Lockhead (1966b), using hue and value, had found no gain when the two dimensions were made separable in the same way, with an absolute judgment task. Thus we had reason to expect this stimulus change to produce a substantial performance change.

Our result here was equally straightforward: No facilitation was obtained when subjects sorted the correlated stimuli, and no interference was found when they sorted the orthogonal stimuli.

Our conclusion so far is clear: When stimulus dimensions are integral, we get the Euclidean metric in direct distance scaling, facilitation in speed of classification when the dimensions are redundant, and interference when single-dimension classification is required with orthogonal decks, that is, when the subject is required to filter or to attend selectively.

Dot Location

We tried a further pair of dimensions, the horizontal and vertical location of a single dot on a card. We felt that if ever two dimensions satisfy the idea of integrality at an intuitive level, certainly these two do. With these two dimensions, we once again obtain the result that seems to go with integral dimensions: facilitation when the dimensions are correlated and interference when they are orthogonal.

However, the first bit of disquiet occurs with these dimensions. The overall result is clearly qualitatively the same that we obtained with integral colors. Even further, the amount of facilitation obtained with correlated dimensions was much the same for both colors and dot locations. But the integral colors caused much more interference than did the dots, nearly five times the actual numerical amount. And this relative lack of interference with horizontal and vertical dot location as dimensions was greater in an experiment by Egeth & Pachella (1969), one of the few experiments using absolute judgments to study interference effects, since they found no interference at all. Thus we appear to need the idea of degrees of integrality. Furthermore we may find that subjects can indeed adjust so as both to use a facilitating effect and also to avoid an interfering effect; that is, they can use a particular pair of dimensions either as integral or separable, depending on the task demands.

Circle and Line

The last pair of stimulus dimensions added to the disquiet about a simple picture. We used the size of a circle and the angle or orientation of a diameter within the circle. Once again we used these because they were similar to dimensions previously found to give a city-block metric, indicating separability, by Shepard (1964) and Hyman & Well (1967) In this case we got different results for the two dimensions. The classification speed for size of circle was neither facilitated with a redundant diameter nor interfered with when the diameter was added as an irrelevant dimension. But when classification by the angle of the diameter was done, there was some facilitation. We think this result came from the fact that the length of the line was correlated with the size of the circle, so that length and angle of the line were operating to some extent as a pair of integral dimensions. Further, however, it is entirely possible for the subject to focus on a particular part of the card and in effect get a redefined stimulus in which the entire circle is ignored, but instead the curvature and location of the end of the diameter are used integrally as a new stimulus dimension. I had previously found evidence for a similar redefinition of stimulus dimensions with pairs of dots as stimuli (Garner, 1969).

WHAT IS INTEGRALITY?

One problem that this and other experiments require us to face is that we have no good operational definition of integrality which is clearly independent of the experimental result to be explained or understood. I do think it possible to have a limiting definition, however, and it is this: Two dimensions are integral if in order for a level on one dimension to be realized, there must be a dimensional level specified for the other. For example, a visual stimulus must have a brightness and a hue and a saturation and a size and a form. That fact makes any pair of these dimensions integral. Notice that things such as brightness may have a value of zero, but zero brightness does not mean that the dimension is not functional; rather, it simply means that one possible value of the dimension is zero.

If, on the other hand, a zero value of a dimension means that the dimension is nonexistent, then the dimensions involved are separable. To illustrate, we may have the letters *A* or *U* appear in either or both of two positions. If nothing appears in one position, that dimension is nonfunctional, but that fact in no way influences the functioning of the other dimension.

Now the reason these can only be limiting definitions, or perhaps idealized definitions, is the very versatility and adaptability of the organism in carrying out information processing I mentioned earlier. The organism can redefine a stimulus dimension to provide optimum processing. This adaptability of the organism does not alter the fact that the most valuable concept in understanding and relating these several results is a stimulus concept. We have not asked whether, for example, processing is serial or parallel, and I sincerely doubt that such a question really makes sense for these experiments, even though they are typically information-processing experiments. What is pertinent is first and foremost whether the stimulus can be redefined into an effectively new dimension, which is the essence of the integrality idea.

REDUNDANCY AND SEPARABLE DIMENSIONS

This discussion so far has suggested that you can get a gain in discrimination performance by adding a redundant stimulus dimension only if the two or more dimensions are integral. Based only on the experiment just described, that is a fair statement. It needs modification, however, to cover a broader base, and that modification itself requires that we make further stimulus distinctions – distinctions that relate to what it is that limits performance when performance is in some sense less than optimum.

Process or State Limitation

John Morton and I (Garner & Morton, 1969), in discussing models of perceptual independence, distinguished between independence of states of the organism and independence of the direct perceptual processes. This distinction between state and process will be useful in the present context.

Consider a discrimination task in which a subject is expected to discriminate between two alternative stimuli, and these stimuli are lines having different angles of orientation. And suppose, for purposes of illustration, that in a particular case the accuracy of discrimination is 75%. The question we want to consider is: What is preventing perfect identification or accuracy of judgment?

There are two clear possibilities: First, the difference in angle of orientation may be too small, so that even if each stimulus is completely visible, we still cannot get perfect accuracy. Second, the difference in angle of orientation is quite big enough so that we can get perfect accuracy on that basis, but the stimuli are presented at such a low contrast, or possibly at such a short duration, that the subject cannot always see the stimulus. We would call the first case one of process limitation and the second case one of state limitation.

Figure 1 illustrates the kinds of ideal functions one might expect for these two situations if we increase the discriminability units in the one dimension on which the two stimuli differ, that is, the dimension to be processed. If performance is only process limited, then as we increase the inherent discriminability of the stimuli on the pertinent dimension, performance should increase to an asymptotic perfect accuracy. On the

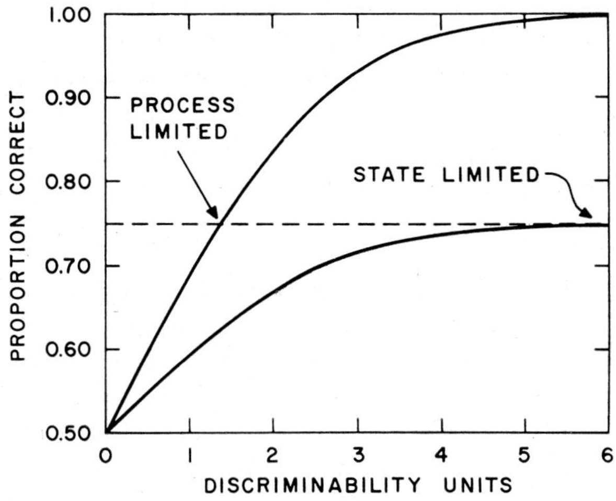

Fig. 1. Idealized discrimination functions contrasting situations where accuracy is limited only by the direct discrimination process, and those in which it is also limited by the state or sensitivity of the organism in receiving stimulus energy input. (The lower curve is derived from the upper on the simple assumption of two states, detect and nondetect, each occurring with probability 0.50. This value gives a state-limited asymptotic performance of 0.75. The discriminability units are with respect to the direct discrimination process.)

other hand, if performance is also limited by the state of the organism or the stimulus which limits performance on a sensitivity basis, then the asymptotic value will be somewhat lower, depending now not on the magnitude of the process discriminability, but on the amount of state limitation. Given these two kinds of situations, I think it is obvious how, in each case, we can change the stimulus so as to get improved performance.

If accuracy is process limited, we need to increase the stimulus discriminability. If we do this by simply increasing the angular difference in our two illustrative stimuli, we will accomplish the result, but would not consider this effect to be due to redundancy. On the other hand, if we can increase discriminability of the pair of stimuli by adding a redundant dimension, then we would say that the increased performance has come about because we added redundancy. This is the sort of situation we have been talking about so far, and dealt with in the Garner-Felfoldy experiment. And it is in this case that integral dimensions are required.

On the other hand, if accuracy is state limited, somehow we must find a way of offsetting the state limitation. One way would be to increase the stimulus duration or contrast, but once again we would not consider any improvement obtained this way as being due to redundancy. Alternatively, we could add redundant stimulus dimensions. Now, however, we need to be sure that the new dimensions increase the probability that the stimulus has been seen, that is, that additional information gets into the organism. The way to accomplish this is to add separable dimensions, so that independent opportunities to experience the stimulus are obtained. This is what happens if we increase the number of elements in space or time. As examples, Eriksen & Lappin (1965) and Garner & Flowers (1969) have shown that the use of multiple stimulus elements, letters in both cases, does improve stimulus discrimination. These letters as stimulus elements, however, are perfectly and easily discriminable if seen, so any limitation in accuracy is due only to state limitation. Thus the use of separable stimulus dimensions as redundancy does improve performance when it is state limited.

SOME PRINCIPLES CONCERNING REDUNDANCY GAIN

We can summarize these experimental findings and conjectures with some principles concerning when stimulus redundancy will aid discrimination:

1. There will be a gain with redundancy if the need for the redundancy is due to a process limitation and if the redundant dimensions are integral.

2. Alternatively, there will be a gain with redundancy if the need for redundancy is due to state limitation and the redundant dimensions are separable.

These two principles state in effect that there are two quite different ways in which dimensional redundancy can aid information processing. In one case, performance is improved by actual information combining, and for this integral dimensions are necessary. In the other case, performance is improved by a multiple-look process, and in this case separable dimensions are required.

Notice that only with separable dimensions is a concept such as perceptual independence (see Garner & Lee, 1962; Garner & Morton, 1969) appropriate to explain when discrimination performance improves with redundancy. Separable dimensions, we can argue, are perceptually independent; but we certainly cannot argue that integral dimensions are. Thus perceptual independence is an asset in information-processing tasks only when performance is state limited, in which case separable redundant dimensions will aid performance. On the other hand, if performance is process limited, then integrality rather than independence of dimensions is needed in order to improve performance by the addition of redundancy.

Our evidence makes it clear that if performance is process limited, then redundant separable dimensions will not aid performance. In fact, a recent apparently confusing result by Keeley & Doherty (1968) can be clarified by this principle. They were comparing multiple form discrimination to single form discrimination, and found that there was a gain in accuracy of discrimination with multiple letters, but not with Landolt rings, which have a gap in one of four positions. These Landolt rings, however, are much less discriminable than the letters, and performance is very possibly process limited rather than state limited, as with the letters. This possible difference in the two kinds of stimuli is strongly suggested by the fact that the exposure duration required to give a fixed accuracy for the letters was approximately half that required for the rings. Thus, with letters, performance was state limited and then improved with redundant separable dimensions. But with Landolt rings, performance was process limited and not improved with redundant separable dimensions.

A point of confusion remains, however, in that there was improvement in performance if the Landolt rings were repeated in time. The fact that Lockhead (1966b) found the same result with hue and value means that this is not an isolated case. There clearly is something different between spatial and temporal separability. Possibly a memory trace allows integration over time.

As one last comment on this aspect of the problem, we should note that if performance is state limited it may also be process limited; that is, these are not mutually exclusive limitations. Thus there might well be a performance gain with redundant integral dimensions even with stimuli that are clearly state limited. In fact, Lockhead (1966a), using length of line and vertical position, found a gain in absolute judgment accuracy under two conditions of state limitation. Since almost certainly these two dimensions are reasonably integral, we must draw the conclusion that performance was both state limited and process limited in his experiment. Insofar as it was process limited, then redundant integral dimensions could provide a gain in accuracy.

SERIAL, PARALLEL, OR NEW DIMENSION?

I mentioned earlier that when two dimensions are integral, the subject in effect combines them into a new stimulus dimension, particularly when the dimensions are correlated. If this is so, then to ask – as is so popular today – whether multidimensional stimuli are processed in parallel or serial fashion is really to bypass the most important question. It is quite meaningless to ask whether integral dimensions are processed in serial or in parallel, because only two or more things can be processed in serial or parallel fashion. So we must ask the logically primary question whether dimensions are separable or integral, and only when we establish that dimensions are separable is it then meaningful to ask whether processing is serial or parallel. Thus the integrality-separability distinction must take priority over the serial-parallel distinction.

I want to emphasize this fact because it is rare today that any attempt is made to answer the integrality question first. Furthermore, several studies requiring same or different judgments of multidimensional stimuli have used stimulus dimensions that are very likely integral, yet the authors of these studies have been primarily concerned with differentiating between serial and parallel processing. Egeth (1966) used color and shape (which are certainly integral) and the tilt of a line within the form (which we have seen can be separable from the shape at least) and found no clear answer concerning the type of processing. But he did not consider the possibility of the dimensions combining into a new dimension. Hawkins (1969), in an elaboration of Egeth's experiment, explicitly noted the possibility of stimulus redefinition, but then essentially rejected it with no further consideration. His stimulus dimensions were color, form, and size – and any pair of these is almost certainly integral. Hawkins likewise arrived at no clear decision concerning mode of processing. Nickerson (1967) also used color, form, and size, and obtained results giving the usual ambiguous answer concerning the nature of the processing. He did, however, specifically mention the possibility that the results he and others have obtained might well be obtained with unidimensional stimuli, and pointed out that an early experiment by Kellogg (1931) with unidimensional stimuli gave similar results.

Certainly at a qualitative level most of the results obtained in these experiments can be duplicated with stimuli varying unidimensionally. But if this is so, where is the question concerning serial vs parallel processing? At the least I must argue that it is not meaningful to draw conclusions concerning processing of separable dimensions until we know that the dimensions are in fact separable. Furthermore, if the same results can be obtained with unidimensional stimuli, then we must exercise real caution in interpreting results with multidimensional stimuli as though the dimensions are separable.

STIMULUS REDEFINITION AS GESTALT

This concept of stimulus integrality has an intriguing similarity to gestalt concepts such as the whole being more than the sum of the parts, or the nonanalyzability of percepts. Egeth (1966) mentioned the possibility of a stimulus being reorganized into a sort of gestalt in order to explain why he obtained faster same judgments for stimuli identical on three dimensions than for stimuli identical on two dimensions – or more accurately where only two dimensions were relevant to the decision. It seems entirely possible that such wholistic phenomena will be experienced wherever possible, and that they can be experienced ordinarily only with integral dimensions.

I say ordinarily, because once again the versatility of the human organism comes into play. Sekuler & Abrams (1968) used visual stimuli consisting of matrices with some cells blackened. They found that judgments of same were much faster if sameness was based on identity rather than similarity, and concluded that the patterns were being processed as gestalt wholes rather than as a set of elements. Thus here we have stimulus dimensions (the cells) that are clearly separable by any reasonable definition, and yet they can be redefined into a form.

Certainly to process information as wholistic or gestalt stimuli rather than as separate elements is an efficient thing for the organism to do – and possibly that is the advantage of gestalt patterns. This result is reminiscent of experiments by Royer (1966) and by Clement & Varnadoe (1967), both showing that pattern discrimination of dots in matrices is better when the dots form good patterns. Possibly James Gibson's (1960) query as to when a pattern is a single stimulus rather than a number of stimuli can only be answered: when the dimensions can be integrated to form a new stimulus. This answer is a long way from being completely satisfactory, but certainly the concept of integrality of dimensions and gestalt concepts do have much in common.

Conclusion

In conclusion, let me reiterate my plea that we pay more attention to the stimulus in information processing. The role of the stimulus needs to be studied, and concepts based on stimulus properties must be evolved before we can truly understand how the organism processes information. For too long we have considered that a stimulus is a stimulus is a stimulus, whose only function is to elicit behavior. But all stimuli are not equivalent, and all information cannot be processed the same way.

I hope, however, that we never make the mistake of ignoring other factors in information processing as much as the stimulus has been ignored. I certainly hope as well that my plea for study of the stimulus is not interpreted to mean that I wish to deny the role of other factors, because I most sincerely do not. It is very clear, for example, that response conflict does operate in some tasks and prevents effective filtering of a stimulus dimension. And Morton (1969) in a recent article has even made a good case for response facilitation with numerosity and numerals as stimulus dimensions. As another example, Bindra *et al.* (1968) have shown the importance of codability of the stimulus as a factor in determining whether same judgments are faster than difference judgments. And there are many studies that make it absolutely clear that stimulus-response compatibility has a great effect on information processing.

It would seem, then, that my real plea is for a greater maturity on the part of psychology, maturity that does not expect our answers to be very simple, that does not seek a single solution. Rather, we must be prepared to ask when and under what circumstances does the organism process information in a particular way. We will find a tremendous diversity of answers, but nevertheless we will be closer to a true understanding of the organism. The answers will be more complex for just one reason: The organism itself is complex.

References

Attneave, F. Perception and related areas. In S. Koch (Ed.), *Psychology: A study of a science*. Vol. 4. New York: McGraw-Hill, 1962.

Bindra, D., Donderi, D. C., & Nishisato, S. Decision latencies of "same" and "different" judgments. *Perception and Psychophysics*, 1968, **3**, 121–130.

Clement, D. E., & Varnadoe, K. W. Pattern uncertainty and the discrimination of visual patterns. *Perception and Psychophysics*, 1967, **2**, 427–431.

Egeth, H. Parallel versus serial processes in multidimensional stimulus discrimination. *Perception and Psychophysics*, 1966, **1**, 245–252.

Egeth, H. Selective attention. *Psychological Bulletin*, 1967, **67**, 41–57.

Egeth, H., & Pachella, R. Multidimensional stimulus identification. *Perception and Psychophysics* 1969, **5**, 341–346.

Eriksen, C. W., & Lappin, J. S. Internal perceptual system noise and redundancy in simultaneous inputs in form identification. *Psychonomic Science*, 1965, **2**, 351–352.

Garner, W. R. *Uncertainty and structure as psychological concepts*. New York: Wiley, 1962.

Garner, W. R. Speed of discrimination with redundant stimulus attributes. *Perception and Psychophysics*, 1969, **6**, 221–224.

Garner, W. R., & Felfoldy, G. Integrality of stimulus dimensions in various types of information, processing. *Cognitive Psychology*, 1970, **1**, 225–241.

Garner, W. R., & Flowers, J. H. The effect of redundant stimulus elements on visual discrimination as a function of element heterogeneity, equal discriminability, and position uncertainty. *Perception and Psychophysics*, 1969, **6**, 216–220.

Garner, W. R., & Lee, W. An analysis of redundancy in perceptual discrimination. *Perceptual and Motor Skills*, 1962, **15**, 367–388.

Garner, W. R., & Morton, J. Perceptual independence: Definitions, models, and experimental paradigms. *Psychological Bulletin*, 1969, **72**, 233–259.

Gibson, J. J. The concept of the stimulus in psychology. *American Psychologist*, 1960, **15**, 694–703.

Handel, S. Classification and similarity of multidimensional stimuli. *Perceptual and Motor Skills*, 1967, **24**, 1191–1203.

Hawkins, H. L. Parallel processing in complex visual discrimination. *Perception and Psychophysics*, 1969, **5**, 56–64.

Hyman, R., & Well, A. Judgments of similarity and spatial models. *Perception and Psychophysics*, 1967, **2**, 233–248.

Hyman, R., & Well, A. Perceptual separability and spatial models. *Perception and Psychophysics*, 1968, **3**, 161–165.

Keeley, S. M., & Doherty, M. E. Simultaneous and successive presentations of single-featured and multi-featured visual forms: Implications for the parallel processing hypothesis. *Perception and Psychophysics*, 1968, **4**, 296–298.

Kellogg, W. N. The time of judgment in psychometric measures. *American Journal of Psychology*, 1931, **43**, 65–86.

Lockhead, G. R. Effects of dimensional redundancy on visual discrimination. *Journal of Experimental Psychology*, 1966, **72**, 95–104. (a)

Lockhead, G. R. Visual discrimination and methods of presenting redundant stimuli. *Proceedings of the 74th Annual Convention of the American Psychological Association*, 1966, **1**, 67–68. (b)

Morton, J. The use of correlated stimulus information in card sorting. *Perception and Psychophysics*, 1969, **5**, 374–376.

Nickerson, R. S. "Same"-"different" response times with multi-attribute stimulus differences. *Perceptual and Motor Skills*, 1967, **24**, 543–554.

Royer, F. L. Figural goodness and internal structure in perceptual discrimination. *Perception and Psychophysics*, 1966, **1**, 311–314.

Sekuler, R. W., & Abrams, M. Visual sameness: A choice time analysis of pattern recognition processes. *Journal of Experimental Psychology*, 1968, **77**, 232–238.

Shepard, R. N. Attention and the metric structure of the stimulus space. *Journal of Mathematical Psychology*, 1964, **1**, 54–87.

Torgerson, W. S. *Theory and methods of scaling*. New York: Wiley, 1958.

ON THE SENSORY EVALUATION OF COMPLIANT MATERIALS

ROLAND HARPER[1]

Department of Food Science, University of Reading

Abstract. The background of the sensory evaluation of compliant materials is outlined, including some of the underlying practical and theoretical issues. A study originally reported by Harper & Stevens (1964) is summarized together with some previously unpublished data. These experiments involved both the evaluation of the hardness and softness of a number of samples of compliant materials using both the methods of magnitude estimation and cross-modal matching. The exponent (n) of the power-law relating hardness (and softness) to a physical criterion was approximately 0.8. Some evidence suggested that hardness and softness were not perfectly reciprocal. Some recent developments in the evaluation of compliant materials are also noted.

The systematic evaluation of the sensory qualities of compliant materials dates back to the first few decades of the present century. Many of the early studies were essentially phenomenological, and included the analysis of such qualities as hardness, softness, roughness, smoothness and stickiness and other touch 'blends'. Names of investigators like those of Bentley, Meenes, Sullivan and Zigler immediately come to mind. One of the most influential persons was Katz (1925), selections from his book on *The World of Touch* having been recently translated from the German by Kreuger (1970). Katz and Stephenson (1937) anticipated the use of heterogeneous matching techniques (later referred to as 'cross-modal') by matching 'elastic pulls' to 'dead weights.' Katz (1938) also studied the skills of traditional bakers who manipulate the raw materials (dough) and exercise an important degree of control of the whole baking process by the 'feel' of the dough. G. W. Scott Blair met Katz about this time and in 1938 he (Scott Blair) initiated a series of psychophysical studies which continued until 1952, apart from an interruption during World War II. These studies arose out of the analogous skills of cheesemakers and cheesegraders who used the 'feel' of the materials as control variables. Fundamental and applied studies were carried out at the National Institute for Research in Dairying, Reading, (England). Cheese curd, hard pressed cheeses, as well as simpler and more stable materials such as samples of vulcanized rubber or stiff liquids of comparable physical properties were studied. The main problems investigated included the usual ones, such as:

1. Identifying and defining the relevant sensory qualities.
2. Determining the powers of discrimination based upon appropriate physical criteria.
3. Matching operations, including both qualitatively similar and qualitatively different samples.
4. Evaluating the degree or extent to which the various qualities are present, usually by employing rating scales.

[1] Leverhulme Senior Fellow.

H. R. Moskowitz et al. (eds.), Sensation and Measurement. 91–98.

5. Investigating the empirical or functional relationships between what is perceived and what is measured.

The Choice of Experimental Variables

The investigator is always faced with the question of the choice of experimental variables. In the simplest examples only two well-defined variables are involved, one sensory and one instrumental. Such examples raise no special problems. However, particularly when the materials handled are complex, like clays, doughs or textiles, for example, there will be several relevant variables, if not many. Examples include a number of multidimensional studies of which some of the earliest involved up to a total of 18 sensory and instrumental tests on Cheshire and Cheddar cheeses. These studies were carried out between 1948 and 1952 and have been summarized elsewhere (Harper, 1956).

Terms and Their Meaning

No discussion of the sensory evaluation of compliant materials would be complete without reference to descriptive terminology and its meaning. A medium-sized English Dictionary containing some 200000 words may include at least 70 terms which refer to the sensory qualities of compliant materials. These include both unipolar and bipolar terms, such as:

Unipolar	*Bipolar*
Oily	Soft – Hard
Greasy	Thick – Thin
Tacky	Rough – Smooth
Sticky	Tough – Tender
etc.	etc.

To these must be added a number of special technical terms, mostly associated either with clearly defined physical properties or with empirical parameters derived from the use of particular instruments. Without going into their actual definitions or origins, examples include viscosity, elasticity, cohesiveness and adhesiveness. The existence of sensory and instrumental terms raises a number of problems. First, there is the question in a particular study whether the terms such as viscosity and elasticity are used in a purely technical sense, or whether they refer to related, though not necessarily identical, sensory qualities. This question is also associated with establishing precisely what the various sensory terms mean. Much still remains to be done, especially in defining the various qualities in terms of (sets of) samples which demonstrate these qualities (i.e. ostensive definition). Another approach is to examine the empirical relationship between the sensory qualities and the objective-instrumental measurements as illustrated by the multidimensional analysis of the network of statistical relationships referred to above. Any conclusions will automatically be influenced by the particular test-samples and experimental variables (both sensory and instrumental) selected in any study.

Even experts may differ in their opinions of the nature of such apparently simple sensory qualities as springiness. Thus in discussions c.1960 Scott Blair emphasized the importance of the *amount of recovery* whereas Harper emphasized the *rate of recovery* in an instrumental test as the most likely determinant of this sensory quality. There are also divergent opinions concerning whether the subject should evaluate some specified physical parameter, or whether he should be concerned exclusively with the sensory qualities. This is inevitably associated with perceptual attitudes and the effects of instructions given to the subject on the results obtained. Perhaps this reflects the old controversy about the 'stimulus error' in a contemporary form. Some investigators (e.g. Szczesniak, or Sherman) have emphasized the importance of instrumentally measured parameters or physical properties and trained their subjects to judge in these terms. Others, including the present author, take the opposite view and consider that the evaluation should be made in terms which the subject himself considers to be appropriate. In the last analysis, however, an appeal to experimental data should be used to determine as precisely as possible the actual basis upon which the judgments are made.

Instrumental Criteria

Instrumental measurements provide the objective criteria against which to compare the sensory qualities of compliant materials. Until fairly recently (i.e. the last few decades) it was common practice to develop special instruments adapted to the task in hand. An increasing number of commercial instruments is now available. Some, like the various types of viscometers, are designed to measure a very limited range of physical behaviour. Others, like the INSTRON, are general-purpose instruments which allow the continuous recording of data in a form suitable for immediate computer analysis. Historically, some of the instruments available simulate the action of the human hand (or the teeth) in probing various materials. Various types of indentation tests have been derived from long-established industrial practices, especially in the petroleum and the rubber industries.

Only in the case of a limited selection of ideal materials can their behavior in conditions of deformation or flow under pressure be specified in terms of a single physical property having a constant value. Most traditional text books of physics dealing with 'Properties of Matter' (e.g. Poynting & Thompson, 1934) restricted themselves to situations involving small deformations or small forces. These ideal systems are best illustrated by the measurement of the (coefficient of) viscosity of Newtonian liquids or the (coefficient of) elasticity of Hookean Solids. The behavior of more complicated materials which deform or flow under pressure is usually discussed in text books on rheology. A number of different (and quasi-independent) properties may be involved; or the relevant tests may be 'empirical' in the sense that the behavior is complex and is not capable of being fitted into a well understood simple theoretical system. Alternatively, whatever is being measured may be altered by the process of testing and the instrumental measurements obtained will vary according to these conditions.

The Method of Magnitude Estimation

The method of magnitude estimation is associated in particular with a paper by Stevens (1956). However, he had already set out the underlying principles some twenty years earlier, as indicated in the following quotation:

> Now, in the case of sensation what we want is a scale for measurement of some aspect of the response of a living organism to a certain class of stimuli. Two conditions should be satisfied. First the scale numbers should be applied to the attribute of sensation in such a way as to make the scale one of true numerical magnitude, which means simply that if the numbers are manipulated according to the rules of arithmetic, the result (and the manipulations) correspond to a set of physical operations. Secondly, although at the outset we could conceivably choose any one of several sets of scales operations as defining the scale, that set will ultimately prove to be most satisfactory for a subjective scale when it leads to a scale number bearing a reasonable relationship to the experience of the observer. Thus a scale would be satisfactory if the magnitude of the attribute of a sensation to which the number 10 is assigned should appear to be half as great to the experiencing individual as that to which the number 20 is given, and twice as great as the magnitude to which the number 5 is given ... (Stevens, 1936, p. 406).

The method usually leads to the well-known power law representing the manner in which what is *perceived* intensity (ψ) grows with the increasing value of the stimulus (ϕ). In its simplest form the power law may be expressed as:

$$\psi = k\phi^n .$$

The exponent (n) is the critical parameter and k is a constant which relates to the size of the unit used on the chosen ratio scale.

Magnitude Estimation of the Hardness of Compliant Materials

A study which has been described in detail elsewhere (Harper & Stevens, 1964) was carried out in the spring of 1962 in the basement of Memorial Hall, a distinctive building on the edge of the Harvard Campus built to celebrate the end of the Civil War. Stevens (1970) has described how he began his war-time investigations there in World War II. In the present investigation a number of samples of vulcanized rubber were prepared by a small firm in the back streets of Cambridge (Mass). The range of hardnesses chosen was based upon previous knowledge and experience. The particular values and intervals were determined largely by trial and error adjusting the various mixtures accordingly. Rubber samples having a Shore Durometer reading greater than 70 were rejected as being too hard for investigations of a sensory nature. The range of hardnesses was extended on the soft side by the addition of a number of foam samples. Details of the final selection are given in Table 1. A simple testing instrument was constructed so as to provide a suitable objective criterion. This instrument consisted of a $\frac{7}{8}''$ steel ball which could be impressed into the surface of the test samples by means of a loaded lever system and the indentation measured.

The values of the ratio of the force (F) to the indentation (I) were calculated for each sample for different applied forces. A series of curves representing the variation of F/I against F was plotted. It was evident that no *single* value of F/I characterized each

TABLE 1

Specification of samples of compliant materials used in magnitude estimation study

Code designation	Material or substance	Objective criterion F/I	Description
II	Light textured sponge rubber	8.3	Feathery and airy yet more compact than V. Finger sinks in at lightest contact.
IIa	Ditto but slightly harder than II	10	Very soft. Fingers sink in with little resistance. Sample 'comes back' but does not actually push the fingers back (like some of the other samples). Can feel the curved surface with the thumb. Tactile component is important here.
IV	Close-textured 'NEOPRENE'	65	Rather soft, but yields bodily rather than at one localized patch. Just a little softer than V, but a different sort of softness. Rather as if it were filled with down or kapok. Unlike V, has no distinct and identifiable surface. Even when pressing hard there seems to be more material between the fingers than V; might be described as having more 'body'.
V	Open-textured sponge rubber with a rough *skin*	83	A peculiar sample. A superficial hardness gives way suddenly to a yielding sensation; although this ceases on further compression, gives a feeling of rounded accommodation to the fingers. Rather like pressing one's fingers into a balloon not too highly inflated. Has no 'body', yet recovery (after compression) clearly identifiable.
20	Solid rubber	230	Very comfortable and pleasant to handle. One's fingers sink in; can just feel the recovery although this is not easy to see.
25	Solid rubber	240	Same as 30 only more readily deformed. Recovery not so detectable as in 30.
30	Solid rubber	315	Deformation and accommodation to the finger and thumb very noticable, more so than for 40. Recovery clearly detectable.
40	Solid rubber	430	Very noticeable deformation. Can feel a bowing of the surface and a comfortable spreading of the material round the finger and thumb. More pleasant to handle than 70. Can also feel the recovery.
70	Solid rubber	970	Dead hard at first. Can just feel it yielding under high pressure between finger and thumb. Mainly aware of a little spreading area of contact. Little deformation; little recovery (resilience or springiness).

Note. The numbers 20–70 are the Shore Durometer Readings provided by the supplier. Reference to tables giving the corresponding Elastic Moduli for rubber samples and comparing these with previous studies involving vulcanized rubber as a material to be handled, an upper limit to *perceptible* deformation would be expected at and above a Shore Durometer Reading of 75. This would correspond to an elastic modulus of about 10^7 dyne cm^{-2}.

sample accurately under all conditions of testing. A compromise was required. A slightly curved line was drawn intersecting each of the individual curves of F/I against F. The points of intersection provided a set of objective criteria in arbitrary units ranging in value from 930 for the hardest sample to 8.3 for the softest.

The samples were presented to the subjects in an irregular order and compressed between finger and thumb. No designated reference standard was used. Magnitude estimates of hardness and of softness were made separately. These ranged from 1.8 to 73.6 for hardness and from 0.65 to 31.4 for softness (median values). A replicate study involving hardness gave results which agreed with the previous investigation. The value of the exponent (n) was approximately 0.8, implying a growth-rate that decreases as the stimulus value increases if both the sensory and the instrumental variables are represented on a linear scale. The slopes of the lines fitted by eye to the data for hardness and for softness differed only slightly. However, the data for softness presented a degree of curvature not evident in the hardness data. This curvature was never fully explained. The heterogeneous nature of the samples could have been a contributory factor, but this should have affected the data for hardness and for softness in a similar way. In some real sense hardness and softness of the same samples do not represent a perfectly reciprocal relation.

Cross-Modal Studies

A series of experiments was included using cross-modal matching procedure. In separate experiments the hardness (or softness) of each sample was matched to:

1. Force of handgrip on a hand dynamometer.
2. Force exerted between finger and thumb on a finger dynamometer.
3. Loudness of a noise.

The *calculated* exponents relating to hardness (or softness) were slightly lower than those determined directly. A distortion from a simple linear relationship was again evident for softness in these cross-modal studies. This was also associated with a num-

TABLE 2

Number of zero settings in instrumental matches

System	Quality	
	Hardness	Softness
1. Handgrip	II (3) IIa (1)	30(1) 40(1) 70(5)
2. Finger Dynamometer	none	70(2)
3. Loudness	none	none

(The figures II, IIa, 30, 40 and 70 represent the individual samples as described in Table 1. The figures in brackets represent the number of ZERO settings in the corresponding instrumental match).

ber of zero settings on the matching continua in the case of the forces (1 and 2 above) but not in the case of loudness. This observation to some extent reflects certain end-effects created by the limited range of perceptual variation available, especially in the case of force of handgrip, and to a lesser extent in the forces which can be exerted between finger and thumb.

In contrast, a wide variation of loudnesses could be achieved with the equipment used. Out of thirty judgments for each condition the number of zero settings as shown in Table 2 were obtained.

Some Recent Developments

A passing reference is now made to some recent developments which might not otherwise have been noted. The evaluation of the 'viscosity' of a number of different fluid samples by Stevens and Guirao (1964) is already well-known, although the question has to be posed whether the term 'viscosity' refers here strictly to a measured property or to a perceived quality which may not necessarily be identical. More recently Wood (1968) used the method of magnitude estimation in evaluating soups of different thicknesses or consistencies and Barry & Grace (1971, 1972) examined the topical application of cosmetic creams. There is some doubt whether the rules essential in magnitude estimation have been followed precisely. Certainly in the case of Barry & Grace (1972) it would be more correct to refer to the particular example as involving a scoring technique. However, this criticism is quite a minor one. More important is the systematic development originally due to Wood but processed further by Barry and Grace and later by Shama & Sherman (1973a, b) in which the zones associated with the variable 'property' of apparent viscosity, relating to a number of different samples, are identified by matching techniques (some physical and some sensory). A rational choice was provided for a single set of physical criteria relating to such different tasks as the evaluation of viscosity by oral methods or the topical application of cosmetic creams of varying consistency.

Reference must be made to the original papers for details. However, in these and other instances, the question whether the subject should direct his attention to the evaluation of the physical properties which it is convenient to measure instrumentally, or whether it is more appropriate to find out precisely what the subject is evaluating, remains to be resolved. Although this can only be resolved by reference to further data, it raises all the familiar problems about the validity of instrumental tests and the ultimate aims involved in developing them.

Selected References

A full bibliography on the evaluation of compliant materials would contain many more items than can be included here. Reference must be made elsewhere for the missing information. For example, fairly comprehensive bibliographies are included in Harper (1952, 1972).

Anonymous. Standard test methods for rubber and rubber-like materials. *ASTM Standards*, 1958, pp. 1297–1310. Philadelphia: American Society for Testing and Materials. See also Shore Durometer. A.S.T.M. Tentative Methods D 676-47 T.

Barry, B. W., & Grace, A. J. Structural, rheological and textural properties of soft paraffins. *Journal of Texture Studies*, 1971, **2**, 259–279.

Barry, B. W., & Grace, A. J. Sensory testing of spreadability: Investigation of rheological conditions operative during application of topical preparations. *Journal of Pharmaceutical Science*, 1972, **61**, 335–341.

Harper, R. Psychological and psychophysical studies of craftsmanship in dairying. *British Journal of Psychology*, Monog. Supplement No. 28, pp. xi + 64, Cambridge University Press, 1952.

Harper, R. Factor analysis as a technique for examining complex data on foodstuffs. *Applied Statistics*, 1956, **5**, 32–48. Reprinted in Frank, R. E. *et al.* (Ed., 1963) *Quantitative techniques in marketing analysis*. Homewood, Illinois: R. D. Irwin Co.

Harper, R. Texture and consistency from the standpoint of perception. pp. 11–39 in *Rheology and texture in foodstuffs*. Monograph Series No. 27. London: Soc. Chem. Ind., 1968.

Harper, R. *Human senses in action*. London and Edinburgh: Churchill Livingstone, 1972.

Harper, R. & Baron, M. Factorial analysis of rheological measurements on cheese. *Nature* (Lond.), 1948, **162**, 821.

Harper, R. & Stevens, S. S. Subjective hardness of compliant materials. *Quarterly Journal of Experimental Psychology*, 1964, **16**, 204–215.

Katz, D. *Der Aufbau der Tastwelt*. Leipzig: Verlag von Johann Ambrosius Barth, 1925.

Katz, D. The judgments of test bakers. *Occupational Psychology*, 1938, **12**, 139–148.

Katz, D. & Stephenson, W. Experiments on elasticity. *British Journal of Psychology*, 1937, **28**, 190–194.

Kreuger, L. E. David Katz's *der Aufbau der Tastwelt* (*The world of touch*): A Synopsis. *Perception and Psychophysics*, 1970, **7**, 337–341.

Poynting, J. H. & Thompson, J. J. *A Text-book of physics: Properties of matter*. London: Charles Griffin and Co. Ltd., 1934, (13th ed.).

Scott Blair, G. W. The subjective assessment of the consistency of materials in relation to physical measurements. *Journal of the Society of Cosmetic Chemists*, 1966, **17**, 45–56.

Shama, F., Parkinson, C., & Sherman, P. Identification of stimuli controlling the sensory evaluation of viscosity. I. Non-oral methods. *Journal of Texture Studies*, 1973, **4**, 102–110. (a)

Shama, F. & Sherman, P. Identification of stimuli controlling the sensory evaluation of viscosity. II. Oral methods. *Journal of Texture Studies*, 1973, **4**, 111–118. (b)

Stevens, S. S. A scale for the measurement of a psychological magnitude: Loudness. *Psychological Review*, 1936, **43**, 405–416.

Stevens, S. S. Direct estimates of sensory magnitudes: Loudness. *American Journal of Psychology*, 1956, **69**, 1–25.

Stevens, S. S. *Notes for a life story 1906 –*. History of psychology in autobiography, 1970.

Stevens, S. S. & Guirao, M. Scaling apparent viscosity. *Science*, 1964, **144**, 1157–1158.

Szczesniak, A. S. Classification of textural characteristics. *Journal of Food Science*, 1963, **28**, 385–389.

Szczesniak, A. S. Correlations between objective and sensory texture measurements. *Food Technology*, 1968, **22**, 981–986.

Wood, F. W. Psychophysical studies on the consistency of liquid foods. pp. 40–49 in *Rheology and texture in foodstuffs*. Monograph Series No. 27. London: Soc. Chem. Ind., 1968.

RATIOS OF MAGNITUDE ESTIMATES[1]

R. DUNCAN LUCE
School of Social Science, University of California, Irvine

and

DAVID M. GREEN[2]
University of California, San Diego

Abstract. Suppose magnitude estimates on successive trials preserve the ratio of random internal representations of the corresponding signals. Then the mean response generally exhibits drift over trials; sequential dependencies usually exist in which case the mean response ratio is not a function of intensity ratio; however, a modified function is if the mean representation is a power function of intensity. Relevant loudness data are cited. The special timing representation is wrong if the sample size is just a function of the signal, but is viable if it is one of two sizes depending on the size of the intensity ratio to the preceding signal. This attention hypothesis is an analogue for intensity of the critical-band notion for frequency.

When using magnitude estimation data in an attempt to infer the underlying psychophysical function, what estimated function should we plot? As we show, the answer is rather more subtle than it first seems.

Until recently the consensus was to follow Stevens' original approach, namely, to plot some central tendency of the responses – either mean, median, geometric mean, or some mixture of these – against some physical measure (usually additive) of the signal variable. Indeed, if one collects but two observations at each signal level from each observer, little else is possible. If, however, one decides to approach magnitude estimation much like the rest of psychophysics – using well practiced observers, collecting many observations at each of many signal levels, and, perhaps, studying more of the response distribution than just its central tendency – then other options become available. In particular, response ratios are a serious possibility.

Three motives underlie the collection of large samples of response ratios. First, magnitude estimation instructions to observers have come, over the years, to be standardized in a way that (*i*) does not assign a standard response to any particular signal and (*ii*) urges them to reflect in their responses the subjective ratio of signals. If we take our own instructions seriously, then surely it is response ratios, not the responses themselves, that matter, and so perhaps we should study them. This point was made by Krantz (1972) in the context of algebraic models for cross-modality matching, by Marley (1972) in his internal state probabilistic model, and by Ward (1973) in analyzing sequential dependencies. The reason Stevens never plotted response ratios was, presumably, because in his view the central tendency of the responses is a

[1] This work was supported in part by National Science Foundation grants to the University of California, Irvine and San Diego.

[2] Present address: Department of Psychology and Social Relations, William James Hall, Harvard University, Cambridge, Massachusetts.

H. R. Moskowitz et al. (eds.), Sensation and Measurement. 99–111.

power function of signal level. The ratio of central tendencies is then the same power function of the corresponding signal ratio. Therefore, it really does not matter which function one plots, and the former is both simpler and requires fewer data. As we will see below, this argument glides over some complications in at least one quite general and moderately plausible model for the response behavior. If, indeed, we elect to study response ratios, then since N signals yield $N(N-1)/2$ unordered pairs of successive signals, we will need many more responses to each signal than we usually collect in order to maintain the same quality of the estimates. An increase in sample size of $(N-1)/2$ is needed just to estimate the mean response ratios, and unless we find a way to collapse the data over signal pairs the problem is much more severe when we wish to study the entire distribution of response ratios.

A second motive for attending to response ratios arises from one account of the existence, in both absolute judgment and magnitude estimation data, of strong sequential effects due to the preceding signal and much weaker effects due to earlier ones (Cross, 1973; Garner, 1953; Holland & Lockhead, 1968; Ward, 1972, 1973; and Ward & Lockhead, 1970, 1971). One suggestion is that they arise from the indirect effect of the observer using the preceding signal and his response to it as the standard against which to compare the present signal. We explore below one version of this hypothesis.

A third motive is an interest in the form of the distribution of response ratios. This arises from the possibility that these distributions contain useful information about the underlying representations of the signals and the decision mechanism that generates the responses. Of course, Stevens (1957, 1959, 1961a, b, 1971) held the view that variability in magnitude estimates is uninformative noise, or at best a second-order phenomenon correlated with the central tendency. As such, it is no more capable of informing us about the underlying perceptual process than the noisiness of a voltmeter is informative about either the voltage being measured or the working of the meter itself. When the variability is small, this position is probably sound; but in magnitude estimation it is not small, either between individuals or for repeated observations on the same individual. An alternative view holds that this variability reflects something basic about the perceptual process itself. If so, then we need accurate estimates of these distributions.

The Response Ratio Hypothesis

Magnitude estimation instructions seem to make sense only if the stimulus attribute causes an internal change that can be represented by a number, and these responses can be chosen so as to maintain (at least some) ratios of these representations. Further, since these responses, like those in the rest of psychophysics, are variable, it seems plausible for the representation actually to be a random variable, with some unknown probability distribution that is a function of the signal presented. To be more specific, let $\mathbf{S}_n$ be a random variable representing the signal presented on trial n – either a numbering of the signals, e.g., 1, 2,..., or a physical measure of the attribute being varied, e.g., 20, 30, 40,... dB, – and let $\mathbf{R}_n$ be the number (a random variable) emitted by the observer. Both of these RVs are observables, with the distribution of the former under the experimenter's control. In addition, we postulate the existence of an internal representation $\mathbf{X}(s)$ when signal s is presented; note that we assume $\mathbf{X}$ does not depend directly on the trial number, n.

The first hypothesis that comes to mind, the one suggested by Ward (1973), is that the observer uses his representation and response on the preceding trial as a standard against which to generate the current response from the current representation, i.e., for all trials n,

$$\mathbf{R}_n = C\mathbf{R}_{n-1}\mathbf{X}(\mathbf{S}_n)/\mathbf{X}(\mathbf{S}_{n-1}). \tag{1}$$

This model is, at best, a first approximation since by induction we see that

$$\mathbf{R}_n = C^{n-1}\mathbf{R}_1\mathbf{X}(\mathbf{S}_n)/\mathbf{X}(\mathbf{S}_1). \tag{2}$$

So, in effect, given the first representation and response, R_n is uniquely determined by the present representation, and no sequential dependencies are predicted. The data showing their existence are overwhelmingly clear.

The failure of this simplest model leads one to consider slightly more complicated alternatives. One idea is that an internal representation of a signal is destroyed when it is used to generate a response. Put another way, a representation of a signal can be stored, but once it is removed from memory to generate a response it is lost. If so and if representations from successive trials are used to generate the responses, then it is necessary to assume that, when signal s is presented, two independent representations, $\mathbf{X}(s)$ and $\mathbf{X}^*(s)$, arise. We do not assume that the distributions of $\mathbf{X}$ and $\mathbf{X}^*$ are necessarily the same. Presumably the quality of these representations is poorer in some sense than when only one is needed as, say, in detection and discrimination experiments. The fact that peripheral neural representations of visual and auditory signals are encoded on a large number of parallel fibers means that it would not be difficult for the nervous system to use one set for $\mathbf{X}$ and another for $\mathbf{X}^*$. Given these two independent representations, the *response ratio hypothesis* takes the form

$$\mathbf{R}_n = C\mathbf{R}_{n-1}\mathbf{X}(\mathbf{S}_n)/\mathbf{X}^*(\mathbf{S}_{n-1}). \tag{3}$$

This hypothesis has been studied by Marley (1973) (with $C=1$ and under strong restrictions on the distributions of $\mathbf{X}$ and $\mathbf{X}^*$) and by Luce and Green (1974). We summarize here the main conclusions of the latter paper. First, we make the following weak assumptions about the distribution functions of $\mathbf{X}$ and $\mathbf{X}^*$:

(i) $F(s)=E[\mathbf{X}^*(s)]$ exists for all signals s.

(ii) $F^*(s)=E[1/\mathbf{X}^*(s)]$ exists for all signals s.

(iii) The distribution function of $\mathbf{S}_n$ is independent of n and $B=E[F(\mathbf{S}_n)\,F^*(\mathbf{S}_n)]$ exists.

Equation 3 together with these three assumptions lead to the following four equations involving expected responses and response ratios:

$$E(\mathbf{R}_n \mid \mathbf{S}_n = s) = (CB)^{n-1}\mathbf{R}_1 F(s), \tag{4}$$

$$\frac{E(\mathbf{R}_n \mid \mathbf{S}_n = s \;\&\; \mathbf{S}_{n-1} = s')}{E(R_n \mid S_n = s)} = \frac{F(s')\, F^*(s')}{B}, \tag{5}$$

$$E\left(\frac{\mathbf{R}_n}{\mathbf{R}_{n-1}} \,\middle|\, \mathbf{S}_n = s \;\&\; \mathbf{S}_{n-1} = s'\right) = CF(s)\, F^*(s'), \tag{6}$$

$$\frac{E\left(\frac{\mathbf{R}_n}{\mathbf{R}_{n-1}} \,\middle|\, \mathbf{S}_n = s \;\&\; \mathbf{S}_{n-1} = s'\right) E(\mathbf{R}_n \mid \mathbf{S}_n = s)}{E(\mathbf{R}_n \mid \mathbf{S}_n = s \;\&\; \mathbf{S}_{n-1} = s')} = CB\,\frac{F(s)}{F(s')}. \tag{7}$$

We discuss each separately. Equation 4 is the expression for the ordinary magnitude function. It exhibits two important features. First, except when $C = 1/B$, this expectation drifts over trials. The existence of drift was shown clearly by Ward (1973) and by Green & Luce (1974) in their data, and it has been noted informally by others; its existence is one of the reasons that many experimenters are hesitant about collecting repeated responses from individual observers. One might anticipate that a well-practiced observer would learn to choose C so as to eliminate the drift, but the process is not completed even after thousands of trials. Obviously, the existence of drift in this model, and in some data, make it difficult to study the distribution of responses to a given signal since the estimated distribution is a mix of the actual distribution and the drift. Second, aside from the drift, the magnitude function is proportional to the mean, $F(s)$, of the $\mathbf{X}(s)$ representation.

Equation 5 is a convenient form in which to study sequential effects. We see that they exist if and only if $F(s)\, F^*(s)$ depends on s; moreover they are assimilative – the response on trial n tends toward the signal on trial $n-$ as in the data (see Figure 1 below) if and only if $F(s)\, F^*(s)$ is an increasing function of s.

Equation 6 is the natural response ratio to study. A desirable feature of this function is that it exhibits no drift; an undesirable one is that the right side depends on two different functions of s and s'. The only case in which they would be the same is if $F^*(s') = D/F(s')$; however, this is equivalent to there being no sequential dependencies, which appears to be empirically false (see the data in the next section, but also the interpretation in the following one).

We would prefer to study a function in which $F(s)/F(s')$ appeared on the right, which is the reason for the peculiar function in Equation 7. Note that to the extent that F is a power function of signal intensity, Equation 7 depends only on the ratio of signal intensities, not on their individual values.

In the context of ratio estimation, Equation 6 has received some attention. Writing $\mathbf{R}(s, s')$ for the ratio judgment when s and s' are presented, the analogue to Equation 1 seems appropriate,

$$\mathbf{R}(s, s') = C\mathbf{X}(s)/\mathbf{X}(s'),$$

also

$$E[R(s, s')] = CF(s)/f^*(s'),$$

where

$$f^*(s') = 1/F^*(s').$$

Comrey (1950) (see Torgerson, 1958, pp. 104–112) suggest the special case $C=1$ and $f^*=F$. Sjöberg (1962), using data from three papers, compared this with $C\neq 1$ and $f^*=F$ and with the general result. He found the first two cases inadequate, as we would expect if there are sequential dependencies. These ideas, along with statistical procedures and further data, are reported in Sjöberg (1971). Svenson and Åkesson (1966a, b; 1967) studied empirically the function

$$E[R(s, s')]\, E[R(s', s)] = C^2 \frac{F(s)\, f^*(s)}{F(s')\, f^*(s')}.$$

Some Data

According to Equation 5, a good way to estimate $F(s')\, F^*(s')$, and so to study sequential effects, is to average $E(\mathbf{R}_n \mid \mathbf{S}_n = s \;\&\; \mathbf{S}_{n-1} = s')/E(\mathbf{R}_n \mid \mathbf{S}_n = s)$ over s. These functions for the data reported by Cross (1973) and Ward (1973), both averaged over observers, and for the six observers studied by Green & Luce (1974) are shown in Figure 1. In each case, the sequential effect is assimilative.

The six observers of Green & Luce and the group data of Cross are all remarkably similar, with relatively slight sequential effects. Ward's group data exhibit a much more pronounced effect.

The model Cross fitted to his data is, in essence, ours with

$$F(s) \sim I(s)^{\beta - b}$$
$$F^*(s) \sim I(s)^{2b-\beta}$$

and so

$$F(s)\, F^*(s) \sim I(s)^b,$$

which means the plotted functions should be straight lines with slope b. In his case $\hat{b}=0.027$; the other estimated slopes are given in the figure caption. Whether the data are best described by power functions is obscure; they do not give a bad fit, but many other functions would be at least equally good.

Since in our data FF^* is nearly a constant, it should not matter greatly whether we plot Equation 6 or 7. They, together with the ordinary magnitude function, all normalized to agree at the left-most point, are shown in Figure 2, and as we anticipated there is little difference between the ratio functions. Note, however, that for observers 2, 4, and 5 the ratio functions differ by as much as 10 dB from the magnitude functions and are considerably closer to power functions. We do not know if this is due to drift or something else.

As we noted earlier, to the extent that these functions appear to be power functions, the quantity of Equation 7 should depend only on the signal ratio, not the individual values. Let $H(s; d)$ denote the left side of Equation 7, where $d=I(s)/I(s')$, and let

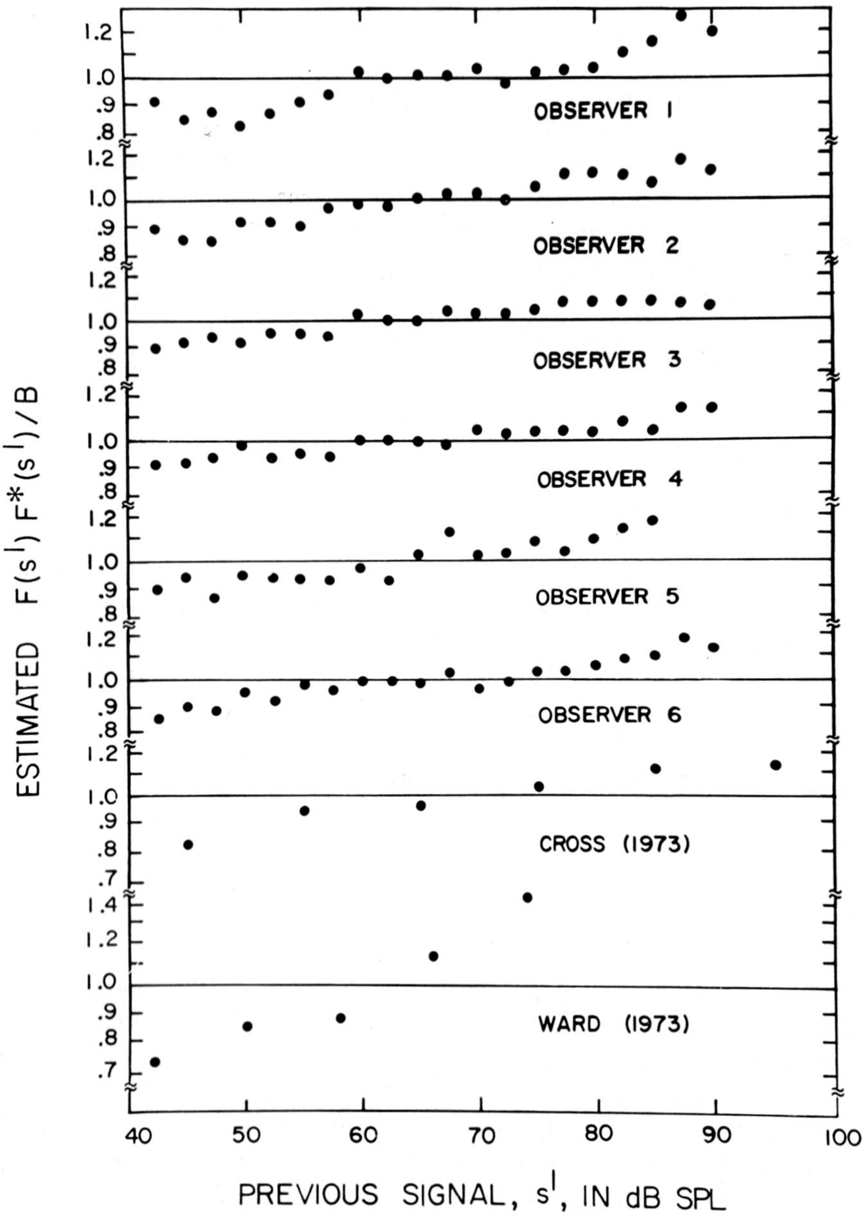

Fig. 1. Estimates of $F(s')\,F^*(s')/B$ using Equation 6 from group data reported by Cross (1973) and Ward (1973) and from individual data reported by Green & Luce (1974). Reading from top to bottom, the exponents of power functions to fit these data are: 0.030, 0.028, 0.019, 0.019, 0.027, 0.022, 0.028, and 0.088. (This is Figure 1 of Luce & Green, 1974.)

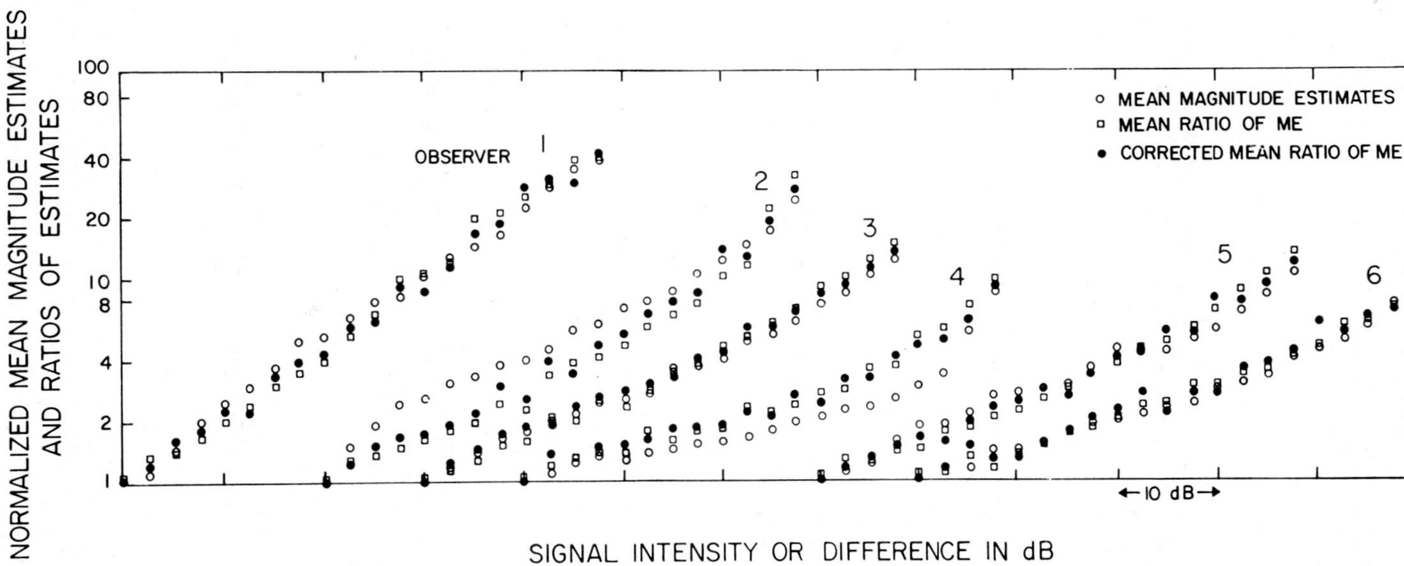

Fig. 2. Plots of mean magnitude estimates, mean ratio of successive magnitude estimates, corrected (Equation 7) mean ratio of successive magnitude estimates versus signal intensity in dB. The first is normalized to be 1 at the lowest signal, 42.6 dB SPL, and the latter two to be 1 at the smallest signal difference, 0 dB. (This is Figure 3 of Luce & Green, 1974.)

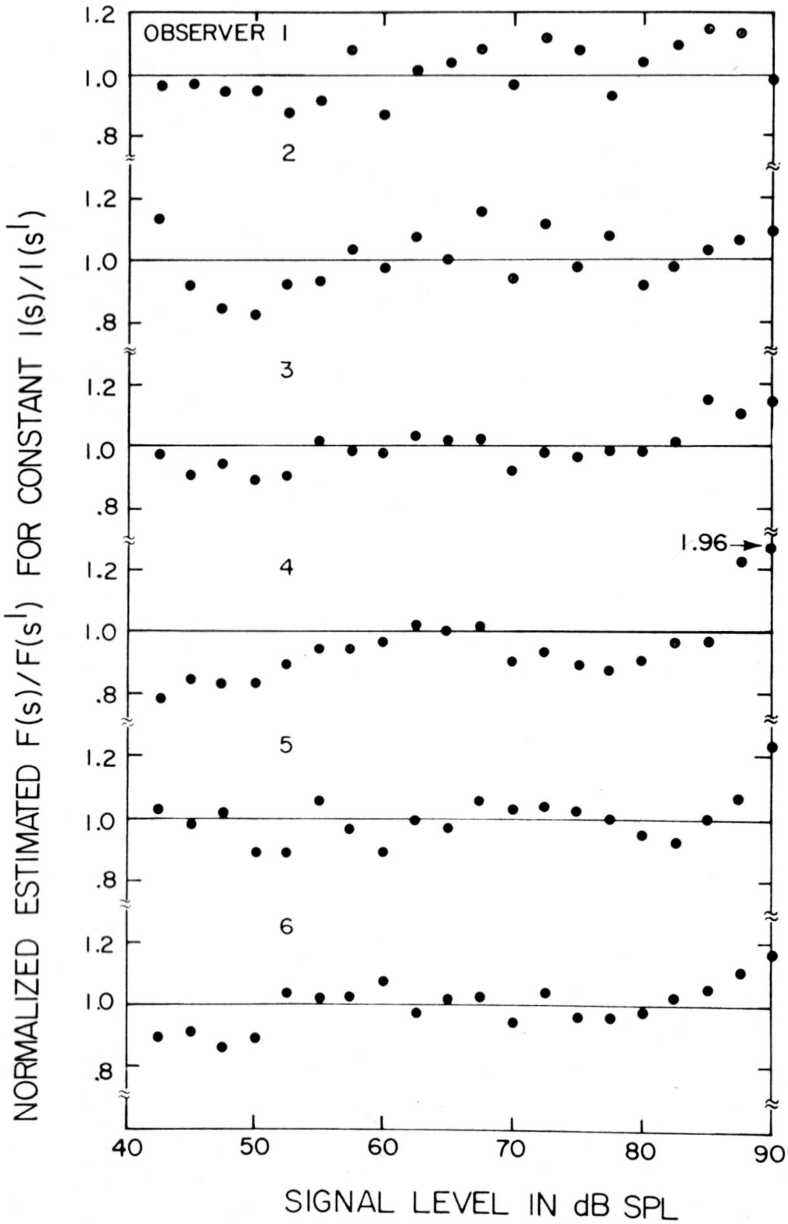

Fig. 3. Estimates of $(1/m)\Sigma_d[H(s; d)/H(\cdot; d)]$ versus $I(s)$. According to Equation 7, this function should be 1 if $F(s)$ is a power function of $I(s)$. (This is Figure 2 of Luce & Green, 1974.)

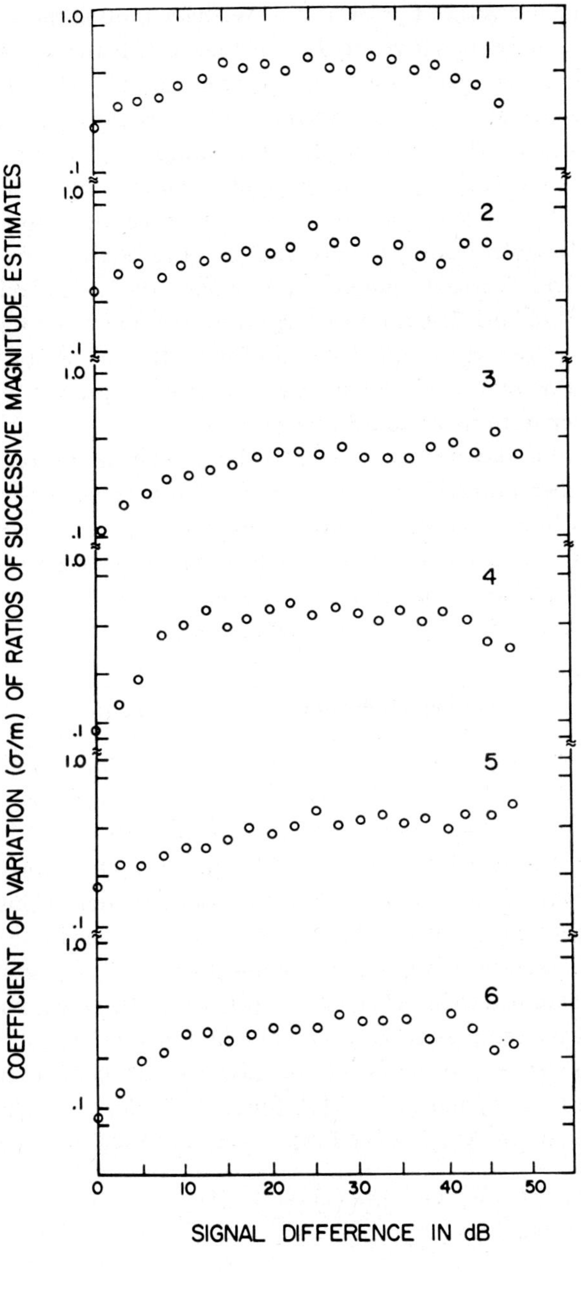

Fig. 4. Coefficient of variation (standard deviation/mean) of response ratio on successive trials as a function of signal ratio (in dB) on those trials. (Adapted from Figure 5 of Green & Luce, 1974.)

$H(\cdot\,; d)$ denote the average of this over all s. We have plotted the average of $H(s; d)/H(\cdot\,; d)$ over all signal ratios d versus $I(s)$ in Figure 3. If the model is correct and F is a power function, then this function should be equal to 1. Although there is a slight tendency for it to increase with $I(s)$ over most of the range and a distinct increase at the most intense signal, which may be due to deviations of F from a power function, to a good first approximation, $H(s; d)$ depends on d and not on s.

Even for our well-practiced observers, there is evidence that response drift occurred, and so it seems advisable to study the distribution of response ratios rather than of the responses themselves. Various studies (Luce & Mo, 1963; Schneider & Lane, 1963) indicate that the standard deviation of magnitude estimates is roughly proportional to the mean, so we elected to plot that ratio for $\mathbf{R}_n/\mathbf{R}_{n-1}$ as a function of $I(s)/I(s')$. This is shown in Figure 4. It is evident that σ/m grows rapidly at first and tapers off to a constant at separations of 20 dB and more.

In some cases, σ/m may decrease again for large intensity ratios. Inspection of the distribution, together with the anomaly in Figure 3 for the 90 dB signal, suggests that the observers may have absolutely identified this extreme case. In contrast, we suspect that the very small variability in the ratio when the signals are close is an important result. In particular, as we discuss in Green & Luce (1974), it may relate to some of the perplexing range effects in absolute identification experiments.

Timing Model and Selective Attention

Luce & Green (1972) proposed a timing model of the following character. When signal s is presented, it activates on each of J channels (not necessarily neural fibers, but some abstraction from them) independent Poisson processes of common intensity $\mu(s)$. The intensity function is assumed to be an increasing function of signal intensity $I(s)$ and, indeed, various data suggest that it is approximately a power function of I. Whenever the observer is to answer a question about $I(s)$, he is assumed to take some sample of these Poisson processes from which he estimates $\mu(s)$. In the timing model, the sample size is assumed to be, $k(s)=J(s)\,\kappa(s)$, where $J(s)$ is the number of channels excited and $\kappa(s)$ is the sample size from an individual channel. The sum $\mathbf{T}$ over channels of the times from the first to the $(\kappa+1)$ st pulse on each channel has a gamma distribution of intensity $\mu(s)$ and order $k(s)$. Since the mean is $k(s)/\mu(s)$, this suggests using the representation $\mathbf{X}(s)=k(s)/\mathbf{T}(s)$. Assuming that, it is easy to show that

$$F(s) = \mu(s)\,k(s)/(k(s)-1)$$
$$F^*(s) = 1/\mu(s),$$

and so

$$F(s)\,F^*(s) = k(s)/(k(s)-1).$$

This implies that if the sample size $k(s)$ is a constant, then the timing model exhibits no sequential dependencies. (Essentially the same result is true for the counting model; see Luce & Green, 1974.)

It is also not difficult to show that the ratio of two such RVs, one with sample size k and the other with k^*, and therefore the ratio of responses on successive trials, is distributed according to the Beta distribution of the second kind with parameters k and k^*. From this it is almost immediate that

$$\left(\frac{\sigma}{m}\right)^2 = \frac{k + k^* - 1}{k^*(k-2)},$$

which means that if the sample sizes are constant, then σ/m is a constant for the timing model.

Both of these statements are clearly contradicted by the data, and so either the timing model is wrong or the sample sizes are not constant. If they are not constant, it is evident that no simple postulate involving a change just with signal intensity is adequate to account for both of these functions. Some rather more subtle idea is needed.

One that appears to account sensibly for these data is the existence of a selective attention mechanism that is the intensity analogue of critical-frequency bands. Specifically, let us suppose that in terms of pulse rates of Poisson processes, there is a band of fixed width in which most attention can be focused in the sense of collecting a large sample, and for all rates outside that band, a considerably smaller sample is collected. For simplicity, we assume $k(s) = k^*(s)$ in both cases, and that the two sample sizes are K and K_0, where $K_0 < K$. Second, we assume that the observer is free to center the band where he wishes in advance of the signal presentation; for this experiment, in particular, he is assumed to center it around the estimated rate of the preceding signal.

Consider first the $F(s)\,F^*(s)$ function. For any pair of trials it is either equal to $K/(K-1)$ or $K_0/(K_0-1)$, where the former is smaller than the latter. Which value it has depends on whether or not the preceding signal, s', was in the region of greater attention. We argue that this is more probable for low intensities than for high, and hence FF^* should grow with intensity The reason is that the band is of constant width in pulse rate, which in turn is roughly a power function of signal intensity; hence, the band width in dB decreases with intensity.[3] Since the signals were equally probable and equally spaced in dB, it follows that it is somewhat more likely for a weak than for a strong signal to lie in the attention span of a randomly presented signal.

Second, consider the σ/m function. Let $P(s')$ denote the probability that the preceding signal s' lay in the region of greater attention. If the current signal, s, is close to s', then with high probability it will lie in the region of greater attention and so the estimated $(\sigma/m)^2$ is simply a probability mix of two terms:

$$P(s')\,\frac{2K-1}{K(K-2)} + [1 - P(s')]\,\frac{K + K_0 - 1}{K_0(K-2)}.$$

[3] To be more formal, suppose the upper and lower intensities of the band of greater attention are I_u and I_l, that $\mu = \alpha I^\beta$, and $\mu_u = \mu_l + \theta$ where θ is a constant. Then,

$$\log I_u/I_l = (1/\beta)\log(1 + \theta/\mu_l)\,.$$

If, for example, $\alpha = 0.1$, $\beta = 0.3$, and $\theta = 50$, the ratio of bandwidths in dB at $I_l = 10^3$ and $I_l = 10^8$ is 3.8.

On the other hand, if the current signal lies sufficiently far from s' so that it is outside the region of greater attention, the estimated (σ/m^2) is the mix:

$$P(s')\frac{K+K_0-1}{K(K_0-2)}+[1-P(s')]\frac{2K_0-1}{K_0(K_0-2)}.$$

It is easy to see that for all $P(s')$ the latter expression is greater than the former. Were the band to be rigidly centered on the true rate of the preceding signal, then for any fixed value of s' there would be a discontinuous shift in σ/m at the boundary of the band. Since, however, the centering is assumed to be on the estimated rate of the preceding signal, which is variable, the transition is smoothed. In addition, the band width in dB varies with s', which also smooths the observed transition.

Third, consider the expected ratio of responses which, by Equation 6, is proportional to

$$F(s)\,F^*(s')=\frac{\mu(s)}{\mu(s')}\left[\frac{k(s)}{k(s)-1}\right].$$

Thus, the factor multiplying $\mu(s)/\mu(s')$ is less when s is near s' than when they are widely separated. This means that if μ actually is a power function of intensity, then the attention model implies that the observed curve in log-log coordinates should be concave up, not a straight line; this appears to be the case (see Figure 2).

Discussion

Let us make explicit where our path has led us. We began with a very simple response ratio hypothesis, embodied in Equation 3, and its predictions, formulated as Equations 4–7. Looking at the data as suggested by this model uncovered evidence of weak sequential effects and of a marked reduction in the variability of the response ratio when the separation between successive signals is small (<20 dB). Other work led us to examine a special case of the response ratio hypothesis suggested by the neural timing model. Neither the version with a constant sample size nor one with a sample size that depends just on the signal presented were consistent with these two empirical functions. For this model to hold, the sample size must depend on both the present and preceding signal. We suggested a two-state attention model in which a large sample is taken if the present signal lies within a band centered about the estimated rate of the preceding one and a smaller one is taken otherwise. This seemed adequate to explain these data. Experiments need to be designed to study this hypothesis more directly.

It is important to realize that if this line of argument is correct, then the nature of the sequential dependencies rests on the relation between the spacing of signals and that of the attention band. It is assimilative when the signals are equally spaced in dB because the band in dB narrows as intensity is increased. Were we to space the signals so that their density increases sufficiently with intensity, this model predicts an ultimate reversal in the nature of the dependencies.

To generalize the attention-timing model, one must reformulate the response ratio hypothesis. In particular, a pair of *RV*s $\mathbf{X}(s)$, $\mathbf{X}^*(s)$ is observed when s is close to s'

and another pair $\mathbf{X}_0(s)$, $\mathbf{X}_0^*(s)$ when s is far from s'. This means that $\mathbf{R}_n/\mathbf{R}_{n-1}$ is one of four possible ratios. The timing model has the special simplifying feature that $E(1/\mathbf{X}^*)=E(1/\mathbf{X}_0^*)$. This general model has not yet been studied.

Bibliography

Comrey, A. L. A proposed method for absolute ratio scaling. *Psychometrika*, 1950, **15**, 317–325.

Cross, D. V. Sequential dependencies and regression in psychophysical judgments. *Perception and Psychophysics*, 1973, **14**, 547–552.

Garner, W. R. An informational analysis of absolute judgments of loudness. *Journal of Experimental Psychology*, 1953, **46**, 373–380.

Green, D. M., & Luce, R. D. Variability of magnitude estimates: A timing theory analysis. *Perception and Psychophysics*, 1974, in press.

Holland, M. K., & Lockhead, G. R. Sequential effects in absolute judgments of loudness. *Perception and Psychophysics*, 1968, **3**, 409–414.

Krantz, D. H. A theory of magnitude estimation and cross-modality matching. *Journal of Mathematical Psychology*, 1972, **9**, 168–199.

Luce, R. D., & Green, D. M. A neural timing theory for response times and the psychophysics of intensity. *Psychological Review*, 1972, **79**, 14–57.

Luce, R. D., & Green, D. M. The response ratio hypothesis for magnitude estimation. *Journal of Mathematical Psychology*, 1974, **11**, 1–14.

Luce, R. D., & Mo, S. S. Magnitude estimation of heaviness and loudness by individual subjects: A test of a probabilistic response theory. *British Journal of Mathematical and Statistical Psychology*, 1965, **18**, 159–174.

Marley, A. A. T. Internal state models for magnitude estimation and related experiments. *Journal of Mathematical Psychology*, 1972, **9**, 306–319.

Schneider, B., & Lane, H. Ratio scales, category scales, and variability in the production of loudness and softness. *Journal of the Acoustical Society of America*, 1963, **35**, 1953–1961.

Sjöberg, L. On ratio estimation. Report 191. Psychological Laboratory, University of Stockholm, 1962.

Sjöberg, L. Three models for the analysis of subjective ratios. *The Scandinavian Journal of Psychology*, 1971, **12**, 217–240.

Stevens, S. S. On the psychophysical law. *Psychological Review*, 1957, **64**, 153–181.

Stevens, S. S. On the validity of the loudness scale. *Journal of the Acoustical Society of America*, 1959, **31**, 995–1003.

Stevens, S. S. Toward a resolution of the Fechner-Thurstone legacy. *Psychometrika*, 1961, **26**, 35–47. (a)

Stevens, S. S. To honor Fechner and repeal his law. *Science*, 1961, **133**, 80–86. (b)

Stevens, S. S. Issues in psychophysical measurement. *Psychological Review*, 1971, **78**, 426–450.

Svenson, O., & Åkesson, C. Å. Fractional and multiple estimates in ratio scaling. Report 202. *Psychological Laboratory*, University of Stockholm, 1966. (a)

Svenson, O., & Åkesson, C. Å. On a relation between fractional and multiple estimates in ratio scaling. Report 220. Psychological Laboratory, University of Stockholm, 1966. (b)

Svenson, O., & Åkesson, C. Å. A further note on fractional and multiple estimates in ratio scaling. Report 224. Psychological Laboratory, University of Stockholm, 1967.

Torgerson, W. S. *Theory and methods of scaling*. New York: Wiley, 1958.

Ward, L. M. Category judgments of loudness in the absence of an experimental-induced identification function: Sequential effects and power functions fit. *Journal of Experimental Psychology*, 1972, **94**, 179–187.

Ward, L. M. Repeated magnitude estimations with a variable standard: Sequential effects and other properties. *Perception and Psychophysics*, 1973, **13**, 193–200.

Ward, L. M. & Lockhead, G. R. Sequential effects and memory in category judgments. *Journal of Experimental Psychology*, 1970, **84**, 27–34.

Ward, L. M. & Lockhead, G. R. Response system processes in absolute judgment. *Perception and Psychophysics*, 1971, **9**, 73–78.

MEASUREMENT, INVARIANCE, AND PSYCHOPHYSICS

RICHARD J. W. MANSFIELD
Harvard University

Abstract. In psychophysics, invariant relations can be grouped into three broad classes: (*i*) invariances in the measurement process, (*ii*) invariances of functional capacity, and (*iii*) invariances in the neural events that code information. An analysis is given of selected examples in each category. In psychophysical measurement, for every scale type there is a characteristic distribution of observations. For example, observers' estimates in direct scaling procedures usually follow lognormal distributions that are typical of ratio-scale variables. In the description of sensory function, ratio scales of sensory magnitude can be related to other behavioral measures that are independent of the matching operation. Over a wide range of conditions, perceived brightness, for instance, can be described by simple power functions with rational exponents similar to those describing visual latency, and temporal and spatial summation. In the analysis of neural mechanisms, a parametric comparison of behavioral and neurelectric measures can often suggest candidate codes. For the visual system such a comparison points to a frequency code of retinal origin for perceived brightness.

The central concern of psychophysics is to determine the invariances that govern the behavior of organisms in their interaction with an environment of impinging energetic stimuli. The sought-for invariances are schemapiric by nature, capable of a stern mathematical perfection, yet reflect empirical laws. The ultimate goal is to relate these quantitative invariances both to the organism's functional capacities and to the mechanisms of its behavior.

Three critical issues have emerged in the search for invariances. First, can an observer's responses to stimuli exhibit a degree of invariance comparable to that of physical measurement? Second, is there an invariant form and structure to the relation between sensory magnitude and physical intensity? Third, how are behavioral measures of sensory function related to neural events? In the last twenty years, the first two issues have been pushed to the point of resolution, but the third constitutes a continuing challenge. The rich complexity of both brain and behavior has left the matter unresolved. The study of these issues, as the present brief essay will outline, has and will continue to illuminate new invariances in the measurement of behavioral systems, in the descriptive psychophysics of sensory function, and in the analysis of information processing in the nervous system.

Scale-Type Invariance and Measurement Distributions

The concept of invariance inherent in the hierarchy of scale types was proposed by Stevens (1946) to counter the notion of Helmholtz and Campbell then prevalent that fundamental measurement depended upon an operation of additivity. From that perspective "sensation was not and could not be measured unless and until additivity could be demonstrated." Stevens' insight was that the particular operation of additivity was irrelevant to physical or what we now term ratio-scale measurement. Rather, the

H. R. Moskowitz et al. (eds.), Sensation and Measurement. 113–128.

important criterion was the degree of invariance obtained in the measurement process. For ratio variables the measurement values obtained by different operations differ by at most a multiplicative constant; to each of the other three basic scale types – interval, ordinal, and nominal – there corresponds a similar defining restriction on the permissible measurement values. From ratio to nominal scale measurement, the degree of invariance that measured values incorporate decreases progressively in a simple hierarchical fashion so that for measurements on a nominal scale the assignment of numbers to objects merely serves the function of identification.

In the more than quarter of a century since its introduction, the seminal concept of invariance has fostered the development of more formal descriptions and models of the measurement process and has created a lively debate concerning the appropriateness of various statistics for different scales of measurement. The basic problem remains that of assessing for a particular system the degree of invariance produced by a measurement process. Since measurement involves both the application of certain operations and the reactions of the system observed, there are at least two approaches to the problem of assessing invariance. The direct approach which has been employed with considerable success is to vary the operational parameters and determine if the measurements retain the invariances appropriate to a given measurement scale. For magnitude estimation, modifications of the wording of the instructions, use of different number assignments to the standard stimulus, different locations of the standard or even the absence of a standard, and variations in the number and spacing of the stimuli all to a first approximation leave the estimates invariant except for a multiplicative factor (Stevens & Galanter, 1957; J. C. Stevens, 1958). However, the question of when all relevant operational parameters have been tried poses a difficult problem. Alternatively, a second approach is to repeat the same operation and examine the fluctuations in the system's response for signs of invariance.

Figure 1 presents six examples of cumulative distributions obtained by repeated measurements in different psychophysical, biological, and physical systems. The data plotted on logarithmic probability paper tend to follow straight lines, indicating that the distributions are approximately log-normal. Skewed distributions such as those shown in Figure 1 are frequently encountered in psychophysical measurements (Stevens, 1955) but are even more frequent in biological and physical data (Aitchison & Brown, 1957). The distributions are typical examples for the measured variables. For instance, the dendritic domains of seven classes of retinal neurons in one or more of five species including monkey, pigeon, and cat (Moreland, 1969) form lognormal distributions. In the business centers of cities such as Tokyo or New York during the day-time or in quiet residential areas, environmental noise exhibits a Gaussian distribution in decibels and hence a lognormal distribution in terms of sound pressure level (Price, 1972). When a light pulse from a laser beam passes through a turbulent medium such as the atmosphere, the irradiances of the scintillation pattern are distributed in a lognormal fashion rather than a Rayleigh distribution as theoretically expected (Mitchell, 1968; Minott, 1972; Bluemel, Norducci, & Tuft, 1972; Kerr & Dunphy, 1973).

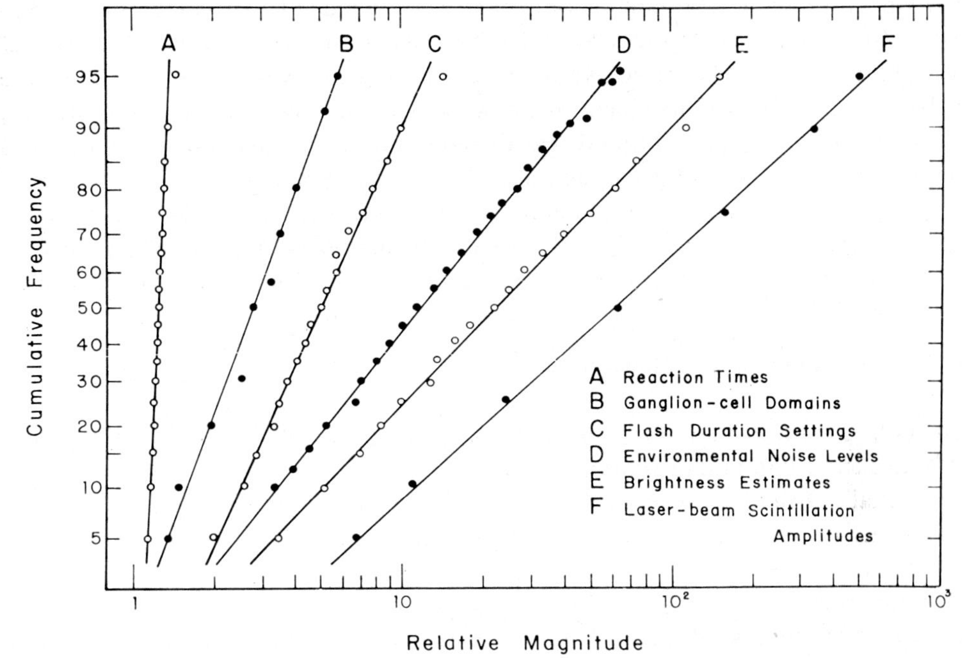

Fig. 1. Distribution functions for measurements in various systems. The straight lines represent lognormal distributions.

The first common feature of these diverse data is the form of the cumulative distributions. In every case the lognormal distribution is an excellent approximation to the data. For an appropriate choice of the parameter, μ and σ, the probability density function

$$p(x) = \frac{1}{x\sqrt{2\pi}\,\sigma}\, e^{-(\log x - \mu)^2/2\sigma^2} \tag{1}$$

describes each of the straight lines. The slope of the line is reciprocally related to σ, and the median, which depends only on μ, is given by e^{μ}. The lognormal distribution has the property that the geometric mean is equal to the median, and for samples the geometric mean is the minimum-variance, unbiased estimator of the median. The coefficient of variation, $(e^{\sigma^2}-1)^{1/2}$, is the ratio of the mean, $e^{\mu+\sigma^2/2}$, and standard deviation, $(e^{\sigma^2}-1)^{1/2}e^{\mu+\sigma^2/2}$. In simply physical systems where fluctuations are small so that σ is small compared to μ, the distribution becomes symmetric and approximates a normal distribution with a mean of e^{μ} and standard deviation of e^{μ}. However, for both simple and complex systems, the coefficient of variation is independent of a measure of central tendency such as the median or geometric mean. One depends upon σ; the other upon μ. When μ varies independently of σ, as often occurs, the resulting constancy of the coefficient of variation with location is expressed by saying that "the relative error remains constant." For instance, Moreland (1969) found that the coefficient of variation for distributions of dendritic spread was constant across classes of neurons and also across species. In psychophysical tasks involving direct scaling, the constancy for observers' judgments is known as Ekman's law (Ekman, 1956; Stevens, 1966). Teghtsoonian (1971) found that the constant in Ekman's law was about 0.03 across nine different perceptual continua. Translated into stimulus terms, the result is Weber's law, the first law in psychology worthy of the term. Perhaps the most interesting characterization of the lognormal distribution is in terms of its entropy.

The entropy for a distribution with probability density function $p(x)$ is defined by the expression

$$\xi(x) = \int p(x) \log p(x) \, \mathrm{d}x . \tag{2}$$

The lognormal distribution has the maximum entropy of all distributions on a semi-infinite metric continuum $(0, \infty)$ for given mean and variance. Conversely, for a lognormal distribution and constant coefficient of variation, the variable must possess ratio-scale invariance. In other words, the lognormal distribution is characteristic of ratio variables.

In confirmation of this observation, it is important to note that the second common feature of the data shown in Figure 1 is that the distributions correspond to ratio variables. The operations shown in Table 1 for measuring duration, length, sound

TABLE 1

Measurement distributions

	Variable	Measurement operation	Number of observations	Reference
A.	Visual latency	Simple reaction time	200	Mansfield (1973b)
B.	Ganglion cell-domains	Length of tangential spread of dendritic tree in Golgi-stained chimpanzee and macaque retinae	25	Moreland (1969) based on Polyak (1941)
C.	Locus of peak brightness	Method of adjustment with magnitude maximization	100	Mansfield (1973a)
D.	Noise level	Meter reading of sound pressure level for residential section at night	20000 [a]	Price (1972)
E.	Brightness	Direct scaling with magnitude estimation	250	Mansfield (1973a)
F.	Light intensity	Meter reading of irradiance with wide aperture target for laser beam in turbulent atmosphere	100 [a]	Kerr & Dunphy (1973)

[a] Estimated.

pressure, and irradiance are clearly sufficient to generate ratio scales for four of the six variables. The ratio invariance of the measurements of flash duration corresponding to maximum brightness for a fixed luminance depends first upon the existence of a maximum (the well-known Broca-Sulzer effect) and secondly upon the existence of an ordinal scale for observer's judgments of brightness (a weak invariance that is commonly accepted). Magnitude estimates of brightness, it can be argued on independent grounds (Mansfield, 1970), can attain ratio scale invariance but for other applications of direct scaling procedures, the criterion of a lognormal distribution may prove a useful guide.

TABLE 2

Characteristic distributions of measurement scales

Scale type	Invariance property	Characteristic distribution
Ratio scale	Invariant up to a multiplicative transformation	Lognormal
Interval scale	Invariant up to a linear transformation	Normal
Ordinal scale	Invariant up to a monotonic transformation	Binomial
Nominal scale	Invariant up to an isotonic transformation	Uniform

Table 2 presents the results of applying the characteristic of maximum entropy to other scale types. The characteristic distribution for interval variables (such as IQ scores or pitch intervals) is the normal or Gaussian distribution. For discrete ordinal variables, a binomial distribution is characteristic; and for nominal variables, the characteristic distribution is a uniform one. For the four basic types of scales, the lognormal distribution is associated only with ratio variables. Ratio variables can be distinguished from logarithmic interval variables by the fact that the coefficient of variation for a lognormal distribution is constant under multiplicative transformations but not constant under power-group transformations. Departures from these characteristic distributions would indicate either intermediate degrees of invariance or further structure in the data, for example periodicities. The brief outline suggests that in addition to the variation of operational parameters, the measured degree of invariance can be assessed by inspection of the distribution functions of the observed system's output.

Invariance Properties of Power-Function Exponents

Stevens' power law describes the major regularity observed in the direct scaling of sensory magnitude on prothetic continua: sensory magnitude varies as a power function of stimulus intensity. Literally hundreds of experiments on more than 40 perceptual continua have shown that sensory magnitude, ψ, is related to stimulus intensity, ϕ, by an equation of the form

$$\psi = k\phi^{\beta}, \tag{3}$$

where k is a constant of proportionality that depends upon the choice of units and β is the power-function exponent. In a review of scaling procedures, Ekman & Sjöberg (1965) commented: "As an experimental fact, the power law is established beyond all reasonable doubt, possibly more firmly established than anything else in psychology." From a preliminary announcement two decades ago (Stevens, 1953), the psychophysical power law has become an accepted empirical fact. The invariance of the power-function form of the psychophysical law prompts the further question: How characteristic are the power-function exponents?

The question of the invariance of the exponent has immediate practical import to all who desire precision in the measurement of human sensory responses, but it also raises important theoretical issues concerning the nature of the measurement involved. If the power-function form is preserved but the exponent values depend upon procedural parameters, then measures of sensory magnitude are invariant only up to a power-group transformation. Since the power-group is the defining group of the logarithmic interval scale, the conclusion follows that measurement of sensory magnitude has fallen short of ratio-scale invariance. Variations of power-function exponents with parameters of the measurement operation have been frequently noted. Stevens & Greenbaum (1966) have pointed out that for a number of sensory continua the two main methods for determining sensory magnitude functions, magnitude estimation and magnitude production, do not yield equivalent results. Subjects tend to shorten the range of their adjustments on whichever variable is under their control, resulting in a regression toward the mean magnitude; hence, the term regression effect. Cross (1973) has shown how sequential response dependencies with different orders of stimuli can modify the exponent obtained in magnitude-estimation tasks. In examining the question of invariance of the psychophysical exponent for a given continuum, Poulton (1968, p. 5) concluded that direct scaling procedures were ill-designed because "experimenters did not compensate for the effects of the different physical ranges...." In his view the exponents are simply artifacts of the stimulus ranges. Indeed, Teghtsoonian (1971) found a correlation of -0.94 between stimulus range in a given experiment and the exponent obtained. Is there but one range for a given continuum that yields the appropriate exponent? If so, the invariance in the data would be fragile rather than robust.

One approach to the problem of exponent invariance is to make these context dependencies explicit. According to Luce & Galanter (1963, p. 283), only then can one ask "... under what conditions is it reasonable to view the magnitude scale as a satisfactory estimate of the underlying invariant psychophysical scale?" Poulton (1968) considers the task a formidable methodological challenge; Stevens (1971, p. 426) has given some examples of how these "sources of deviation and perturbation" could be counterbalanced and their effects assessed. In many instances a more direct approach can be taken. The reality of a construct, as Quine observed, depends upon the number of independent operations that can be used to define it. If the power law describes a basic sensory response, then it should be possible to relate the results of direct scaling procedures to other measures of sensory response that are independent of the matching

TABLE 3

Exponents of the power functions for brightness, latency, and temporal integration.[a]

Stimulus parameters			Transient brightness exponent $[\psi = kE^{\alpha}]$ α	Steady-state brightness exponent $[\psi = kI^{\beta}]$ β	Flash duration exponent $[\tau = kI^{\gamma}]$ γ	Latency exponent $[L - L_{\infty} = kI^{\delta}]$ δ
Retinal Locus	Target size	Spectral composition				
fovea	0.05°	white	0.94 ± 0.1	0.52 ± 0.02	-0.48 ± 0.01	-0.49 ± 0.02
fovea	0.72°	white	0.50 ± 0.03	0.33 ± 0.01	-0.32 ± 0.02	-0.33 ± 0.01
fovea	2°	white	0.50 ± 0.03	0.34 ± 0.02	-0.32 ± 0.02	-0.31 ± 0.01
fovea	4°	white	0.53 ± 0.03	0.34 ± 0.02	-0.29 ± 0.03	-0.32 ± 0.01
fovea	1.5°	480 nm	0.51 ± 0.02	0.33 ± 0.03	-0.30 ± 0.03	-0.33 ± 0.02
fovea	1.5°	498 nm	0.50 ± 0.03	0.34 ± 0.03	-0.30 ± 0.03	-0.33 ± 0.01
fovea	1.5°	575 nm	0.52 ± 0.02	0.33 ± 0.01	-0.32 ± 0.04	-0.31 ± 0.01
20° temporal	2°	white	0.48 ± 0.03	0.32 ± 0.03	-0.30 ± 0.04	-0.31 ± 0.01

[a] Each value is the least-squares estimate of the exponent $\pm$ the standard error.

operation. For perceived brightness, the approach is particularly successful and yields some surprising dividends.

For a representative set of stimulus conditions involving luminous targets of varying size, location, spectral composition, brightness functions were determined for groups of ten or more dark-adapted observers under conditions that minimized the effects of most of the procedural biases such as sequential order and range effects (Mansfield, 1973a). In addition, two other independent measures of visual function, latency and an index of temporal integration (the location of the Broca-Sulzer peak) were determined as functions of luminance for the same set of eight representative conditions (Mansfield, 1970; 1973a; 1973b). The data for all three measures were well-fit by power functions. For the eight conditions, Table 3 displays the power-function exponents for four relations (*i*) brightness as a function of luminous energy in the Bloch region; (*ii*) brightness as a function of luminance in the steady-state region; (*iii*) flash duration corresponding to maximum brightness as a function of luminance; (*iv*) latency of response in a simple reaction time task as a function of luminance. The striking feature of the power functions is the regularity of their exponents. The precise values closely approximate simple fractions: 1, $\frac{1}{2}$, $\frac{1}{3}$, $-\frac{1}{2}$, $-\frac{1}{3}$.

The simple invariances disclosed in Table 3 together with the results of other studies can be summarized in schematic form as a map of the determinants of brightness and latency. Target area, flash duration, and luminance are the essential parameters so the map shown in Figure 2 can be drawn as a plane through the parameter space for a

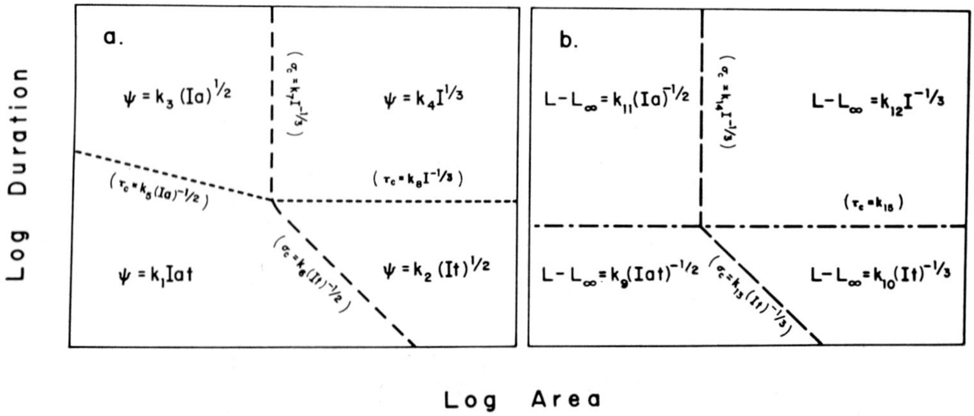

Fig. 2. Schematic representation of the determinants of perceived brightness and visual latency. (a) Brightness. The distinction between brief- and long-flash brightness and between point sources and extended sources led to four distinct regions of brightness, each with a specific function: the boundaries of the regions can be specified in terms of space and time constants that are reciprocally related to the brightness of the adjoining region. (From Mansfield, 1973a.) (b) Latency. The distinction between latency for brief- and long-flashes and that for point sources and extended sources led to four distinct regions of latency, each with a specific function. The time constant, τ_c, for latency is approximately 10 msec and is independent of target size and luminance level. The boundary between target sizes, however, can be specified in terms of a time constant that is reciprocally related to the latency of the adjoining region.

given luminance level. In the area-duration plane there are four sectors for both brightness and latency where a single power function prevails. For long flashes from large targets, brightness is reciprocally related to latency but in other sectors the relation is more complex. The complexity results from differences in the effect of duration on latency and on brightness. The variable component of visual latency is determined at an early stage in the response of the visual system. In fact, the variable component depends only upon the energy or quantum catch contained in the first 10 msec of a flash. Brightness, on the other hand, continues to depend upon flash duration up to 50 or 500 msec depending upon luminance level. In spite of the complex nature of the relation, the similarity in the set of rational exponents in the simple power functions describing brightness and latency suggests that brightness determined by direct scaling procedures does reflect an invariant index of visual function. An examination of the boundaries between the sectors in the brightness schema settles the question.

The boundary between two regions that differ in their brightness determinants can be measured by a variety of psychophysical methods including some that involve only threshold settings. Alternatively, the boundary can be calculated from the expressions for brightness on either side (Anglin & Mansfield, 1968). Both procedures lead to exactly the same simple results shown in Figure 2a, namely, that the space or time constant is reciprocally related to the brightness of an adjoining region. The reciprocity rules out the possibility that brightness has the invariance properties of a logarithmic interval variable rather than of a ratio variable. In summary, the regularity of the exponents, the similarities between brightness and latency, and the reciprocal relation between brightness and its adjoining boundary all support the view that brightness exponents are invariant indices of visual function. Perceived brightness provides a fine example of a sensory magnitude that can be measured on a ratio scale by direct scaling methods.

Neurobiological Invariances and the Neural Quantum of Sensory Discrimination

Stevens' law describes a relation between an observer's behavior and stimulus intensity but refrains from assigning loci to or mechanisms for the intervening transformations. The orderly analysis of the psychophysical function involves first establishing the form of the function and the invariance properties of the principal parameter, the exponent, before turning to the question of interpretation. But the question of whether the exponents refer to receptor organ characteristics, refer only to central characteristics, or have both peripheral and central components, has been a source of speculation and controversy since the psychophysical power law was first proposed in 1953.

As would be expected from the pattern of scientific revolutions (Kuhn, 1962), many of the proposed interpretations were attempts to reconcile the conflicting paradigms of Fechner and Stevens. Ekman (1964) took the extreme view that the power law was simply a special case of Fechner's law. In his view, both subjective magnitude and subjective number vary as logarithmic functions of the corresponding physical stimuli, and as a result both magnitude estimation and cross-modality matching would give rise to power functions. In a similar but more ingenious attempt to eliminate an explicit power function, MacKay (1963) proposed a model that would retain a logarithmic response characteristic for the receptors but could account for the observed differences in exponent for various modalities by differences in coupling coefficients of an internal comparator. In MacKay's model no explicit exponentiating function was postulated as in Marimont's schema (1962). More recent attempts (Treisman, 1965; Treisman & Irwin, 1967; Lipetz, 1969; 1971) to reconcile power-law performance with presumed Fechnerian logarithmic response characteristics have postulated nonlinear central transformations often invoking hypothetical neural mechanisms.

Although the use of hypothetical neural mechanisms may appear to reduce the question to one of neurophysiology, the interpretation of exponents and the issue of central linearity cannot be resolved entirely on the neurophysiological level. As Mountcastle (1967) has stressed, effective quantification at the behavioral level is necessary for the determination of stimulus correlates at the neural level that have behavioral relevance. Numerous neural events can be described by power functions (Stevens, 1970). By a comparison of precisely defined parametric effects, it may be possible to determine which of many possible physiological events is the appropriate element of a neural code for sensory magnitude. In vision, for example, effective quantification of brightness can be used to interpret power-function exponents in terms of neurobiological invariances.

NEURAL CODING OF BRIGHTNESS

Figure 3 compares photopigment absorption, neurelectric responses of different retinal neurons, and a segment of the perceived brightness function over the same intensity range. A sequence of compressive transformations in the retina reduces the linear absorption of quanta in the photoreceptors to a nonlinear cube-root response at the ganglion-cell level. Rushton & Henry (1968) found that the half-bleaching point for cone pigments was similar to that for rod pigments, about 10^9 above absolute threshold, so that over a wide range, absorption increases linearly with the intensity of a steady background. Below a semi-saturation point of the same order of magnitude as that of the photopigments, the receptor potential of foveal cones in primates approximates a power function with an exponent close to $\frac{2}{3}$ (Boynton & Whitten, 1970). Stone & Fabian (1968) found that the frequency of discharge of action potentials in cat retinal ganglion cells could be described by a power function of luminance with an exponent of 0.34 ± 0.03. The brightness data (Mansfield, 1973a) for a white light target of similar size lie essentially parallel to the response function for the ganglion cells and are best fit by a power function with an exponent of 0.32 ± 0.03. At the retinal level the assumption of cross-species functional similarity between man and cat is probably valid because of the similarity of retinal anatomy. Therefore the quantitative similarity between ganglion-cell response and the behavioral measure of perceived brightness does suggest a candidate code. Frequency of neural discharge in ganglion cells and in subsequent neuronal populations may form a neural basis for the encoding of brightness information. The extension or qualification of the proposed code requires further

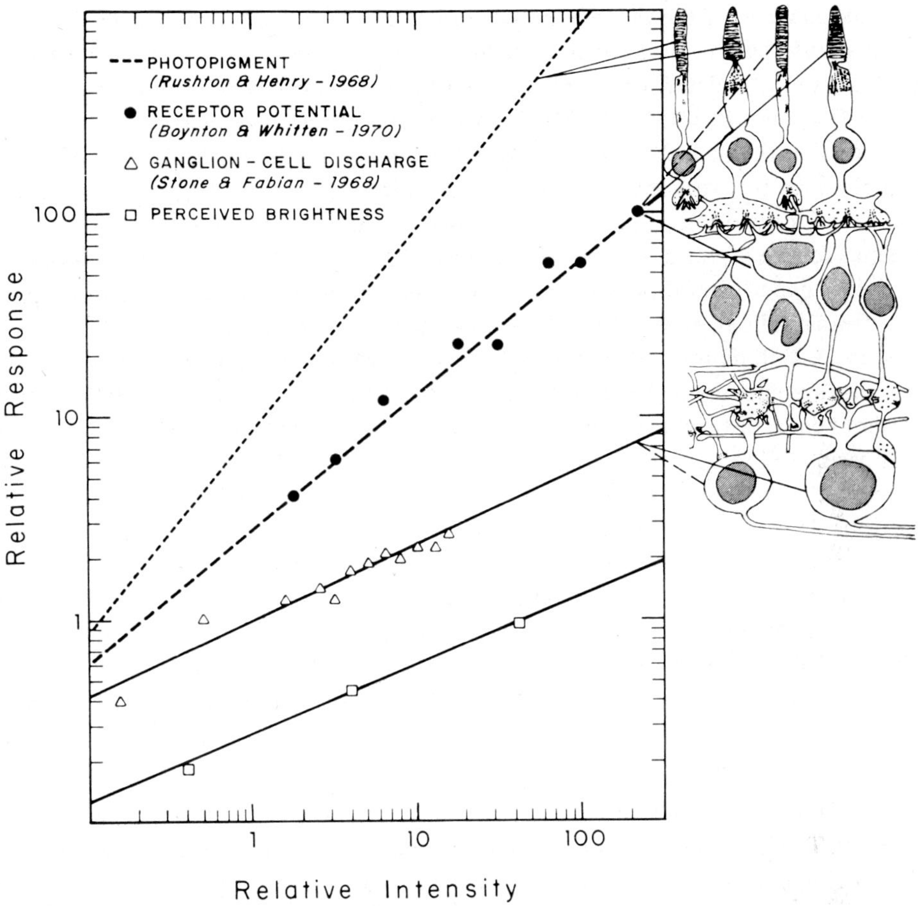

Fig. 3. Response functions at different locations in the retina. In the logarithmic coordinates the straight lines represent power functions. The lines drawn to the schematic diagram of the retina (after Dowling & Boycott, 1966) indicate neurons where the response function has been experimentally determined (solid lines) or is probably similar (dashed lines). The lower set of data points represents a segment of a perceived brightness function for a foveal target (data from Mansfield, 1973a).

comparisons for different stimuli such as brief flashes; at different recording locations, for example in the primary visual cortex; and in different species, for instance in the macaque monkey whose visual system and visual behavior closely resemble that of man. At present the simplest view consistent with the observations is that the neural code for brightness is established at the retinal level and is transmitted without essential modification to the behavioral response by linear central transformations.

NEURAL QUANTUM OF VISUAL DISCRIMINATION

A neural code for brightness in terms of the frequency of action potentials provides an opportunity to consider the concept of a neural quantum of sensory discrimination.

One consequence of the discrete gating function of neurons is that their all-or-none action should lead to a sharp boundary in terms of sensory discrimination between detection and non-detection when the behavioral response is determined by one or at most a few neurons (Boring, 1926). Since its inception controversy has consistently swirled about the neural quantum concept, for step-like threshold functions have not been obtained by every investigator. However, in seeking critical points, the observer is asked to function at the limit of his capacities and under these conditions any extraneous source of noise or variability may well disrupt and obscure the phenomenon. The initial experimental evidence in favor of neural quanta in sensory discrimination came from auditory experiments involving pitch and loudness (Békésy, 1930; Stevens, Morgan, & Volkmann, 1941; Miller & Garner, 1944). However, in a number of ways the visual system may be better suited to reveal neural quanta. Stevens (1972) analyzed threshold data for brightness increments from small foveal targets (Mueller, 1951) and from peripheral targets (Blackwell, 1953) as well as data for brightness increments of striped patterns (Sachs, Nachmias, & Robson, 1971) and found 39 step-like threshold functions. In addition to a steep threshold function, the neural quantum concept for vision predicts how threshold should increase with background level.

Consider the visual response produced by adding a luminance increment to a steady background. For backgrounds of low and moderate luminance below the region of significant bleaching of visual pigment, the perceived brightness of the background, ψ_b, grows as a power function of background intensity, I_b, according to the expression

$$\psi_b = kI_b^{\beta}, \tag{4}$$

where k is a scale factor and β is the exponent for the appropriate target size (see Figure 2). The increase in brightness, $\Delta\psi$, produced by an increment in target intensity, ΔI, superimposed on the background would be given implicitly by

$$\psi_b + \Delta\psi = k(I_b + \Delta I)^{\beta}.$$

Then for a fixed neural quantum corresponding to a criterion increment of perceived brightness, $\Delta\psi_c$, increment threshold, ΔI_c, would be implicitly defined by the expression

$$\Delta\psi_c = k(I_b + \Delta I_c)^{\beta} - kI_b^{\beta}. \tag{6}$$

For threshold values that are small in comparison with the magnitude of the background luminance, that is to say, $\Delta I_c \ll I_b$, a condition that holds except near absolute threshold, Newton's approximation of the binomial expansion in Equation 6 together with a rearrangement of terms yields the following analytical expression for increment threshold:

$$\Delta I_c = (\Delta\psi_c/k^{\beta})\, I_b^{1-\beta}. \tag{7}$$

Formally, increment threshold varies as a power function of background intensity, but consideration needs to be given to the domain of validity for such an expression. Near absolute threshold the approximation applied to Equation 6 would be invalid if the brightness function were nonlinear, but experimental evidence indicates that near absolute threshold the brightness function steepens and becomes linear (Ekman & Gustafsson, 1968). A linear brightness function ($\beta=1$) would result in a constant increment threshold ($\Delta I_c = \Delta\psi_c/k$), that is to say, one that is independent of background level. At high intensity levels, as Stevens (1957) pointed out, a fixed neural quantum of discrimination would be swamped by the noise and variability that give rise to the Weber-Fechner relation. Figure 4 puts these expectations to empirical test.

The results of three separate determinations of increment threshold for extended source targets are shown in Figure 4. Blackwell (1946) employed a group of 18 trained observers and computed threshold by the method of constant stimuli. Barlow (1957) used a single trained observer and made repeated determinations with the method of adjustment. For twelve cat retinal ganglion cells, Sakmann & Creutzfeldt (1969) employed as a threshold criterion a fixed increase in firing rate for flashes superimposed on a background field and presented to the central excitatory region of each

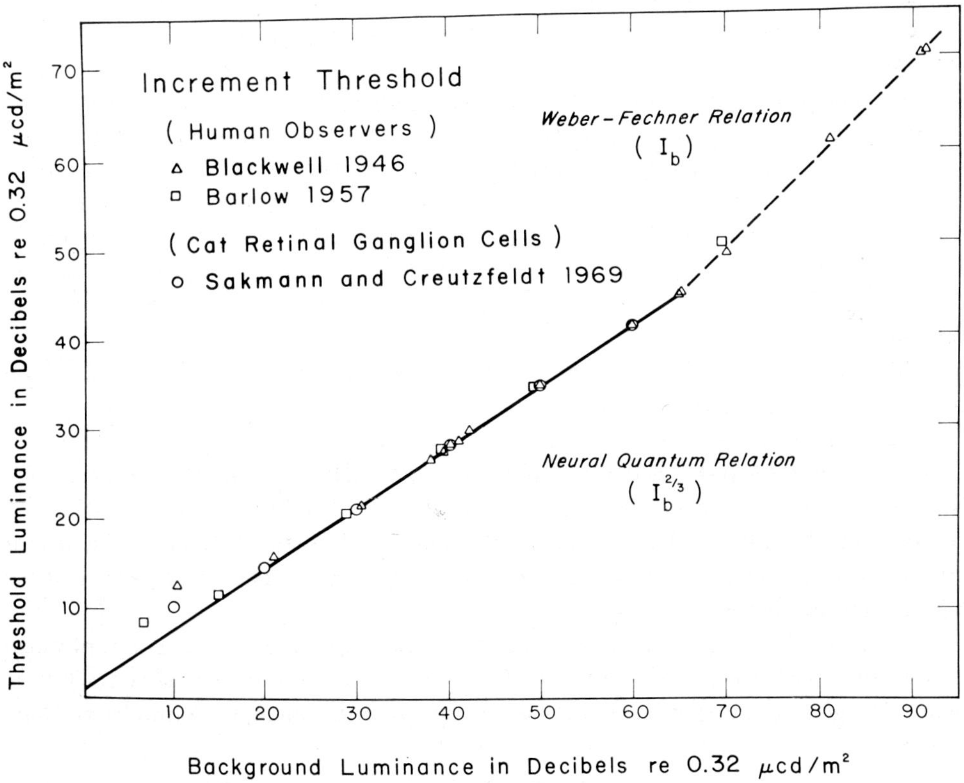

Fig. 4. Increment threshold as a function of background luminance. The solid line drawn through the lower portion of the data represents the relation, $\Delta I_c = kI_b^{2/3}$, predicted by the neural quantum model. The dashed line drawn through the upper portion of the data represents the Weber-Fechner relation, $\Delta I_c = kI_b$. The neurophysiological data for cat retinal ganglion cells was determined by a constant criterion and for purposes of comparison has been uniformly lowered by 3 decilogs.

cell's receptive field. For an extended target, the exponent, β, is approximately equal to $\frac{1}{3}$ for both psychophysical and neurelectric responses, so according to Equation 6 threshold should rise as the two-thirds power of the background intensity. In each case the data closely approximate the predicted neural quantum relation over the considerably range of five log units. Three principles are affirmed by the result: (1) the cube root relation between brightness and luminance; (2) the existence of a fixed neural quantum of sensory discrimination and (3) the neural coding of brightness at the retinal ganglion-cell level.

Summary and Conclusion

The orderly analysis of invariants in psychophysics involves the resolution of issues concerning the measurement properties of direct scaling procedures, the specification of the psychophysical function, and the establishment of neural codes for sensory function.

1. Direct procedures give rise to lognormal distributions with constant coefficients of variation that are characteristic of ratio-scale variables. To each scale type a signature distribution can be assigned by choosing the distribution possessing the maximum entropy.

2. A comparison of the results of direct scaling procedures with other measures of sensory response that are independent of the matching operation can reveal fundamental properties of sensory systems. Perceived brightness, visual latency, and the limits of areal and temporal summation can be described by power functions with simple rational exponents: $1, \frac{1}{2}, \frac{1}{3}, -\frac{1}{2}, -\frac{1}{3}$. The simplicity, regularity, and similarity of the exponents suggests that a remarkably simple mechanism underlies the encoding of brightness information and that brightness exponents are invariant indices of visual function.

3. The comparison of parametric effects can be used to discern which of several physiological events is the appropriate element of a neural code. A comparison of the ratio scale of perceived brightness with retinal response functions suggests a frequency code for brightness established at the retinal ganglion-cell level. The coding scheme for brightness and the existence of a neural quantum for brightness discrimination are confirmed by the finding that increment thresholds for human observers and constant criterion thresholds in cat retinal ganglion cells varied as the two-thirds power of the background luminance.

The issues of measurement and of the form and structure of the psychophysical power law have been essentially resolved. The determination of neural codes by the neurobiological analysis of behavior is where the present challenge lies and from which future discoveries will come.

References

Aitchison, J., & Brown, J. A. C. *The lognormal distribution.* Cambridge: Cambridge University Press, 1957.

Anglin, J., & Mansfield, R. J. W. On the brightness of short and long flashes. *Perception and Psychophysics*, 1968, **4**, 161–162.

Barlow, H. B. Increment thresholds at low intensities considered as signal/noise discriminations. *Journal of Physiology*, 1957, **136**, 469–488.

Békésy, G. von. Über das Fechnersche Gesetz und seine Bedeutung für die Theorie der akustischen Beobachtungsfehler und die Theorie des Hörens. *Annalen der Physik*, 1930, **7**, 329–359.

Blackwell, H. R. Contrast thresholds of the human eye. *Journal of the Optical Society of America*, 1946, **36**, 624–634.

Blackwell, H. R. *Psychophysical Thresholds*. Ann Arbor: Engineering Research Institute, University of Michigan, Bulletin no. 36, 1953.

Bluemel, V., Narducci, L. M., & Tuft, R. A. Photon-count distributions and irradiance fluctuation of a lognormally distributed light field. *Journal of the Optical Society of America*, 1972, **62**, 1309–1314.

Boring, E. G. Auditory theory with special reference to intensity, volume, and localization. *American Journal of Psychology*, 1926, **37**, 157–188.

Boynton, R. M., & Whitten, D. N. Visual adaptation in monkey cones: Recording late receptor potentials. *Science*, 1970, **170**, 1423–1426.

Cross, D. V. Sequential dependencies and regression in psychophysical judgments. *Perception and Psychophysics*, 1973, **14**, 547–552.

Dowling, J. E., & Boycott, B. B. Organization of the primate retina: Electron microscopy. *Proceedings of the Royal Society* (London), 1966, **B166**, 80–111.

Ekman, G. Discriminal sensitivity on the subjective continuum. *Acta Psychologica*, 1956, **12**, 233–243.

Ekman, G. Is the power law a special case of Fechner's law? *Perception and Motor Skills*, 1964, **19**, 720.

Ekman, G., & Gustafsson, U. Threshold values and the psychophysical function in brightness vision. *Vision Research*, 1968, **8**, 747–758.

Ekman, G., & Sjöberg, L. Scaling. *Annual Review of Psychology*, 1965, **16**, 451–474.

Kerr, J. R., & Dunphy, J. R. Experimental effects of finite transmitter apertures on scintillations. *Journal of the Optical Society of America*, 1973, **63**, 1–8.

Kuhn, T. S. *The structure of scientific revolutions*. Chicago: The University of Chicago Press, 1962.

Lipetz, L. E. The transfer function of sensory intensity in the nervous system. *Vision Research*, 1969, **9**, 1205–1234.

Lipetz, L. E. The relation of physiological and psychological aspects of sensory intensity. In W. R. Lowenstein (Ed.), *Principles of receptor physiology*. New York: Springer-Verlag, 1971, pp. 191–225.

Luce, R. D., & Galanter, E. Psychophysical scaling. In R. D. Luce, R. R. Bush, & E. Galanter (Eds.), *Handbook of mathematical psychology*. New York: Wiley, 1963. Vol. 1, pp. 245–307.

MacKay, D. M. Psychophysics of perceived intensity: A theoretical basis for Fechner's and Stevens' laws. *Science*, 1963, **139**, 1213–1216.

Mansfield, R. J. W. Intensity relations in vision: Analysis and synthesis in a nonlinear sensory system. Unpublished doctoral dissertation, Harvard University, 1970.

Mansfield, R. J. W. Brightness function: Effect of area and duration. *Journal of the Optical Society of America*, 1973, **63**, 913–920. (a)

Mansfield, R. J. W. Latency functions in human vision. *Vision Research*, 1973, **13**, 2219–2234. (b)

Marimont, R. B. Model for visual response to contrast. *Journal of the Optical Society of America*, 1962, **52**, 800–806.

Miller, G. A., & Garner, W. R. Effect of random presentation on the psychometric function: Implications for a quantal theory of discrimination. *American Journal of Psychology*, 1944, **57**, 451–467.

Minott, P. O. Scintillation in an earth-to-space propagation path. *Journal of the Optical Society of America*, 1972, **62**, 885–888.

Mitchell, R. L. Permanence of the log-normal distribution. *Journal of the Optical Society of America*, 1968, **58**, 1267–1272.

Moreland, J. D. The distribution of dendritic domains of retinal neurons. *Vision Research*, 1969, **9**, 529–535.

Mountcastle, V. B. The problem of sensing and the neural coding of sensory events. In G. C. Quarton, T. Melnechuk, & F. C. Schmitt (Eds.), *The neurosciences*. New York: Rockefeller University Press, 1967, pp. 393–408.

Mueller, C. G. Frequency of seeing functions for intensity discrimination at various levels of adapting intensity. *Journal of General Physiology*, 1951, **34**, 463–474.

Polyak, S. *The retina.* Chicago: The University of Chicago Press, 1941.

Poulton, E. C. The new psychophysics: Six models for magnitude estimation. *Psychological Bulletin*, 1968, **69**, 1–19.

Price, A. J. Community noise survey of greater Vancouver. *Journal of the Acoustical Society of America*, 1972, **52**, 488–492.

Rushton, W. A. H., & Henry, G. H. Bleaching and regeneration of cone pigments in man. *Vision Research*, 1968, **8**, 617–631.

Sachs, M. B., Nachmias, J., & Robson, J. G. Spatial-frequency channels in human vision. *Journal of the Optical Society of America*, 1971, **61**, 1176–1186.

Sakmann, B., & Creutzfeldt, O. D. Scotopic and mesopic light adaptation in the cat's retina. *Pflügers Archiv*, 1969, **313**, 168–185.

Stevens, J. C. Stimulus spacing and the judgment of loudness. *Journal of Experimental Psychology*, 1958, **56**, 246–250.

Stevens, S. S. On the theory of scales of measurement. *Science*, 1946, **103**, 677–680.

Stevens, S. S. On the brightness of lights and the loudness of sounds. *Science*, 1953, **118**, 576 (Abstract).

Stevens, S. S. On the averaging of data. *Science*, 1955, **121**, 113–116.

Stevens, S. S. On the psychophysical law. *Psychological Review*, 1957, **64**, 153–181.

Stevens, S. S. A metric for social consensus. *Science*, 1966, **151**, 530–541.

Stevens, S. S. Neural events and the psychophysical law. *Science*, 1970, **170**, 1043–1050.

Stevens, S. S. Issues in psychophysical measurement. *Psychological Review*, 1971, **78**, 426–450.

Stevens, S. S. A neural quantum in sensory discrimination. *Science*, 1972, **177**, 749–762.

Stevens, S. S., & Galanter, E. Ratio scales and category scales for a dozen perceptual continua. *Journal of Experimental Psychology*, 1957, **54**, 377–411.

Stevens, S. S., & Greenbaum, H. Regression effect in psychophysical judgment. *Perception and Psychophysics*, 1966, **1**, 439–446.

Stevens, S. S., Morgan, C. T., & Volkmann, J. Theory of neural quantum in the discrimination of loudness and pitch. *American Journal of Psychology*, 1941, **54**, 315–335.

Stone, J., and Fabian, M. Summing properties of the cat's retinal ganglion cells. *Vision Research,* 1968, **8**, 1023–1040.

Teghtsoonian, R. On the exponents in Stevens' law and the constant in Ekman's law. *Psychological Review*, 1971, **78**. 71–80.

Treisman, M. Sensory scaling and the psychophysical law. *Quarterly Journal of Experimental Psychology*, 1965, **16**, 11–22.

Treisman, M., & Irwin, R. J. Auditory intensity discriminal scale 1. Evidence derived from binaural intensity summation. *Journal of the Acoustical Society of America*, 1967, **42**, 586–592.

LISTEN AND HEAR[1]

GEORGE A. MILLER
The Rockefeller University

Abstract. The English verbs 'listen' and 'hear' are contrasted and compared semantically to 'look' and 'see.'

"I want you to listen and tell me what you hear." Over the years this request, or some more detailed paraphrase of it, must have been made thousands of times by auditory psychophysicists, yet little analysis has been made of this step in the experimental procedure. What analysis there has been relates either to the listener's motivational state or to the difficulties of posing the request to inarticulate animals or children. It is generally assumed that when one is dealing with a cooperative, intelligent adult who understands and uses the English language, such requests automatically put him into the receptive condition that the experimenter desires.

The surprising thing is that the request nearly always works. Because it nearly always works, most of those who use it need never pause to reflect how surprising their success really is. In order to put the request into proper perspective, one has to think how it could be phrased for a computer. Before we could think seriously about such a project the task would have to be better defined, but, however it was defined, it is obvious that months of detailed programming would be required before a computer could be expected to do anything resembling what a person will do after receiving a simple verbal instruction to "listen and hear." The difference, of course, is that those months of programing have already been done by (or to) the person before he reaches the laboratory – done as part of that process we call "learning to speak English."

To carry the analogy a step further, it is obvious that the computer's subsequent performance would be critically dependent on the program provided to it. We can assume that a person's performance is similarly dependent, yet we take the human program for granted, as if we knew all about it. In one sense, of course, the experimenter does understand a listener's program, because he himself is similarly programmed. But in the sense that implies scientific understanding – the sense in which an experimenter should understand his equipment, the acoustic properties of the stimuli, the response characteristics of the auditory system – he is woefully ignorant. He does not understand in a principled way the difference between listening and hearing, or why two different verbs are used, or what kind of computer program would enable a machine to perform these two related but apparently different functions.

[1] Preparation was supported in part by Grant No. GM16735 to The Rockefeller University. I am indebted to Philip N. Johnson-Laird and Aravind Joshi for helpful discussions of the English verbs of perception. My interest in analyzing the meanings of words originated many years ago in luncheon conversations with Edwin G. Boring and S. S. Stevens, both of whom were close students of the dictionary.

H. R. Moskowitz et al. (eds.), Sensation and Measurement. 129–135.

There is no compelling reason why a psychoacoustician must understand this complicated cognitive organ, any more than he must understand the workings of the equally indispensible heart, lungs, and liver. He is protected by the fortunate fact that it does work. The claim here is merely that its working is surprising. The suggestion would be that the program might be worth analyzing in its own right, even for someone convinced in advance that none of the variance in his psychophysical observations could be attributed to it.

But how can such an analysis be undertaken?

In 1967 Jeffrey Gruber published a speculative article entitled "Look and See." In order to analyze the syntactic and semantic aspects of the program that enables speakers of English to use these two verbs, he tried substituting them into a variety of sentences. For example, "John looked toward the house" is acceptable, but "John saw toward the house" is not; "The bird saw the nest" is acceptable, but "The bird looked the nest" is not; "John looked through the glass carefully" is acceptable, but "John saw through the glass carefully" is not. And so on. After marshaling such observations in the manner of a good linguistic analyst, Gruber offered the following facts and hypotheses to account for his observations:

– 'See' can be used either transitively or intransitively; 'look' is used only intransitively.

– Both 'see' and 'look' behave like motional verbs (e.g., 'go,' 'run,' 'fly,' 'slide') with respect to the prepositions that can follow them. 'See' takes prepositions that would be used with motional verbs to indicate the goal of the motion; 'look' takes prepositions that would indicate direction of motion.

– 'Look' is an agentive and 'see' is a nonagentive verb – "What he did was look at the bird" is acceptable, but "What he did was see the bird" is not.

– 'Look' is used freely in the progressive; 'see' is subject to restrictions

– "John was looking at the tree" is acceptable, whereas "John was seeing the tree" is not. (This test is generally used to distinguish stative verbs like 'be' or 'know' from active verbs like 'buy' or 'move,' but since Gruber thought 'see' was a motional verb, he could not draw that conclusion.)

– 'Look' can occur in affirmative sentences with 'until,' but 'see' cannot – "He looked at the lake until noon" is acceptable, but "He saw the lake until noon" is not. ('See' resembles 'arrive,' which has momentary aspect, whereas 'look' is like 'move,' which has continuative aspect.)

Although Gruber's attempt to treat 'look' and 'see' syntactically as motional verbs was probably misguided, his work indicates the kind of evidence available for analysis. The same method can be applied to verbs of hearing. But first we should note another line of inquiry that may be relevant to the enterprise.

When linguistic philosophers turned their attention to theories of empiricism, they were struck by the differences between such verbs as 'see' and 'watch.' For example, Gilbert Ryle (1949) comments that verbs like 'see,' 'hear,' 'detect,' 'discriminate,' are generally used to record observational success, whereas verbs like 'watch,' 'listen,' 'probe,' 'scan,' 'savor,' are used to record observational undertakings whose success may still be in question. "Hence it is proper to speak of someone watching carefully and successfully, but not of his seeing carefully or successfully" (p. 222). Ryle proposes a distinction between "achievements" and "activities": to see something is an achievement, to look at something is an activity. The difference can be recognized by the fact that achievements ('see,' 'hear,' 'win,' 'find') happen at a particular moment, whereas activities ('watch,' 'listen,' 'run,' 'fight') may last through an interval of time. Moreover, Ryle noticed a difference between those achievements that necessarily involve an associated task and those that can be purely lucky – you cannot win a race without competing, but you can find things without searching. Seeing and hearing are lucky achievements. Ryle's distinctions were later elaborated by Anthony Kenny, Zeno Vendler, and other philosophers, and have also received attention from linguists interested in verbal aspect (Dowty, 1972).

Philosophical observations about perceptual verbs are generally insightful and important, although extracting them from the epistemological or metaphysical arguments in which they occur runs some risk of misrepresentation. There is a prevailing emphasis on vision in these discussions; audition is usually mentioned more or less as an afterthought to demonstrate the generality of the argument, on the assumption that 'hear' resembles 'see' and 'listen' resembles 'look.' This favoritism for vision may reflect nothing more than the fact that examples involving verbs of seeing may come more readily to mind; English has between fifty and a hundred (depending on how one counts) verbs of seeing, but only five to ten verbs of hearing. At least one philosopher, however, has indicated that there is more to it than that.

For Peter Strawson the world consists of particular things and events that we can talk about to one another. In order to talk about them, however, a listener must be able to identify the particular thing or event a speaker is referring to. Language must, therefore, provide ways to identify particulars. The most convenient way to identify any particular is by its location in the unique spatiotemporal system that speaker and listener share; Strawson argues that such locative identification is in some sense basic to all the alternative ways a particular might be identified. Where does this unique, shared, spatiotemporal system come from? It comes from our visual perception of material objects arrayed in space. Material bodies constitute the framework of our conceptual scheme. Particular material objects can be identified without referring to events, processes, states, or particulars of any other kind, but it is not possible to identify other classes of particulars without referring to material objects. Material objects, therefore, are basic to particular-identification.

Being a philosopher, Strawson was not content to leave this as a description of the conceptual scheme we *do* have. He wished to convince himself that it is the only conceptual scheme we *could* have. So he tried to imagine a No-Space world based on auditory experience alone. He asked: Could a being whose experience was purely auditory have a conceptual scheme that provided for objective particulars – that is, for particulars distinguished by that being from himself and regarded as actual or possible objects of those experiences? Strawson concluded that the idea of space, and with it the idea of a spatial system of objects, cannot be given meaning in purely auditory terms. Without the idea of space, there would be no sense in which sounds might be thought to exist when we were not hearing them. It might be possible to identify the recurrence of particulars in a nonspatial scheme, but it would not be possible to imagine one's self as an immaterial agency acting in this world. Such a being could make no distinction between private and public; he would be a true solipsist.

If Strawson's opinions are representative, the philosopher's emphasis on vision, or on visual access to the spatial arrangement of objective particulars, may be more than fortuitous. Whatever one makes of the No-Space fantasy, however, it forces to one's attention the lack of objective particulars in our language of audition. Of course, we do say such things as "I can hear an airplane" and an airplane is certainly a tangible particular. But such sentences are elliptical; what we mean is "I can hear the sound of an airplane." An airplane and the sound it makes are not the same; we see the one and we hear the other. "I can see an airplane" is not an elliptical version of "I can see the sight of an airplane." The language of audition is a language of processes and events; the language of vision is a language of objects.

Thousands of English words denote objects we can see, but our vocabulary for events we can hear is limited. Compare, for example, the rich variety of color terms in English with the terms available for pitch: 'high,' 'low,' 'deep,' 'shrill.' Even people with absolute pitch must draw on some special language of music or acoustics for identifying phrases. Why this discrepancy? The auditory "objects" whose recurrence we are most attuned to are spoken words. Perhaps our potential capacity for identifying auditory particulars has been sacrificed in the service of a more important social function.

If there is anything to these speculations, we should find differences between the way we use 'listen' and 'hear' and the way we use 'look' and 'see.' So our analysis should have two goals; first, to characterize differences between 'listen' and 'hear' and, second, to compare those differences with corresponding differences between 'look' and 'see.' The simplest way to proceed is to take Gruber's observations as our outline.

– 'Hear' can be used either transitively or intransitively; 'listen' is used only intransitively. In this respect, they parallel 'see' and 'hear.' The major difference has already been noted. When 'hear' is used transitively, there is usually an implicit 'the sound of' between the verb and its object, owing to our lack of words for denoting acoustic particulars. The only exceptions arise when the object of the verb is a noun denoting a speech act – "I can hear the instructions" is not the same as "I can hear the sound of the instructions." To say "John can hear the sound of what you are saying" suggests that John does not understand what is being said. Apparently we think of ourselves as hearing through the speech signal to the message itself, just as we think of seeing through the optical image of a tree to the tree itself.

– 'Hear' and 'listen' do not behave like motional verbs with respect to the prepositions that can follow them. (It would not be difficult to make the case that 'see' and 'look' are not as motional as Gruber claims, but that is another argument.) Note that "He could hear into the cup" sounds odd, although the same sentence with 'see' is perfectly acceptable. Or, again, "He looked about the room" sounds more natural than "He listened about the room." A better phrasing of Gruber's observation would be that verbs of seeing and moving both presuppose a spatial manifold in which to see and move, so locative prepositions denoting spatial relations are appropriate to both. Hearing and listening, on the other hand, are only derivatively spatial; they presuppose a temporal continuum in which events and processes happen. The difference is illustrated by a comparison of "He looked for the mailman," which suggests active spatial exploration, and "He listened for the mailman," which suggests quiet waiting. It is possible to search through space in a way that we cannot search through time.

– 'Listen' is agentive and 'hear' is not, which parallels 'look' and 'see.' Several tests are used to establish agency. Agentive verbs can take a purpose phrase beginning 'in order to': "He listened to the chimes in order to find out the time' is acceptable, but "He heard the chimes in order to find out the time" is odd. Agentive verbs can appear with 'do' phrases: "What he did in the experiment was listen" is acceptable, but "What he did in the experiment was hear" is odd. Agentive verbs can take certain manner adverbials like 'carefully': "He listened carefully" is acceptable, but "He heard carefully" is not. Agentive verbs can occur in the complement of 'persuade' sentences: "He persuaded John to listen" sounds more acceptable than "He persuaded John to hear." Agentive verbs can take an instrumental phrase: "He listened with his stethoscope" is better than "He heard with his stethoscope." Agentive verbs can occur in imperatives: "Listen to the motor" is better than "Hear the motor," although this distinction may have been eroded by exposure to the military announcement, "Now hear this!".

Semantic analysis of agentive verbs indicates that they can be paraphrased roughly as: '*x* does something *y* and *y* causes *z* to happen.' For example, "She moved the cup" would correspond to 'She did something that caused the cup to change location.' Since 'listen' is an agentive verb, it can be paraphrased the same way: "She listened to the music" corresponds to 'She did something that caused her to hear the music.' If we analyze 'hear' as 'perceive by ear,' then it becomes 'She did something that caused her to perceive the music by ear.' Agency is the major semantic difference between 'listening' and 'hearing.'

If this analysis of 'listen' is applied to 'look,' however, the result is incorrect. For example, it would suggest that "She looked at the picture" should correspond to 'She did something that caused her to perceive the picture by eye.' But you can look at something without perceiving it. It is perfectly acceptable to say "She looked at the picture, but she didn't see it," whereas to say "She listened to the music, but she didn't hear it" sounds odd. In the case of 'look,' therefore, we must assume that what she was to direct her eyes toward the picture; whether she attended to what she was looking at involves an additional assumption.

A visual agent has many tactics at his disposal to control what he will see; he can move around, change his point of fixation, attend selectively, even close his eyes. An auditory agent can withdraw or try not to pay attention, but he is more vulnerable to whatever sounds occur around him. In general terms, the difference between hearing and listening is more subjective than the difference between seeing and looking. It is easier for an observer to tell what a person is looking at than to tell what he is listening to. In terms of the agentive-nonagentive distinction, therefore, there is a greater difference for seeing verbs than for hearing verbs. None of the test sentences involving 'hear' that were given above are completely out of bounds; they sound slightly odd, perhaps, but they might pass in informal discourse. Thus, although agency is important to the distinction between 'listen' and 'hear,' it is less important than to the distinction between 'look' and 'see.'

– 'Listen' can be used more freely in the progressive than 'hear' can, although again the difference seems weaker than in the case of 'look' and 'see.' One test for stative verbs is that they make unacceptable answers to the question, "What happened?" For example, "He was knowing English" or "He was being dead" would be unacceptable. "He was seeing the tree" is less unacceptable, but would be odd in most situations. "He was hearing the airplane" is only mildly strange, however, and "He was hearing testimony" is well within bounds. The subtlety of the difference between the state of hearing and the activity of listening may be reflected linguistically in greater tolerance for violations of the usual stative-active distinctions.

– 'Listen' can occur in affirmative sentences with 'until' more naturally than 'hear' can. For example, "I will listen until noon" is more acceptable than the same sentence with 'hear.' Once more, the distinction seems weaker here than for verbs of seeing, but the situation is complicated for both 'see' and 'hear.' When these verbs are used to denote the enduring capability of perceiving, they do not go well with any temporal locatives; when they are used to denote a momentary perceptual success, they go with momentary temporal locatives ('at noon,' 'before lunch'), but not so well with temporal duratives ('until noon,' 'for three days'). Among the verbs of seeing are those, like 'glimpse' or 'glance at,' that denote a momentary success, and such sentences as "I glimpsed (glanced at) John until noon" are clearly unacceptable. Verbs of hearing are less well differentiated: "I heard the crash until noon" is unacceptable, not because hearing must be momentary, but because crashes are; "I heard the motor until noon" is not unacceptable, because motor noises need not be momentary.

On balance, there are more similarities than differences between 'look-see' and 'listen-hear.' Considering the enormous differences in the physical stimuli, the perceptual experiences, and the adaptive functions of the two sense modalities, the remarkable thing is that we talk about them both in so nearly the same way – that so little modulation of linguistic form is required to accommodate such important differences of content.

The critical semantic distinction between 'listen' and 'hear' is that listening is an activity under the voluntary control of an agent who does something in order to hear, whereas hearing is an involuntary perceptual consequence of listening successfully. When an experimenter asks his friend to listen, therefore, he is relying on a kind of psychological preprogramming far more complex than we are likely to understand from linguistic evidence. Fortunately, the person usually understands what we want him to do – whatever it is – and on that pragmatic basis the science of auditory psychophysics proceeds.

References

Dowty, David R. Studies in the logic of verb aspect and time Reference in English. Ph.D. Dissertation Department of Linguistics, University of Texas at Austin, 1972.

Gruber, Jeffrey S. Look and see. *Language*, 1967, **43**, 937–947.

Kenny, Anthony. *Action, emotion, and will.* New York: Humanities Press, 1963.

Ryle, Gilbert. *The concept of mind.* New York: Barnes and Noble, 1949.

Strawson, P. F. *Individuals: An essay in descriptive metaphysics.* London: Methuen, 1959.

Vendler, Zeno. *Linguistics in philosophy.* Ithaca, N.Y.: Cornell University Press, 1967.

ON THE ORIGIN OF "SCALES OF MEASUREMENT"

EDWIN B. NEWMAN
Harvard University

Abstract. Stevens proposed that measurement in psychology should employ one of four scales, nominal, ordinal, interval and ratio, each characterized by a mathematical operation that defines the group of which the scale is an example. Isomorphic with the mathematical scale, there is an appropriate psychological operation which if employed warrants the use of the corresponding scale. The development of this proposal is traced.

That measurement is a central aspect, indeed the very core, of science seems almost a commonplace. A little reflection, however, reminds one that the relation has not always been clear, nor easy to capture in a simple statement. During the last century our ideas both about what is science and about what is measurement have changed profoundly. In psychology, for example, we once depended on Fechner's psychophysics. As an alternative, we turned to Galton's estimates of human abilities, and to mental tests and the IQ. There followed the development of statistics, plain and fancy, and methods of scaling and estimation. Finally, behavioral psychologists introduced a variety of quite uncertain measures. Which of these are the "right" measures? Do not the measurements themselves constrain the very facts that we record and bias thereby our attempts to explain them? To understand our science we must understand measurement; it is not just an ancillary tool.

For many of us the account of scales of measurement given by Stevens in the first chapter of the *Handbook of Experimental Psychology* (Stevens, 1951) has stood like the Decalogue. It is certainly the fixed point around which most recent psychophysics has been built. No single more recent statement has replaced it. Where did it come from? What was its history? The account which follows is intended not so much as a discussion of the issues inherent in a theory of measurement, but rather as some historical notes which may throw modest light on this subject.

"Scales of measurement" is taken here to mean the description of four ways in which numerals can be used in psychology. The scales are the (1) nominal, (2) ordinal, (3) interval, and (4) ratio scales. For each there is a defining mathematical characteristic, a group-structure, and for the use of each there must be at least one empirical operation isomorphic with the group structure. Finally, there are statistical operations appropriate to each scale. This is the heart of the matter which is to be examined.

The Background

That measurement was important was a view which required no apology in Harvard's Emerson Hall in 1932. I would not claim this was the universal view, but Boring (1929) had written recently, speaking of Fechner, that without psychophysics "there would ... have been little of the breath of science in the experimental body, for we hardly

H. R. Moskowitz et al. (eds.), Sensation and Measurement. 137–145.

recognize a subject as scientific if measurement is not one of its tools [p. 286]." Psychology, like chemistry, had a course in quantitative methods. Statistics as a course appeared for the first time in 1933. The twig was bent.

But all was not well. A modest but growing understanding of statistics did not offer great solace, as was clear in Boring's (1920) dissatisfaction with the normal law of error. More serious was our recognition that the measurement of a genuinely psychological variable had not been convincingly established. In talking about "The Data of Psychology" in Boring's 1934 seminar, Holway and McGregor reviewed the arguments against Fechner's assumptions. At the end of the semester Boring concluded,

> Psychology lacks true measurement of direct experience because there are not additive units. The limen is measurable in units of the stimulus, but all limens are not equal.... These facts accord with the definition of consciousness by the operation of discrimination.[1]

The judgment was a harsh one, but I am persuaded we all more or less agreed. For one thing there was the "quantity objection" which really no one had answered: there was no introspective sense in which a large sensation consisted of so many little ones. James was right. All the pinks in the world don't add up to red. For another thing, psychophysics had become preoccupied with method and had produced little hard fact. One has only to reread the history of tonal volume to understand how fruitless was that approach. Finally, we had a great suspicion that Fechner's fundamental assumption, that JNDs are equal, was simply not true introspectively.

As a reflection of the mood, I wrote a short paper testing the Fechnerian scale across different hues and different pitches (Newman, 1933). Relatively complete data had recently become available on intensive JNDs in hearing. There was also Kingsbury's determination of equal-loudness contours. It required only a little work to show that a tone eight JND's above threshold at 80 Hz was judged equal in loudness to one 116 JND's above threshold at 4000 Hz. The same case could be made easily in vision using heterochromatic matches of brightness and early measures of intensity discrimination by König. I submitted this as a term paper to Whitehead who explained to me in the most friendly fashion that he had no idea what I was talking about.

What were we to do? The obvious answer was some kind of more direct approach to estimates of magnitude. But before coming to this, let me list three other things that were in the air:

1. The 1930's were a period during which there was a good deal of ferment in logic and related parts of philosophy. I have commented on operationism elsewhere (Newman, 1973). My own recollection is of Professor Sheffer's course in symbolic logic for which, as an exercise, I produced a new postulational system for Boolean algebra. Huntington had done it with ten postulates, Sheffer with five, Nicod with two (see Jørgensen, 1931). My system required four postulates, about three pages of text and seven of footnotes! It was a short step, although not altogether an easy one, to books and courses in the foundations of mathematics. What I am suggesting is that

[1] Mimeographed notes, unpublished.

we understood many things about mathematics which were far beyond what was accessible to Fechner and James and G. E. Müller and Titchener.

2. New tools were at hand in psychophysics. Using a method of equivalents that actually had some little history, Kingsbury (1927) had determined equal-loudness contours. Stevens (1934a, 1934b, 1934c) had capitalized on the technique to give the first clear demonstration of the reality of tonal volume and tonal density. The emphasis is reversed from that of the usual procedure of measurement. In a multidimensional manifold the emphasis is now on invariance across some complex set of transformations. This alone is not measurement, but on the experimental side it has much the same feeling as does the definition of a group in mathematics. And a group in mathematics is the first step toward the definition of a number.

3. Finally, at this point we had encountered some relatively sophisticated discussion of the problems of measurement in other sciences. I have described elsewhere our encounter with operational concepts. In 1935 McGregor (1935) published a paper on measurement which contains, I believe, more or less the position argued in Boring's seminar. His argument derives largely from Campbell (1920), a British physicist, and in turn from what Russell (1919) calls "mathematical philosophy." The mathematical part starts with primitive definitions of the operations which have to do with a determination of equality. There is a class defined by those instances for which neither $a<b$ nor $b<a$. There are definitions of order and number. Campbell's position is then that there is in physics a set of "fundamental magnitudes" to which numerals may be applied because one applies experimental operations which correspond to the mathematical ones. He adopts a narrow concept of number, one which obeys all the rules of arithmetic. This limits him to physical operations which have just those properties which his numbers have. This is easy and obvious for length and weight. McGregor argues that there are equally obvious cases in psychology, e.g., visual extent.

Let me sum up by saying Fechner was dead, the statistical approach begged the question, a more sophisticated approach to measurement was emerging in the physical sciences, and in logic and mathematics as well.

A Direct Approach to Scaling

Independently of the more general discussion of scales of measurement there had developed rather practical concern about a scale of loudness. The use of decibels, a logarithmic scale that should reflect Fechner's law, made it rather evident that something else was required. The simplest way to put it is that no one would say that a 40 dB sensation-level was half as loud as an 80 dB sensation-level. It was far too low. So what was half as loud?

The concept of the equal sense-distance had been around, of course, for some time. Technically, it had been hard to implement. But now came a fresh look. The logic which inheres in the use of equal sense-distance is not too different from the logic of the Weber-Fechner Law. In the theory, one Δs (increment in sensation) is like another. Psychologically, however, the two experiments are very different. There is something very explicit that feels like a magnitude when you sound three tones in succession and adjust one to be midway between the other two. With the much improved control of the physical stimulus, several people tried this early in the 1930's. The most successful measurements were by Churcher (1935), at Metropolitan-Vickers in England. He had subjects judge half-loudness. The Weber-Fechner Law was wrong. Churcher proposed an empirical scale which made loudness proportional to the fifth power of sound intensity in decibels. Factually the scale was beautiful; as a mathematical expression, it was monstrous.

Fletcher (Fletcher & Munson, 1933) had made an elaborate attack on the same problem but used rather different and less comfortable psychological assumptions. One was that loudness in the two ears adds exactly. The other was that loudness of tones differing widely in pitch will also add exactly. He developed empirically something he called a *G*-function, which happily agreed roughly with Churcher's curve.

A third piece of evidence came from the measurements of cochlear potentials by Stevens & Davis (1936). With the characteristic Stevens' (1936) touch all three sets of data were combined, a convenient unit was defined and named the "sone," and thus, in 1936, the sone scale was born. Two things are to be noted. First, it was a purely empirical scale. Second, from the psychological point of view, the most persuasive measurements were Churcher's. The convergence of the other data was happy, but less necessary to the argument.

If fractionation worked for loudness, could it not also be applied to pitch? There was a good deal of disagreement on the issue. After all one did have the musical scale and intervals (psychological distances?) which seemed to answer the question. But, if nothing else, the musical scale with its harmonic relations completely leapt over the issue of empirical thresholds. JNDs for pitch clearly were very unequal in size if expressed in musical terms. If the Fechnerian assumption was correct, fractions of tones should have been equally discriminable, and they are not. So we tried making judgments of "half" pitch. McGregor, with some little musical sophistication, remained skeptical throughout. Volkmann, Stevens, and I were convinced it would work. In six weeks the mel-scale was born (Stevens, Volkmann, & Newman, 1937).

Once more the scale found support from other directions. The most notable was its coincidence with the map of the cochlea that Stevens, Davis, & Lurie (1935) had produced by physiological experiments. Also, the fit to data from differential sensitivity was quite good, in very sharp contrast with the loudness function. Some years later we were to discover that it also matched Fletcher's (1940) measure of the "critical band" in hearing, as well as the related data on speech comprehension (French & Steinberg, 1947). The point here is not what ultimately happened to the mel-scale, but rather that a fractionation procedure produced a scale on which there was a convergence of reasonably related supporting evidence.

The Critique: Is This Measurement?

The issue of the proper rules for measurement was alive in another quarter. In 1932 the British Association for the Advancement of Science had appointed a joint committee of its sections on physical sciences and psychology which brought together eight or nine distinguished British psychologists and an equal number from mathematics and physics. One of the latter was N. R. Campbell whose book (1920) *Physics, the Elements* was widely accepted as the authority on measurement, quoted, we have noted, by McGregor. Seven years and many meetings later, the Committee (Ferguson, 1940) reported its fundamental disagreement and was discharged. In their final effort they had chosen the sone scale as an example, and Campbell, among others, found it wanting.

This is hardly the place to recapitulate the argument. It depends roughly on a number of assertions that I will simply list:

1. The quantity argument: since no meaning can be given to the cutting up of a single sensation into parts, which can in turn be added together again to form the original whole, there is not measurement.
2. There exists no other definition for addition. Without the operation of addition no numerical scale can be constructed, and without this operation the concept of magnitude is meaningless.
3. The assertion that a sound in two ears is twice as loud is pure assumption. It has no factual (operational?) meaning.
4. Physical concepts are universal; psychological facts are particular to the individual observer and may be idiosyncratic.
5. Physical facts are true because great care is taken to free them from unwanted contamination.
6. Different procedures give different measurements of the same presumed psychological magnitude. Since we do not know which is correct we cannot choose among them.

It is obvious that some of the physicists on this Committee were unfamiliar with either what Russell had called the philosophy of mathematics or the whole tradition in physics from Mach to Planck to Einstein to Bridgman. That there are no assumptions involved when one unites two weights in a scale pan, or successively applies a ruler to a distance, or counts ticks of a clock seems a trifle naive. It is hard not to admit that the strictures about psychological measures are partly true; it is equally difficult not to point out the beam in their own eyes.

The counterposition would be simply this:

1. There exist several logical structures, each of which represents an example of "numbers" or "arithmetic" or "geometry." No one is more correct than another. They will, of course, differ in elegance and utility.
2. There exist a large number of presumed facts in psychology most of which can, sometimes with effort, be specified in terms of operational definitions.
3. By setting some mathematical structure in relation to a subset of the facts, we come out with a product that constitutes measurement within that limited universe.
4. The test of whether such measurement makes "sense" depends upon the power of the measurement.

The fault of psychological measurement in the past is not that it is wrong or nonsensical (as a rule!) but that it has been weak and trivial.

Stevens did not give this rebuttal. (See, however, Reese, 1943.) We talked about it but practical matters pressed and the outcome was rather the development in more general terms of the requirements for psychological measurement. This treatment of scales of measurement bypassed the narrow view of the Campbell committee.

The Answer: Scales of Measurement

A glance at the early statement of Campbell, at the McGregor paper of 1936, at the report to the British Association, and at two or three other publications in the same period, makes clear that there was no evident way out of the confrontation. The Campbell position was narrow. In 1939 Stevens (1939) proposed three types of scales, ordinal, intensive, and extensive, but these did not quite do the trick. Finally, in a paper read before the International Congress for the Unity of Science in September, 1941, he proposed the fourfold classification that is familiar to everyone.[2] This statement becomes the kernel, relatively unchanged in later presentations, of Stevens' position on measurement.

The first statement of the 1941 paper repeats what Campbell had said, often in fact, "Measurement ... may be defined as the assignment of numerals to objects or events according to rules." The second sentence is the kernel of what was added. "The fact that numerals can be assigned under different rules leads to different kinds of scales and different kinds of measurement."

What are these different kinds of scales? There are four types to be distinguished, nominal, ordinal, interval, and ratio. The effective definition of each type is in terms of a mathematical group-structure, that is, by stating those transformations which may be performed on the elements of a class while leaving invariant all other relations or properties which may exist among the elements in the class. Each such scale can be set into correspondence with at least one empirical operation such that the results of that operation are assumed to be isomorphic with the structure of the scale. There are listed, in the familiar 4×4 table, certain statistical procedures permissable for each of the scales.

So far as I can discover this classification is a relatively pure invention. It brings together two or three things which are crucial. First of all, it is responsive to one fact that every psychologist knows, i.e., how useful is quantification as an aid to clear thinking, without that quantification requiring elaborate mathematics. Why one should argue that counting of instances is not measurement, albeit primitive measurement, is hard to conceive. The second point was the avoidance of the operation of addition as the alpha and omega of measurement. It is curious how strong is our belief

[2] This paper corresponds rather closely to the second part of the 1946 paper (Stevens, 1946) in *Science*. It contains the four scales with their new names. So far as I know it was read to the International Congress for the Unity of Science in Cambridge, Massachusetts, in September, 1941. It was mimeographed and given limited distribution.

in that view, and yet probably far more practical measurements depend on ratio devices, potentiometers, bridges, beam balances, photometers, than depend on addition. Most of geometry, as opposed to algebra, is built on ratio concepts.

From the more formal point of view the key difference from earlier treatments lies in the use of a particular set of relationships to define the group structures corresponding to each scale. The traditional treatment which regarded natural numbers as something very special did not need this approach. But in the more sophisticated treatment of irrational or imaginary numbers, the concept of group structure is fundamental. Stevens' choices were more modest, but they still contrasted with the usual treatment of the cardinal numbers. It requires a trivial demonstration to prove that the two structures, one based on addition, the other on multiplication, are equivalent. On the other hand, so far as I know, a detailed formal demonstration, starting from familiar postulates, of just this set of group-structures has never been carried out. It would be a delightful exercise.

In a substantial sense, the scales of measurement as a theory were complete in the 1941 paper. There may remain some question of whether all the methods developed later were fully congruent with that model. As a guess, they are. There is also a good deal of evidence, particularly in the 1949 draft of the Handbook chapter on measurement, that Stevens continued to search in Russell, in Bell, in Haskin and other sources for other simple formulations that might accomplish the same purpose.[3] The evidence is that he found none. What came out, rather, was a moderately sophisticated setting for the rough diamond. Interest in a theory of measurement lagged, and by the 1950's issues in empirical psychophysics took the center of the stage.

Epilogue

In his discussion of mathematical philosophy, Bertrand Russell makes the point that it is the task of philosophy to move from those things which are open and obvious, concepts such as number and measurement, to less obvious but perhaps more fundamental concepts. The creation of *Principia Mathematica* is the evident example. Perhaps the time has come to ask this question about measurement. What we have done is to show that there are certain kinds of numbers of arithmetic which can be set down in correspondence to scientific operations in the realm of psychology. We are asserting thereby that there exists a significant isomorphism between the two, the mathematics on the one hand and empirical science on the other. Yet if they are isomorphic they are both instances of some common structure. This should tell us something. What is the larger class of which these are instances? For want of a better term we simply have to label it scientific theory – or in this case, a theory of measurement. In a sense, both Stevens and Campbell stopped short of asserting this. Perhaps the time has come to go on.

[3] This draft was widely circulated in mimeographed form. Except for very minor additions, it is identical with Stevens (1951).

Campbell said simply that "measurement may be defined as the assignment of numerals to things so as to represent facts about them ..." Numerals accomplish this purpose because "the primary function of numerals [is] to represent number, a property of all groups." (Ferguson, 1940, p. 340) Numerals and number have a rather fixed place in this firmament.

Stevens, as we have said, cast the net much more broadly. "Measurement ... may be defined as the assignment of numerals to objects or events according to rules ... different rules lead to different kinds of scales and different kinds of measurement." (1946, p. 677)

Let me close by adding my own definition:

A theory of measurement is the logical structure which makes it possible to express psychological (more generally, scientific) *facts in quantitative terms.* It is the conjunction, not the juxtaposition, of mathematics and psychology.

References

Boring, E. G. The logic of the normal law of error in mental measurement. *American Journal of Psychology*, 1920, **31**, 1–33.

Boring, E. G. *A history of experimental psychology*. New York: Century, 1929.

Campbell, N. R. *Physics, the elements*. Cambridge: University Press, 1920.

Churcher, B. G. A loudness scale for industrial noise measurements. *Journal of the Acoustical Society of America*, 1935, **6**, 216–226.

Ferguson, A. (Chm.) Quantitative estimates of sensory events. Final report of the Committee to consider and report upon the possibility of quantitative estimates of sensory events. *The Report of the British Association for the Advancement of Science*, 1940, No. 2, 331–349.

Fletcher, H. Auditory patterns. *Review of Modern Physics*, 1940, **12**, 47–65.

Fletcher, H., & Munson, W. A. Loudness, its definition, measurement and calculation. *Journal of the Acoustical Society of America*, 1933, **5**, 82–108.

French, N. R., & Steinberg, J. C. Factors governing the intelligibility of speech sounds. *Journal of the Acoustical Society of America*, 1947, **19**, 90–119.

Jørgensen, J. Treatise of formal logic. Copenhagen: Levin & Munksgaard, 1931.

Kingsbury, B. A. A direct comparison of the loudness of pure tones. *Physical Review*, 1927, **29**, 588–600.

McGregor, D. Scientific measurement and psychology. *Psychological Review*, 1935, **42**, 246–266.

Newman, E. B. The validity of the just noticeable difference as a unit of psychological magnitude. *Transactions Kansas Academy of Sciences*, 1933, **36**, 172–175.

Newman, E. B. Stevens's operationism. *Journal of the Acoustical Society of America*, 1973, **54**, 864–866.

Reese, T. W. The application of the theory of physical measurement to the measurement of psychological magnitudes, with three experimental examples. *Psychological Monographs*, 1943, **55** (3, Whole No. 251).

Russell, B. *Introduction to mathematical philosophy*. London: Allen and Unwin, 1919.

Stevens, S. S. The attributes of tones. *Proceedings National Academy of Sciences*, 1934, **20**, 457–459. (a)

Stevens, S. S. Tonal density. *Journal of Experimental Psychology*, 1934, **17**, 585–592. (b)

Stevens, S. S. The volume and intensity of tones. *American Journal of Psychology*, 1934, **46**, 397–408. (c)

Stevens, S. S. A scale for the measurement of a psychological magnitude: Loudness. *Psychological Review*, 1936, **43**, 405–416.

Stevens, S. S. On the problem of scales for the measurement of psychological magnitudes. *Journal of Unified Science (Erkenntnis)*, 1939, **9**, 94–99.

Stevens, S. S. On the theory of scales of measurement. *Science*, 1946, **103**, 677–680.

Stevens, S. S. Mathematics, measurement, and psychophysics. In S. S. Stevens (Ed.), *Handbook of experimental psychology*, New York: Wiley, 1951.

Stevens, S. S., & Davis, H. Psychophysiological acoustics: Pitch and loudness. *Journal of the Acoustical Society of America*, 1936, **8**, 1–13.

Stevens, S. S., Davis, H., & Lurie, M. H. The localization of pitch perception on the basilar membrane. *Journal of General Psychology*, 1935, **13**, 297–315.

Stevens, S. S., Volkmann, J., & Newman, E. B. A scale for the measurement of the psychological magnitude pitch. *Journal of the Acoustical Society of America*, 1937, **8**, 185–190.

THE NEW YORK STUDY OF PHYSICAL CONSTITUTION AND PSYCHOTIC PATTERN[1]

WILLIAM H. SHELDON
University of Oregon Medical School

Abstract. The paper provides a short history of somatotyping, including the early indices that were based upon 17 different measurements, and a subsequent system that was simpler, and comprised three primary parameters. From longtudinal studies of students, and experiments in starvation in which the individual's weights changed markedly during the starvation regimen, it appears that the individual's somatotype remains constant during the trajectory of life. The paper also shows the necessity for these three basic parameters to determine a somatotype, and illustrates how the somatotyping procedure has been made an objective method.

There is one apparently urgent need common to all doctors. Whether physician, surgeon or psychiatrist, the doctor needs to comprehend the distinctive, characteristic and persisting individuality of the person with whom he is confronted. Against some familiar frame of reference with which he is as intimately at home as a rat must be at home with his immediate geography, a doctor needs to be alertly aware of the underlying biological predisposition of his patient. It may be the psychiatrist's main job to promote and use this awareness. If so, he has a primary need to be grounded in a constitutional taxonomy.

The first imperative for such a taxonomy was that of discovering first order criteria for the classification of human physiques. We had obvious criteria for differentiating man from the rest of the animal kingdom and for separating one sex from the other. All members of the same sex are not alike, however. They differ in innumerable ways, and in terms of a host of indices they could be sorted and classified. The challenge lay in finding those variables for sorting physiques which would produce the most fruitful and meaningful schema. These would be our first order variables.

Three primary aspects of bodily constitution were selected for study because they behave in bodily morphology as though each were a *component* of structure – something which enters universally but in different amounts into the making of every organism. Identification of these three is simple and straightforward. In order to facilitate the procedure and standardize the technique, the subjects are photographed from the three angles – front, back and side. From a series of several thousand photographs of young men of college age it thus became an easy task to select those which showed the most extreme variations in the components under examination. Study of these extreme examples led to objective measurements which ultimately set each polar group apart from the other poles.

Three primary components were identified. The name of the first component, endomorphy, is derived from the fact that the digestive viscera, which (in endomorphs)

[1] Reprinted from *Journal of the History of the Behavioral Sciences* (1971) 7, pp. 119–126.

H. R. Moskowitz et al. (eds.), Sensation and Measurement. 147–155.

tend to dominate the bodily economy, develop essentially from the *endoderma.* embryonic layer. The second component, mesomorphy, means predominance of bone, muscle and connective tissue – the three principal *mesodermal* tissues. The third component, *ectomorphy*, appears to define a radical biological departure involving sacrifice of bodily mass in favor of surface. In proportion to his mass, an ectomorph has the greatest surface area and hence the greatest exposure to the outside world. Relative to his mass he therefore has the largest investment in skin and in sensory exteroceptors together with central nervous system and brain – all of which come from the *ectodermal* embryonic layer.

The somatotype is simply a three digit formula expressing the strength of each of these three primary components on a 7 point scale. The somatotypes 117, 171 and 711 are excessively rare polar extremes. The 444, a common somatotype in the male, is near the midpoint in all components.

It will readily be seen that both endomorphy and mesomorphy describe compactness of body (the pyknic physique in Kretschmer's terms), but two *very different kinds* of compactness. For an endomorph, the abdominal segment – the boiler room, as we sometimes say, seems to be dominant and to overshadow the thoracic segment, or engine room. Endomorphs are digestive athletes, as it were. They are champion processors of food, easily producing surplus fat for storage throughout the body. Therefore they tend to assume roundness of form, and to become spherically compact when they are overly nourished. The abdominal segment is king. Mesomorphs, on the other hand, are compact because they invest heavily in the supportive framework of the body – the somatic hard substance, bone and muscle, with connective tissue. The mesomorphic extremities become powerfully developed, and the thoracic segment is king, prevailing strongly over the boiler room. Mesomorphy means athletic potential in the conventional sense and the suggestion of squareness, cuboidal ruggedness, and chestiness.

Ectomorphy defines an opposite to both kinds of compactness. This condition is really stretched-outness. An ectomorphic creature, of any kind, appears to be one who has abandoned the obvious biological securities of compact massiveness in favor of a pursuit, presumably, of some other kind of advantage which may accrue from an adventurous extension into what, for the growing organism, is unknown space and danger. The ectomorphic way would seem to be a dangerous way, perhaps like the danger of falling from a height. This may be why ectomorphs, when they break mentally, tend to break irreparably. One of the oldest and most constant observations in constitutional psychiatry emphasizes the tendency of ectomorphs toward that pattern of schizophrenia which used to be called hebephrenic – and almost always with a poor prognosis. It has been suggested that for ectomorphs the term schizophrenia should be translated, not split mind but fractured mind. Ectomorphy may be a high priced luxury, with fracturability a part of the cost. But such a luxury may be worth its cost. In the field of constitutional *values* we are appallingly ignorant.

The method of somatotyping, when first presented in *Varieties of Human Physique*, in 1940, involved four rather simple steps. First, calculate the ratio height over the cube root of weight, using a nomograph prepared for the purpose. Second, record 17 transverse measurements, each expressed as a ratio to stature.

The first four measurements are of the head and neck; the next three thoracic; the third group of three are arm measurements; the fourth group are abdominal; and the last group of four are leg measurements. Third, inspect the photograph and, referring to the table on which all the known somatotypes are distributed against the criterion height over the cube root of weight, make your estimate as to the somatotype. Normally one has available a file of correctly somatotyped photographs for comparison. Fourth, now turn to the 17 transverse measurements that you've recorded under the five appropriate bodily regions, and for each of the 17 consult the table on which the distribution of known somatotypes is plotted against the range of scores for that measurement. What one actually is doing, in each of these 17 instances, is measuring any deviation from the tentative somatotype estimate that was just recorded (step three).

At Harvard, in 1940, Professor S. S. Stevens built a machine which greatly facilitated this process by wiring into an illuminated switchboard the measurement patterns for each of the known somatotypes. With this machine, after the measurements were available, it was possible to determine the nearest somatotype in two or three minutes. The Harvard somatotyping machine also eliminated the need for step three, as presented above, since the switchboard included the height over cube root of weight ratio as an eighteenth measurement.

However, as matters turned out, this method of somatotyping from 17 measurements and a ponderal index was eventually to be superseded by a much simpler although more comprehensive procedure.

Some Recurrent Objections to Somatotyping, and Further Objectification

As the theory of somatotyping was published in the first volume of the Human Constitution series, a number of major problems were doubtless over-simplified and some were left unexplored – or even worse, unmentioned. Hundreds of critical papers have resulted, some excellent and constructive; a few voicing mere emotional protest at the vulgar corruption of psychiatry with organic considerations. Space does not permit a review of this commentative literature here, but there are at least four specific objections which have been so cogently expressed or so widely discussed that it is almost mandatory for a serious presentation of the somatotyping idea to mention them. These are the main objections: (1) The somatotype changes. (2) Somatotyping is not objective. (3) There are only two, not three primary components. (4) Somatotyping omits the factor of size.

The objection that the somatotype changes has been regarded academically as a most damaging criticism. It has been possible to test this objection only by longitudinal studies carried out over respectably long periods. The real problem, of course, lies in the definition of the somatotype, and in the selection of the determining criteria. It will be recalled that in the very earliest beginnings somatotypes were determined by subjective inspection of photographs. This appeared to be the only possible way to make a sensible start. At the University of Chicago, with the help and guidance of Dr L. L. Thurstone, who was mentor to my Ph.D. thesis, we had tried to use cluster analysis – later called factor analysis – in half a dozen attempts to identify primary factors in physical constitution. The results varied remarkably with different sets of measurements, although when I finally tried transverse measurements only – 32 of them – Thurstone decided that four primary factors were demonstrated, and that one of these factors was size. When we expressed all the measurements as ratios to stature, thus eliminating size, three factors remained. These apparently were expressions of the same three primary components that were later used in somatotyping. At any rate, the 17 measurements which were later used were selected from the original 32.

In the first laying out of the somatotypes, with 4000 sets of pictures, after deciding to try a 7 point scale and three primary components, we were confronted with the question, how many somatotypes shall there be? That would have been easy to answer if at the outset there had been available objective and unchanging criteria for determining the somatotype. But, of course, the purpose of the study was to find precisely those criteria. The question would have been self-answering if I could have assumed that the three primary components were completely orthogonal – zero correlations with one another. Then there could be 343 somatotypes, the cube of 7. At the other extreme, a critical threshold of high negative correlations would demand that the three components add up to a constant. This would be a *reductio ad absurdum*, for then the somatotypes would be plottable only on a plane surface, would have no third dimensional existence, and in fact would not exist as three structural components at all, but as only two. For if the sum of three units is a constant the third has no independent existence; and in that case the outcome of our experiment in three dimensional description of the human organism would simply have been a paper-thin man, two-dimensional. Since I had never encountered a two-dimensional man it seemed reasonable that a scientific classification of men had better rest its case on at least three primary structural dimensions.

Clearly it was necessary to steer between the Scylla of complete dependence and the Charybdis of complete independence among the primary dimensions. After a series of soul-searching discussions with Dr. Thurstone, who still played the kindly role of statistical mentor for my project, it was decided that in the absence of any advance knowledge of the probable correlations among our presumptive three primary dimensions, there could be no way of setting up *a priori* a correct set of boundaries for the somatotype matrix. It was like cutting a suit of clothes for a man you couldn't see, and whose measurements had never been taken. The only thing to do was to cut the suit by guess and common sense, try it out, and remodel – perhaps repeating the process many times.

At this point I recalled my first conversation with Kretschmer, and his patient answers to my then youthfully impatient academic insistence that *his* primary components of human constitutional variation ought to be mathematically objectified. "Yes, I would like that too," he said, "but that may be a long way off yet. Perhaps it will be done in another generation. Now it would be like dressing a baby in men's clothes".

Well, by 1940 it seemed time to try out a suit for the somatotype matrix, and we made up one. By then we had for years been "recognizing" such somatotypes as 711 and 444 – 9-totals and 12-totals, as well as tens and elevens. Thurstone had agreed that since men are structurally three-dimensional, surely *that* much "thickness" must be present in the somatotype matrix – *that* much independence among the components. So I postulated a matrix of 76 somatotypes, almost immediately added three more in the endomorph-mesomorph "Northwest", and *Varieties of Human Physique* went to press with 9-totals, 10-totals, 11-totals, and 12-totals. (No 8-totals and no 13-totals.)

For our purpose this matrix "worked" in the sense that it seemed feasible and fitting – by subjective criteria at this stage – to include all of the available cases within the 79 categories. And the distribution was 3-dimensionally continuous. There were examples for each category. The garment *appeared* to fit the contours, so far as a sizable population of college youths was concerned. I was well aware, as were several of my associates, that there were problems. The intuition grew that the material in that garment just might be more suggestive of stretchable elastic than of good English worsted, and by the mid-nineteen fifties that intuition had become a certainty. But more of this in a few minutes.

In laying out the original schema, we had of course visualized the somatotype as a dynamic, not a static concept. The height-weight ratio constituted one of the principal determining criteria, but this ratio travels through time as a trajectory, not as a straight line. From the data of the Actuarial Society of America, we had the "normal curve" for height over cube root of weight, from age 18 to 65, for 221 819 men who had been accepted for life insurance. From many cross-sectional (non-longitudinal) somatotype studies of men and women of various ages I had been able to construct approximately accurate trajectories of this sort for all of the common somatotypes, and for the rare ones by interpolation or extrapolation.

In 1954, in *Atlas of Men*, we published these trajectories for each of the 88 somatotypes which by then had been included in the putative somatotype matrix. Also by 1954, all of my associates had for more than a decade been teaching that for somatotyping purposes, just as a person's height is the maximal height of record, the somatotyping ponderal index (SPI) must likewise be based on the heaviest ponderal index of record. By this rule, for somatotypic purposes, just as a person gets credit for his greatest achieved investment in linearity, so also he gets credit for his greatest achieved investment in mass. Otherwise the somatotype would indeed be a mere phenotypic concept, subject to change with any change in nutritional status.

By 1956 several normal, clinical and psychiatric populations had been followed, some of them for nearly 20 years. It had become very clear that despite nutritional changes the fundamental constitutional pattern remains stubbornly constant through life. We were searching for a set of parameters which both reflect the basic pattern accurately and remain constant. Certainly more than one hundred anthropometric measurements, ratio and indices had been explored – only to be found inadequate to that assignment. However, working with the Berkeley Growth Study at the University of California, we turned up an index that looked promising.

This was simply the area of the thoracic trunk over the area of the abdominal trunk, measured with a planimeter on a standard somatotype photograph. The trunk was divided at the nearest possible approximation to the plane of the anatomical waist – this is the plane midway between the lowermost plane of the ribs and the uppermost plane of the pelvis, with the individual standing fully erect. For the purposes of deriving and standardizing this index – now called the *trunk index* – the TT (thoracic trunk) is the numerator and the AT (abdominal trunk) the denominator. The upper limit of the TT is defined by a line connecting the points where the sterno-cleido-mastoids cross the trapezii. The lower limit of AT is at the photographic center of the angle of the sub-gluteal fold. A specially constructed rectangular frame is used for holding the three photographs – frontal, lateral and dorsal – at exactly the same level with reference to one another while the areas are marked off.

The trunk index turned out to be a singularly valuable ratio, solving three of our difficult somatotyping problems. First, it provided an apparently dependable parameter for differentiating quantitatively between endomorphy and mesomorphy. Second, it has proved to be a constant, at least from the third year of life to old age, and is completely independent of nutritional state. That is to say, it is unaffected even by extreme variations in fatness or leanness, and in this last characteristic is unique among the almost countless measurements and ratio with which I have experimented. Third, it opened the way to a complete objectification of somatotyping.

At the University of California in 1929, a long term growth study and follow-up study of almost 1000 children was initiated. The subjects were about equally divided between the two sexes. Nearly half of them were born during the year 1928–29. For approximately 400 of this series, somatotype photographs were taken at least once a year until the subjects were fully grown. Many of them were followed through their twenties, and some through their thirties. The 400 who stayed with the California project until they were fully grown are being studied intensively in connection with our project on the development of the somatotype in children. For all of the 400 the trunk index remained constant from the first photograph to the last. The TI may not be altogether a genetically determined characteristic, but it certainly is a pattern which stays constant through childhood, except for cases developing major pathology.

At the University of Minnesota, during World War II, a "starvation experiment" was carried out on a group of 34 subjects. Under mild starvation conditions these men lost from 25% to 40% of their total weight. Somatotype photographs of them were taken before and after the weight loss. All of these photographs were somatotyped during 1958 at the Texas Instruments Branch of the Constitution Laboratory, and at this time the trunk indices were calculated. The starvation changed none of the trunk indices (and, therefore, actually, none of the somatotypes.)

Somatotype photographs were taken of the class entering the United States Military Academy at West Point in 1946, and again on graduation in 1950. These boys had the advantages of closely supervised body conditioning and muscle developing exercises for four years at West Point. Many of them changed remarkably in their general appearance of physical competence and in the surface manifestations of muscular definition. But for all of them the trunk index remained a constant.

At Columbia University, somatotype photographs of the entering freshmen were taken regularly in the years between 1912 and 1917. In 1955 we re-photographed 208 of these Columbia graduates at the Constitution Laboratory in the Columbia Medical Center. None of the trunk indices had changed, although weight in a few instances had nearly doubled, and in a few other cases had decreased.

In a series of 46 pairs of identical twins of both sexes studied at the Constitution Laboratory during the same period, the trunk indices were identical within each pair, although in a few cases there were dramatic nutritional differences.

At this time we were running a follow-up study of 412 women and 22 men who had been attending the Columbia Medical Center Nutrition Clinic for purposes of supervised weight reduction. Some of the women succeeded in shedding – very temporarily – as much as 150 pounds. But the photographs at maximal and at minimal weight showed no detectable changes in trunk index. This remained constant despite nutritional changes.

In brief, then, the trunk index appears to remain unchanged from early childhood through late middle life – in both sexes. From the point of view of both objectification and standardization of somatotyping, this was news of some importance.

The next experiment was that of running the trunk index on a sample of 2000 young men and 2000 young women from our file of "standard examples" of all of the "recognized common somatotypes". It will be recalled that these collections had necessarily been built up from photographs somatotyped by the older partially objective – partially subjective procedure. It was soon discovered that in somatotyping, one thing we had learned to do was in large measure to make a surprisingly accurate subjective estimate of the trunk index – long before this index had been "discovered."

When the trunk indices for all the then available somatotypes were plotted, three facts almost literally jumped out from the page. (1) This ratio was manifestly a constant for those somatotypes in which endomorphy and mesomorphy were in balance. (2) Its variation was completely independent – zero correlation, in fact, for both sexes – with ectomorphy. (3) There was strongly positive correlation with mesomorphy, strongly negative correlation with endomorphy. In mesomorphy the thoracic segment really *is* king, and in endomorphy the abdominal segment is king.

Even more remarkable was the fact that the progression from endomorphic dominance to mesomorphic dominance, in both sexes, advanced in a series of progressive increments in trunk index. In somatotypes with the first component (endomorphy) at 7 and the second component (mesomorphy) at 1, the TI (trunk index) falls at 0.85 – and in those rare extreme asymptotic endomorphs who may weigh 600 pounds or more, at an even lower level. (I have one case of a 700 pound woman with a TI of 0.65, but in our experience only one in about 4500 women, and one in about 13000 men reaches this asymptotic tail of the distribution on TI).

In somatotypes with both of the first two components at 4, or at any other level, from 1 to 7, the TI falls at 1:45. When the first component is at 1, and the second at 7, the TI is 2.05. Here again there is an extreme asymptotic tail where the TI reaches still higher levels. We have two cases at 2.25 and one at 2.35. These men look like comic strip characters with gigantic chests and shoulders, and beanpole abdominal segments. They suggest Al Capp's L'il Abner.

We now had an operational procedure for objectively fixing the relative strengths of endomorphy and mesomorphy; and also, in the ponderal index taken at maximal mass, a second objective parameter – if we could just find a way to make effective use of it. But a third such parameter was needed. By definition the somatotype is a point in three-dimensional space. Such a point is actually the crossing point for three distributions, or three parameters.

I finally woke up, after twenty years of somewhat feeblemindedly making a hobby of this problem. The third parameter was, of course, stature. Maximal height is simply the degree of extension into space. When the other two parameters are known, that is precisely what ectomorphy is. First we have to have a measure of maximal massiveness (SPI); then a separator for the two kinds of mass (TI); finally, a measure of the degree of stretched-outness into space (MH or maximal height).

Even back in 1954 I had published, in *Atlas of Men*, a table listing the mean height we had found for each somatotype in the male. For many years I had *used* height in somatotyping, but had not standardized its use as a determining parameter. The final move was just that step of standardization. We found that, as in the case of TI, the old subjective somatotyping had also made remarkably systematic use of this third parameter without fully appreciating what it was doing. The final step was to work out the systematic and realistic distribution of somatotypes on maximal stature. This was done, and a final set of basic tables for somatotyping was prepared.

In studies carried out since these tables have been available, it has been found that the matrix of somatotypes which originally we set up, and published in 1940, was almost shockingly too conservative. In this later work, by letting our three objective parameters *themselves* determine what somatotypes exist, we have now found it necessary to deal with a matrix far thicker than that originally postulated. Previously we had assigned somatotypes totalling 10, 11, and 12 with a few 9s. With the now fully objective procedure we find, in addition, somatotypes totalling 7 and 8, with all of the 9s; also 13, 14 and 15. Instead of the original matrix of 76 somatotypes, gradually expanded to 88, we now have a matrix of 267 7-point scale somatotypes, or 1713 13-point scale somatotypes. This results, of course, from the fact that the inter-correlations among the three objectively determined components are far lower than we originally dared suppose. TI yields zero correlations – orthogonality – with stature and with ectomorphy. The correlations between endomorphy and mesomorphy approach zero in both sexes. In males the mean for this correlation hovers around −0.05; in females, around +0.05. The ectomorphy-endomorphy correlations, and the ectomorphy-mesomorphy correlations, always negative, now average about −0.40 in both instances.

Return now to the four critical objections regarding the somatotype:

1. The somatotype changes. It cannot change, since maximal stature and maximal massiveness are simply items of historical fact, and TI is constant through life.

2. It is not objective. Now it is completely objective. It can be derived on a computer as a function of three parameters, thus providing an operational definition of the procedure.

3. There are only two, not three primary components. This difficulty no longer exists. It arose from the fact that the negative correlations among the primary components were too high. That condition has been corrected, thus permitting us to live and operate in three spatial dimensions again.

4. Omits the factor of size. Size has been restored by using stature as a determining parameter.

FAMILIES OF CONVERGING POWER FUNCTIONS IN PSYCHOPHYSICS[1]

JOSEPH C. STEVENS

John B. Pierce Foundation and Yale University

Abstract. Thirteen families of psychophysical power functions from the auditory, visual, proprioceptive, warmth, and cold modalities, are shown to have the property that the members of each family intersect at a common point. In some cases this point corresponds to a very strong stimulus level that approximates the threshold of pain and maybe the ceiling level for the modality.

Early statements of the psychophysical power law tended to highlight the variation of the shape of the input-output curve from one sense-modality to the other in the face of the invariance of the power relation. As one after another modality came under investigation each appeared to give a power function, but also to have its own "characteristic exponent." Summary statements spread the information that the exponent ranges from about 0.33 for subjective brightness to about 3.5 for 60-Hz electric current passed through the fingers.

Although it was useful and interesting to point out this variation among modalities, there were those who erroneously took it to mean that the exponent for a given modality is a single, fixed quantity (not counting measurement variance). This is not so. The exponent can vary enormously (though systematically) with the sundry dimensions of stimulation – the level of adaptation, the stimulus duration, the locus and areal extent of stimulation of the sensory surface, the frequency of a tone or vibration, the presence of inhibitory stimulation, and the like. In fact, a most useful feature of the direct scaling methods is that they can be put to use to generate, often conveniently and quickly, entire families of power functions, whose parameters (slopes and intercepts) abound in information about the dynamic, functional properties of a sense modality.

It happens also that a number of such families (but by no means all) display the interesting feature that when plotted as straight lines in log-log coordinates they converge on a point corresponding to some intense stimulus level. The properties of this particular class of psychophysical families furnish the subject of this paper.

Apparent Heaviness: An Illustration of how to Analyze the Data

As the first example (Figure 1) consider a family for apparent heaviness obtained by magnitude estimation of lifted objects that varied in both weight (abscissa) and volume (parameter) in the same test session. The plot shows that for any constant volume, estimated heaviness grows as a power function of weight; but the larger the volume,

[1] This research was supported by Grant AFOSR 70-1950 from the United States Air Force Office of Scientific Research.

H. R. Moskowitz et al. (eds.), Sensation and Measurement. 157–165. *All Rights Reserved.*

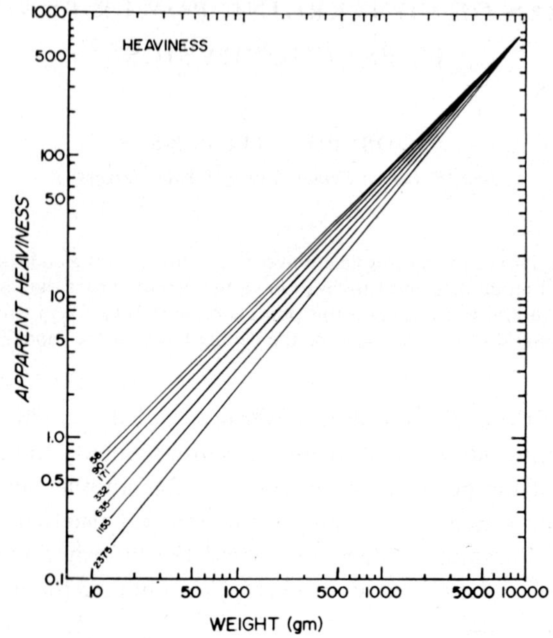

Fig. 1. The family of power functions for the apparent heaviness of lifted weights. The parameter is the volume of the weights in milliliters. Constructed from the data plotted in Figure 2.

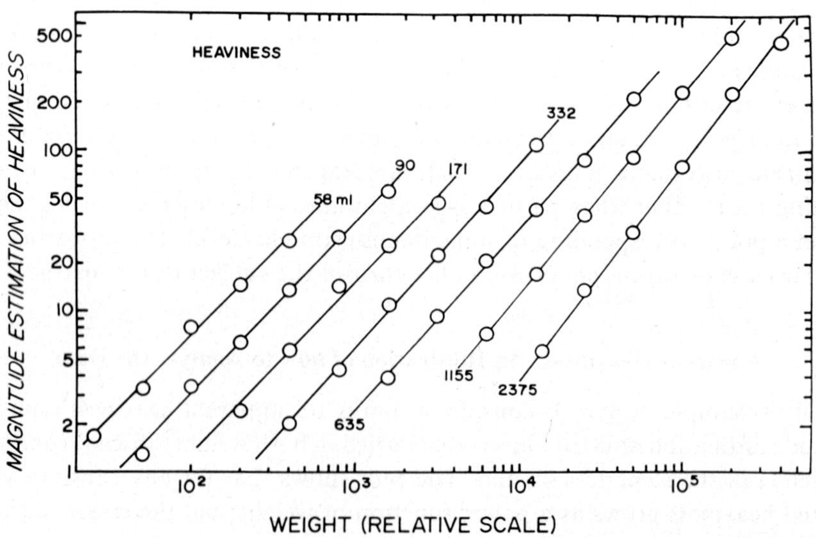

Fig. 2. Apparent heaviness as a function of weight. The abscissa is a relative scale only. For clarity the horizontal positions of the seven functions were arbitrarily adjusted.

the steeper the log-log function. Note that for any given weight, the larger the volume over which it is distributed, the lighter the weight feels. This is the famous size-weight illusion. (In fact a horizontal cut through Figure 1 serves to specify the combinations of weight and volume that produce a given constant degree of heaviness.) Figure 2 shows the data (geometric means from 14 observers) from which the idealized picture in Figure 1 was constructed. (For clarity, the power functions in Figure 2 were spread apart horizontally so that the convergence is not obvious here as it is in Figure 1.)

These results with lifted weights brought to light a convenient and interesting property of a convergent family of functions having the generic power formula

$$\psi = k\varphi^{\beta}, \tag{1}$$

where ψ is subjective magnitude and φ is physical magnitude, namely that the size of β must relate to the size of k by a logarithmic function. Consider the family in its logarithmic form

$$\log\psi = \beta \log\varphi + \log k, \tag{2}$$

and assume that the members intersect at the point $\log\psi = a$, $\log\varphi = c$. Then by substitution and rearrangement of terms

$$a = c\beta + \log k \quad (\text{or } \log k = a - c\beta). \tag{3}$$

Figure 3 (semi-log coordinates) illustrates this point (using the constants β and k

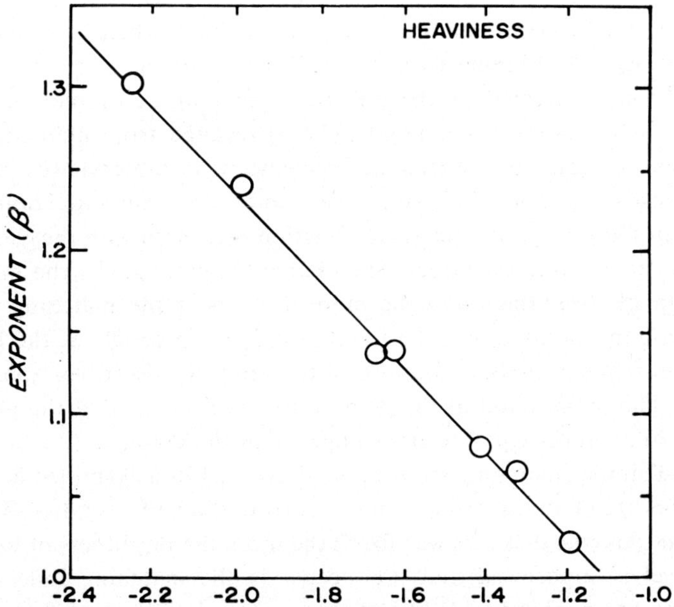

Fig. 3. Showing the relation between β and k for the power function for heaviness.

obtained by the method of least squares applied to the data of Figure 2) in that β approximates a log function of k.

A plot like Figure 3 not only signifies that we deal with a convergent family, but it also can furnish a good objective estimate of the intersection point. You simply fit the best log function, then take the antilogarithm of the slope of the line. The result gives the stimulus level at which the functions "ideally" intersect. A proof goes as follows. From any pair of intersecting functions $\psi = k_1\varphi^{\beta_1}$ and $\psi = k_2\varphi^{\beta_2}$ it follows from equality of ψ at the intersection point that

$$k_1\varphi^{\beta_1} = k_2\varphi^{\beta_2}. \tag{4}$$

Algebraic rearrangement of Equation 4 gives the expression

$$\frac{\log k_1 - \log k_2}{\beta_2 - \beta_1} = \log \varphi, \tag{5}$$

which is equivalent to the slope of the log function (as in Figure 3). For lifted weights the point of intersection turned out to lie at about 8 kg, or approximately the maximum weight that the average subject can lift under the experimental conditions (for details, see J. C. Stevens & Rubin, 1970).

Visual Brightness

Other examples of convergent families are listed in Table 1, which gives several relevant summary features of 13 families from five sensory continua.

All families were generated by the method of magnitude estimation, except two. One of these, S. S. Stevens & Diamond's (1965) resulted from matching a criterion light (dependent variable) to a target light (independent variable) viewed in the presence of a small intense glare. The family comprises some 14 matching functions that plot as straight lines in log-log coordinates, each function measured with the glare at a particular angular distance from the target. The smaller the glare angle, the more the glare disrupts the target brightness and the more it steepens the matching function. As Stevens & Diamond pointed out, the family intersects precisely at the luminance of the glare (a subsequent analytic solution of the kind just described above confirmed the obvious). The intersection at the glare luminance means that the glare does not inhibit target luminances equal to or stronger than the glare.

A somewhat similar matching study (J. C. Stevens, 1967) examined how brightness depends on the size of an inhibiting annulus surrounding a target disk. The larger the area of the annulus (the disk size was fixed) the more the brightness of the disk at any luminance level is suppressed and the steeper is the matching function (in other words, the area of an inhibiting field and glare angle play similar roles). As expected, the family intersects at the luminance of the surround (i.e., no inhibition) regardless of the size of the annulus.

TABLE 1

Families of converging power functions

Continuum	Source	Independent variable	Parameter	Approximate convergence	Possible significance
Auditory volume	S. S. Stevens & Terrace (1962)	sound pressure	frequency	140 dB SPL	tickling & pain
Auditory density	Guirao & S. S. Stevens (1964)	sound pressure	frequency	130–150 dB SPL	tickling & pain
Heaviness	J. C. Stevens & Rubin (1970)	weight	volume	8 kg	maximum heft
Brightness	J. C. Stevens & S. S. Stevens (1963)	luminance	level of light adaptation	10^9 cd m^{-2}	solar luminance
Brightness	S. S. Stevens & Diamond (1965)	luminance	glare angle	2×10^5cd m^{-2}	glare luminance
Brightness	J. C. Stevens (1967)	luminance	size of inhibitory surround	32 cd m^{-2}	surround luminance
Cold	Marks & J. C. Stevens (1972)	lowering of irradiance from neutral	duration	1 W cm^{-2} below neutral	pain threshold?
Warmth	J. C. Stevens & Marks (1971)	3-s irradiation of forehead	areal extent	0.8 W cm^{-2}	pain threshold
Warmth	J. C. Stevens & Marks (1971)	3-s irradiation of back	areal extent	0.8 W cm^{-2}	pain threshold
Warmth	Marks & J. C. Stevens (1973)	0.5-s irradiation of forehead	areal extent	2.3 W cm^{-2}	pain threshold
Warmth	J. C. Stevens & Marks (unpublished)	3-s irradiation of forearm	areal extent	1.0 W cm^{-2}	pain threshold
Warmth	J. C. Stevens & Marks (unpublished)	3-s irradiation of cheek	areal extent	0.9 W cm^{-2}	pain threshold
Warmth	J. C. Stevens, Marks, & Simonson (unpublished)	3-s irradiation of calf	areal extent	0.9 W cm^{-2}	pain threshold

Another brightness study (J. C. Stevens & S. S. Stevens, 1963) called for magnitude estimates of targets viewed alternately by the dark-adapted (left) eye and the light-adapted (right) eye. A family of power functions was obtained relating brightness to luminance for several different levels of light adaptation. These functions extrapolate to a convergence point at a luminance level approximating that of the sun. The correctness of this extrapolation remains subject to direct test. Also, its meaning is not obvious, except to say that it is fortunate that strong lights have a relatively small adapting effect on the brightness of intense targets. Else we would fast grow used to intense stimulation at the peril of our eyes.

Audition

Two dimensions of hearing yielded convergent families: auditory volume (S. S. Stevens & Terrace, 1962) and density (Guirao & S. S. Stevens, 1964). Both grow as power functions of sound pressure, the slope (exponent) varying greatly with tonal frequency; the volume slope increases with frequency, the density slope decreases with frequency. In the present context the important finding is that both families extrapolate to an intersection point at about 140 db re 0.0002 μbar. This level is the threshold of "tickle" and pricking pain in the ear (not to be confused with a kind of general "discomfort" threshold some 20 dB lower). (For a discussion, see Licklider, 1951.) It is tempting to conjecture that this pain threshold may also mark the practical ceiling on the growth of auditory experience per se (as opposed to sensations of tickle, pain, burning, dizziness, etc. which may continue to grow with increases in pressure beyond 140 dB).

Warmth and Cold

Next, we turn to the thermal continua. To study cold, (Marks & J. C. Stevens, 1972) the observer lay unclothed and supine in very cold, dry air (3–4 °C) beneath a panel of infra-red heat lamps regulated so as to keep him comfortable by offsetting the conductive loss to the cold air (Gagge & J. C. Stevens, 1968). Periodically this panel was abruptly displaced by another panel set at some lower radiance, thereby causing an immediate sensation of cold. Cold sensations grow markedly stronger over time as the skin cools. In this experiment the observers estimated the cold felt at the *end* of an exposure. Both the magnitude and the duration (4 to 31 s) of the exposure varied in the same test session.

For each duration a power function related the estimated cold to the change in the irradiance from the neutral level; the longer the duration, the larger the intercept k and the smaller the exponent β, such that the family extrapolates to an intersection at a level corresponding to a rate of heat loss of 1 W cm^{-2} (very roughly for the average male subject this means a heat loss from the ventral body surface of about 6.5 kW, which is approximately 75 times the basal metabolic heat rate). This finding eludes sure interpretation, but so rapid a heat loss would certainly feel painful within a few seconds.

Finally we turn to six families of warmth functions obtained with infrared irradiation of various areal extents of the skin of five body regions: forehead, back, forearm, cheek, and calf. Stimulations lasted three sec each, except that the forehead was stimulated for three and 0.5 s in two separate studies. As we shall see, the duration of stimulation has to do with the intersection point.

These studies of warmth all touch on the property of spatial summation, or ability of the warmth sense to integrate the neural effects of stimulation over large portions of the skin – up to anyway several hundreds of square centimeters. For all practical purposes a person cannot distinguish between a large area of weak stimulation and a small area of strong stimulation. In fact, Cain (1973) has demonstrated that a person cannot even distinguish a split field of irradiation from a unitary field, even when the field was split by as much as the anatomy of the back or the forearm would allow. In short, the warmth sense is geared primarily to gauge the total heat load on the skin and correspondingly fails at good spatial discrimination and localization. Therefore, the variation in area in these experiments rarely, if ever, actually registers itself as anything but a variation in subjective warmth.

One of the six families appears in Figure 4 (0.5-s stimulation of six different areal extents of the forehead). Three features of the family stand out. First, for any constant level of irradiance, the larger the area, the warmer the irradiation feels, i.e., spatial summation takes place; however, the degree of summation falls off with increasing level of irradiance and finally becomes zero at the convergence point. (This makes

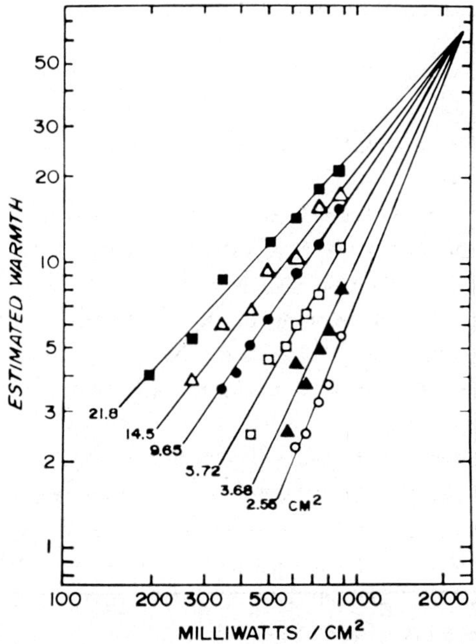

Fig. 4. Apparent warmth as a function of level of 0.5-s irradiance of the forehead. The parameter is the areal extent of stimulation in square centimeters.

sense, because measurements of the pain threshold show that there is no summation of thermally aroused pain [Greene & Hardy, 1958].) Second, each stimulus area yields a power function, and the smaller the area, the larger is the function's exponent. Third, the level at which convergence takes place, 2300 mW cm^{-2}, approximates the threshold of burning pain. Note in Table 1 that the convergence level of the other warmth families (3-s stimulations) is about 900 mW cm^{-2}, which also approximates the threshold of burning pain – i.e., the longer the stimulus, the smaller the irradiance level needed to heat the skin to the threshold of pain (approximately 45 °C).

As another example of how the convergence point can be estimated graphically, Figure 5 shows the constants of the psychophysical power functions in Figure 4, each calculated by the method of least squares. The result accords well with Equation 3, namely β is a log function of k. The intersection point, 2300 mW cm^{-2}, was computed with Equation 5.

Why do all the warmth functions, regardless of the areal extent, the body locus, and the duration of stimulation, consistently intersect near (or at) the pain threshold? It may well be that the pain threshold marks the terminus of warmth sensation per se. Of course, increasing the irradiance beyond this point will augment the degree of *pain*. According to J. D. Hardy (personal communication), author of the dol scale of pain, pain aroused by heat irradiation *lacks* the quality of warmth. Moreover, the firing rate of warmth receptors, measured by Hensel & Kenshalo (1969) in the cat, plunges to baseline when the stimulating temperature exceeds approximately 45 °C. Perhaps the

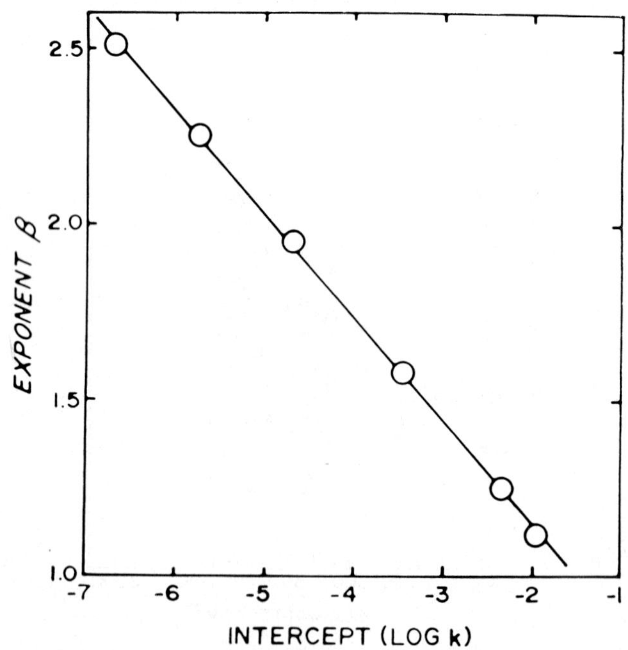

Fig. 5. Showing the relation between β and k for the power functions for warmth.

warmth sensation not only reaches a ceiling but also declines or even vanishes beyond the pain threshold.

The last column in Table 1 lists the possible significance of the convergence points. In some instances it seems to coincide roughly with the appearance of pain, possibly signaling that a ceiling on the continuum has been approached. Ceilings on most sensory continua are, needless to say, difficult, maybe impossible, to demonstrate directly. (For one thing it is hard to conscript subjects for such experimentation.) Convergence may, however, tell us where to look for a ceiling.

In some cases convergence is easier to interpret. The intersection of the brightness functions at the level of an inhibitory glare field is consistent with a whole body of psychophysical knowledge about visual inhibition. In the case of lifted weights, the convergence seems to be determined simply by the maximum that muscles can do.

It is true that the meaning of convergence remains partly a matter of speculation. It is nevertheless indisputably a common phenomenon in recent psychophysical investigation, and the psychophysicist may well want to be on the lookout for fresh occurrences of it.

References

Cain, W. S. Spatial discrimination of warmth. *American Journal of Psychology*, 1973, **86**, 169–181.

Gagge, A. P., & Stevens, J. C. Thermal sensitivity and comfort. In D. R. Kenshalo (Ed.), *The skin senses*. Springfield, Ill.: Charles C. Thomas, 1968, pp. 345–367.

Greene, L. E., & Hardy, J. D. Spatial summation of pain. *Journal of Applied Physiology*, 1958, **13**, 457–464.

Guirao, M., & Stevens, S. S. Measurement of auditory density. *Journal of the Acoustical Society of America*, 1964, **36**, 1176–1182.

Hensel, H., & Kenshalo, D. R. Warm receptors in the nasal region of cats. *Journal of Physiology*, 1969, **204**, 99–112.

Licklider, J. C. R. Basic correlates of the auditory stimulus. In S. S. Stevens (Ed.), *Handbook of Experimental Psychology*. New York: Wiley, 1951, pp. 985–1039.

Marks, L. E., & Stevens, J. C. Perceived cold and skin temperature as functions of stimulation level and duration. *American Journal of Psychology*, 1972, **85**, 407–419.

Marks, L. E., & Stevens, J. C. Spatial summation of warmth: Influence of duration and configuration of the stimulus. *American Journal of Psychology*, 1973, **86**, 251–267.

Stevens, J. C. Brightness inhibition re size of surround. *Perception and Psychophysics*, 1967, **2**, 189–192.

Stevens, J. C., & Marks, L. E. Spatial summation and the dynamics of warmth sensation. *Perception and Psychophysics*, 1971, **9**, 391–398.

Stevens, J. C., & Rubin, L. L. Psychophysical scales of heaviness and the size-weight illusion. *Perception and Psychophysics*, 1970, **8**, 225–230.

Stevens, J. C., & Stevens, S. S. Brightness function: Effects of adaptation. *Journal of the Optical Society of America*, 1963, **53**, 375–385.

Stevens, S. S., & Diamond, A. L. Effect of glare angle on the brightness function for a small target. *Vision Research*, 1965, **5**, 649–659.

Stevens, S. S., & Terrace, H. S. The quantification of tonal volume. *American Journal of Psychology*, 1962, **75**, 596–604.

ON FACTS AND THEORIES IN PSYCHOPHYSICS: DOES EKMAN'S LAW EXIST?

ROBERT TEGHTSOONIAN[1]

Smith College

Abstract. A classical treatment of JND has been to make some assumption about its subjective size in order to construct a scale relating sensation to stimulus intensity; Fechner's law is one result of this tactic. Ekman's law asserts that sensations one JND apart define a constant ratio, and leads to the conclusion that sensation is a power function of stimulus intensity. However, reconsideration of the cited evidence suggests that Ekman's law is tautological with Weber's law.

An alternative approach regards matching experiments as involving two physical continua. Given Weber's law for both continua and cross-modal equivalence of JND, the matching continuum is a power function of the target continuum. Further, the exponent is inversely related to the Weber fraction on the target continuum. This second approach makes measures of resolving power compatible with cross-modal-matching data but avoids assumptions about the subjective size of the JND.

Prudence dictates the achievement of a clear distinction between the verified facts of a discipline, and the theoretical concepts that serve to organize, predict or summarize those facts. Regardless of one's personal taste for each of these aspects of a science (and it is well known that preference for one can engender considerable distaste for the other), it is essential to know and to recognise which is which; a failure to do so may generate two kinds of errors and it is hard to say whether it is more disagreeable to have theoretical concepts represented as facts, or to have empirical relations advertised as theories.

Since the emergence of the "new psychophysics" in the 1950s this fundamental distinction has been often blurred, and only gradually has an awareness of the problem emerged. (See for example Treisman, 1964a, 1964b; Savage, 1966; Stevens, 1964, 1966b.) At the theoretical level one may conceive of sensations, their magnitudes and discriminabilities, but that is quite different from the empirical enterprise of determining the relation between matched intensities on two (or more) physical continua and the ability of observers to resolve differences on those continua. I do not intend to advocate or disparage either of these activities but to suggest that on occasion we write about sensations as if they were public, empirical facts, and refer to our measurements as if they were made directly on sensation. More is at issue than precision or carelessness in the choice of words, although that in itself is not trivial. Of greater conse-

[1] This paper was written while the author was a visitor in the Psychological Laboratories of the University of Stockholm, and was prepared with support from Grant GB 38292 from the National Science Foundation. I wish to thank Hannes Eisler, Gunnar Goude and Martha Teghtsoonian for their valuable comments on an earlier version.

I take satisfaction in noting that this paper grew out of a talk presented on 22 October 1972, to a group in which S. S. Stevens was a vigorous participant. On that occasion Stevens, happily wearing his Fechner Day button, debated psychophysical issues with even more enthusiasm than usual, so I remember vividly the opportunity to present to him in person the beginning of what I now write here in his memory.

H. R. Moskowitz et al. (eds.), Sensation and Measurement. 167–176.

quence is the possibility that a preoccupation with the concept of sensation and the illusion that it is directly measurable may obscure important empirical relations evident in matching behavior, and I believe that such a result has occurred in the case of the just noticeable difference.

Subjective Size of the JND: Two Hypotheses

The historical background is a familiar story and requires only the briefest review. Weber's law, asserting proportionality between JND and stimulus intensity (plus a constant), is generally accepted as a good first-order description of results for many continua. (See, for example, Stevens, 1957). Fechner, adding the premise that JND define constant intervals on a corresponding scale of sensation, concluded that sensation is a log function of stimulus intensity. (See Luce & Edwards, 1958, for a detailed discussion of this argument.) But Fechner's supposition about the subjective size of the JND is not the only possibility, nor perhaps the most reasonable one. According to Stevens (1957), Brentano proposed the equally plausible premise that sensations produced by stimuli one JND apart define not a constant interval but a constant ratio on the scale of sensation. And Fechner himself did the mathematics to show that, if Brentano was correct, then the result must be a power relation between sensation and stimulus intensity; for the arch-protagonist of the logarithmic law that consequence seemed sufficient proof of the falsity of Brentano's premise, and it received little further attention.

Only much later, with the establishment of the psychophysical power law on the basis of magnitude estimation data, was Brentano's premise revived as the necessary concomitant of Weber's law and a power law. (see, for example, Stevens, 1957). That is, if sensation is a power function of stimulus intensity, and JND are proportional to stimulus intensity, then the subjective size of JND must, as Brentano proposed, be proportional to subjective magnitude. Ultimately, Stevens (1966a) proposed that Brentano's premise be renamed Ekman's law on the grounds that "it seems more important to have established the empirical generality than merely to have conjectured it as Brentano did ... (p. 533)." The principle, further described as the "analog to Weber's law," is said to state "that variability measured in psychological units is linearly related to psychophysical magnitude measured in the same units (p. 533)." That is, precision (or error) is thought to follow the same rule for sensation as for stimulus intensities.

Stevens' suggestion seems to have won some acceptance and references to Ekman's law have begun to appear in the literature (for example, Engen, 1971, and Teghtsoonian, 1971). Since it is not every day that a new law is acquired in psychology, a closer examination of the supporting evidence is warranted.

Evidence for Ekman's Law

Most frequently cited are two studies (Ekman, 1956, 1959) that develop essentially the same reasoning. Empirical estimates of the JND for a given continuum are transformed to "subjective" equivalents by means of a psychophysical function such as the veg scale developed by Harper & Stevens (1948), and are then plotted as a function of the standard which has also been translated to the veg scale. The results led Ekman to conclude that he had discovered evidence for linearity between "discriminal sensitivity on the subjective continuum ... and subjective scale values (p. 233)." But is this really a finding or is it a tautology? If the measured values of the JND obey Weber's law, and if the psychophysical function follows the power law, then Ekman's result is mathematically necessary. (Since Weber's law specifies that JND define constant intervals on a logarithmic scale, and the power relation is linear on logarithmic coordinates, it is evident that the transformed JND will still constitute constant intervals on a logarithmic scale.) And given the strong evidence supporting both Stevens' law and Weber's law, it seems clear that at most Ekman's results must be regarded as confirmation of those principles and not as evidence for a new empirical principle. In fairness to Ekman, it should be noted that he proposed his technique without regard to the form of the psychophysical relation, or for the exact form of the relation between JND and stimulus intensity. Yet, since for prothetic continua these functions are closely approximated by Stevens' and Weber's laws respectively, the outcome of Ekman's tactic could hardly be in doubt. Thus, even if it were accepted that the veg and similar scales accomplish a transformation from stimulus to sensation (in itself a dubious argument; see below), Ekman's application of them to JND and standard intensities and the resulting linear relation is not evidence for "the empirical generality" of Brentano's premise.

But other evidence is cited. Eisler (1962, 1963a, 1963b) has reported (with some qualification) a linear relation between standard deviations and means of magnitude estimations for a variety of continua. That is, the variability in magnitude estimations grows in the same way that the region of uncertainty grows in measurement of the JND. Doesn't this indicate that the ability to distinguish one subjective magnitude from another is governed by the same principle of relativity that applies to stimulus intensities? Doesn't it support the view that there is a subjective analog to Weber's law? I believe that the answer is yes only on the assumption that the numerical udgments obtained in Eisler's experiments are linear with sensation, or at least that the transformation rule is such that the proportionality observed for numerical judgment holds for sensations as well. Such an assumption is clearly essential to justify the leap from properties of the observer's judgments to conclusions about his sensations.

For many, including myself, the linearity assumption is a very appealing, even seductive idea.[2] It makes excellent introspective sense as an account of the observer's

[2] In some earlier papers (Teghtsoonian, 1971, 1973), I have referred to numerical judgment as if it were a direct measure of subjective magnitude, and have used the terms interchangeably. I believe that little if any harm results in those cases and the reader is free to select the terms he prefers. However, I have also employed sensation as a theoretical concept in those papers in reference to a central mechanism introduced to account for certain observations. In that case, it is regarded as standing in the same type of relation to number as to all other continua.

experience: He hears a particular loudness and tries to describe it numerically, and when he doubles his judgment he means that the new loudness sounds twice as great. But, I think it essential to realise that, as Treisman (1964b) made very clear, it *is* an assumption, and that when it is made, two important considerations should be recalled. First, it is by no means the only possible assumption. Among others, Attneave (1962) has proposed a specific departure from linearity and has attempted to explore its implications (in, for example, Curtis, Attneave, & Harrington, 1968). And Treisman (1964b) has suggested that the arithmetic of sensations may take even more radically different forms. Second and more generally, it can be argued that no measurement can determine the relation between sensation, a theoretical event, and stimulus intensity. The relation must of necessity be a matter of supposition whose merit can only be determined by the success of the theoretical structure to which it belongs. In the absence of compelling theoretical support for the linearity assumption, Eisler's results cannot be regarded as any more persuasive than Ekman's that Brentano's premise has been verified empirically.

However, since the establishment of cross-modal matching (CMM) as the more general procedure of which magnitude estimation and magnitude production (or more simply, number matching) are particular cases, assumptions about the relation of numbers to sensations are no longer essential. In this framework, the dependent variable as well as the independent variable is a physical continuum, and the only assumption concerns the ability of the observer to match intensities across continua.

JND in the Context of CMM

What does this shift in emphasis from an effort to measure sensation to a study of matching behavior have to do with Brentano's premise? Simply that in the context of CMM procedures, the question of the subjective size of the JND is irrelevant. We need not opt for either Fechner's or Brentano's guess about subjective JND because we do not need to accept their shared belief that the ultimate task is to relate sensation to stimulus intensity. If instead, we accept a view of empirical psychophysics as limited to the relations applying within and between matching continua, no assumptions about sensation are needed at all. In this context, only Weber's law is required to derive the power relation between matching continua. For if Weber's law holds, then it applies to *both* the target continuum plotted on the abscissa, *and* the matching continuum plotted on the ordinate. If it is further assumed that changing two matched intensities by the same number of JND will produce two new matching intensities, then the relation between the matching continua must be a power function The proof is no different from that employed by Fechner to show that sensation would be a power function of stimulus intensity given Weber's law for the latter, and its equivalent (Brentano's premise) for the former. If stimuli at constant interval steps on a logarithmic scale (Weber's law) produce matching values separated by constant interval steps on a logarithmic scale of the matching continuum, the matching function must be linear on those logarithmic coordinates, i.e., a power function.

There is however one important difference between the argument relating sensation to stimulus intensity and that relating two continua of stimulus intensities. In the first case, the matching of units on the ordinate (subjective JND) to units on the abscissa (physical JND) is a matter of definition, and permits no direct test. In the second case however, the assumed equivalence of JND across continua is certainly open to empirical test in a variety of ways. For example, an observer could be asked to select matching intensities on two continua. A second intensity could then be specified on the target continuum at some fixed number of JND from the first. It is predicted that a match to this second stimulus will be separated by the same number of JND from the first stimulus on the matching continuum. But other, less tedious tactics are possible.

Support for the intermodal equivalence of JND has been previously reported by Teghtsoonian (1971), and the logic of that evidence can be briefly recapitulated. If JND constitute constant intervals on a log scale (Weber's law), and if a single JND on any arbitrarily selected reference scale would be matched by one JND on any other matching scale, it is clear that the size of the latter (in log units) will be inversely proportional to the exponent of the power function relating the two continua. Auerbach (1971) has provided a clear mathematical account of this interdependence of the two Weber fractions and the exponent of the matching power function. (If continuum ϕ is a power function of continuum λ with an exponent β, $\phi = c\lambda^{\beta}$, and if

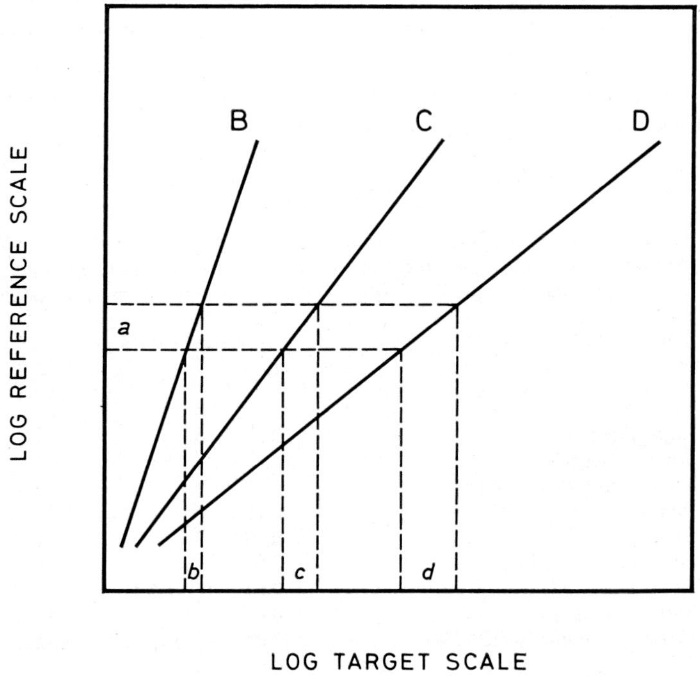

Fig. 1. The cross-modal equivalence of JND for continua related by a power function.

the two Weber fractions are W_ϕ and W_λ respectively, then $\beta = \log(1+W_\phi)/\log(1+W_\lambda)$). The relation is illustrated in Figure 1 where the interval a on the ordinate represents one JND and is matched by one-JND intervals b, c, and d for three continua all of which are related by power functions to the reference continuum but with differing exponents. Or, arguing in the opposite direction, the size of the JND in log units for the scales plotted on the abscissa multiplied by the slope of the linear matching function (on log-log coordinates), should yield an invariant estimate of the JND on the reference scale. For nine continua with Weber fractions ranging from 1.3% to 8.3% the technique just described yielded estimates of the Weber fraction for number (as the reference scale) tending toward an invariant 3.0%. The data shown in Table 1 are adapted from Teghtsoonian (1971), where sources for all of the tabled values are also given.

Of course the important feature of these estimates is not their absolute value but their relative invariance. Perhaps exceptions to the rule represented in Table 1 will be found; but the value of an empirical invariant is very great and warrants, I think, careful scrutiny of seeming counter-examples before it is abandoned. For example, faced with the gross discrepancy between McBurney's (1966) exponent for saltiness of 0.41 (the value listed in Table 1) and Stevens' (1969) value of 1.3, one may suspect that the former is the appropriate value to pair with the JND estimate obtained with the same technique by McBurney, Kasschau, & Bogart (1967). Indeed, Meiselman (1972) has shown convincingly that the methods employed by Stevens (sip-and-spit) and by McBurney (flow) differ fundamentally and that the difference in exponents is the result. It remains to be seen whether, given the sip-and-spit method and the resulting high exponent, there is the marked superiority in resolving power which would be predicted from the relation represented in Table 1, with a Weber fraction around 2% instead of the 8% obtained by McBurney *et al.*

TABLE 1

The invariance of $1 + W_N$ as estimated by $(1 + W_\phi)^\beta$ where W_ϕ is the Weber fraction for some continuum, β is the exponent for that continuum obtained by magnitude estimation, and W_N is the Weber fraction for numerical judgment

Continuum	Empirical values		Predicted
	W_ϕ	β	W_N
Light intensity	0.079	0.33	0.026
Sound intensity	0.048	0.6	0.029
Thumb-to-finger interval	0.022	1.30	0.029
Weight	0.020	1.45	0.029
Length	0.029	1.04	0.030
NaCl concentration	0.083	0.41	0.033
Saturation (red)	0.019	1.7	0.033
Shock intensity	0.013	2.5	0.033
Vibration intensity (125 Hz)	0.046	0.67	0.031
Mean	0.040		0.030
Variance	6.09×10^{-4}		5.11×10^{-6}

The interdependence of Weber fractions and power-law exponents seems to hold also for odor strength. Engen (1973), summarizing the work of Stone and his associates on DL measurement, suggests that the nose requires a change of about 25% in intensity of odorant to detect it. This is an overall figure derived from findings with several different odorants, but it is apparent by reference to Table 1 that on the basis of differential sensitivity such a value puts the sense of smell at the bottom of the list. On this basis, very low exponents would be expected to occur with magnitude estimations of odor strength. Such a prediction is borne out in a study reported by Berglund, Berglund, Ekman & Engen (1971): the median exponent for 26 odorants was 0.15. Combined with the Weber fraction of 0.25 the prediction of the Weber fraction for number is 0.34, not very far from the mean of 0.30 reported in Table 1. This use of values averaged over odorants can provide only a rough-and-ready indication, since it is likely that there are important differences among odorants. However, until further evidence becomes available, the picture of poor resolving power and relatively low exponents seems a fair description for the sense of smell. The rule reflected by the data in Table 1 may be false, but it is certainly testable![3]

At least brief comment should be made about the meaning of a Weber fraction near 3% for number. Obviously it cannot mean that an observer will not notice the difference between, say, 100 and 101 any more than he would confuse a weight of 100 g with one of 101 g if each carried a label bearing its name. Evidently, the 3% value must allude to unnamed numerical quantity as defined by an aggregate of objects. But just how such aggregates should be defined without the introduction of confounding spatial variables (as in experiments on numerosity) is far from clear. More generally, there is the problem of the relation between the number continuum (as used in magnitude estimation and production) and the other target and matching continua. Although I have lumped them all together in the preceding discussion under the catch-all title of 'physical continua', it is clear that there are important differences among them, and that number in particular stands apart from the rest. A distinguishing feature (to name just one) that has received relatively little attention is the ease with which numerical judgments can be stored and recalled by the observer. It seems likely that estimates of judgmental variability based on numerical responses are low in comparison to results for more physical, less easily-coded response continua. However, such differences should not obscure our view of the important similarities. Number, like many other continua, is manipulable by the observer in a public and recordable fashion. And the results ob-

[3] After this paper was written I have discovered that the Weber fraction for number appears to be near 3% as estimated from yet another continuum. Hardy, Wolff, & Goodell (1947) measured JND for intensity of pain induced by thermal radiation of the skin and concluded that "the range of intensities between 220 and 320 mCal s^{-1} cm^{-2} represents the stimulation of a type of cutaneous pain for which $\Delta I/I = \text{constant} = 0.03$ (p. 1156)." Adair, Stevens, & Marks (1968) scaled the apparent intensity of such thermally induced pain by the method of magnitude estimation, using similar equipment and for approximately the same range of intensites. The power law proved to be an appropriate description (given a stimulus correction for threshold), and the authors summarize their results as follows: "The exponent β was approximately 1.0 for all four experiments (p. 164)." Taken together these two values yield an estimate of W_N which is exactly 0.03!

tained with numbers are consistent with and predictable from results obtained with other continua (Stevens, 1968). Despite its distinctive features, the number continuum behaves in important respects like other continua.

Summary and Conclusions

There are two central features of the foregoing analysis and each deserves some concluding comment. First, it seems that JND measurements are intimately related to the power relation between matching continua, and to the specific exponents obtained. Second, the framework that achieves this harmony can be constructed without reference to the subjective size of the JND.

The compatability of measured resolving power with power law exponents illustrated in Table 1 stands in marked contrast to the many reports (e.g., Stevens, 1957, 1961) purporting to show the failure of JND data to conform to the results obtained by magnitude estimation. But this failure now seems uniquely attributable to the Fechnerian premise concerning the subjective size of the JND, not to some basic flaw in the logic of JND measurement or its use in scale construction. If Brentano's premise were adopted in place of Fechner's, it is clear that an integrated JND function would be approximately linear with a magnitude estimation scale. It is unfortunate that the inadequacies of the logarithmic relation as a model for the psychophysical matching function, led to the concurrent (but unnecessary) argument that those matching functions were unrelated to measures of resolving power. One may have justifiable qualms about the efficiency of JND measurement as an approach to scaling, and about the biases associated with threshold measurement, but that is a very different matter from the claim that the results conflict with those obtained in matching experiments. The latter does not appear to be true.

Turning finally to the important proposal that JND are equivalent across continua, and that demonstration of this equivalence requires no assumption about the subjective size of the JND, a similar point has been made concerning the relation between cross-modal power functions and theoretical sensation-stimulus functions. Ekman (1964) noted that the latter could be a Fechnerian log function and that the cross-modal function would then have to be a power function. In the same year, Treisman (1964a, 1964b) showed that the same result occurs on assuming either a log function *or* a power function for the relation between sensation and stimulus. Finally, Phillips (1964) pointed out that there were in fact an infinite number of possible sensation-stimulus functions given the power relation for the stimulus-stimulus function. The criteria offered thus far for choosing among them seem at best vague, and whether there is merit in making any choice at all seems a moot point. It is clear that such a choice has no bearing on the empirical fact of a power relation between matching continua.

And finally, what can be said of Ekman's law? If it is a statement about sensations, then it must be regarded as unproved, but unnecessary to empirical psychophysics. If on the other hand it is a statement about the continuum manipulated by an observer to produce a match, then it would seem to be more than an "analog to Weber's law," it *is* Weber's law.

Despite the disagreements over the subjective size of the JND, certain conclusions about empirical psychophysics seem warranted:

1. Evidence supports the plausible assumption of cross-modal equivalence for JND.
2. Given Weber's law on matching continua and the cross-modal equivalence of JND, the result must be a power relation.
3. Stimuli separated by one JND have the same property as any other pair of stimuli: the constant ratio so defined will be matched by a corresponding constant ratio on a matching continuum.
4. There is no conflict between the measurement of resolving power and the determination of cross-modal matching functions. The two Weber fractions and the exponent of the power relation are interrelated so that given two of these values, the third can be calculated.

References

Adair, E. R., Stevens, J. C., & Marks, L. E. Thermally induced pain, the dol scale, and the psychophysical power law. *American Journal of Psychology*, 1968, **81**, 147–164.

Attneave, F. Perception and related areas. In S. Koch (Ed.), *Psychology: A study of a science*, Vol. 4. New York: McGraw-Hill, 1962.

Auerbach, C. Interdependence of Stevens' exponents and discriminability measures. *Psychological Review*, 1971, **78**, 556.

Berglund, B., Berglund, U., Ekman, G., & Engen, T. Individual psychophysical functions for 28 odorants. *Perception and Psychophysics*, 1971, **9**, 379–384.

Curtis, D. W., Attneave, F., & Harrington, T. L. A test of a two-stage model of magnitude judgment. *Perception and Psychophysics*, 1968, **3**, 25–31.

Eisler, H. Empirical test of a model relating magnitude and category scales. *Scandinavian Journal of Psychology*, 1962, **3**, 88–96.

Eisler, H. How prothetic is the continuum of smell? *Scandinavian Journal of Psychology*, 1963a, **4**, 29–32.

Eisler, H. Magnitude scales, category scales, and Fechnerian integration. *Psychological Review*, 1963b, **70**, 243–253.

Ekman, G. Discriminal sensitivity on the subjective continuum. *Acta Psychologica*, 1956, **12**, 233–243.

Ekman, G. Weber's law and related functions. *The Journal of Psychology*, 1959, **47**, 343–352.

Ekman, G. Is the power law a special case of Fechner's law? *Perceptual and Motor Skills*, 1964, **19**, 730.

Engen, T. Psychophysics II. Scaling methods. In J. W. Kling & L. A. Riggs (Eds.), *Woodworth & Schlosberg's experimental psychology*, 3rd ed. New York: Holt, Rinehart and Winston, 1971.

Engen, T. The sense of smell. In P. H. Mussen & M. R. Rosenzweig (Eds.), *Annual Review of Psychology*, Vol. 24. Palo Alto: Annual Reviews, Inc., 1973.

Hardy, J. D., Wolff, H. G., & Goodell, H. Studies on pain: Discrimination of differences in intensity of a pain stimulus as a basis of a scale of pain intensity. *Journal of Clinical Investigation*, 1947, **26**, 1152–1158.

Harper, R. S., & Stevens, S. S. A psychological scale of weight and a formula for its derivation. *American Journal of Psychology*, 1948, **61**, 343–351.

Luce, R. D., & Edwards, W. The derivation of subjective scales from just noticeable differences. *Psychological Review*, 1958, **65**, 222–237.

McBurney, D. H. Magnitude estimation of the taste of sodium chloride after adaptation to sodium chloride. *Journal of Experimental Psychology*, 1966, **72**, 869–873.

McBurney, D. H., Kasschau, R. A., & Bogart, L. M. The effect of adaption on taste JNDs. *Perception and Psychophysics*, 1967, **2**, 175–178.

Meiselman, H. L. Human taste perception. *Chemical Rubber Companies Critical Review in Food Technology*, April 1972, 89–119.

Phillips, J. P. N. A note on Treisman's model. *Quarterly Journal of Experimental Psychology*, 1964, **16**, 386.

Stevens, S. S. On the psychophysical law. *Psychological Review*, 1957, **64**, 153–181.

Stevens, S. S. To honor Fechner and repeal his law. *Science*, 1961, **133**, 80–86.

Stevens, S. S. Concerning the psychophysical power law. *Quarterly Journal of Experimental Psychology*, 1964, **16**, 383–385.

Stevens, S. S. A metric for the social consensus. *Science*, 1966a, **151**, 530–544.

Stevens, S. S. Operations or words? *Psychological Monographs*, 1966b, **80** (15, whole No. 627, part 2).

Stevens, S. S. Tactile vibration: Change of exponent with frequency. *Perception and Psychophysics*, 1968, **3**, 223–228.

Stevens, S. S. Sensory scales of taste intensity. *Perception and Psychophysics*, 1969, **6**, 302–308.

Savage, C. W. Introspectionist and behaviorist interpretations of ratio scales of perceptual magnitudes. *Psychological Monographs*, 1966, **80**, (15, whole No. 627, part 1).

Teghtsoonian, R. On the exponents in Stevens' law and the constant in Ekman's law. *Psychological Review*, 1971, **78**, 71–80.

Teghtsoonian, R. Range effects in psychophysical scaling and a revision of Stevens' law. *American Journal of Psychology*, 1973, **86**, 3–27.

Treisman, M. Sensory scaling and the psychophysical law. *Quarterly Journal of Experimental Psychology*, 1964a, **16**, 11–22.

Treisman, M. What do sensory scales measure? *Quarterly Journal of Experimental Psychology*, 1964b, **16**, 387–391.

A QUANTAL MODEL FOR PSYCHOLOGICAL MAGNITUDE AND DIFFERENTIAL SENSITIVITY

JOHN VOLKMANN
Mount Holyoke College

Abstract. The model assumes a series of quantal elements, divided into successive subseries. Within each subseries, the quanta are equal in psychological magnitude. Between subseries, they may differ in magnitude; if they differ, they do so by some integral ratio. The quanta of any subseries may thus be converted into the units of the subseries with the smallest quanta. The total converted value of all of the quanta excited determines the psychological magnitude. The converted value of any quantum divided by the total converted value of all of the preceding quanta in the series determines the relative differential sensitivity; this ratio is analogous to the Weber fraction. When the ratio is plotted against its denominator, analogous to a plot of $\Delta R/R$ against R, the result is a set of reciprocal functions that resemble visually a Weber-law plot. The model also has consequences for the measurement of magnitudes, for the relations governing latency and confidence, and for certain issues in systematic psychology.

In his effort to measure psychological magnitudes, Fechner proposed the simplest model for relating magnitude to differential sensitivity. He saw the just noticeable difference (JND) as a natural unit of sensation; to measure a magnitude, one needed only to begin at the absolute threshold and to count up the number of JNDs to the level in question. The JNDs were specifically assumed to be equal. (If that assumption is to be of any use, it must mean that the JNDs are equal in psychological magnitude.) But Fechner's effort failed. The JND came to be recognized as a statistical construct with an arbitrary statistical definition; not a natural unit at all. Further, psychological magnitudes came to be scaled independently, first in the tradition of Delboeuf and then in the tradition of Stevens. When measured against scales of magnitude, the JNDs of most sensory variables are definitely not equal. The JNDs at higher levels of magnitude contain much more magnitude than JNDs at lower levels. To take a single example, Stevens (1936) computed the subjective size of JNDs for loudness, and found that this size might increase with their successive number above threshold by as much as 30 times, depending on the frequency of the tone. So psychophysics is left with a basic problem: how to relate magnitude and differential sensitivity.

Development of a Model

The first step toward solution seems obvious, and surely not novel. It follows directly from Fechner's simplest model, mentioned above. Weber-law plots have usually looked to me like reciprocal functions, having in common with them an initial sharp drop and a long approach to some asymptote. With this minor inspiration, we can look back at Fechner's hypothetical natural units, and see that a differential discrimination requires the addition of one unit to the number of units already present (or, of course, the subtraction of one unit from the number already present). Stevens

H. R. Moskowitz et al. (eds.), Sensation and Measurement. 177–184. *All Rights Reserved.*

and Davis say that this idea is "attractive for its simplicity" (1938, p. 151). Psychological magnitude is given by the total number of units. So relative differential sensitivity (analogous to the Weber fraction, and not stated in terms of a stimulus variable) is $1/N$ in which N is the total number of units. A plot of $1/N$ against N is analogous to a plot of $\Delta R/R$ against R; it shows a familiar reciprocal form, asymptotic to zero.

This basic argument has been obscured for a variety of reasons. In the first place, psychophysical operations typically include the manipulation and control of stimulus variables. As a result, the stimulus-relations of magnitude and of differential sensitivity have entered the argument somewhat too soon. In the second place, Fechner himself took a very different course. On the basis of much less evidence than we now have, he rejected the sharp initial drop as being due to the difficulty of attending to weak stimuli, and adopted Weber's Law as a firm assumption. In the third place, the argument so far must be only a beginning, if it is any good at all. For it assumes the equality of the natural units in terms of magnitude, and thus arrives immediately at the wrong answer to our problem; the JNDs, at any rate, are usually not equal in magnitude. Next, the zero asymptote appears implausible; differential sensitivity is limited, not infinite. And next, some psychophysicists have seemed willing to view the Weber-law relation as reflecting an ill-defined relativity of sensation; it is a "fact of nature," as inevitable as tomorrow's sunrise. The actual data of differential sensitivity are not well fitted by Weber's Law, and would not seem to encourage this view. Lastly, the hypothetical natural units were all too hypothetical; at any rate, they were not the JNDs.

Logically considered, the next step in the development of the model was taken by von Békésy (1930) in his discovery of the quantum of discrimination. Here was indeed a natural unit, not at all arbitrary in definition or size. His model was clear and verifiable, and received independent experimental support (Stevens, Morgan, & Volkmann, 1941). Stevens (1972) in one of his last major publications, examined a mass of psychophysical data for evidence of second-quantum discrimination, and concluded that there was a great deal of evidence to support a quantal model. (See also the criticism by Corso, and the reply by Norman, in Corso & Norman, 1973.) My own view is slightly different from all of these; I feel that we have yet to identify and produce the experimental conditions that would yield excellent quantal data; data that would satisfy both the supporters and the critics of quantal models. Nevertheless, I also feel that it can and will be done.

On this optimistic note, we turn to a system that might be a useful analog for psychological magnitudes. On the edge of a long table, lay in a single, continuous row the following U.S. coins: 100 pennies, 20 nickels and 4 quarters. The row (or series) is discontinuous at two points, which divide it into 3 subseries. Within each subseries, the members are equal. Between adjacent subseries, the members are unequal, but they are related by statable conversion ratios of 5 or $\frac{1}{5}$. Going from pennies to quarters, the ratios are integral; that is, the ratios are 5.0 rather than 5.392 or the like. A complete downward conversion would produce the equivalent of 300 pennies, although there are only 124 coins. The idea of conversion is important, because it is the converted number rather than the sheer number of coins that is the analog of psychological magnitude. Note that the system is a quantal system: there are no coins other than whole pennies, whole nickels, and whole quarters. Note also that confining the three subseries in a fixed order removes some of the flexibility normally associated with coinage. For example, one could produce 98 pennies or 99 pennies, and the converted values of 105 or 110, but not the converted values of 101–104 or 106–109, etc. Nevertheless, much flexibility remains; the number of possible values, including converted values, equals the number of coins (124).

In the example above, the three subseries have equal converted values (of 100 pennies each), and the number of members varies from series to series. In another example, we might have 100 pennies, 100 nickels, and 100 quarters: an equal number of members in each series. Then there would be 300 coins, with a total converted value of 3100 pennies. If the example contained pennies, dimes, and silver dollars the conversion ratios would change from 5 to 10. If it contained pennies, nickels, and silver dollars, the ratios would expand, and be 5 and 20 respectively.

Passing now from analog to model, we may list the following principal assumptions:

1. A psychological magnitude and the corresponding differential sensitivity are both determined by an ordered series of subseries in which each subseries is composed of ordered quantal units. The order referred to here is the order in which the quantal units are excited by a continuously varying stimulus.

2. Within each subseries, the quantal units are equal in psychological magnitude.

3. Between subseries of a single series, the quantal units may differ in psychological magnitude. When they do so, they differ by ratios of whole numbers. That is, the units of subseries II may be 2, 3, 4 ... times the units of subseries I; correspondingly, the units of subseries I will be 1/2, 1/3, 1/4,... times the units of subseries II. When the ratios are known, the units of any subseries may thus be converted to those of any other subseries, most conveniently to the units of the subseries that has the smallest units.

4. This conversion of all the excited units into the smallest units of the whole series we may call the *converted number*. It is to be distinguished from the *excited number*, the sheer number of quantal units (of any size) that are excited. Psychological magnitude is determined by the converted number, not by the excited number.

5. Under quantal conditions, the discrimination of differences will be controlled by the size of the quanta in the subseries in which the excitation falls. The size of the difference, in terms of the number of quanta (1, 2, 3 ...) will determine some features of the discrimination; subseries boundaries or whole subseries may also be determining.

Consequences and Discussion

The model aims at some generality, and might be used in describing the quantitative structure of many different psychological variables: both the variables in which the JNDs are approximately equal (e.g. auditory pitch), and those in which they are very unequal (e.g. auditory loudness); both the variables subject to sensory compression, in which a huge range of stimulus intensities is represented by a manageable range of phenomenal intensities (e.g. loudness, visual brightness) and those in which the stimulus variable is "adequately" represented, with a Stevens exponent of approximately 1.0 (some visual spatial variables). Note that those two oppositions are not the same; these visual spatial variables approach adequacy, but their JNDs are far from equal. Conversely, auditory pitch has JNDs nearly equal, but a complex relation to stimulus frequency.

Because it aims at generality, the model does not specify particular conversion ratios or the number of quantal units in subseries. These quantities would presumably be determined empirically. Nor does the model specify particular stimulus relations for either magnitude or differential sensitivity. Nevertheless, if one assumes that the overall relation between a psychological magnitude and a stimulus variable is given by some increasing monotonic function, some consequences appear. First, an instantaneous view of the relation, permitting no variability, would show steps. The size of the steps would change discontinuously from one subseries to the next; larger magnitudes would come in larger lumps. Under most circumstances the steps would be obscured by variability, especially if variability were also related to the stimulus by an increasing monotonic function. The subseries boundaries might be more important, both in the theory and the practice of scaling magnitudes. For it might be necessary to describe the growth of a magnitude by a separate function for each quantal subseries; the successive functions being discontinuous (at least in slope) at the subseries boundaries. In practice, magnitude judgments are subject to anchoring effects and other perturbations; the subseries boundaries would be another possible source of perturbations. Or the basic difference between excited number and converted number might produce difficulties in the judgment of magnitude. To the degree that the subject's reports depended upon the converted number alone, they could yield stable and internally consistent scales: down to the level set by the coarseness of a quantal series, the internal relations of magnitude could be approximately preserved in spite of wide variations in quantum size.

The assumptions listed above have some definite consequences for functions of (relative) differential sensitivity, analogous to Weber-law plots. In the first example, we assume five subseries of ten quanta each; a conversion ratio of two, at each subseries boundary; and first-quantum discrimination throughout.

In Figure 1, the ordinate values are the ratios between the converted number of first-series quanta in each successive quantum (N_{qc}), and the lower boundary of that quantum expressed as a total converted number ($\sum N_{qc}$). Thus each subseries yields a set of ratios; for the first subseries, 1/0–1/9, for the second subseries, 2/10–2/28, and so on. The abscissa values are the lower boundaries of the same quanta, still expressed as a converted number. The result is a set of reciprocal curves, one for each subseries, with the form $a \cdot 1/n$ as a function of n; each curve has a vertical asymptote of infinity and a horizontal asymptote of zero. The asymptotes would seem to present no problem, because the functions contain a limited number of points, and are soon interrupted by the adjacent subseries, or by the stimulus limen, or by a terminal limen.

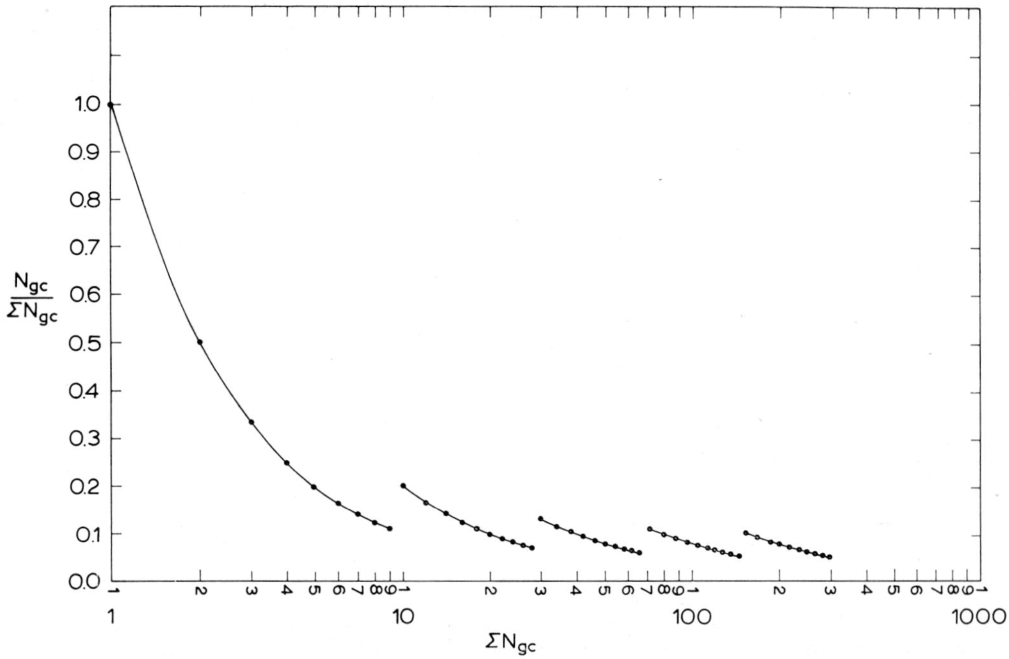

Fig. 1. The ratio of the converted number of units in each quantum to the total number of converted units in the preceding quanta, plotted as a function of this total number. Coordinates are semi-logarithmic. Uniform conversion ratios of two are assumed.

Figure 1 has a marked resemblance to the typical Weber-law plot of $\Delta R/R$ against R: the sharp initial drop, the long levelling off. The resemblance appears in spite of the fact that the coordinates of the curve are not expressed in units of the stimulus. There may be two reasons. First, like the ratio $N_{qc}/\sum N_{qc}$, the ratio $\Delta R/R$ is a pure number, although both ΔR and R are expressed in stimulus units (and the *same* stimulus units). Secondly, regarding the abscissae, it is quite reasonable to assume that the converted number will vary with an appropriately chosen stimulus variable according to some increasing, monotonic function.

Just as Weber's Law is a useful first approximation to many sets of experimental data, so it would be to the theoretical values of Figure 1. The Weber fraction would be about 10%. Why does Weber's Law have such general application to data? The model implies that the obvious reasons may not be the correct ones. It is not because of stimulus relations or the properties of sensory systems. It is because of a basic reciprocal relation between the quanta of magnitude on one hand and relative differential sensitivity on the other.

Figure 2 presents a model-variation on Figure 1. The coordinates are the same; there are still five subseries of ten quanta each. But now the conversion ratios expand (linearly) as we pass from the first subseries to the ones above, being respectively 2, 3, 4, 5. For the five subseries the ratios are as follows: 1/0–1.9; 2/10–2/28; 6/30–6/84;

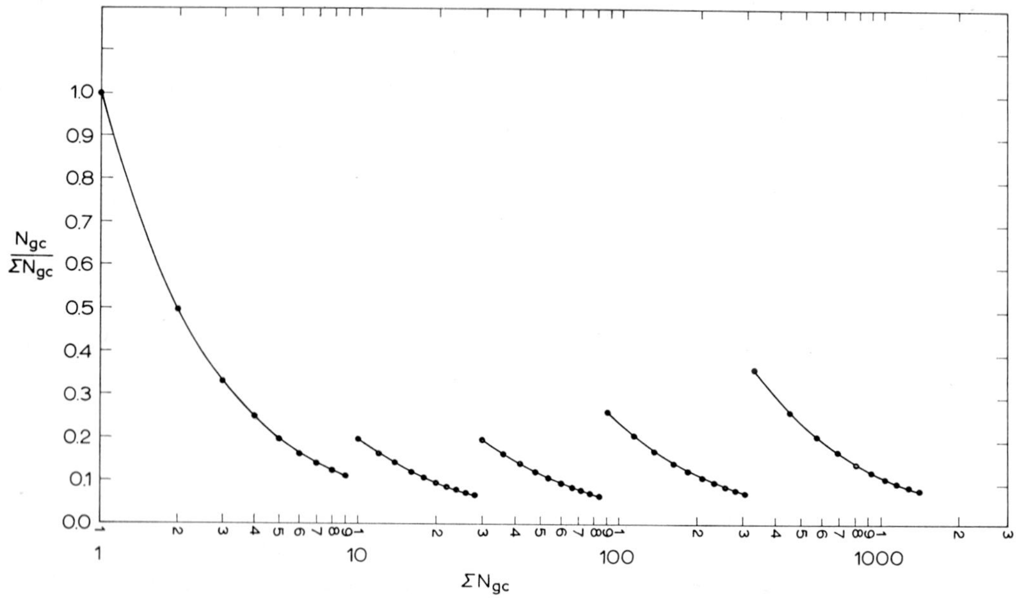

Fig. 2. The ratio of the converted number of units in each quantum to the total number of converted units in the preceding quanta, plotted as a function of this total number. Coordinates are semi-logarithmic. A (linearly) expanding conversion ratio of 2, 3, 4, 5 is assumed.

24/90–24/306; 120/330–120/1410. The converted values of the individual quanta in the five subseries are 1, 2, 6, 24, 120 respectively. Figure 2 is interesting because it exhibits another familiar feature of Weber-law plots: a tendency to turn upward at high values of the abscissa. The implication is that some sensory variables may have expanding conversion ratios.

The quantal models have consequences for two important variables of human judgment, namely latency and confidence. Johnson (1939) has shown how these vary with stimulus difference in a two-category judgment, in the framework of classical psychophysics. His description begins with a sigmoid poikilitic function. It might be possible to produce quantal conditions and rectilinear poikilitic functions; then latency should vary inversely with the number of quanta excited by the stimulus difference, down to some minimum latency (approximately 0.1 s). Confidence should vary directly with this same number, up to maximum confidence. Both sets of data should show characteristic discontinuities, reflecting the action of each additional quantum excited by the stimulus difference. Note that we are dealing here with the excited number of quanta rather than any converted number. The contrast between the two may account for the differences between the psychophysics of liminal differences and the psychophysics of much larger, supraliminal differences.

In order to work out the quantal organization of a psychological variable, one would need to locate each of the subseries boundaries, and to measure quantum size (in terms of the stimulus) immediately above and immediately below each such boundary.

Over such short distances one might be justified in assuming that the conversion ratio in stimulus units would equal the conversion ratio in psychological magnitudes. On the basis of the boundary locations and the conversion ratios, it should be possible to estimate closely the number of quanta in each subseries, and to work out the entire quantal series. Some modification of this plan could be used to verify the model in the first place.

The model has implications for systematic psychology, particularly for the "representational" view, which holds that the sensory systems and a central display-system reproduce or code various features of the external and internal environments. The display operates to bring together large amounts of information, some of which is rapidly changing. Troland held such a view; Wooldridge (1963) has more recently advocated it; Attneave (1972) considers it with reference to three-dimensional visual space. One obvious difficulty with this view is the enormous number of representational elements that it apparently requires. Our model would reduce the number somewhat. The first example give above, with a uniform conversion ratio of 2, employs 50 quanta to represent a magnitude of 296. The second example, with an expanding conversion ratio, employs 50 quanta to represent 1410.

Perhaps the least plausible feature of the model is its prediction of numerous discontinuities in the curves for magnitude, differential sensitivity, latency, and confidence. The presumption of continuity is both widely and firmly held; experimenters naturally hesitate before the great labor required to demonstrate either continuity or the opposite. Yet it is very unlikely that only two discontinuities need concern the experimental psychologist: the rod-cone discontinuity in dark-adaptation, and the subitizing-estimating discontinuity in the visual perception of number. (For the latter, see Kaufman, Lord, Reese, & Volkmann, 1949.) The discovery of numerous other discontinuities waits on four conditions: (*a*) increased reliability of measurement, (*b*) more cautious averaging of data, (*c*) the use of many more values of the variables, and (*d*) the disposition to look for discontinuity as well as for continuity. The requirement of more values of the variables is particularly important. Consider what the points in Figures 1 and 2 would look like if there were only 8 or 10 of them instead of 50, covering the same range; any slight evidence of discontinuity would be charged off to unreliability of the data, and the plot would soon show one smooth curve drawn through a scatter of points.

The model is not a psychophysiological model, but rather a relatively abstract one. Its terms have only those properties that we wish to assign to them. For this reason, I see little advantage in calling the model-units "neural quanta." If psychophysical operations verify one or more quantal models, psychophysiological operations will discover the necessary neural mechanisms, and will most probably not be far behind.

Those who seek an effective antidote for this dose of quantum psychophysics can surely find it in the neural timing model of Luce & Green (1972). The model explicitly avoids quantal assumptions, and is based on the statistics of a specific physiological variable, the interarrival times of sensory impulses at a central decision-point. At a constant intensity and in a single channel, the distribution of these times is assumed to be of the Poisson variety. The stimulus relations of sensory intensity are assumed to be power functions. The authors derive Weber's Law from their assumptions, for intensities well above absolute threshold I_0. As intensities decrease and approach absolute threshold, the authors invoke two effects to explain the observed increase in $\Delta I/I$ (the "rapid initial drop" as *I increases*, referred to in the present article).

(1) "Most obviously, I_0 can no longer be neglected and $\Delta I/(I-I_0)$ is constant only if $\Delta I/I$ is increasing" (Luce & Green, 1972, p. 24). (2) As I decreases, the number of inter-arrival times available for decision is effectively reduced; the reduction necessitates a higher Weber ratio. The neural timing model and the quantal model outlined in the present article are plainly very far apart.

At the present time, quantum psychophysics needs experimental support more than it needs theoretical elaboration. Nevertheless, there is some value in seeing what quantal models could do to solve the basic problems of psychophysics. The prospect of attaining exact solutions, however remote that prospect might be, would surely have interested my friend Smitty Stevens. He devoted most of his life to advancing the science of psychophysics, and not a little of it to quantum psychophysics.

References

Attneave, F. The representation of physical space. In A. W. Melton (Ed.), *Coding process in human memory*. Washington, D.C.: Winston, 1972, pp. 283–306.

Békésy, G. von. Über das Fechnersche Gesetz und seine Bedeutung für die Theorie der akustischen Beobachtungsfehler und die Theorie des Hörens. *Annalen der Physik*, 1930, **7**, 329–359.

Corso, J. F., & Norman, D. A. Neural quantum controversy in sensory psychology. *Science*, 1973, **181**, 467–469.

Johnson, D. M. Confidence and speed in the two-category judgment. *Archives of Psychology*, 1939, No. 241.

Kaufman, E. L., Lord, M. W., Reese, T. W., & Volkmann, J. The discrimination of visual number. *American Journal of Psychology*, 1949, **62**, 498–525.

Luce, R. D., & Green, D. M. A neural timing theory for response times and the psychophysics of intensity. *Psychological Review*, 1972, **79**, 14–57.

Stevens, S. S. A scale for the measurement of a psychological magnitude: loudness. *Psychological Review*, 1936, **43**, 405–416.

Stevens, S. S. A neural quantum in sensory discrimination. *Science*, 1972, **177**, 749–762.

Stevens, S. S., & Davis, H. *Hearing: Its psychology and physiology*. New York: Wiley, 1938, p. 151.

Stevens, S. S., Morgan, C. T., & Volkmann, J. Theory of the neural quantum in the perception of loudness and pitch. *American Journal of Psychology*, 1941, **54**, 315–335.

Wooldridge, D. E. *The machinery of the brain.* New York: McGraw-Hill, 1963, pp. 219–220.

A POWER FUNCTION FOR SENSORY RECEPTORS[1]

JOZEF J. ZWISLOCKI

Institute for Sensory Research, Syracuse University

Abstract. An attempt is made at demonstrating that receptor potentials and the neural spike rates they produce can be related to stimulus intensity by a couple of rather simple equations, independent of sensory modality. The equation describing the spike rate differs from that for the receptor potentials only by an additive threshold constant. Both equations imply that sensory receptors perform a power-function transformation of stimulus intensity. The transformation is modified by a saturation effect and, in the instance of spike rates, a threshold effect. It is possible that receptors of all sensory modalities obey one of only two power exponents. Their numerical values amount approximately to 0.5 and 1.0. Thus far, the power of 1.0 has been found applicable only to gustatory and thermo-receptors. Some experimental evidence is presented suggesting that psychophysical intensity functions parallel the receptor functions when the psychophysical intensity range is narrow. When the range is broad, as in vision and audition, the psychophysical power exponent tends to be smaller than that for sensory receptors.

Some human senses cover an unbelievably wide range of stimulus intensity. They achieve it with the help of strong compression of the adequate stimulus magnitudes. Both audition and vision compress a physical intensity range of twelve orders of magnitude into a subjective range of only about three or four orders. How do they accomplish this feat? Biological economics suggests that the compression occurs as near the interface between the organism and its environment as possible to minimize the processing of the full physical range. Sensory receptors appear to provide the earliest opportunity for the requisite nonlinear transformation, and their input-output characteristics have been investigated for decades. Some of the investigators were induced by their results to believe that the receptor characteristics completely determined the nonlinear relationship between subjective magnitudes and their physical correlates. When Fechner's logarithmic law was in vogue neurophysiologists tended to interpret their early results in its terms. So, for instance, Matthews (1931) found that the neural firing rate produced by single stretch receptors followed the logarithm of the weight loading a muscle fiber. Hartline & Graham (1932) saw a similar relationship between light intensity and the spike output of single photoreceptors of the horseshoe crab. As Stevens' power law gradually gained acceptance at the expense of Fechner's law, neurophysiologists began to cautiously change horses. Mountcastle (1967) successfully approximated intensity characteristics of cutaneous touch receptors by power functions, and Borg, Diamant, Ström, & Zotterman (1967) could do the same for nerve fibers ending on gustatory receptors. However, Stevens (1970) warned us against an oversimplified view of sensory psychophysiological relationships.

Intensity Characteristics of Sensory Receptors

When intensity characteristics of sensory receptors are recorded over a sufficient range

[1] This research was supported by NIH Grant NS-03950.

H. R. Moskowitz et al. (eds.), Sensation and Measurement. 185–197.

of stimulus intensities, they do not fit either a logarithmic or a power function but take an *S*-shaped form, whether plotted on linear, semilogarithmic, or double-logarithmic coordinates. Only when the range is sufficiently restricted, can they be approximated by either a logarithmic or a power function (Zwislocki, 1973). Since the psychophysical range either equals or exceeds the corresponding receptor range, it appears desirable to describe explicitly the complete receptor characteristics before comparing them to the psychophysical ones.

In a preceding article, I could show that the intensity characteristics of many, perhaps all sensory receptors can be fitted by one mathematical expression (Zwislocki, 1973). It was derived with the help of the characteristic plotted in Figure 1 on double-logarithmic coordinates. The crosses indicate the spike rates recorded from a single fiber of the auditory nerve by Kiang (1968); the star shows the average spontaneous activity (SPA) of the unit. When the spontaneous firing rate is subtracted from the total firing rate, the resulting values can be approximated by the intermittent curve of

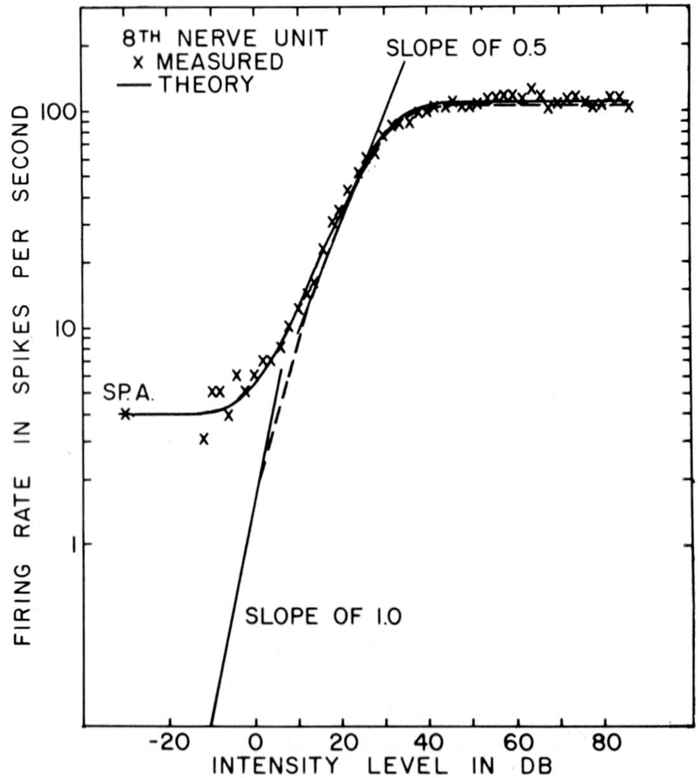

Fig. 1. A typical intensity characteristic of an auditory-nerve unit. Crosses – data of Kiang (1968). SPA – spontaneous activity. Solid curve – theoretical approximation of the data. Intermittent curve – theoretical driven firing rate equal to total firing rate less the spontaneous firing rate. Solid straight lines indicate tangents to the intermittent curve. Reference point on the intensity level scale coincides with $S/N_I = 1$ (see text).

the figure. The curve has two asymptotes. The lower one, indicated by a solid straight line, has a slope of 1.0 meaning a direct proportionality between the firing rate and stimulus intensity. The higher asymptote has a slope of zero and reflects a saturation effect. In its midcourse, the curve has a slope of 0.5 indicated by another solid straight line.

If we assume that the spontaneous activity is produced by an intrinsic noise, we can express the total firing rate at low intensity levels as

$$R^*(S) = A(S + N_I), \tag{1}$$

where S means stimulus intensity, N_I – intrinsic noise intensity, and A – a proportionality constant. At somewhat higher intensity levels, the firing rate follows approximately the square root of stimulus intensity. This can be accounted for by taking the square root of the sum in Equation 1:

$$R(S) = A(S + N_I)^{1/2}. \tag{2}$$

By taking N_I before the parenthesis, we obtain

$$R(S) = AN_I^{1/2}\ (1 + S/N_I)^{1/2}, \tag{3}$$

or

$$R(S) = R_0(1 + S/N_I)^{1/2}, \tag{4}$$

with $R_0 = AN_I^{1/2}$ denoting the spontaneous firing rate. The latter equation approximates fairly well the empirical data of Figure 1 up to an intensity level of about 20 dB. It should be pointed out in particular that its plot converges toward a slope of 1.0 at low intensity levels when the spontaneous activity R_0 is subtracted. This is so because, for $S/N_I \ll 1$, the expression under the square root can be approximated by the first two terms of its series expansion. We have

$$R(S) \simeq R_0(1 + 0.5\ S/N_I), \tag{5}$$

and, after subtraction of spontaneous activity,

$$R_D(S) \simeq 0.5\ R_0 S/N_I, \tag{6}$$

where R_D means driven firing rate.

The direct proportionality between driven firing rate and stimulus intensity at low stimulus levels has far-reaching implications. It suggests that sensory receptors respond fundamentally to stimulus energy even though this energy may be integrated over extremely short time intervals. It is consistent with a number of psychophysical relationships. Detection of acoustic signals depends directly on their energy within a critical frequency band (Gässler, 1954) and within a time interval of about 200 msec (Garner, 1948; Zwislocki, 1960). The magnitude of acoustic masking is proportional to the intensity of the masking sound within a critical band (Feldtkeller & Zwicker, 1956). The loudness level of sounds whose spectra are confined to a critical band depends on total sound intensity irrespective of its frequency distribution (Zwicker, Flottorp, & Stevens, 1957; for review, see Scharf, 1970). Last but not least, loudness as a function of stimulus intensity approaches a slope of one at low stimulus levels (Hellman & Zwislocki, 1961). As a matter of fact, the whole loudness function may be approximated by the equation

$$L = L_0(1 + S/N_I)^\theta - L_0 \tag{7}$$

(Zwislocki, 1965) which becomes analogous to Equation 6 for driven firing rate when $S/N_I \ll 1$.

At sufficiently high stimulus levels, the firing rate deviates from Equation 4 and saturates. Various suggestions were made for the mathematical description of the saturation function (see Lipetz for review, 1971), but an exponential function appears to fit the empirical data best. An appropriate one could be derived on the basis of neurophysiological evidence and reasonable assumptions. The derivation has led to the following expression for the firing rate as a function of stimulus intensity (Zwislocki, 1973):

$$R(S) = R_m(1 - e^{-(R_0/R_m)(1+S/N_I)^{1/2}}), \tag{8}$$

with R_m standing for the saturation firing rate. The solid curve approximating the empirical data in Figure 1 is the plot of Equation 8.

It should be pointed out that the exponent of the exponential function in Equation 8 is directly proportional to Equation 4 and, consequently, is a power function of the sum of extrinsic and intrinsic stimulus intensities. The exponential form of the relationship between the firing rate and stimulus intensity is required only near saturation levels. At lower levels, the exponential function can be approximated by its series expansion, and Equation 8 converges toward Equation 4. As a consequence, Equation 4 may be regarded as the fundamental transformation between the stimulus and the receptor response.

The function expressed in Equation 8 has been shown to fit most intensity characteristics of single auditory-nerve fibers. It also fits the characteristics of other mechanoreceptors, such as touch receptors of glabrous and of hairy skin, and muscle spindles. Furthermore, it fits the intensity functions of receptor potentials of Pacinian corpuscles, ampulla Lorenzini organs and photoreceptors, and of the potential of the olfactory epithelium (Zwislocki, 1973). The equation seems to apply generally to the intensity functions of receptor potentials and to the firing-rate functions they produce, provided a sufficient spontaneous activity is present. When the spontaneous activity is low or absent, a threshold constant corresponding to the neural firing threshold must be introduced. Under such conditions, Equation 8 takes the form (Zwislocki, 1973)

$$R(S) = R_m(1 - e^{-(R_0/R_m)(1+S/N_I)^{1/2}}) - T \quad [R(S) \geqslant 0], \tag{9}$$

where T means the threshold constant, and R_0 and R_m now stand for the spontaneous and maximum firing rates that would occur in the absence of the threshold.

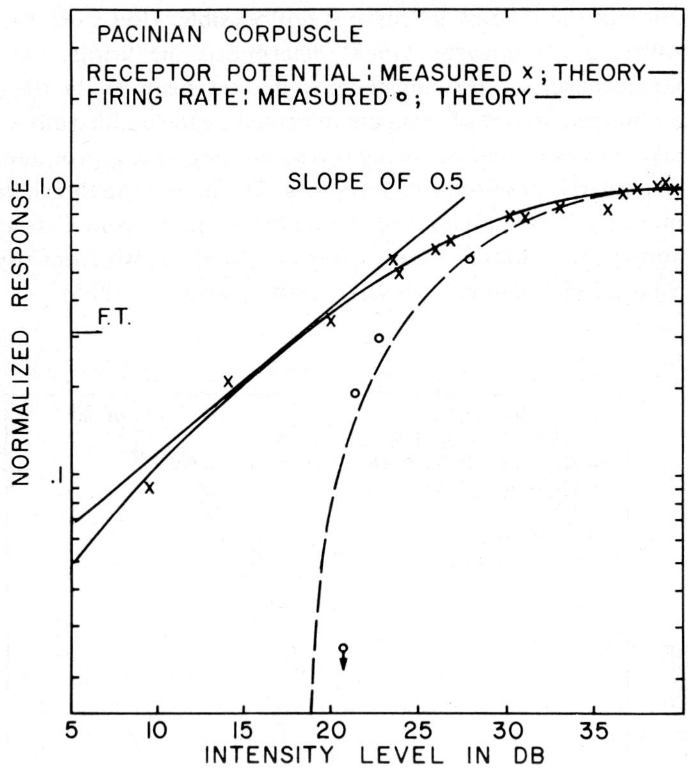

Fig. 2. Receptor potential and firing rate of Pacinian corpuscles. Crosses – receptor potential according to Loewenstein & Mendelson (1965). Horizontal line marked FT – firing threshold of the same corpuscle. Circles – firing rate of another Pacinian corpuscle according to Talbot *et al.* (1968). The curves obey Equation 9; the solid curve corresponds to a small threshold constant T, the intermittent curve to a threshold constant equal to FT.

A prominent threshold effect is shown in Figure 2 for the intensity characteristics of Pacinian corpuscles. The crosses indicate the receptor potential as a function of stimulus intensity according to measurements of Loewenstein & Mendelson (1965). The solid line represents the plot of Equation 8 with a small threshold correction resulting from some noise evident in the recordings. The correction affects the response at the lowest stimulus intensities only. Without it, the theoretical curve would asymptote on the straight line marked "slope of 0.5." As can be seen, both the curve and the straight line lie within the scatter of the experimental points so that the correction is not essential. Loewenstein & Mendelson measured the firing threshold of the corpuscle and found it to be quite high. It is indicated by the short line segment on the left side of the graph and marked FT. When the numerical value of the threshold is subtracted from the curve approximating the receptor potentials, the curve indicated by the intermittent line is obtained. It should reflect the firing rate produced by the Pacinian corpuscle. Unfortunately, Loewenstein & Mendelson omitted to measure it so that a direct validation of the theoretical curve is not possible. However, Talbot, Darian-Smith, Kornhuber, & Mountcastle (1968) determined the firing characteristics of several Pacinian corpuscles and found them to be very steep, as the theoretical curve suggests. Data obtained on one of them are indicated by the unfilled circles. The curves of Figure 2 make it evident that the firing threshold may have a pronounced effect on the intensity characteristics of sensory receptors. The higher the threshold the steeper becomes the intensity characteristic and the more it departs from a straight line on a double-logarithmic plot. Similar relationships are well known from psychophysical studies (for instance, Hellman & Zwislocki, 1964; Zwislocki, 1965).

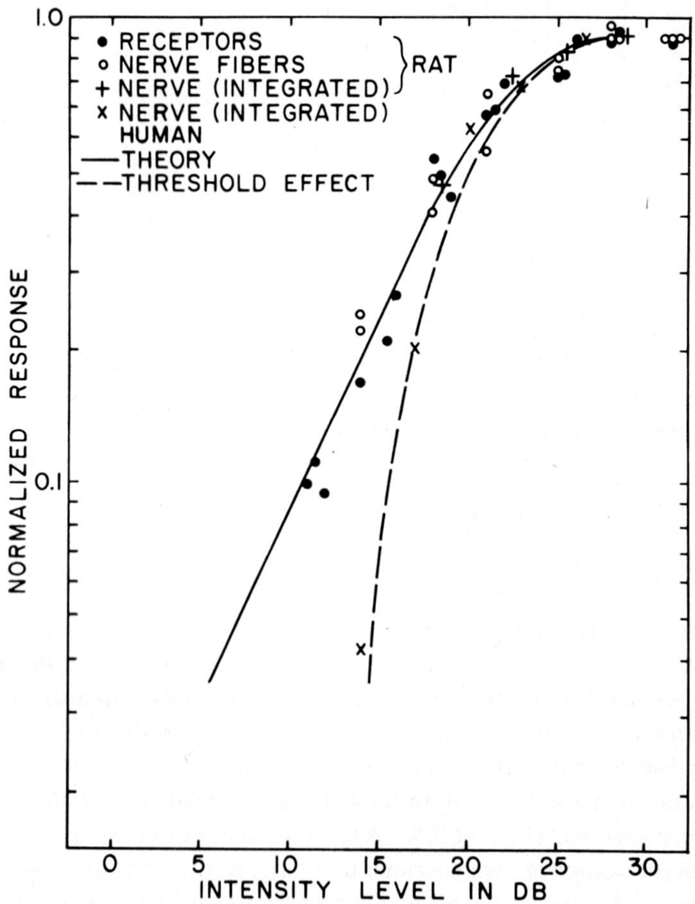

Fig. 3. Intensity characteristics of gustatory receptors and chorda-tympani nerve in response to NaCl. Filled circles – receptor potentials of three units according to Kimura & Beidler (1961). Unfilled circles – responses of three nerve fibers, vertical crosses – whole-nerve responses, both according to Fishman (1957). Slanted crosses – human whole-nerve responses according to Borg *et al.* (1967). Solid curve – plot of Equation 8, intermittent curve – plot of Equation 9, both with a power exponent of 1.0. Intensity scale proportional to concentration.

The equations introduced thus far imply four functional steps in stimulus processing by receptor units:

1. energy summation;
2. power-function transformation;
3. saturation; and
4. a threshold effect.

The power-function transformation is of main interest here because of its analogy to psychophysical power functions. Application of Equations 8 and 9 to several sensory modalities has indicated that most receptor units follow a power of approximately 0.5 with respect to stimulus intensity. For mechanoreceptors, this means a response proportional to the effective amplitude. However, the same exponent appears to hold for photoreceptors and olfactory receptors. Perhaps surprisingly, gustatory receptors and thermoreceptors appear to respond in a different manner and obey a power of 1.0. We could construe this to mean that the two receptor classes miss the square-root operation that other receptors seem to perform. Intensity characteristics of several gustatory receptors are shown in Figure 3. The filled circles refer to receptor potentials recorded from three receptors by Kimura & Beidler (1961) and the unfilled circles, to firing rates determined on three fibers of the chorda-tympani nerve by Fishman (1957). The solid curve approximating the empirical data is a plot of Equation 8 with a power of 1.0 rather than 0.5. The remaining entries in Figure 3 are explained in the following section.

Our investigations summarized here and described more fully in a preceding article (Zwislocki, 1973) lead to the conclusion that, with respect to the power-function transformation, there are only two classes of receptors – one that follows a linear function of stimulus energy and one that performs a square-root operation. Additional modifications of the apparent intensity characteristics can be accounted for by the effects of threshold and saturation. For instance, a low saturation level together with strong spontaneous activity may make the characteristic appear quite flat. On the other hand, a high threshold produces a steep characteristic and may conceal the power-function transformation.

Psychophysical vs Receptor Intensity Characteristics

By contrast to the receptor characteristics, the psychophysical intensity functions seem to be governed by an almost continuous spectrum of power exponents. But are they? As things look presently, the psychophysical intensity functions sometimes parallel the receptor functions and sometimes do not. Can we find a rule for the dichotomy? Let us consider two cases of congruence.

Mountcastle and his coworkers (Mountcastle, 1967) depressed the surface of monkeys' hands by means of a small probe and recorded impulses from nerve fibers innervating the underlying skin. They found that the firing rate increased linearly with skin indentation (square root of energy). An almost identical stimulus was given to human observers who were asked to estimate the subjective pressure. An approximately linear function of skin indentation resulted. A more direct psychophysiological comparison was achieved by Borg *et al.* (1967) in gustation on patients undergoing middle-ear surgery. Through an evolutionary peculiarity, the gustatory receptors in the anterior part of the tongue are innervated by the chorda tympani, a nerve crossing freely the cavity of the middle ear and readily accessible during the surgery. Borg and his coinvestigators were able to record the integrated activity of the nerve and obtain gustatory magnitude estimations from the same individuals. They found that the individual psychophysical curves paralleled the corresponding physiological ones. One set of their physiological results for a sodium-chloride stimulus is shown in Figure 3 by means of slanted crosses. They trace a substantially steeper curve than single-fiber recordings taken from the analogous nerve in rats and shown in the same figure by means of unfilled circles. The difference does not seem to stem from integration over many fibers, since integrated responses of the rat nerve parallel the single-unit responses, as shown by vertical crosses. It seems to be produced by a high threshold of the human nerve. When a threshold constant amounting to about 15% of the maximum response is subtracted from the theoretical curve approximating the rat data, the intermittent curve is obtained which agrees with the responses of the human nerve. As a consequence, the human intensity function obeys a power of 1.0, like the rat function, but appears to be steeper as a result of a high threshold. Because of the psychophysiological congruence found by Borg and his associates, the power of 1.0 should also apply to the subjective magnitude of saltiness, although the corresponding intensity function appears steeper, presumably, as a result of the threshold effect.

Additional recordings obtained by Borg *et al.* on individual gustatory nerves are shown in Figure 4. The stimuli consisted of citric acid, sucrose, and sodium chloride in varying concentrations. Magnitude estimations of acidity, sweetness, and saltiness evoked by the same stimuli could be approximated by the same functions. As can be seen in Figure 4, the sensitivity to citric acid was the greatest and the data points follow the flattest course. The curve approximating them obeys Equation 8 with a power of 1.0 instead of 0.5. Two simple corrections of the curve suffice to achieve an approximate fit to the data for sucrose and sodium chloride. They consist of the subtraction of a threshold constant and of a parallel horizontal shift representing a change in sensitivity. Both corrections leave the power transformation invariant, although the responses to sucrose and sodium chloride appear to grow much faster on the double-logarithmic plot than responses to citric acid.

Examples of Figures 3 and 4 open the possibility that all gustatory intensity functions, whether neural or psychophysical, obey a power of 1.0 when appropriate corrections are made for threshold and saturation. Perhaps the same is true for thermoreceptors and the sensations of cold and warm, although a power of 1.0 is currently assigned only to the growth of cold and a higher one to the growth of warmth (Stevens, 1970). Perhaps all the other sensations that seem to parallel the peripheral neural output follow the power of 0.5 of stimulus energy or concentration. This seems to be true for touch and smell. But, if all sensory receptors can be divided in two classes according to the power of their intensity characteristics, at least one additional class

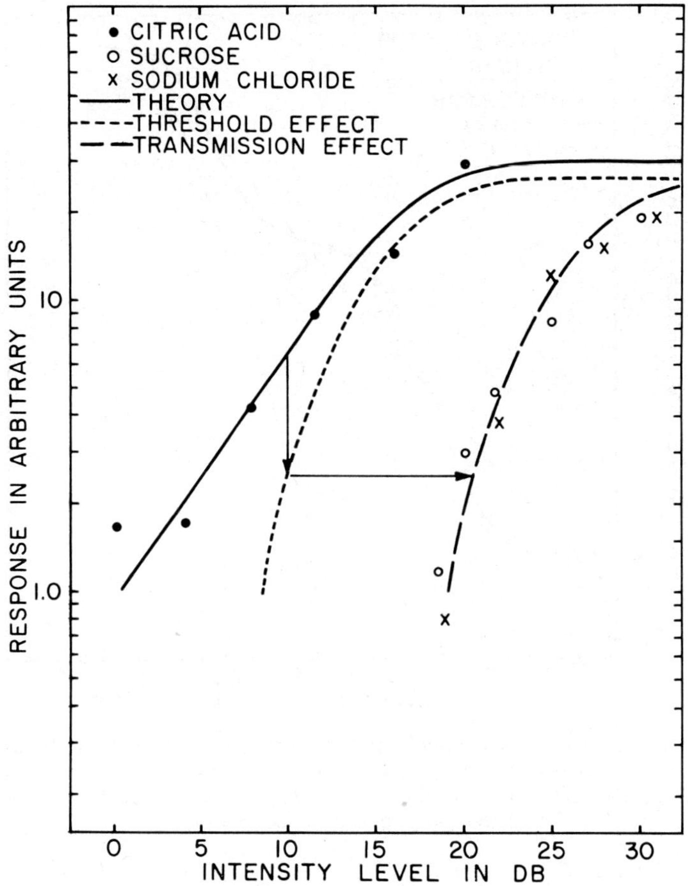

Fig. 4. Intensity characteristics of the human chorda-tympani nerve in response to three substances, according to Borg *et al.* (1967). Solid curve – plot of Equation 8 with the power of 1.0. Left intermittent curve – same as solid curve except for a threshold correction according to Equation 9. Right intermittent curve – same as left intermittent curve but shifted by 20.5 dB. Intensity scale proportional to concentration.

is required for the psychophysical intensity functions. It includes vision and audition which cover dynamic ranges exceeding by several orders of magnitude the ranges of single receptor cells. The wide ranges seem to be achieved with the help of additional compression resulting from a smaller power. How the additional compression may be achieved is illustrated in Figure 5 on the example of the primitive eye of the horseshoe crab. The eye consists of many individual receptor units, the ommatidia. Each unit comprises on the order of 14 retinular cells surrounding an eccentric cell which sends an axon to the animal's optic ganglion. When the eye is kept in a good biological condition, and impulses are recorded from one of the axons, their rate increases with light intensity, as indicated by the filled circles in Figure 5 (Barlow & Kaplan, 1971, 1972). The course of the data points may be approximated by Equation 8 by applying

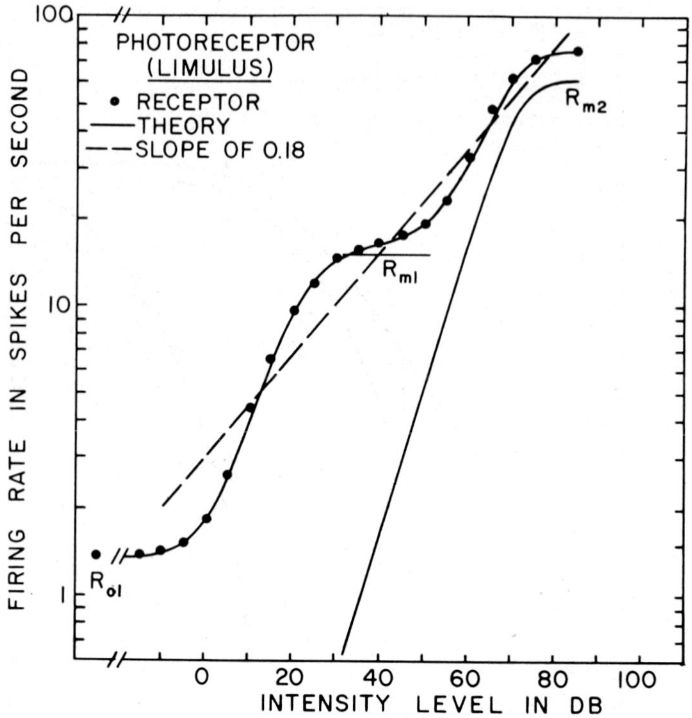

Fig. 5. Intensity characteristic of a *Limulus* photoreceptor in the lateral eye. Experimental points according to Kaplan & Barlow (1972). Thin lines follow Equation 8 with two different sets of parameters for spontaneous and maximum firing rates. Heavy line results from linear superposition of the values traced by the thin lines.

it twice (Zwislocki, 1973). The component functions are indicated in the figure by thin lines. The lower one is based on the actual spontaneous activity R_0, and on an assumed saturation rate R_{m1} (the lower component is not obvious because it partially coincides with the heavy curve drawn through the data points); the upper one is based on a negligible spontaneous activity, consistent with a smaller sensitivity, and on the saturation rate R_{m2} equal to the actual saturation rate less R_{m1}. Both functions obey a power of approximately 0.5. The heavy curve which goes through the data points results from a linear superposition of the component functions. The agreement with the empirical points suggests that the intensity characteristic is produced by two processes staggered along the intensity axis. The staggering extends the physical energy range of the receptor unit to about 90 dB. If we tried to approximate the empirical data of Figure 5 with a power function, as indicated by the intermittent straight line, an exponent of only 0.18 would result. The more highly developed human eye achieves an even greater psychophysical intensity range with an exponent of about 0.3.

Perhaps an analogous process takes place in the human ear through the interaction of many outer and inner hair cells. Some of the relevant numerical relationships are illustrated in Figure 6. The solid curve follows the loudness function for 1000 Hz

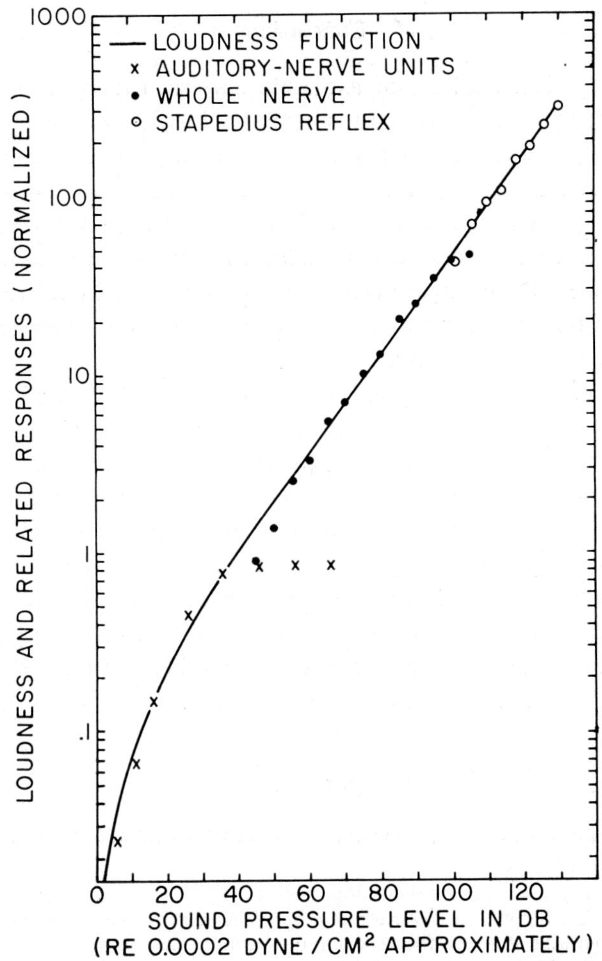

Fig. 6. Loudness function for 1000 Hz according to Hellman & Zwislocki (1961) and related variables. Crosses – driven firing rate of a typical auditory-nerve unit according to Zwislocki (1973). Filled circles – N_1 response of the auditory nerve according to Teas *et al.* (1962). Unfilled circles – stapedius-muscle response according to Zwislocki & Shepherd (1972).

(Hellman & Zwislocki, 1961), the crosses indicate the driven firing rate of a typical auditory-nerve unit (Zwislocki, 1973), the filled circles, the integrated N_1 response of the auditory nerve (derived from the data of Teas, Eldredge, & Davis, 1962), and the unfilled circles, the change of the acoustic compliance at the eardrum produced by the stapedius-muscle contraction (Zwislocki & Shepherd, unpublished data). The latter set of data shows that the output of the auditory nerve increases beyond what can be demonstrated by means of a macroelectrode. It is clearly evident that the auditory periphery is capable of covering an intensity range that exceeds the intensity range of single receptor units by 9 orders of magnitude.

Conclusions

A simple mathematical analysis of available empirical data suggests that sensory receptors perform a power-function transformation on the sum of extrinsic and intrinsic energies impinging upon them. Only two power-function exponents appear to be utilized: 1.0 and 0.5. Of course, these exponents are not accurately observed in all units and deviations of as much as 20% can be encountered. The basic power-function transformation is more or less concealed by effects of neural saturation and threshold; however, it becomes clearly apparent in receptor units with a relatively wide dynamic range. Such units have low thresholds and exhibit a high ratio between the saturation response and spontaneous activity.

In sensory modalities with a small dynamic range, the functions of subjective intensity appear to parallel the receptor intensity functions, and it is possible that they also obey only two power exponents. The almost continuous spectrum of powers encountered in the literature may be the result of saturation and threshold effects. In sense modalities with a wide dynamic range, such as vision and audition, the psychophysical power exponent is beyond any reasonable doubt smaller than the power exponent of the receptor units. The added compression seems to result from interaction of two or more units or processes whose sensitivities are staggered along the intensity scale. If these conclusions are true, the simplicity of the sensory metrics may be even greater than S. S. Stevens (1962) anticipated.

References

Barlow, R. B., & Kaplan, E. *Limulus* lateral eye: Properties of receptor units in the unexcised eye. *Science*, 1971, **174**, 1027–1029.

Barlow, R. B., & Kaplan, E. Personal communication, 1972.

Borg, G., Diamant, H., Ström, L., & Zotterman, Y. The relation between neural and perceptual intensity: A comparative study on the neural and psychophysical response to taste stimuli. *Journal of Physiology*, 1967, **192**, 13–20.

Feldtkeller, R., & Zwicker, E. *Das Ohr als Nachrichtenempfänger*. Stuttgart: S. Hirzel, 1956.

Fishman, I. Y. Single fiber gustatory impulses in rat and hamster. *Journal of Cellular and Comparative Physiology*, 1957, **49**, 319–334.

Garner, W. R. The loudness of repeated short tones. *Journal of the Acoustical Society of America*, 1948, **20**, 513–527.

Gässler, G. Über die Hörschwelle für Schallereignisse mit verschiedenem breitem Frequenzspektrum. *Acustica*, 1954, **4**, 408–414.

Hartline, H. K., & Graham, C. H. Nerve impulses from single receptors in the eye. *Journal of Cellular and Comparative Physiology*, 1932, **1**, 277–295.

Hellman, R. P., & Zwislocki, J. J. Some factors affecting the estimation of loudness. *Journal of the Acoustical Society of America*, 1961, **33**, 687–694.

Hellman, R. P., & Zwislocki, J. J. Loudness function of a 1000 cps tone in the presence of a masking noise. *Journal of the Acoustical Society of America*, 1964, **36**, 1618–1627.

Kiang, N. Y.-S. A survey of recent developments in the study of auditory physiology. *Transactions of the American Otological Society*, 1968, **66**, 108–116.

Kimura, L., & Beidler, L. M. Microelectrode study of test receptors of rat and hamster. *Journal of Cellular and Comparative Physiology*, 1961, **58**, 131–139.

Lipetz, L. E. The relation of physiological and psychological aspects of sensory intensity. In W. R. Loewenstein (Ed.), *Handbook of sensory physiology*. Vol. 1. Berlin: Springer-Verlag, 1971.

Loewenstein, W. R., & Mendelson, M. Components of receptor adaptation in a pacinian corpuscle. *Journal of Physiology (London)*, 1965, **41**, 377–397.

Matthews, B. H. C. The response of a single end organ. *Journal of Physiology*, 1931, **71**, 64–110.

Mountcastle, V. B. The problem of sensing and the neural coding of sensory events. In G. C. Quarton, T. Melnechuk, & F. O. Schmitt (Eds.), *The neurosciences*. New York: The Rockefeller University Press, 1967.

Scharf, B. Critical bands. In J. V. Tobias (Ed.), *Foundations of modern auditory theory*. New York: Academic Press, 1970, pp. 157–202.

Stevens, S. S. The surprising simplicity of sensory metrics. *American Psychologist*, 1962, **17**, 29–39.

Stevens, S. S. Neural events and the psychophysical law. *Science*, 1970, **170**, 1043–1050.

Talbot, W. H., Darian-Smith, I., Kornhuber, H. H., & Mountcastle, V. B. The sense of flatter-vibration: Comparison of the human capacity with response patterns of mechanoreceptive afferents from the monkey hand. *Journal of Neurophysiology*, 1968, **31**, 301–334.

Teas, D. C., Eldredge, D. H., & Davis, H. Cochlear responses to acoustic transients. *Journal of the Acoustical Society of America*, 1962, **34**, 1438–1459.

Zwicker, E., Flottorp, G., & Stevens, S. S. Critical bandwidth in loudness summation. *Journal of the Acoustical Society of America*, 1957, **29**, 548–557.

Zwislocki, J. J. Theory of temporal auditory summation. *Journal of the Acoustical Society of America*, 1960, **32**, 1046–1060.

Zwislocki, J. J. Analysis of some auditory characteristics. In R. D. Luce, R. B. Bush, & E. Galanter (Eds.), *Handbook of mathematical psychology*. Vol. 3. New York: John Wiley and Sons, 1965, pp. 1–97.

Zwislocki, J. J. On intensity characteristics of sensory receptors: A generalized function. *Kybernetik*, 1973, **12**, 169–183.

Zwislocki, J. J., & Shepherd, D. C. Unpublished data, 1972.

PART II

HEARING, SPEECH

AUDITORY MASKING AND SIGNAL DETECTION THEORY[1,2]

JAMES P. EGAN

University of Texas, Austin

Abstract. The contributions of signal detection theory to the study of auditory masking are examined from two points of view.

1. *Theory:* In a given masking situation, the theory of signal detectability specifies the limitation imposed upon the performance of an observer by the characteristics of the signal and of the masking noise. The limitation upon performance imposed by a particular environment is represented by the limiting ROC. The theory of limiting ROCs is the theory of ideal observers. Each masking situation determines a particular ideal observer. Factors that degrade performance relative to the appropriate ideal observer, such as filter bandwidth and methods of processing, may then be investigated.

2. *Methods:* The fundamental detection experiment, that is, the single-interval paradigm with a *yes-no* response, must provide data for the estimation of two, formally independent, conditional probabilities. One probability is the hit rate, and the other probability is the false-alarm rate. These probabilities determine a point in ROC space. Both probabilities must be estimated, because the decisions of the real observer may be influenced by nonsensory factors that are not subject to direct experimental control. The advantages of a two-interval task are discussed.

I would like to give an overview of the general theory of signal detectability. This general theory is a natural development from two separate areas of thought. One of these areas is statistical decision theory. In its simpler forms, this theory is concerned with the two types of errors in the testing of hypotheses, and it shows how a decision may be evaluated in terms of the outcomes, or consequences, of that decision. The other area involves the probability distributions associated with signals and with noises. This area deals with the statistical characteristics of ensembles of noise waveforms. So, the general theory of signal detectability consists of the application of decision theory to the probability distributions that must be used to specify the characteristics of noise. In this general theory, one important question is that of signal existence: Did the received waveform consist of signal-plus-noise or of noise alone? In the most interesting cases, the evidence used for the decision varies from trial to trial, and this fact makes it possible for the observer to adjust his criterion for signal existence according to the demands of some decision goal. This general theory describes the methods for the collection of data so that it is possible to secure measures of sensitivity that are relatively independent of the observer's criterion for the positive response, 'Yes, the signal was present.'

The introduction of the receiver operating characteristic (ROC) is a major contribution to the study of signal detection. The ROC shows how the hit rate is related to the false-alarm rate as the criterion of the observer is varied from one set of trials to the next. The ability of an observer to detect a masked signal may be defined by some measure that is related to the degree of difference between the obtained ROC and the

[1] Reprinted from *Audiology*, 1971, **10**, 41–47.

[2] Paper presented at the Round Table on Auditory Masking at the Tenth International Congress of Audiology in Dallas, Tex., on October 14, 1970.

H. R. Moskowitz et al. (eds.), Sensation and Measurement. 201–205.

line for chance performance. The entire curve characterizes the sensitivity of the observer for some constant signal-to-noise ratio, whereas that point on the curve at which he happens to operate for a set of trials reflects his criterion for saying 'Yes.'

Another functional relation used in the study of masking is called the psychometric function. In such studies, this function usually shows the relation between some measure of the detectability of the signal and signal strength. If the measure of signal detection is the hit rate, or the probability of saying 'Yes' given that the signal occurred, then in order to be easily and meaningfully interpreted, the function must have a constant parameter, the false-alarm rate.

The two functions mentioned above may be described in statistical parlance. In the test of two hypotheses, H_0 and H_1, there are two types of errors. If H_0 is rejected when in fact it is true, then a type I error is committed. If H_0 is accepted when in fact it is false, then a type II error results, and the power of the statistical test is defined as one minus the probability of a type II error. Now, other things being equal, the power, or the hit rate, depends upon two factors: (*a*) the probability of a type I error, or the false-alarm rate, and (*b*) the degree of difference between H_0 and H_1, or the signal-to-noise ratio. In this statistical terminology, the ROC is a plot of the power of a statistical test against the probability of a type I error. For such a relation to be meaningful, all other factors in the situation must be held at constant, average values. Also, the psychometric function corresponds to the power function of a statistical test, that is, the psychometric function is a plot of the power of the test against the degree of difference between the two hypotheses with the probability of a type I error held at some constant value.

The concept of the ideal observer concerns the limitation upon performance imposed by the statistical characteristics of the signal and of the noise. The detectability of a particular signal is limited by the statistical properties of the masking noise. If all information concerning the statistical properties of the signal and of the noise are known to an observer, and if that observer is able to process the input waveform so as to extract all relevant information contained in the received waveform, then the observer is ideal, and his ROC is a limiting ROC. This limiting ROC places an upper bound upon the performance of any real observer.

There is an ideal observer for each type of signal and for each type of noise. Thus, when the signal is specified exactly to an ideal observer who must detect this signal in Fourier-series, band-limited, Gaussian noise, then the limiting ROC is based upon two normal curves of equal variance. (The signal must be bandlimited in the same way as the noise.) However, if a sinusoidal signal is specified except for phase, then the limiting ROC is based upon Rayleigh-Rice distributions. And, as a final example, if both the signal and the noise are samples of the output of a narrow-band filter that is excited by Gaussian noise, then the limiting ROC is based upon two Chi-square distributions with the appropriate number of degrees of freedom.

The concept of the ideal observer emphasizes two basic aspects of the detection process: optimal processing of the received waveform and optimal decision processes. As would be expected, the performance of the human observer is inferior to that of the ideal. Three principal factors have been proposed to account for the inferiority of the human observer. These are: (*a*) inferior processing, (*b*) internal noise, and (*c*) noisy decision processes. It is my guess that the manner in which the received waveform is processed accounts for a fairly large part of the inefficiency of the human observer.

The above summary is based primarily upon the contributions of: Tanner & Swets (1954), Egan (1957), Licklider (1959), Green (1960a, 1960b), Swets, Tanner, & Birdsall (1961), Jeffress (1964, 1968), Egan & Clarke (1966), and Green & Swets (1966).

In this brief survey, it may be well to turn to the contributions of signal detection theory to the body of psychophysical methods that are used by the auditory scientist. It is unfortunate that the methods prescribed by signal detection theory are time-consuming and tedious. But, in the final analysis, the measure of the detectability of a weak signal must rest upon the estimation of two probabilities, the hit rate and the false-alarm rate, and in order to estimate these probabilities with reasonable accuracy, many trials must be conducted. To be sure, in some situations, both clinical and experimental, the false-alarm rate may be adequately handled by training and by instructions. Nevertheless, it should be appreciated that such techniques provide only an indirect method for the control of the listener's criterion. It might be thought that a measure of the listener's criterion is relatively unimportant if large changes in the independent variable are accompanied by comparably large changes in the dependent variable. For example, if you increase the level of the masking noise by 60 dB, you must increase the signal level by about 60 dB in order to maintain the same level of performance. But some time ago, two prominent hearing laboratories disagreed about whether this masking function is in fact linear at high levels, and I am convinced that the discrepancy resulted from the different psychophysical methods used. It is better to know, than to assume, that the criterion of the listener has not changed along with a change of the independent variable. Also let us note that for some types of problems, a change in the detectability of a signal corresponding to 3 dB may be very significant. For example, such a change of 3 dB might double the estimated width of a critical band of masking.

I want now to report the results of a simple experiment (Egan, Emmerich, & Viemeister). This experiment shows that the estimate of the masked threshold as measured with the method of constant stimuli can change by at least 8 dB when the listener is trained to adopt extreme criteria. Four listeners were first trained to adopt the three criteria of *strict*, *medium*, and *lax* in a single-interval, *yes-no* task. The principal part of each trial consisted of a single observation interval which was marked off by a light, and during this interval the sinusoidal pulse (400 Hz, 250 msec) was presented on one-half of the trials. The other half of the trials were 'noise alone' trials. The masking noise was continuous with a spectrum level of 45 dB re 2×10^{-5} $N\,\mathrm{m}^{-2}$, and practice was given at three signal levels spaced 2 dB apart. Typical ROCs resulted from these six sessions of practice each lasting 1.5 h, and during this extensive training the listeners successfully learned to adopt the three criteria for 'hearing a tone'.

The procedure was then changed to that called the method of constant stimuli. The sequence of events during a trial was the same as that in the training sessions.

However, during each block of 80 trials, the sinusoidal signal was presented at five levels, ranging from $10 \log_{10}(E/N_0) = 6$ to 14 dB in 2-dB steps. Furthermore, the signal was presented on the average on 90% of the trials, and the remaining 10% consisted of noise-alone, or 'catch trials.' For a given block of trials, the listeners were instructed to adopt one of the three criteria: strict, medium, or lax.

The results of the experiment are presented in Figure 1. The horizontal axis is the signal level in decibels, and the vertical axis is the probability of a response of 'Yes' given a signal occurrence. The vertical axis is the hit rate, and it is sometimes confusingly called the 'probability of hearing.' Please note the large displacement between the two extreme psychometric functions; it is about 8 dB. If the threshold be defined as the level of the signal that can be 'heard' on 50% of the trials, then our observers changed their masked thresholds by 8 dB simply by changing their criterion from strict to lax.

Let me conclude with a few comments on the procedure called the two-interval, forced-choice method. With this method, there are two observation intervals during

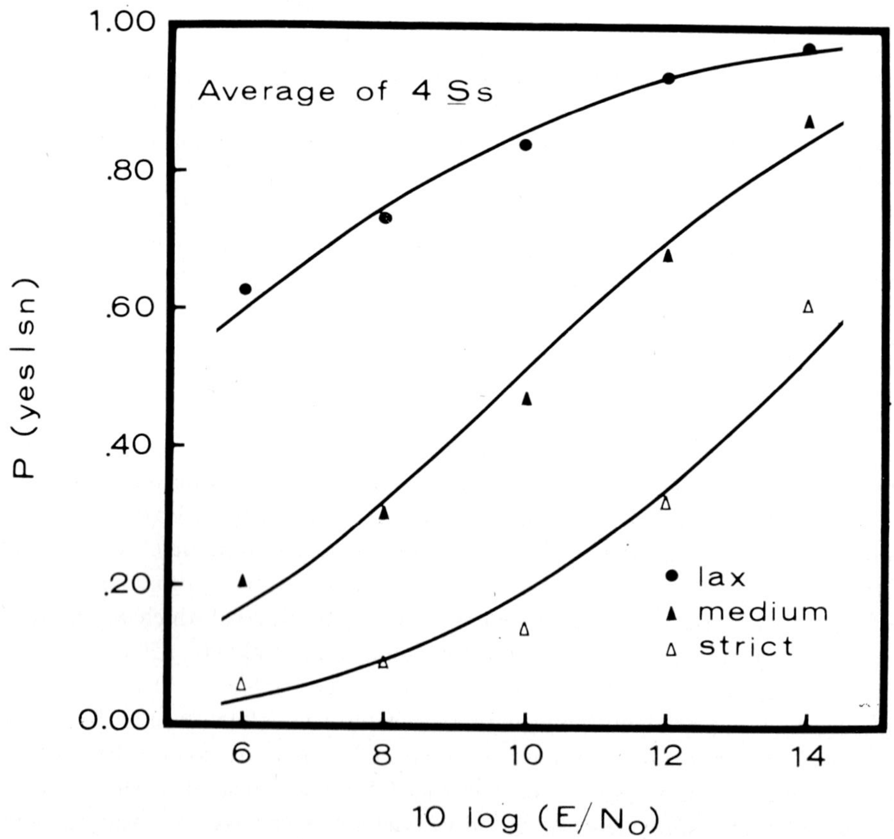

Fig. 1. Psychometric functions determined by the method of constant stimuli. The parameter is the degree of confidence required for a response of 'Yes.' ● = lax; ▲ = medium; △ = strict.

each trial, and the signal always occurs in either the first or the second interval, but not in both. The listeners are forced to select one of the two intervals as the one most likely to have contained the signal. This method has been used in psychophysical investigations for a long time, and in many cases it is one of the best methods for the determination of a psychometric function. Typically, the human observer has little or no bias toward one or the other of the two observation intervals, and consequently a criterion-free measure of the detectability of a signal can be readily secured.

References

Egan, J. P. Message repetition, operating characteristics, and confusion matrices in speech communication. Indiana University: Hearing and Communication Laboratory, 1957, Technical Report No. AFCRC-TR-57-50.

Egan, J. P., & Clarke, F. R. Psychophysics and signal detection. In J. B. Sidowski (Ed.), *Experimental methods and instrumentation in psychology*. New York: McGraw-Hill, 1966.

Egan, J. P., Emmerich, D. S., & Viemeister, N. Psychometric functions determined by the method of constant stimuli. Unpublished data.

Green, D. M. Auditory detection of a noise signal. *Journal of the Acoustical Society of America*, 1960, **32**, 121–131. (a)

Green, D. M. Psychoacoustics and detection theory. *Journal of the Acoustical Society of America*, 1960, **32**, 1189–1203. (b)

Green, D. M., & Swets, J. A. *Signal detection theory and psychophysics*. New York: Wiley, 1966.

Jeffress, L. A. Stimulus-oriented approach to detection. *Journal of the Acoustical Society of America*, 1964, **36**, 766–774.

Jeffress, L. A. Mathematical and electrical models of auditory detection. *Journal of the Acoustical Society of America*, 1968, **44**, 187–203.

Licklider, J. C. R. Three auditory theories. In S. Koch (Ed.), *Psychology: A study of a science*. Vol. 1. New York: McGraw-Hill, 1959.

Swets, J. A., Tanner Jr., W. P., & Birdsall, T. G. Decision processes in perception. *Psychological Review*, 1961, **68**, 301–340.

Tanner Jr., W. P., & Swets, J. A. A decision-making theory of visual detection. *Psychological Review*, 1954, **61**, 401–409.

AN AUDIOGRAM FORMAT CONVEYING THE PSYCHO-PHYSIOLOGY OF HEARING

GORDON FLOTTORP

The Institute of Audiology, University of Oslo

Abstract. Because its scales for frequency and hearing threshold level are rather arbitrarily chosen, the traditional audiogram inadequately portrays the handicap associated with a hearing loss. Therefore, a new format has been developed. The frequency scale is based upon a compromise between the observed tonotopical representation along the basilar membrane and the assumption that equal numbers of JNDs for pitch correspond to equal lengths on the basilar membrane. On the hearing loss scale, equal distances are associated with equal numbers of JNDs for loudness. This new format is more logically correlated with the psychophysiology of hearing than the old one. Examples of hearing losses mapped on the traditional audiogram format are compared with the same examples on the new psychophysiological format.

When the Western Electric Company 2A Audiometer was designed in the Bell Telephone Laboratory in the early 1920s, there seemed to be little doubt about the format for recording the results of the hearing tests. The two basic stimulus parameters in hearing tests were frequency and intensity. A Cartesian co-ordinate system with frequency on the abscissa and intensity on the ordinate was the obvious choice. No problems other than those of a practical nature seemed to exist in the choice of a frequency scale and the range of test frequencies. The only serious decision required was the choice of zero level on the ordinate. From the engineering point of view the dyne per square centimeter was the correct physical solution. However, the otological consultant to the project, Edmond P. Fowler, considered the instrument a new diagnostic tool for the otologist, and recommended that the ordinate should feature the deviation from normal hearing (Davis & Silverman, 1970). The decibel, as the unit of stimulus intensity, was the obvious unit of hearing loss. At that time little consideration was given to subjective magnitude, i.e., to loudness.

The format of the audiogram has been determined by international recommendation; at first the ratio between the intensity and frequency scales was arbitrary, but in recent years the ratio has been fixed at 20 dB:1 octave. This format does not give a visual impression that readily conveys the subjective effects of the hearing loss. The audiogram must be interpreted by a person with a good command of psychoacoustics and auditory physiology. The audiogram should, for instance, be compared with the frequency range of speech, and with the information-receiving capacity of the ear in various frequency and intensity ranges. Normal and pathological relations between intensity and loudness should also be taken into consideration.

If the frequency and intensity axes were scaled in accordance with corresponding subjective and physiological variables, the audiogram pattern would reflect better the handicap resulting from a hearing loss. The development of such an audiogram was the goal of the work reported here.

H. R. Moskowitz et al. (eds.), Sensation and Measurement. 207–213.

Procedure

Since the mel scale (Stevens & Volkmann, 1940) corresponds fairly well, but not perfectly, to the tonotopical representation in the cochlea, it seems logical to base the abscissa of a new audiogram format on a compromise between the mel scale and the observed frequency distribution along the basilar membrane.

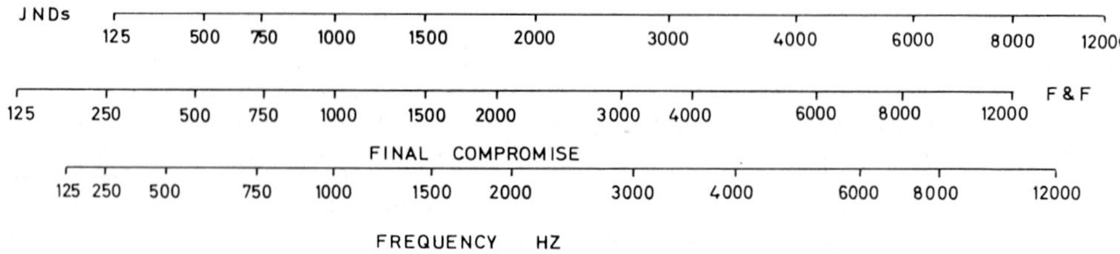

Fig. 1. Frequency scales based on psychoacoustical data (upper line), physiological data (middle line), and a compromise (third line) between the two.

Information theory makes attractive the concept of an equal number of just noticeable differences (JNDs) for pitch representing equal lengths on the frequency axis. Since the number of JNDs does not vary substantially with intensity above a sensation level of about 40 to 50 dB, and since it is the ratio between adjacent frequency intervals that is important in this connection, it was possible to construct a scale reflecting this concept of JNDs (the scale shown at the top of Figure 1).

The scale is based on data from Stevens & Volkmann (1940) and Stevens & Davis (1938), together with some of my own measurements of the JND for frequency (Flottorp, 1950). These last data agree better with the differentiated pitch function than do the results that Stevens & Volkmann had available (Knudsen, 1923; Shower & Biddulph, 1931).

The second line of Figure 1 presents the frequency distribution along the basilar membrane, with the locus of 1000 Hz unchanged from the upper line. This second line is based on a review by Foss and Flottorp (1974) of the data on the localization of frequencies along the basilar membrane and on the topography of the blood supply. The third line of Figure 1 is a compromise between the two upper scales. Between 500 and 3000 Hz the correlation between the upper two scales is very good; outside these limits the correlation is fair. Below 250 Hz and above 8000 Hz the tonotopical representation is probably less valid than at the middle frequencies. Similarly, psychoacoustic experiments yield uncertain results at the extreme ends of the scale. My compromise between the two sets of data is not a straightforward averaging, but rather a kind of extrapolation from the middle range.

Clinical audiometers usually have 125 Hz as the lowest frequency, and therefore the present audiogram will only suggest where the half octave below 125 Hz might be located. Although the highest frequency on clinical audiometers often is 8000 Hz, growing interest in the higher frequencies (Fletcher, 1973; Flottorp, 1973; Lipscomb, 1973) led me to go up to 12000 Hz in the new audiogram format. The correlation

between the psychoacoustic and physiological data is better in this high-frequency range than in the lowest frequency range.

For several reasons the standard loudness scale in sones cannot be used directly to indicate hearing loss. Based upon a similar philosophy as used for the frequency scale, I decided to apply the concept of equal numbers of JNDs for loudness to represent equal distances on the ordinate. The idea and the basic data stem from the division of the auditory area into small cells as drawn by Stevens & Davis (1938) for the purpose of calculating the number of distinguishable tones.

For the most important frequencies, I calculated graphically the function relating JNDs to normal sensation level in dB. A single function adequately serves for frequencies between 500 and 2000 Hz, but not for lower and higher frequencies. The possibility of representing each frequency on the audiogram by its own JND function was rejected in favor of an orthogonal, two-coordinate plot of hearing loss against frequency. I therefore chose to base the hearing-loss scale on a compromise between the function representing the range from 500 to 2000 Hz and the function for 4000 Hz. (See Figure 2.) This solution seemed reasonable since the area corresponding to the

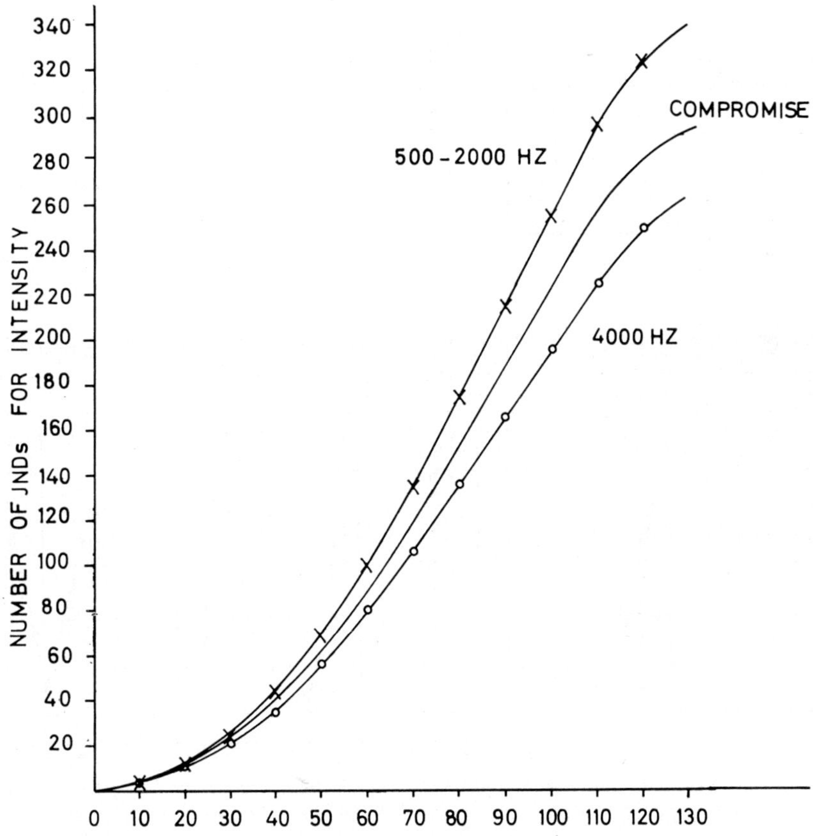

Fig. 2. Intensity functions based on JNDs for loudness.

frequency range below 250 Hz and above 6000 Hz is rather small. Although the resulting ordinate scale at the low and high frequencies on the audiogram is about twice the correct length, the visual impression is not correspondingly distorted, because the incorrect ranges are of limited extent.

Results

Figure 3 presents examples of the new audiogram format. It seems natural to retain the hertz as the unit for frequency on the abscissa and the decibel as the unit for hearing

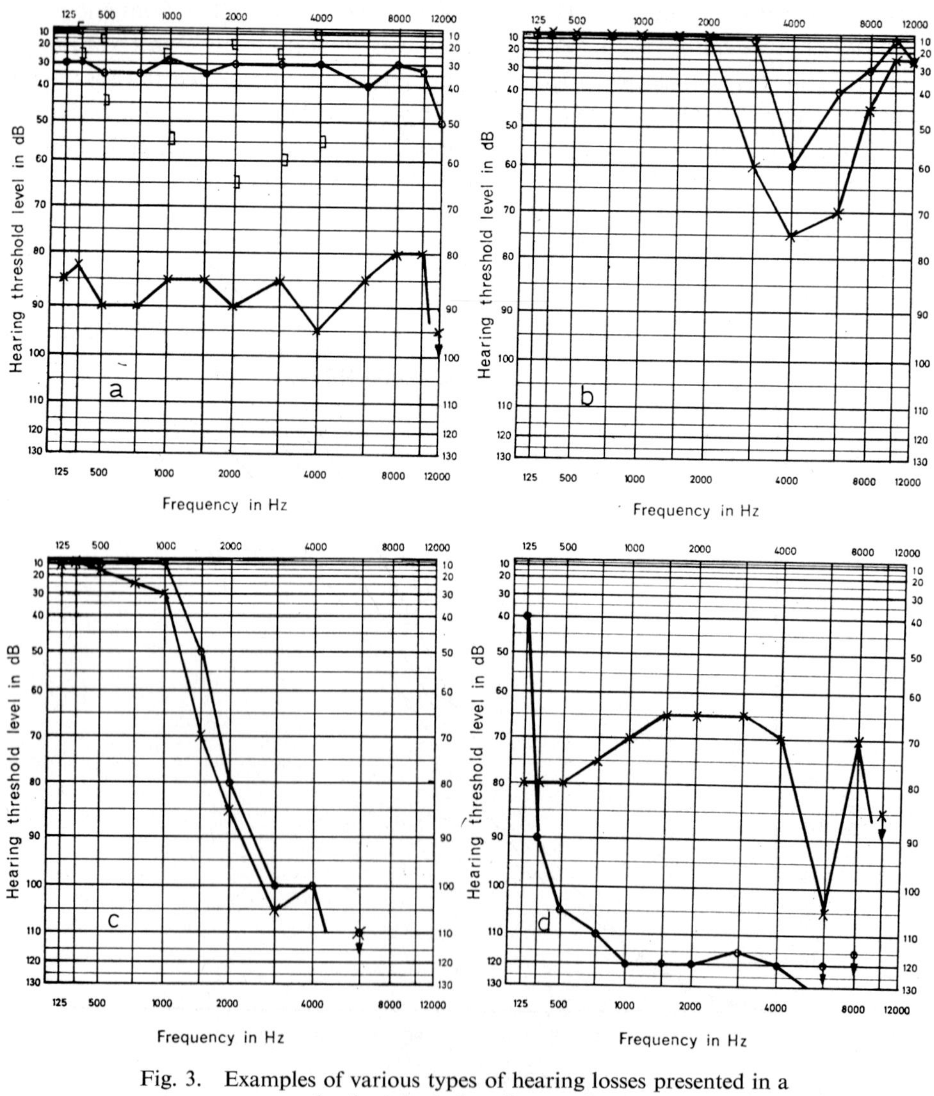

Fig. 3. Examples of various types of hearing losses presented in a psychophysiological audiogram format.

loss on the ordinate because all audiometers are designed with hertz and decibel as the main parameters. It is the unequal weighting along the frequency and intensity scales that provides the new picture of the curve on the audiogram.

The central position is now occupied by 2000 Hz instead of 1000 Hz so as to emphasize frequencies above 2000 Hz. This new format represents the information channel capacity of the auditory system quite well, as shown by its compatibility with Pimonow's (1965) division of the auditory area into units of equal channel capacity (equal number of bits). Some of the advantages of the new audiogram format may be judged by comparing the four examples presented in Figure 3 with the same four in Figure 4 under the traditional format.

(*a*) Hearing loss due to otosclerosis in an early stage in one ear and in an advanced stage in the other ear.

(*b*) Hearing loss due to acoustic trauma of moderate type in one ear, and of a more serious type in the other ear.

(*c*) Hearing loss due to acoustic trauma of a severe type in both ears.

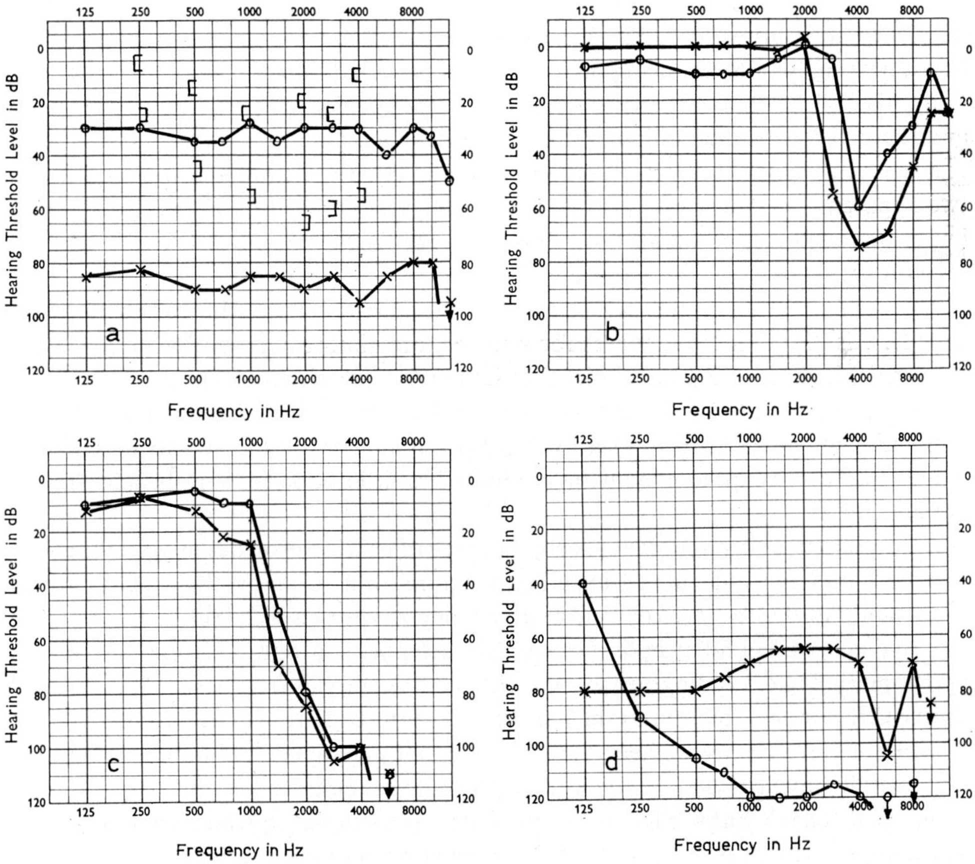

Fig. 4. The examples of Figure 3 presented in the traditional audiogram format.

(*d*) Hearing loss of congenital type in two different patients, one with a very severe loss, the other with a moderate to severe loss.

Discussion

The experienced audiologist is able to judge the audiogram in its traditional form both for diagnostic and therapeutic purposes. The somewhat distorted visual picture may, however, affect the judgments in certain directions. A small hearing loss of 40 to 50 dB is easily overestimated. In the new psychophysiological format the same loss will probably be more correctly estimated. The old format would lead the clinician to expect little benefit to a person with a hearing loss of 80 to 90 dB, whereas the new audiogram makes a possible hearing reserve more easily recognized. I know quite a few cases where the audiologist deemed the hearing loss too severe for a hearing aid, yet a strong aid proved to be unexpectedly helpful. The increasing ability of the ear to utilize information above a threshold of 80 dB, as emphasized in the psychophysiological format of the audiogram, may account for these good results.

Even more obvious is the lack of emphasis given by the traditional audiogram to the frequency range above 2000 Hz. The frequency range considered important in evaluating a hearing loss due to acoustic trauma has been 500–2000 Hz (ISO recommendation), which is located only in the upper half of the cochlea. The redundancy of speech and the division of the audiogram along an octave scale are probably the principal reasons for this limitation. It is 2000 Hz and not 1000 Hz that divides the cochlea into two apparently equally important parts. For the clear perception of speech – the most important task of the human hearing organ – the frequency range above 2000 Hz is much more important than is usually realized.

The audiogram in Figure 3C is from a retired army officer who served in World War II. His discrimination curves for numbers are almost normal; for monosyllabic PB-words, he has a 20% discrimination loss and a speech-reception threshold 20 to 30 dB above normal. The patient himself considers his hearing handicap to be much more severe than reflected by these values. His audiogram in the new format demonstrates the severity quite convincingly and offers little hope for any benefit from a hearing aid.

In addition to understanding speech, the sense of hearing provides us with the ability to "feel" the environment, to experience nature, and to enjoy the musical world. These abilities depend heavily on the frequency range above 2000 Hz, as shown by experiments with blind people wearing ear defenders (Monrad-Krohn, 1960). The psychophysiological audiogram format with its shift of focus from 1000 Hz to 2000 Hz should direct more attention to the importance of the frequency range above 2000 Hz.

I do not consider my rendering of the psychophysiological audiogram to be final. However, it may provoke a search for a better format than the one now used. Once we realize that today's knowledge makes possible a new format in which an audiogram's visual impression gives more and better information about the patient's hearing, there should be little reason to adhere to the traditional form of the audiogram.

References

Davis, H., & Silverman, S. R. *Hearing and deafness.* (3d ed.) New York: Holt, Rinehart and Winston, 1970.

Fletcher, J. L. High frequency hearing and noise exposure. Paper presented at International Congress on Noise as a Public Health Problem, Dubrovnik, 1973.

Flottorp, G. The sensitivity of the ear to changes in frequency. (In Norwegian) *Fra Fysikkens Verden*, 1950, **12**, 49–65.

Flottorp, G. Effects of noise upon the upper frequency limit of hearing. *Acta Otolaryngologica*, 1973, **75**, 329–331.

Foss, I., & Flottorp, G. A comparative study of the development of hearing and vision in various species commonly used in experiments. *Acta Otolaryngologica*, 1974, **77**, 202–214.

Knudsen, V. O. The sensibility of the ear to small differences in intensity and frequency. *Physical Review*, 1923, **21**, 84–103.

Lipscomb, D. M. Theoretical considerations in the rise of high frequency hearing loss in children. Paper presented at International Congress on Noise as a Public Health Problem, Dubrovnik, 1973.

Monrad-Krohn, G. H. Distance perception of the blind. *Tidsskrift for Den Norske Lægeforening*, 1960, **80**, 1–8.

Pimonow, L. La parole synthétique et son application dans la correction auditive. *Annales des Télécommunications*, 1965, **20**, 151–187.

Shower, E. G., & Biddulph, R. Differential pitch sensitivity of the ear. *Journal of the Acoustical Society of America*, 1931, **3**, 275–287.

Stevens, S. S., & Davis, H. *Hearing. Its psychology and physiology.* New York: John Wiley & Sons, 1938.

Stevens, S. S., & Volkmann, J. The relation of pitch to frequency: A revised scale. *American Journal of Psychology*, 1940, **53**, 329–353.

THE HUMAN AUDITORY EVOKED RESPONSE

ROBERT GALAMBOS

Dept. of Neurosciences, University of California, San Diego

> I would like to believe that the knowledge that can be gleaned about sensory systems by studying evoked potentials is greater than zero.
>
> S. S. Stevens, *Science* 1971, **172**, 502.

The messages in this paper will be transmitted mainly by its four figures. Smitty would have liked these figures, I think, because they show electrical responses generated in the brains of people as they listen to sounds and make auditory discriminations. In 1947, when he hired me to get some auditory physiology going at the Psycho-Acoustics Laboratory, there was no such thing as an averaging computer, and so it was technically impossible to create pictures like these. If it had been possible to make them I think Smitty would have wanted them made, because his admiration for the cat auditory system I worked on in his laboratory came nowhere near his love for the auditory system of man. And since what Smitty wanted he usually got, and what he liked to believe in he did something about, the experiments these figures summarize could very well have been done a quarter century ago in the basement of Memorial Hall.

The first of them shows the normal human auditory evoked response (AER). For many years *E*s have pasted electrodes to *S*s scalp, connected them to amplifiers, stimulated *S* with clicks or tone bursts, and recorded the AER, which is the brain wave activity timelocked to the stimulus. An AER produced in this way appears at the bottom of Figure 1. At the left-hand side of this bottom record one sees small unresolved deflections which emerge for inspection in the middle record, where the time base has been changed so it displays only the first 50 msec of the AER. And at the left-hand edge of this middle record one sees still more poorly resolved waves which stand out very nicely on the even shorter time base of the top record. All-told, then, the AER actually consists of some 15 different waves.

In the past most *E*s have worked with the big, long latency waves visible in the bottom record; a few have worked mainly with the middle latency group (10–100 msec), while a very few, and these only very recently, have focussed upon those in the 1–10-msec epoch. Figure 1 presents, for the first time to my knowledge, a comprehensive view of the entire response, as accurate in details as we know how to make it in our laboratory. It appears in a 1973 doctoral thesis by Terence W. Picton and in a paper now in press.[1] Picton has labelled the waves in Figure 1 according to the conventions of the *E*s who discovered them or who have worked with them most.

The earliest of the 15 AER deflections peaks at about 1.5 msec after the stimulus and is generated by the auditory nerve; the latest, N_2 at about 300 msec, represents activity in cortex as far away from the primary auditory pathway (in time at least) as one can get. The group bearing Roman numerals originate in the brainstem, and thus trace the passage of nerve impulses away from the cochlea and up through the brainstem enroute

H. R. Moskowitz et al. (eds.), Sensation and Measurement. 215–221.

to the cortex. The middle group (10–50 msec) are the ones most argued about; they probably originate in cortex, but not in auditory cortex, and only with care can *E* visualize them uncontaminated by muscle artifacts. The group with longest latency, N_1–P_2–N_2, are almost certainly cortical in origin.

Any stable, reproducible phenomenon, like the thirsty rat that presses a bar, or the series of waves in Figure 1, can be used in experiments, even though one does not know precisely what causes it, and how desirable this additional information might be. For instance, one can ask, as we have, what happens to our thing when listeners attend to the auditory stimuli that create it.[2] To do this we present a train of clicks

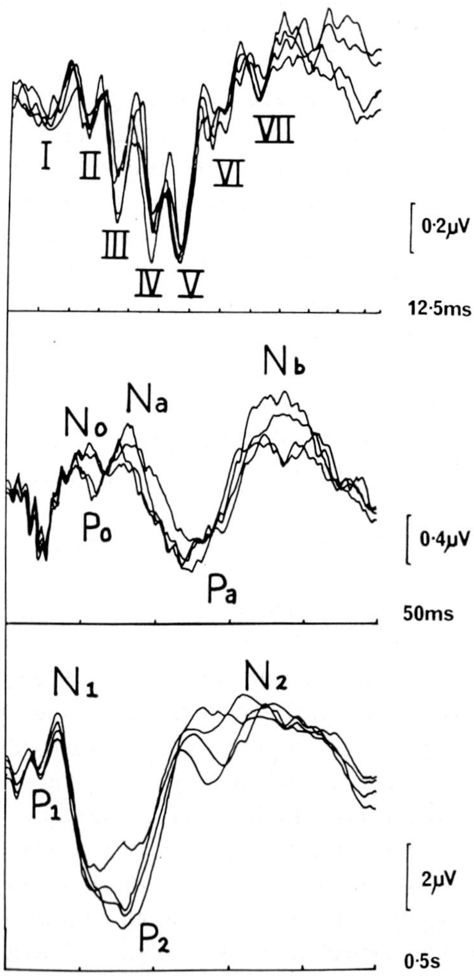

Fig. 1. Components of the human auditory evoked response. Each tracing is the average of 1024 responses to 60 dB SL clicks delivered once per second to the right ear. Electrodes: vertex and right mastoid. Responses initially embedded in the EEG recorded on tape were later extracted by an averager (Fabritek 1052) on the three different time bases.

(or tone bursts), at 1 per sec or so, in which an occasional member of the train (the odd-ball) is different in intensity (clicks) or frequency (tones). *S* hears these signals under 2 conditions: (*a*) he counts the occasional odd-balls, and (*b*) he pays no attention to the sounds (we have *S* read a book). The odd-balls can be adjusted so as to be very easy or very hard to detect. Under both attend and non-attend conditions *S*'s AER, as this appears between a reference (usually the linked mastoids) and one or more scalp electrodes, is extracted from his EEG by conventional computer-averaging techniques. ("Conventional" today, but seen only in the mind's-eye of dreamers like Walter Rosenblith in 1947.) Figure 2, identical in format to Figure 1, shows the results of such an experiment. One sees significant differences between "attend" and "ignore"

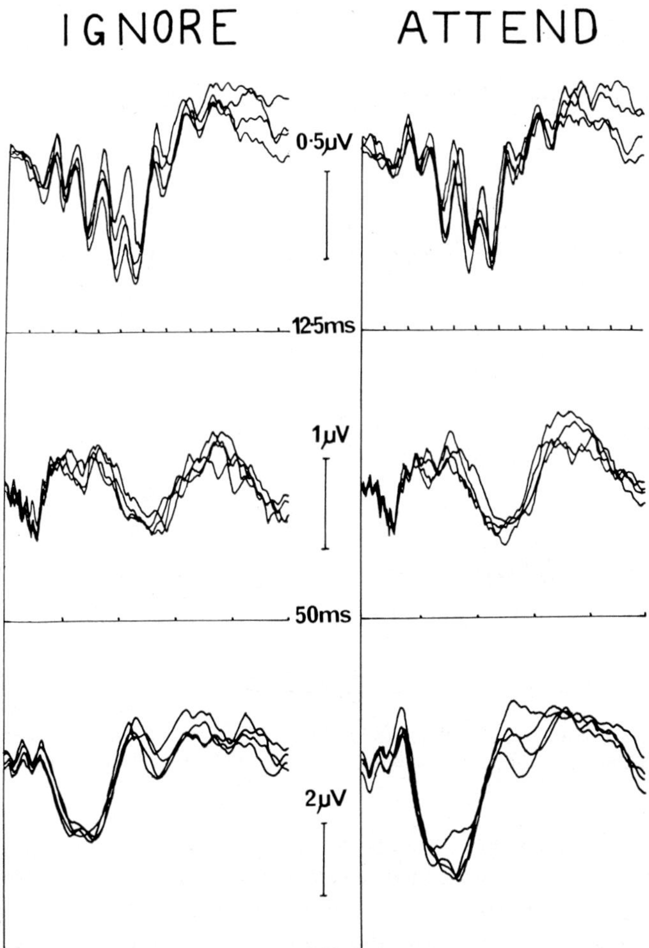

Fig. 2. All details as in Figure 1. In the "attend" condition *S* counted an occasional faint click interspersed among 1024 of them presented at 60 dB SL. In the "ignore" condition he was reading a book. Only responses to the 60 dB SL clicks appear here. Subject S.V.

only in the bottom row. Here large amplitude differences in the N_1–P_2–N_2 wave complex are obvious to the naked eye, and they are consistent, since the results from four replications of the experiment virtually superimpose. Some differences between ignore-attend can be seen in the earlier components of the response (top and middle records), as those of you with a ruler and sharp eyes can confirm; these, however, are not consistent across or within subjects, and they lie at the limit of reliability of the method.

Figure 2 tells us, then, that what we call "attention" in this paradigm does put its mark upon the AER but not until about 0.1 s post-stimulus. So "knowledge ...

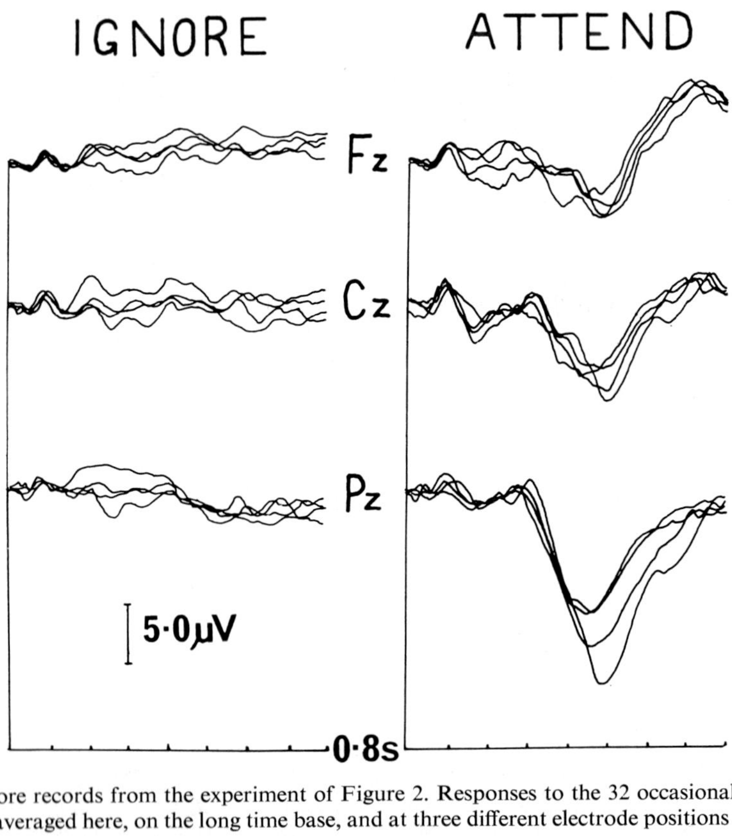

Fig. 3. More records from the experiment of Figure 2. Responses to the 32 occasional faint clicks are shown averaged here, on the long time base, and at three different electrode positions on the scalp.

gleaned ... by studying evoked potentials" is indeed greater than zero, since it has settled a question psychologists have asked for nearly 20 years: Does the efferent auditory pathway, those feedback fibers running from brain to cochlea, act as a gating mechanism which allows a given stimulus to arouse more auditory nerve activity when *S* is in the attentive state? The answer is NO, because there are no changes in that very first wave of the AER, and this is generated by auditory nerve activity.[3]

Recall that occasionally *S* received an odd-ball to count. His responses to these special targets of attention appear in Figure 3 where AERs at three different points on his head ranging from front (Fz) to back (Pz) in the midline are written out on the long-time base. In the "ignore" condition the N_1–P_2 deflections are everywhere present but very small, for the stimulus was weak. In the "attend" state they are larger, which is what we have just learned should happen. But the N_1–P_2 change is trivial compared to what comes later – that huge downward-going wave. This big wave is entirely new, it peaks between 300–600 msec post-stimulus in various experiments, and it is positive

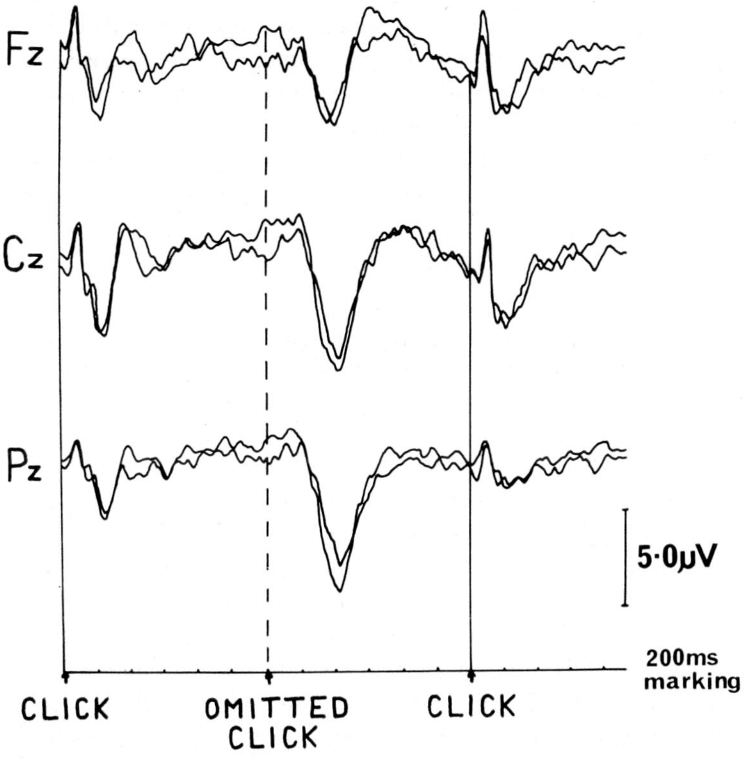

Fig. 4. Recordings from an experiment like that of Figure 2 except that the faint click in the train there was simply omitted here. Interclick interval 1.1 s, *S* counted the number of omissions. Computer was triggered by the click prior to the omitted one; each tracing represents the average of 64 responses. Subject T.P.

in polarity. Sutton and his colleagues first described it in *Science*, in 1965. *E*s now call it the P_3 (or P_{300}) and in the last 5 years more and more of them have been finding it to turn up in association with more and more kinds of interesting behavior.

In our experiment of Figures 2 and 3, P_3 appears only when *S* discovers the weak target-sound he is hunting for. What if his target was nothing at all; would P_3 still be there? Suppose, for instance, the intensity of the odd-ball was attenuated still more, so that it becomes simply an absent click in a regularly repeating train of them. We now have what amounts to the temporal conditioning paradigm in which we make *S* expect a certain interstimulus interval and have him keep track of the number of times his expectation is not met. Figure 4 shows the huge P_3 he generates when his odd-ball target is no stimulus whatsoever.[4]

The main message in Figure 4 is that P_3 can index wholly endogenous brain events – no physical change at a receptor is required to set it off. Here P_3 must be the electrical sign of something going on exclusively inside the skull – a perception, a recognition of difference, unconscious inference, the "aha moment" upon finding what has been looked for. But whatever one calls this brain-business engaging *S* during the Figure-4 experiment one sees in P_3 its electrical signature, uncontaminated by anything else. E. G. Boring would, I think, have had a good time with this *experimentum crucis*, for by simple logic a brain wave invariably associated with the perception of a stimulus not delivered must be a sign of the perception itself.

Some of us believe the P_3 of Figure 4 indexes the same brain processes that yielded the P_3 of Figure 3. If this is correct, you look at the electrical sign of a purely subjective event whenever you see a P_3. In a recent review[5] my colleagues collect 19 P_3 papers by 43 authors, consider what these *E*s think their *S*s were doing, and conclude as follows:

> *P_3 is evoked by signals that deliver information being sought, thereby "resolving" prior uncertainty.* Accordingly an enhanced P_3 is seen to follow 1) a signal which confirms or disconfirms a prior guess... 2) solution of an auditory discrimination... 3) the detection of a threshold-level auditory signal... 4) a signal for a simple choice reaction... 5) an occasional stimulus change... 6) a signal to shift sensory-motor set and 7) a letter which completes a word.[6]

In our laboratory (*a*) P_3 accompanies HITs in the auditory signal-detection task, where its size varies directly (as does the N_1–P_2 amplitude) with *S*'s confidence in his decision: here it is the wave of confidence, if you like. (*b*) If *S*, having made his decision in an auditory discrimination task, is then informed by one of two lights whether he was correct, the response evoked by the light signalling "incorrect" has the larger P_3: a wave of disappointment is bigger than a wave of satisfaction, so to speak. (*c*) If *S* in a visual task is hunting for his odd-balls and suddenly receives an entirely irrelevant one, the P_3 to it is unusually large: the "what the devil was *that*" wave, if you will. Also (*d*) P_3's generated in reasonably comparable visual, auditory and tactile tasks look very much alike, or, waves that signal the same thing equal each other. I overdo the hyperbole, perhaps, but the experimental results do make you wonder what *S* has in mind, and so bring you face-to-face with psychology's best unanswered questions.

What does seem clear is this: when *S* delivers his P_3 to *E*, he tells *E* he has engaged in a conscious process. He has been aware, gotten the message, made up his mind. The language he uses is as ancient as man himself, since cavemen produced P_3's too, but we have only just recently found out how to read it.

I wonder what Smitty would have done after perusing this story of mine. Perhaps lean back in that big chair of his, put the feet on the desk, small smile on his face cocked a little to the left, and say "That's just the kind of thing I had in mind when I hired him in 1947"[7].

NOTES

[1] Picton's thesis consists of 3 chapters, each now a paper in press. "Habituation and attention in the auditory system" is scheduled for *Handbook of sensory physiology*, vol. 5, which Keidel and Neff are editing for Springer-Verlag the publisher. "Human auditory potentials", both "I: Evaluation of components" and "II: Effects of attention" will appear in *Electroencephalography and Clinical Neurophysiology*. His Ph.D. thesis didn't quite come up to Smitty's ideal – a package of papers already published – but he almost made it. (Note added in proof: for the *EEG Journal* papers see **36**, 179, 1974.)

[2] Steven A. Hillyard, a 1968 Ph.D. in psychology (Yale) has been the most persistent asker, and the most successful answerer of these questions in the laboratory. His bibliography lists 28 such successes, 11 on the AER and 10 on the related CNV, a brain-generated slow potential wave that indexes people's expectations. He is a co-author in each of Picton's upcoming publications.

[3] An early variant of this experiment appears in 'Human auditory attention: A central or peripheral process? in *Science*, 1971, **173**, 351–353. We discuss there the possibility that we may have been led astray by the limitations of the method.

Space is not available here for more on those waves given Roman numerals in Figure 1. They are strictly stimulus-bound, varying in amplitude and latency so precisely with change in stimulus intensity that one who knows the rule can predict within a few dB the strength of unknown clicks *E* delivered to *S*. Furthermore, these properties change systematically with age between birth and 18–24 months, as they might if progressive myelination were proceeding in this period. For the data, the argument that these waves provide a means for objective hearing testing in children and adults, and a list of the publications available on these brainstem bumps, see Hecox (K) and Galambos 'Brainstem auditory evoked responses in human infants and adults'. *Archives of Otolaryngology*, 1974, **99**, 30–33.

[4] I believe Rusinov discovered this P_3, if one agrees his EEG recordings of 1958 show it; see them on p. 312 in Jasper & Smirnov (Eds.) *The Moscow colloquium*, suppl. 13, 1960, *Electroencephalography and Clinical Neurophysiology* or on p. 254 in Brazier (Ed.) *The central nervous system and behaviour*. 1959. Josiah Macy Jr. Foundation. In 1971 Picton, Hillyard and I were delighted to send the findings of experiments like that in Figure 3 to Moscow for inclusion in a Festschrift in his honor. The Russians have problems with publication lag too; it is now said to be coming out this fall (1973) in M. N. Livanov (Ed.) *Major problems of brain electrophysiology*, U.S.S.R. Academy of Sciences.

Credit for the visual variant, the missed-flash experiment, goes to J. S. Barlow, who in 1968 precisely described the P_3 from a platform in New York; his abstract appears in *Electroencephalography and Clinical Neurophysiology* 1969, **27**, 545. A prior description had appeared in a house journal of limited circulation: Barlow, L., & Morrell, F. *On Evoked responses in relation to temporal conditioning to paired stimuli in man. Massachusetts Institute of Technolology Research Laboratory Electron., QPR*, 1965, **78**, 263–272.

The somesthetic variant, a missed tap of the finger, was reported by Klinke, R., Fruhstorfer, H., & Finkenzeller, P. in *Evoked responses as a function of external and stored information. Electroencephalography and Clinical Neurophysiology*, 1968, **25**, 119–122.

[5] Squires, K. C., Hillyard, S. A., & Lindsay, P. H. Cortical potentials evoked by confirming and disconfirming feedback following an auditory discrimination. *Perception and Psychophysics*, 1973, **13**, 25–31.

[6] *References*. For 1): *Evoked potential correlates of auditory signal detection*. Hillyard, S. A., Squires, K. C., Bauer, J. W., & Lindsay, P. H., *Science* **172**, 1971, 1357–1360. 2): See Note 5. 3): Eric Courchesne is presently working up his material on this for his Ph.D. thesis. 4): Unpublished evidence from our lab, and an inference gleaned from the publications listed in the bibliography of the paper cited in Note 5, where the various *E*s used one or another input modality.

[7] *Acknowledgements*. The many co-workers named in the notes above will each recognize the ideas and experiments peculiarly his own in what I have written. So too will co-workers in the laboratory whose experiments have not yet reached manuscript form, and the many authors around the world whose publications are listed in the bibliographies of the papers cited above. My grateful thanks to them all. The cost of the experiments reported here was paid in part by grants from NASA, NIH and the Sloan Foundation.

IS THE POWER LAW SIMPLY RELATED TO THE DRIVEN SPIKE RESPONSE RATE FROM THE WHOLE AUDITORY NERVE?[1]

JULIUS L. GOLDSTEIN

School of Engineering, Tel-Aviv University

Abstract. The frequently hypothesized proportionality between loudness and driven spike rate from the whole auditory-nerve bundle is examined with available auditory-nerve data. Salient features of the auditory-nerve data are represented by a mathematical model. It is shown that a neural driven rate for simple tones that is proportional to approximately the square root of sound pressure above about 40 dB sound-pressure level is compatible with auditory nerve data. In consequence of the saturation of firing rate from single auditory-nerve fibers at moderate levels, the recruitment of neural firings from fibers with characteristic frequencies above the stimulus frequency plays a decisive role in the computed power law. The expected dependence of the loudness power law upon masking at frequencies above the stimulus frequency is not supported by psychophysical data.

Stevens as well as other pioneer investigators of auditory perception (Fletcher & Munson, 1933; Stevens, 1970; Stevens & Davis, 1938; Zwislocki, 1969;) have proposed that loudness of sounds could be determined by the magnitude of neural activity along the auditory tract. This viewpoint could be satisfied by neural activity at any one particular neural level from auditory nerve to auditory cortex or, perhaps, by all levels taken together. Mammalian auditory nerve physiology has been sufficiently documented (Kiang, 1965, 1968) to permit a rough examination of the relationship between whole-nerve spike responses to simple tones and Stevens' power law for loudness (Stevens, 1955).

The salient and relevant properties of auditory nerve-fiber responses to simple tones are the saturation of action-potential firing rate at moderate sound-pressure levels, the bandpass sensitivity to frequency with a broad distribution of characteristic frequencies among the different fibers, and the uniformity of the population of fibers with similar characteristic frequency (f_c). We examine here whether data from single auditory-nerve fibers could predict a whole-nerve response rate to simple tone stimuli whose dependence upon sound level is proportional to Stevens' (1955) power law for loudness.

For single auditory-nerve fibers, the dependence of neural rate R, upon the rms sound pressure, P, of a simple stimulus tone of frequency f, is well described by the empirical formula in Equation 1 (Kiang, 1968). The rate-dip phenomenon reported by Kiang and coworkers (Kiang, Baer, Marr, & Demont, 1969; Kiang & Moxon,

[1] The substance of this report was presented at a meeting of the Harvard Psychophysics Colloquy at Smitty Stevens' Laboratory of Psychophysics on 3 June 1971. The motivation, forum, and comments provided by Smitty on this and other occasions are deeply appreciated.

H. R. Moskowitz et al. (eds.), Sensation and Measurement. 223–229.

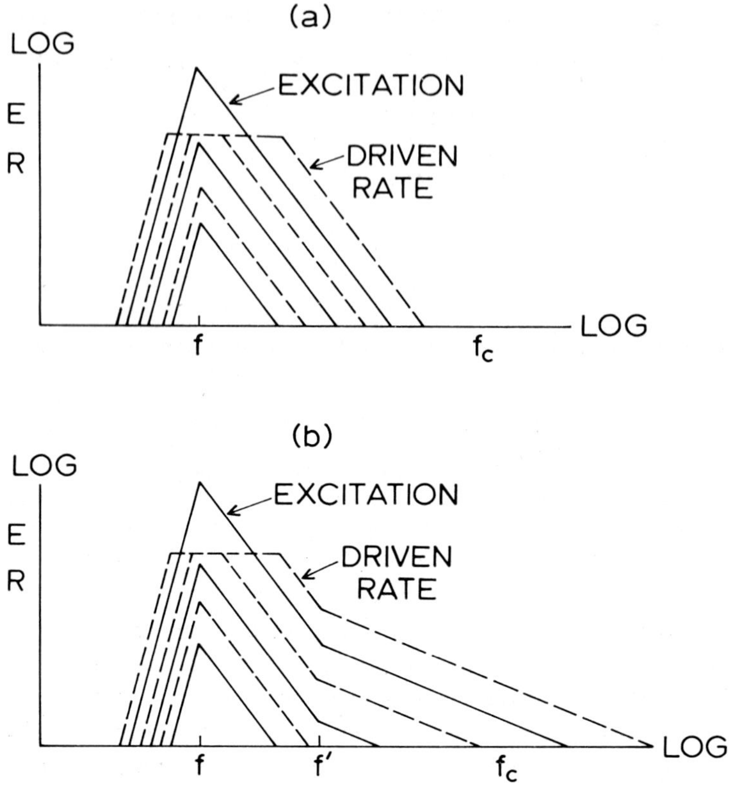

Fig. 1. Two models for the distribution of excitation, E, for a simple tone stimulus. The excitation is the driving signal, P·H, of the auditory nerve-fiber rate model of Equation 1. The distribution of the driven rate, R, of spike response is shown schematically to illustrate the effects of saturation.

1972) is ignored here; we presume its effect would be washed out after summing over the whole population of auditory nerve fibers.

$$R(f_c, f, P) = (r_m - r_s)\{1 - \exp - P \cdot H(f_c, f)\} + r_s, \tag{1}$$

where r_m and r_s are the maximum and spontaneous rates, respectively.

For convenience, we refer to the argument, $P \cdot H$, in the exponential of the model rate function as excitation. Figure 1 shows two models for the dependence of excitation upon characteristic frequency. The simpler model has the form given in Equation 2 and has been found adequate to represent some aspects of auditory data (e.g. Goldstein, Baer, & Kiang, 1971; Siebert, 1968).

$$\begin{aligned} H(f_c, f) &= A_0 (f_c/f)^{S_2}, \quad f_c < f, \\ &= A_0 (f/f_c)^{S_1}, \quad f_c \geqslant f, \end{aligned} \tag{2}$$

where A_0 is the maximum value of H, and the exponents S_n give the piecewise slopes of H on a logarithmic scale as in Figure 1.

Siebert (1968) has already noted on the basis of Equation 2 that if one takes the approximation that auditory nerve fibers are uniformly distributed with the logarithm of characteristic frequency (Schuknecht, 1960; Spoendlin, 1972), then the driven response rate from the whole auditory nerve approaches a logarithmic dependence upon sound pressure (i.e., changes in response rate are proportional to decibel changes in sound pressure). This prediction is easily visualized from Figure 1a. At low stimulus levels the pattern of driven firing rates across characteristic frequencies will be proportional to the triangular excitation pattern. At higher stimulus levels, fibers with characteristic frequencies near the stimulus frequency will saturate, and the pattern of driven firing rates will be trapezoidal. With further increase in stimulus intensity, the height of the trapezoidal pattern of driven firing rate remains substantially unchanged while its width broadens in direct proportion to decibel changes in stimulus level (Whitfield, 1967). It is clear that at these higher levels, the tails of the excitation pattern are responsible for the growth of firing rate.

The second model for the excitation pattern (Equation 3 and Figure 1b) incorporates evidence from wide-range tuning curve data (Kiang, Sachs, & Peake, 1967) that the excitation spreads more rapidly toward higher frequencies than is accounted for with the first model of excitation. This model leads to the prediction that the whole-nerve driven rate increases faster than the logarithm of rms sound pressure, in qualitative agreement with Stevens' (1955) power law.

$$\begin{aligned} H(f_c, f) &= A_0 (f_c/f)^{S_2}, && f_c < f \\ &= A_0 (f/f_c)^{S_1}, && f \leqslant f_c < f' \\ &= A_0 (f/f')^{S_1} (f'/f_c)^{S_3}, && f' \leqslant f_c. \end{aligned} \tag{3}$$

The second model of excitation (Equation 3) is used to formulate the whole-nerve driven rate, since it includes the first model as a special case. We want to combine Equations 1 and 3 and sum the driven rates from a discrete sum of single fibers that are uniformly distributed with the logarithm of characteristic frequency. According to Rasmussen (1940), the number of fibers in man is large, being about 30000, therefore justifying the approximation (Siebert, 1968) for the discrete sum by an integral over a continuous distribution of "fibers" (Equation 4),

$$R_T \sim \int_{f_{c\,\min}}^{f_{c\,\max}} \{R(f_c, f, P) - r_s\}\, N \frac{\mathrm{d}f_c}{f_c}. \tag{4}$$

Substituting Equations 1 and 3 into 4 and changing the variable of integration to excitation, $E \equiv P \cdot H(f_c, f)$, yield the desired whole-nerve driven rate (Equation 5).

$$\begin{aligned} R_T \sim N(r_m - r_s) \Bigg\{ \frac{1}{S_2} \int_{E_1}^{E_{\max}} (1 - \exp - E) \frac{\mathrm{d}E}{E} + \\ + \frac{1}{S_1} \int_{KE_{\max}}^{E_{\max}} (1 - \exp - E) \frac{\mathrm{d}E}{E} + \frac{1}{S_3} \int_{E_2}^{KE_{\max}} (1 - \exp - E) \frac{\mathrm{d}E}{E} \Bigg\}, \end{aligned} \tag{5}$$

where $E_{max} = P \cdot A_0$ is the maximum excitation, E_1 and E_2 are the excitations at the lowest and highest characteristic frequencies, and KE_{max} is the excitation at the break frequency f' (Equation 3). The exponential integral is tabulated in Abramowitz & Stegun (1968).

On the basis of known physiological data, we can assign reasonable values to the variables in Equation 5 and evaluate the dependence of whole-nerve rate upon stimulus level. The form of this function is not affected by the variables N, r_m, and r_s, but values are assigned for concreteness. To obtain N we assume the approximately 30000 auditory nerve fibers are uniformly distributed with logarithm of characteristic frequency over the frequency range 20 Hz–20 kHz. Thus

$$\int_{20}^{20\,000} N \, \mathrm{d}f_c / f_c = 30\,000,$$

whence $N \sim 4500$.

A representative number for the dynamic range of rate for a single fiber is $r_m - r_s = 100$. Representative values for the slopes of the excitation functions (Goldstein *et al.*, 1971; Kiang, 1965; Kiang *et al.*, 1967) in the middle range of stimulus frequencies (say $f_c \sim 1-6$ kHz) are $S_2 = 30$ ($=180$ dB oct^{-1}), $S_1 = 10$ ($=60$ dB oct^{-1}) and $S_3 = 1$ ($=6$ dB oct^{-1}). The attenuation at the break frequency f' for the excitation model (Equation 3) is taken as $K = 0.01$. Next we make the assumption, which is justified for stimulus frequencies in the middle range, that the end excitations, E_1 and E_2, are negligibly different from zero. The whole-nerve driven rate can now be evaluated as a function of the excitation maximum E_{max} (Figure 2).

The final step is to relate the excitation maximum, E_{max}, to the rms pressure, P, of the stimulus tone. The quantity to be determined is A_0 in Equation 3; i.e., $E_{max} = P \cdot A_0$. We relate A_0 to available data by treating it as the product of two transfer functions: $A_0 = H_m(f) \cdot H_r(f)$. H_m is the middle-ear linear transfer function for the ratio of stapes displacement to outer-ear drum pressure (Guinan & Peake, 1967). $H_r(f)$ is a transfer function representation for the frequency dependence of the stapes displacement that is required for a given rate of response from a single fiber (Wiederhold, 1970, Figure 13). We determine H_r at 5.83 kHz by fitting the rate function model for a single fiber (Equation 1) to Kiang's (1968) data, whence $H_r(5.83 \text{ kHz}) = 7 \times 10^4$ per micron peak-to-peak stapes displacement ($\mu p - p$). Turning to the middle-ear transfer functions reported by Guinan & Peake (1967), we obtain (from the left ordinate) H_m (5.83 kHz) $\sim 1.25 \times 10^{-3}$ $\mu p - p$ μbar^{-1}.

Figure 2 shows the calculated whole-nerve driven rate (Equation 5) for the two excitation models of Equations 2 and 3. The horizontal axis is calibrated both in units of the theoretical excitation maximum and the corresponding sound-pressure level (SPL) for a stimulus frequency of 5.83 kHz. Sound-pressure levels for other stimulus frequencies can be obtained by allowing for the frequency dependence of the two transfer functions $H_m(f)$ and $H_r(f)$. According to the data cited, the effects of frequency upon these transfer functions are nearly mutually cancelling over the middle frequency

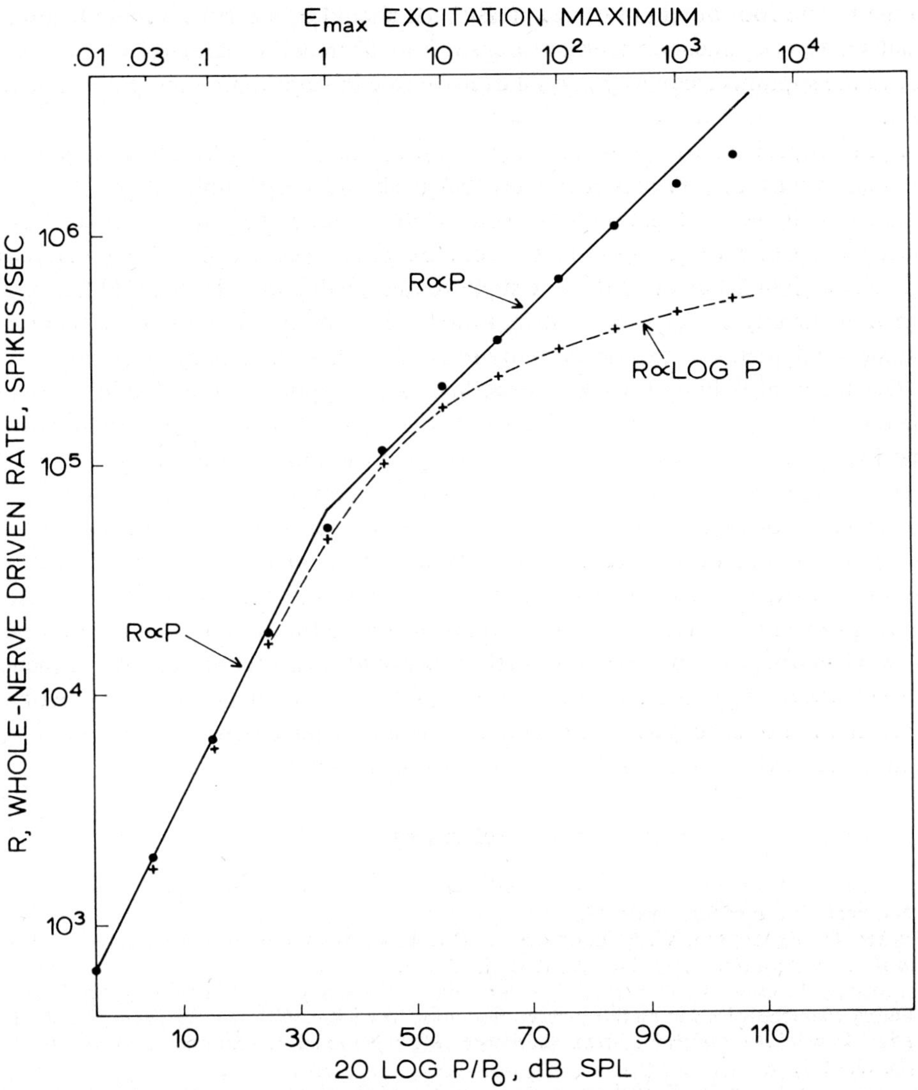

Fig. 2. Calculated driven response rate from the whole auditory nerve in response to a simple tone stimulus. Dashed line curve is for the simple excitation model of Equation 2. Solid line curve is for the more accurate excitation model of Equation 3.

region. Thus, the sound-pressure levels given in Figure 2 would also apply approximately to stimulus frequencies down to about 1 kHz.

Both excitation models yield a linear dependence of whole-nerve driven rate upon stimulus rms pressure at low SPL. At higher levels, the simple excitation model (Equation 2) yields rate changes that are proportional to decibels SPL. In contrast, the more accurate excitation model (Equation 3) yields a rate that is nearly proportional to the square root of stimulus rms pressure. It should be clear from these theoretical results that recruitment of neural responses from fibers with characteristic frequencies above the stimulus frequency plays a decisive role in determining the power-law relation.

If, indeed, driven firing rate from the whole auditory nerve mediates loudness, then the auditory nerve rate model implies that it should be possible to grossly modify loudness judgments of simple tones with relatively modest masking signals that are located in the high frequency tail region of the excitation curve. Masking data reported by Scharf (1964), however, do not support this prediction. Hellman addresses this question directly in another contribution to this volume and finds the course of loudness judgments to be unexpectedly resistant to high-frequency masking.

The apparent failure of masking experiments to support the recruitment model for the power law should not be considered as conclusive evidence against the hypothesis that loudness is proportional to the driven spike response rate from the whole auditory nerve. This reservation reflects particularly the everpresent uncertainty in the completeness of available physiological data and afortiori in the representativeness of idealized mathematical models of these data. For example, it may be reasonable to question whether the data reported by Wiederhold (1970), showing that auditory nerve fibers with similar characteristic frequency have thresholds within a total range of about 20 dB, justify our idealization that fibers with similar characteristic frequencies have identical sensitivities. That is, should $H_r(f)$ in the model be a single function or a distribution of functions with magnitudes spanning 40–60 dB? If new physiological data proved the latter, then the role of recruitment would be secondary.

References

Abramowitz, M., & Stegun, I. A. *Handbook of mathematical functions.* Washington D.C.: U.S. National Bureau of Standards, 1968.

Fletcher, H., & Munson, W. A. Loudness, its Definition, Measurement and Calculation. *Journal of the Acoustical Society of America*, 1933, **5**, 82–108.

Goldstein, J. L., Baer, T., & Kiang, N. Y. S. A theoretical treatment of latency, group delay, and tuning characteristics for auditory-nerve responses to clicks and tones. In Sachs, M. B. (Ed.), *Physiology of the auditory system.* Baltimore, Md.: National Educational Consultants, 1971, pp. 133–141.

Guinan, J. J. & Peake, W. T Middle-ear characteristics of anesthetized cats. *Journal of the Acoustical Society of America*, 1967, **41**, 1237–1261.

Kiang, N. Y. S. *Discharge patterns of single fibers in the cat's auditory nerve.* Cambridge, Mass.: The M.I.T. Press, 1965.

Kiang, N. Y. S. A survey of some recent developments in the study of auditory physiology. *Annals of Otology, Rhinology, and Laryngology*, 1968, **77**, 656–675.

Kiang, N. Y. S., Sachs, M. B., & Peake, W. T. Shapes of tuning curves for single auditory-nerve fibers. *Journal of the Acoustical Society of America*, 1967, **42**, 1341–1342.

Kiang, N. Y. S., Baer, T., Marr, E. M., & Demont, D. Discharge rates of single auditory-nerve fibers as functions of tone level. *Journal of the Acoustical Society of America*, 1969, **46** (A), 106.

Kiang, N. Y. S., & Moxon, E. Physiological considerations in artificial stimulation of the inner ear. *Annals of Otology, Rhinology, and Laryngology*, 1972, **81**, 714–730.

Rasmussen, A. T. Studies of the eighth cranial nerve of man. *Laryngoscope*, 1940, **50**, 67–83.

Scharf, B. Partial Masking. *Acustica*, 1964, **14**, 16–23.

Schuknecht, H. F. Neuroanatomical correlates of auditory sensitivity and pitch discrimination in the cat. In Rasmussen, G. L. & Windle, W. (Eds.), *Neural mechanisms of the auditory and vestibular system*. Springfield, Ill.: Chs. C. Thomas, 1960.

Siebert, W. M. (1968). Stimulus transformations in the peripheral auditory system. In Kolers, P. A. & Eden, M. (Eds.), *Recognizing patterns*. Cambridge, Mass.: The M.I.T. Press, 1968, pp. 104–133.

Spoendlin, H. Innervation densities of the cochlea, *Acta Otolaryngology*, 1972, **73**, 235–248.

Stevens, S. S. The measurement of loudness. *Journal of the Acoustical Society of America*, 1955, **27**, 815–829.

Stevens, S. S. Neural events and the psychophysical law. *Science*, 1970, **170**, 1043–1050.

Stevens, S. S. & Davis, H. *Hearing, its psychology and physiology*. New York: Wiley, 1938.

Whitfield, I. C. *The Auditory pathway*. London: Edward Arnold and Co., 1967.

Wiederhold, M. L. Variations in the effects of electric stimulation of the crossed olivocochlear bundle on cat single auditory-nerve-fiber responses to tone bursts. *Journal of the Acoustica Society of America*, 1970, **48**, 966–977.

Zwislocki, J. J. Temporal summation of loudness: An analysis. *Journal of the Acoustical Society of America*, 1969, **46**, 431–441.

CRITICAL BANDWIDTH IN MAN AND SOME OTHER SPECIES IN RELATION TO THE TRAVELING WAVE ENVELOPE

DONALD D. GREENWOOD
University of British Columbia

Abstract. The hypothesis was offered some years ago (Greenwood, 1961) that critical bandwidth in man was an exponential function of distance on the basilar membrane. Integration of the function yielded a frequency-position curve fitting Békésy's data. Scale relations between frequency-position functions of a few species and between displacement envelopes (Greenwood, 1962) suggest that critical bandwidth may correspond to scale-related distances and may be proportional to the apical segment of the traveling wave envelope. A revision of the critical-bandwidth function (Greenwood, 1971), in which critical bandwidth corresponds to about 1.25 mm in man, is reviewed; functions, based on distances scale related to 1.25 mm, are suggested for cat and squirrel monkey. Analysis of data on basilar-membrane motion in squirrel monkey and guinea pig (Johnstone, 1969/70; Kohllöffel, 1972; Rhode, 1970, 1971) indicates that the apical segments of the displacement envelopes closely agree in length with the respective distances to which critical bandwidth may correspond in these species and would imply an apical segment length close to 1.25 mm in man.

Historically, students of hearing have sought to relate the findings of psychoacoustics to the physical and physiological properties of the auditory system. Stevens was a major contributor to this objective. His early physiological work and the influential book, *Hearing*, written with H. Davis in 1938 are well known. But a contribution of perhaps more far-reaching importance was his constant insistence on the fundamental need to search for basic psychophysical relationships possessing a sufficient generality and precision that we might know more clearly what had to be explained. These psychophysical relationships, essentially expressing what the system can do, would be necessary before an explanation of hearing in terms of the physiological properties and mechanisms of the auditory system could be constructed.

One such relationship, that of critical bandwidth to other basic measures of auditory function such as the pitch scale and to an approximately constant distance on the basilar membrane, interested Stevens for many years. The present paper takes the latter relationship as its point of departure and is presented with the hope that it would have aroused Stevens' interest – along with his usual skepticism. It is also hoped that the ramifications of this empirical relationship will lead to the establishment of more links between psychoacoustics and auditory physiology.

Critical Bandwidth in Relation to Position on the Basilar Membrane

Critical bandwidth refers to a frequency interval – either bounding the spectral components of a stimulus or separating them, depending on the experiment in question – that has been empirically determined to be critical to the observation of certain effects. The frequency interval increases with stimulus frequency and takes similar values in several types of experiment.

A previous paper described a function relating some of the critical-bandwidth

H. R. Moskowitz et al. (eds.), Sensation and Measurement. 231–239.

measurements in man to position on the basilar membrane (Greenwood, 1961). The development of the function assumed that critical bandwidth was an exponential function, $CB = 10^{ax+b}$, of distance, x, along the basilar membrane, and corresponded to a constant distance on the basilar membrane. The latter hypothesis had been advanced by Zwicker, Flottorp, & Stevens in 1957. This paper will be concerned (*a*) with the relation of the function to Békésy's (1960) frequency-position data for man, (*b*) with a recent revision of the function, and (*c*) with a consideration of critical-bandwidth functions for some other species. In addition, a possible relation of critical bandwidth to the dimensions of the traveling wave envelope will be examined further (Greenwood, 1971).

Correspondence of critical bandwidths to equal, although unknown, distances on the basilar membrane would imply proportionality to the derivative of a frequency-position function for the membrane since the derivative is the slope, or change of frequency per unit distance. Thus the paper of 1961 pointed out that it was necessary only to integrate the suggested critical-bandwidth function to obtain a frequency-position function, in which position on the membrane was measured in critical-band units. The length of a critical-band unit in physical units could then be determined by dividing the length of the membrane by the number of critical bands required to subtend the audible frequency range. By coincidence, about 35 critical bands subtended 35 physical units, millimeters. The convenient effect of this adventitious correspondence of one critical bandwidth to the unit distance employed was that the frequency-position function obtained by integration could be compared directly to Békésy's plot of frequency vs position on the membrane without any change of constant required to allow distance, x, to be expressed in millimeters. The coincidence thus meant that critical bandwidth was proportional to the derivative with a constant of 1 rather than with some other constant, as would have resulted from the use of a different unit of measure or been implied by correspondence to a different distance in millimeters, such as the larger distance used in the revised critical-bandwidth function for man to be discussed later. The important outcome was that the frequency-position function closely agreed with Békésy's data, thus appearing to support the two ideas that critical bandwidth might obey an exponential function and correspond to a constant distance, which seemed in man to be about 1 mm by this calculation.

POSSIBLE CORRESPONDENCE OF CRITICAL BANDWIDTH TO A SCALE-RELATED DISTANCE

In the 1961 paper (Greenwood), critical bandwidth was considered only for man, the one species for which critical-bandwidth measurements existed. But in addition some interspecies comparisons of the functions that relate position of maximum amplitude to frequency were made that revealed the possibility of scale relationships among some of the species considered. Left unexplored was the question of how critical bandwidth might be related among the species, mainly because an adequate basis was lacking for associating the distance in man to which critical bandwidth corresponded with any obvious measure of distance based on physical or physiological properties of the cochlea. However, if critical bandwidth were scale related among the species, it would correspond by definition to different distances in cochleas of different lengths; and independent of any scale relations it was unlikely to correspond to the same distance.

Partly in an effort to find evidence that might bear generally on the possibility of a scale-related critical-band distance, while addressed more specifically to the question of other potential scale relations among cochleas, an approximate analysis was made of the dimensions of the traveling wave envelopes (Greenwood, 1962) as they could be calculated from Békésy's data for four species (Békésy, 1960). This calculation revealed (*a*) that the apical segment of the displacement envelope was approximately constant in length over the portion of the basilar membrane observed – roughly the apical half – and (*b*) that the apical segments of the traveling wave envelopes corresponded to nearly the same proportion of the basilar membrane in elephant, man, guinea pig, and chicken. This approximate scale relation in respect to the dimensions of the traveling wave envelopes occurred even among cochleas that were not scale related in respect to the total frequency range to which they were responsive (except for one pair of species: man and elephant).

The possible relevance of envelope dimensions to critical bandwidth is twofold. First, critical bandwidth in man also appears to correspond to an approximately constant distance. Second, whether critical bandwidth is taken simply as some measure of an auditory filter characteristic or, more specifically, as directly related to the pattern of neural excitation produced by a stimulus, it is reasonable to think that the distance corresponding to critical bandwidth ought to be related to the dimensions of the traveling wave envelope. The traveling wave envelope is, after all, a direct reflection of the filtering properties of the basilar membrane, and the traveling wave and attendant shearing forces closely precede neural excitation. It is suggested that critical bandwith – as a distance – should be proportional to the pattern of mechanical excitation and should correspond, in light of Békésy's data, to scale-related distances on the basilar membranes of scale-related species.

Assuming that critical bandwidth corresponds to different distances in different species, we can calculate those distances for scale-related species, starting from the distance for man. As noted above, this distance in the earlier paper appeared to be about 1 mm in man, but later evidence has led to a revised estimate.

A Revised Critical-Bandwidth Function for Man

On the basis of extensive data on masking and combination tones, a revised critical-bandwidth function for man has been proposed, according to which critical bandwidth corresponds to a distance on the basilar membrane of 1.25 mm (Greenwood, 1971).[1]

[1] This revised estimate of the distance to which critical bandwidth corresponds is in near agreement with the average distance of about 1.3 mm associated with critical bandwidth (*Frequenzgruppe*) by Feldtkeller & Zwicker (1956) and again by Zwicker & Feldtkeller (1967), although the functions relating critical bandwidth in hertz to position along the membrane and to frequency are somewhat different.

Moreover, the critical bandwidth associated with a tone at a particular frequency is seen as extending *downward* from that frequency, for an interval in hertz corresponding to the distance of 1.25 mm. Thus a total of 28 critical bands subtends 35 mm and man's audible frequency range.

The reason for revising the critical-bandwidth function will be reviewed in the context of one example. In the simplest case, critical-bandwidth measurements have been obtained in experiments involving two tones. In one type of such experiments, critical bandwidth has been found to be related to a feature of masked audiograms. The feature is a notch which occurs on the immediate high-frequency side of the masking tone. At frequencies in the notch, a signal, as its intensity is lowered, falls below *its* masked threshold before some of the combination tones produced by masker and signal fall below *their* masked thresholds on the *low*-frequency side of the masker. Since the listener continues to hear these signal-related events, the combination (difference) tones, primarily $2f_{\text{masker}}-f_{\text{signal}}$, determine masked threshold in the region of the notch. The low-point of the notch is reached when $2f_m-f_s$ below the masker reaches the low-frequency foot, or a region of reduced slope near the foot, of the masking pattern.

The frequency interval between the masker frequency and signal frequency at the low-point of the notch corresponds to a distance of about 1 mm, which is the "old" critical-bandwidth distance. But the *same* frequency interval on the lower side of the masking tone corresponds to 1.25 mm. Since it is *not* the *signal* that is heard at threshold in the notch on the high-frequency side of the masker but instead a combination tone on the *low* side, the critical band measured in this type of experiment is associated with the interval below the masker and with the distance of 1.25 mm. The interpretation offered is that at this point $2f_m-f_s$ no longer reaches its position of maximum amplitude within the zone of mechanical or neural excitation produced by the masker and exits also from the critical-bandwidth interval associated with the masker. A similar analysis applies to two-tone consonance experiments (Greenwood, 1971).

To revise the critical-bandwidth function so that the critical frequency interval corresponds to 1.25 mm, it is necessary only to change a constant, the b, in the original function, $CB=10^{ax+b}$. In addition, if the bandwidth calculated is to be associated with the point on the membrane corresponding to the *upper* frequency limit of the interval, convenience would dictate that the choice of constant be made accordingly. Hence the two functions given below express critical bandwidth as a function of the position, x in millimeters, corresponding to the upper end-point of the interval, or alternatively, as a function of the frequency, f in hertz, at the upper end-point:

$$\text{CB} = 26.23\,(10^{0.06x}) = 26.23\,(0.0060465f + 1)$$

Scale-Related Critical-Bandwidth Functions for Cat and Squirrel Monkey

Given 35 mm as the length of the basilar membrane in man, 22 mm as the length in cat (Schuknecht & Neff, 1952; Schuknecht & Sutton, 1953), and 20 mm in squirrel monkey (Igarashi, Mahon, & Konishi, 1968), then the scale-related distances corresponding to the critical band are easily calculated if the distance in one species is known. Assuming 1.25 mm in man, we calculate a critical-band distance of about 0.78 mm in cat and about 0.71+ mm in squirrel monkey. The critical-bandwidth functions, analagous to those offered for man, follow:

$$\text{Cat: CB} = 66.4\ (10^{0.0954x}) = 66.4\ (1 + f/418.6)$$
$$\text{Squirrel monkey: CB} = 80.3\ (10^{0.105x}) = 80.3\ (1 + f/506.5)$$

where x in mm is the point corresponding to the upper end-point of the band and f is the frequency in hertz corresponding to x.[2]

The frequency-position function for the cat was published in 1961 and closely fits Schuknecht's data. Support for the squirrel monkey's frequency-position function is discussed in the next section. Both functions appear below:

$$\text{Cat: } f = 418.6\ (10^{0.0954x} - 1)$$
$$\text{Squirrel monkey: } f = 506.5\ (10^{0.105x} - 1)$$

where f is in hertz and x is the point of maximum amplitude in millimeters from the apex.

Apical Segment of the Displacement Envelope in Squirrel Monkey and Guinea Pig

It was previously noted (Greenwood, 1962, 1971) that in Békésy's results the apical segment of the displacement envelope was approximately constant over the observed portions – about the apical halves at least – of the basilar membranes of four species. Kohllöffel's (1971) study of the *basal* half of the guinea pig cochlea would support a similar conclusion, one strengthened by the observation that the nearly parallel apical slopes of the displacement envelopes in living and post-mortem preparations normally remain parallel despite the progressive reduction in their steepness that ensues after death. Kohllöffel's most extensive data were apparently obtained from post-mortem preparations, but slope data from both dead and living preparations would seem to indicate that in both cases apical segments of the envelope are roughly constant, or do not strongly vary, in length over the basal half of the cochlea. Thus, his findings complement Békésy's data derived from the apical half and support the possibility that approximate constancy holds in living as well as in dead preparations.

[2] The critical-bandwidth function for the guinea pig can be calculated also, but with the difference that the guinea-pig cochlea cannot be considered more than a partial scale reduction of man's, since its audible frequency range is not increased by as much as a complete scale reduction would require (i.e. by the square of the scale factor). However, as noted above, Békésy's data would indicate that displacement envelope dimensions in the guinea pig are approximately scale related to those of other species, as data considered in the next section also indicate. Discussion of the guinea pig's critical-bandwidth function is deferred, but the calculated distance to which critical bandwidth would correspond is included in the next section.

It was previously noted (Greenwood, 1971) that the tuning curves of individual points obtained by Rhode (1970, 1971) and Johnstone (1969/70) with the Mössbauer technique implied that traveling waves *in vivo* in the squirrel monkey and guinea pig, respectively, damped from maximum to minimum in *less than* 1 mm. In Kohllöffel's (1971c) data from the guinea pig (obtained with a laser technique), the frequency sensitivity curve *in vivo* of a basal point yields a frequency interval corresponding to a comparably short distance. It will be shown that more precise estimates of these distances are approximately scale-related between the two species and would indicate a scale-related distance close to 1.25 mm for man.

The analysis of Rhode's data will be reported more fully elsewhere, but must be sketched here. Rhode (1971 and personal communication) recorded from points very near the mid-point of the basilar membrane in the basal turn of the cochlea near the beginning of the second turn. The points vibrated maximally to frequencies of about 6.5–7.5 kHz. The squirrel monkey's upper frequency limit is probably about 60 kHz if the monkey, a fellow primate, has an audible frequency range that is scale related to man's, as do the less closely related cat and elephant (Greenwood, 1961). A scale-related frequency-position function yields a near mid-point position, 11.15 mm from the apex, for the frequency of 7 kHz given by Rhode as typical for his mid-point position, and the upper frequency limit is about 63 kHz. Since this scale-related function gives reasonable results, it was used to convert frequency intervals obtained from Rhode's data to distances on the basilar membrane.

It was a straightforward procedure to read from 11 tuning curves and 11 cumulative phase curves (Rhode, 1970, 1971) the frequencies corresponding to certain recognizable points on the curves (and also from all points on the curves intersected by a systematic system of gridlines superimposed on the graphs). Two points from the tuning curves marked the frequencies at maximum and minimum amplitude and specified the frequency interval between them. But not all Rhode's tuning curves extended down to the minimum amplitude point, and the phase curves were needed to provide a related point. This point from the phase curve is one closely identified with the *minimum* amplitude point on the tuning curve in those cases where both are available. The point from the phase curve can be more accurately read and for this and other reasons will be taken as representing also the frequency at the minimum amplitude point. The means of identifying recognizable points on the phase curve require special description and a figure.

Figure 1, left side, presents one of Rhode's phase curves (Rhode, 1970). Each phase curve shows an almost straight section following a brief shoulder in the very low frequencies. The straight section then bends fairly discernably into another identifiably separate curved section which leads downward to a final and approximately constant section. If we convert the cumulative phase measurements to time ($T=\theta/2\pi f$) and plot the logarithm of time against log-frequency, we obtain easily recognizable points of intersection of the separate sections.

Figure 1, right side, presents the replotted data from the left side. To determine the frequencies at the points of intersection was no more difficult in any other case. (The

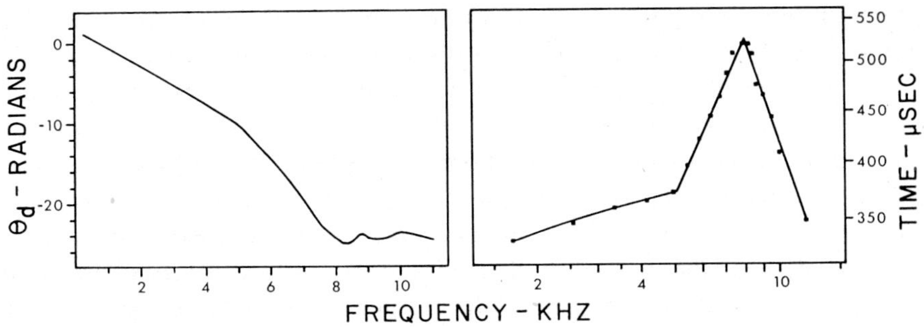

Fig. 1. Left panel: Phase differences, θ_d, between the motion of the basilar membrane and the motion of the malleus. Negative numbers signify that the motion of the basilar membrane lags the motion of the malleus. At low frequencies the curve approaches a phase lead of about $\pi/2$ rad. Data from animal 69-460. Curve adapted from Rhode (1970).
Right panel: Travel time from a point on the membrane at the stapes position to the recording location, calculated from the phase measurements as corrected by $\pi/2$ rad. The points on the graph are not Rhode's original data points. They represent the points of intersection of the original phase curve, as drawn by Rhode, with a system of grid lines superimposed on his curves and used to extract numerical data from the graph (see text).

significance of such figures for determining travel-time relationships will be discussed elsewhere.) For eight of the 11 recording locations, the data cover a sufficient frequency range to permit determination of the frequency at the point of maximum time on the phase curve – taken also as the point of *minimum* amplitude of the tuning curve. The interval between this frequency and the frequency at the point of *maximum* amplitude on the tuning curve corresponds to an average distance of about 0.74 mm, with a standard deviation of about 0.18 mm. Since a tuning curve is measured at a fixed spot as the traveling wave envelope is shifted basally by raising stimulus frequency, this distance corresponding to the interval between frequencies at the maximum and minimum amplitude of the tuning curve is also an estimate of the apical segment of the traveling wave envelope. *If* the corresponding apical segment in man were about 1.25 mm and the two species were scale related, we would expect to have found a distance of about 0.71+ mm in the squirrel monkey. The agreement is close, and the distance of about 0.71 mm is also the proposed scale-related distance corresponding to critical bandwidth in the squirrel monkey.

The Mössbauer data of Johnstone and his colleagues (1967, 1969/70, 1970) from points near the stapes of the guinea pig cochlea bear further on this matter. The tuning curves do not provide minimum points, but Johnstone's constructions of traveling wave envelopes from his data are such (1969/70, Figure 6) that the apical segment falls to about 8% of maximum in a distance of approximately two-thirds of a millimeter. Other estimates of this distance are provided by the data of Kohllöffel (1971c, Figure 4) who illustrates frequency-sensitivity curves *in vivo* from two basal points (same location in two preparations). The distance corresponding to the frequency interval between the points of maximum and minimum sensitivity on the curves is about 0.54 mm in one case and about 0.62 mm in the other. Depending on the length of the basilar membrane in an individual guinea pig, a distance scale-related to 1.25 mm in man would vary from about 0.66 mm for a 18.5-mm membrane to about 0.59 mm for a 16.5-mm membrane (a variation of about 10%). These distances are in approximate agreement with the lengths of the apical segment indicated by the data. Thus near the stapes in the guinea pig the apical dimension of the envelope is approximately scale related both to a distance of 1.25 mm in man and to the corresponding distance in the squirrel monkey near the mid-point. These interrelations are consistent with an approximate constancy of this segment of the envelope over much of the basilar membrane, as inferred above from the data of Békésy and Kohllöffel and as now adopted as a working assumption.

Concluding Comments

In respect to the relation of the apical segment to the distance to which critical bandwidth corresponds, we have seen that about 1.25 mm would be the length, *in vivo*, of the apical segment in man if scale relations held between man, squirrel monkey, and guinea pig in respect to displacement envelopes. This distance of 1.25 mm is, of course, the proposed distance corresponding to critical bandwidth, and in both cases it extends apically from the point of maximum amplitude of a stimulus. There are only partial indications of how critical-bandwidth measurements may be related to the apical segment and to this distance, which poses a difficult question. But it is more specific and limited than the question with which we are faced in any event: "How can critical bandwidth be related to the physics and physiology of the auditory system?"

We do not have *direct* evidence as to the dimensions of displacement envelopes in the living human cochlea nor of their relation to phenomena we wish to explain. However, it would seem accepted that our eventual determinations in this respect must be indirect – taking the form of estimates and inferences based on converging evidence from psychoacoustics and physiology. If the relationships suggested here represent a partial convergence of such evidence and are used as working assumptions permitting species comparisons, it should be possible to conceive other testable relationships between physiological and psychophysical data – even without further experimentation.

References

Békésy, G. von *Experiments in hearing*. New York: McGraw-Hill, 1960.

Feldtkeller, R. & Zwicker, E. *Das Ohr als Nachrichtenempfänger*. (1st ed.) Stuttgart: Hirzel Verlag, 1956.

Greenwood, D. D. Critical bandwidth and the frequency coordinates of the basilar membrane. *The Journal of the Acoustical Society of America*, 1961, **33**, 1344–1356.

Greenwood, D. D. Approximate calculation of the dimensions of traveling wave envelopes in four species. *The Journal of the Acoustical Society of America*, 1962, **34**, 1365–1369.

Greenwood, D. D. Aural combination tones and auditory masking. *The Journal of the Acoustical Society of America*, 1971, **50**, 502–543.

Igarashi, M., Mahon, R. G., & Konishi, S. Comparative measurements of cochlear apparatus. *Journal of Speech and Hearing Research*, 1968, **11**, 229–235.

Johnstone, B. M. & Boyle, A. J. F. Basilar membrane vibration examined with the Mössbauer technique. *Science*, 1967, **158**, 389–390.

Johnstone, B. M., Taylor, K. J., & Boyle, A. J. F. Mechanics of the guinea pig cochlea. *The Journal of the Acoustical Society of America*, 1970, **47**, 504–509.

Johnstone, B. M. Mechanical aspects of cochlear function. In R. Plomp & G. F. Smoorenburg (Eds.), *Frequency analysis and periodicity detection in hearing*. Leiden, Holland: Sijthoff, 1969/70.

Kohllöffel, L. U. E. Studies of the distribution of cochlear potentials along the basilar membrane. *Acta Oto-Laryngologica*, 1971, Supplement 288.

Kohllöffel, L. U. E. A study of basilar membrane vibrations I. Fuzziness-detection: A new method for the analysis of microvibrations with laser light. *Acustica*, 1972, **27**, 49–65. (a)

Kohllöffel, L. U. E. A study of basilar membrane vibrations II. The vibratory amplitude and phase pattern along the basilar membrane (post-mortem). *Acustica*, 1972, **27**, 66–81. (b)

Kohllöffel, L. U. E. A study of basilar membrane vibrations III. The basilar membrane frequency response curve in the living guinea pig. *Acustica*, 1972, **27**, 82–89. (c)

Rhode, W. S. Personal communication, 1970.

Rhode, W. S. *The measurement of the amplitude and phase of vibration of the basilar membrane using the Mössbauer effect*. (Doctoral dissertation, University of Wisconsin) Ann Arbor, Michigan: University Microfilms, 1970. No. 70-11853.

Rhode, W. S. Observations of the vibration of the basilar membrane in squirrel monkeys using the Mössbauer technique. *The Journal of the Acoustical Society of America*, 1971, **49**, 1669–1677.

Schuknecht, H. F. & Neff, W. D. Hearing losses after apical lesions in the cochlea. *Acta Oto-Laryngologica*, 1952, **42**, 263–274.

Schuknecht, H. F. & Sutton, S. Hearing losses after experimental lesions in basal coil of cochlea. *Archives of Otolaryngology*, 1953, **57**, 129–142.

Stevens, S. S. & Davis, H. *Hearing*. New York: Wiley, 1938.

Zwicker, E. & Feldtkeller, R. *Das Ohr als Nachrichtenempfänger*. (2nd ed.) Stuttgart: Hirzel Verlag, 1967.

Zwicker, E., Flottorp, G., & Stevens, S. S. Critical bandwidth in loudness summation. *The Journal of the Acoustical Society of America*, 1957, **27**, 155–161.

EFFECT OF SPREAD OF EXCITATION ON THE LOUDNESS FUNCTION AT 250 Hz[1,2]

RHONA P. HELLMAN

Laboratory of Psychophysics, Harvard University, Cambridge

Abstract. The loudness of a low-frequency 250-Hz tone was measured in quiet and in the presence of an adjacent band-pass noise. Loudness measurements were obtained by loudness matching, magnitude estimation, and magnitude production. Comparisons were made among the effects on loudness of the following noise bands: 390–2400 Hz, 345–2400 Hz, and 300–2400 Hz. The noise increased in intensity with the tone so that during a given listening session the signal-to-noise ratio remained constant at +10, 0, or −10 dB. The data suggest that, when the high-frequency tail produced in the ear by the tone is completely masked, the effect of the noise is to decrease by 20% the slope (exponent) of the loudness function above 70 dB SPL. Otherwise, the loudness functions of the 250-Hz tone in noise and in quiet are essentially the same. The results are consistent with data available in the literature.

Stevens' power law for loudness holds up to a sound pressure level (SPL) of at least 100 dB (Stevens, 1955). However, the mechanisms that allow the ear to cover the whole loudness range are not well known.

Since Fletcher & Munson (1937) published their paper that relates loudness and masking, it has been widely assumed that the magnitude of loudness is controlled by both the height and spread of the excitation pattern produced by an auditory stimulus. Excitation patterns can be derived from masking patterns which at high intensities spread much more toward high than toward low frequencies (cf., Luscher & Zwislocki, 1949; Munson & Gardner, 1950; Wegel & Lane, 1924; Zwicker, 1958, 1963). Moreover, Zwislocki (1971, 1972) has demonstrated a direct correspondence between the asymmetrical shape of masked audiograms measured in central masking and the shape of physiological tuning curves obtained from eighth-nerve units (Kiang, 1965) as well as from units of the cochlear nucleus (Kiang, Pfeiffer, Warr, & Backus, 1965). Once again, psychophysics proves itself extremely useful for suggesting indirectly how the ear functions.

The psychophysical experiments described in this article arose from discussions with J. L. Goldstein concerning the possible bearing on loudness of the skewed shape of tuning curves from units of the auditory nerve (Kiang, 1965; Kiang, Sachs, & Peake, 1967). The relation between the spread of excitation and the growth of loudness is not yet fully understood, and few available data bear directly on this problem (Scharf, 1964; Zwicker, 1958). One approach to this problem is to limit the spread of excitation by means of a band-pass masking noise that increases in intensity with the stimulus tone without masking the tone itself. Accordingly, the loudness of a 250-Hz

[1] Parts of this paper were presented in April 1973 at the 85th meeting of the Acoustical Society of America.

[2] This research was supported by Grant NS-02974 from the National Institute of Health. I wish to thank J. L. Goldstein for valuable conversations at the inception of this study.

H. R. Moskowitz et al. (eds.), Sensation and Measurement. 241–249. *All Rights Reserved.*

tone was measured in the presence of an adjacent band-pass masking noise. Both the low-frequency cutoff of the noise and its intensity were varied systematically.

Procedure

Loudness measurements spanning a range close to 100 dB were made at 250 Hz in quiet and in noise. From six to ten listeners, out of a pool of fifteen people, participated in each experiment. Loudness was measured both indirectly – by loudness matches between a 250-Hz tone in quiet and a 250-Hz tone in noise – and directly – by magnitude estimation and magnitude production, methods first used and described by Stevens (1958). Direct measurements made possible the determination of the absolute form of the loudness function at 250 Hz (Stevens, 1959).

All listening was binaural through TDH-39 earphones mounted in MX-41/AR cushions. The earphones were calibrated on a standard 6-cm^3 coupler and showed an essentially flat response between 100 and 2500 Hz. The high-frequency cutoff of the masking noise was fixed at 2400 Hz, and the low-frequency cutoff was set at 390, 345, or 300 Hz. The noise bands were produced by passing a wide-band Gaussian noise through a continuously variable constant-K network Allison filter (Model No. 2AB). The noise was increased in intensity along with the tone so that during a given session the signal-to-noise ratio remained constant at +10, 0, or −10 dB. Root-mean-square voltages were measured with a Ballantine rms voltmeter.

The experimental setup was the same for all three methods. The listeners sat in a soundproof booth. They turned the stimulus on and off at will by means of a manual switch. For loudness matching, both the 250-Hz tone in noise and the 250-Hz tone in quiet served in different sessions as the standard. The listeners were asked to disregard the noise and to adjust the loudness of the variable stimulus by means of bracketing (Zwicker, Flottorp, & Stevens, 1957) until it equalled the loudness of the standard tone, set at one of eight to ten predetermined sensation levels (SLs). During each session, a listener made two separate matches to each standard, using a sone potentiometer to adjust the variable. In order to eliminate possible effects of adaptation, the listeners were permitted either to listen to the variable stimulus or to adjust its intensity, but not to do both at the same time. The final averages were obtained by first determining the geometric means of each individual's two judgments and then computing the group geometric mean.

Magnitude production always followed the completion of magnitude estimation, for reasons given elsewhere (Hellman & Zwislocki, 1963). In the magnitude estimation series, the listeners were simply asked to assign numbers to the loudness of the tone so that the subjective magnitude of the two continua, loudness and number, appeared equal. The procedure for magnitude production was similar to that for loudness matching between tones, except that the listeners were asked to adjust the sone potentiometer to produce a loudness that matched the subjective magnitude of numbers assigned by the experimenter. The numbers were derived from the range used in magnitude estimation.

For both magnitude estimation and production, no standard was designated. Either ten SLs or ten numbers were presented to each listener three times in an irregular order that differed from listener to listener. The final two judgments were geometrically averaged, and the individual means were used, without normalization, in computing group geometric means.

Threshold Determinations

In order to measure the masking produced by each noise band, the method of limits was used to obtain individual thresholds for tones at 250, 400, 700, 1000, and 2000 Hz both in quiet and in the presence of noise at 40, 60, and 80 dB SPL. Masked threshold data obtained on four to six listeners agree very well with the extensive measurements of Hawkins & Stevens (1950). The obtained results, coupled with the shape of recently published masked audiograms (Greenwood, 1971; Scharf, 1971; Zwislocki, Buining, & Glantz, 1968), indicate that a signal-to-noise ratio of -10 dB is large enough to obliterate completely the high-frequency tail produced in the auditory system by a 250-Hz tone. At the same time, masked loudness measurements by Stevens & Guirao (1967) show that, when a 250-Hz tone is centered in a wide-band noise, a signal-to-noise ratio of -10 dB produces very little reduction in loudness of the tone. Hence, we can safely assume that, when the 250-Hz tone is masked by an adjacent noise band, the loudness of the tone is not appreciably affected by the noise.

In addition to the measurements of masking at threshold, prior to each set of loudness determinations, individual thresholds for the 250-Hz tone were measured in quiet. The average group threshold based on eighteen sessions was 23 dB SPL. This value, arrived at by correcting the measured threshold SPL by the 7-dB difference in SPL produced in the ear canal and in a 6-cm^3 coupler (Shaw, 1966), is in excellent agreement with previous threshold measurements at 250 Hz (e.g., Hellman & Zwislocki, 1968).

Effect of Signal-to-Noise Ratios of +10 and 0 dB

The results of magnitude estimation and magnitude production in quiet and in noise at a constant signal-to-noise ratio of $+10$ dB are shown in Figure 1. The cutoff frequencies of the masking noise band were 390 and 2400 Hz. Each point is the geometric mean of 18 to 20 loudness judgments by nine to ten listeners. The filled circles are for magnitude estimation; the unfilled circles are for magnitude production. All original measurements were made in terms of individual SLs, which were later converted to SPLs by adding to each SL the median threshold value in quiet of 23 dB. Typically, the curves resulting from magnitude production are steeper than those from magnitude estimation (Stevens & Greenbaum, 1966). The middle thin-line curves, called the curves of magnitude balance, were obtained by computing the geometric mean of the experimental curves along the abscissa. (Essentially, the same functions are obtained by averaging along the ordinate.)

Figure 1a shows the loudness data obtained for the 250-Hz tone in quiet. The curve

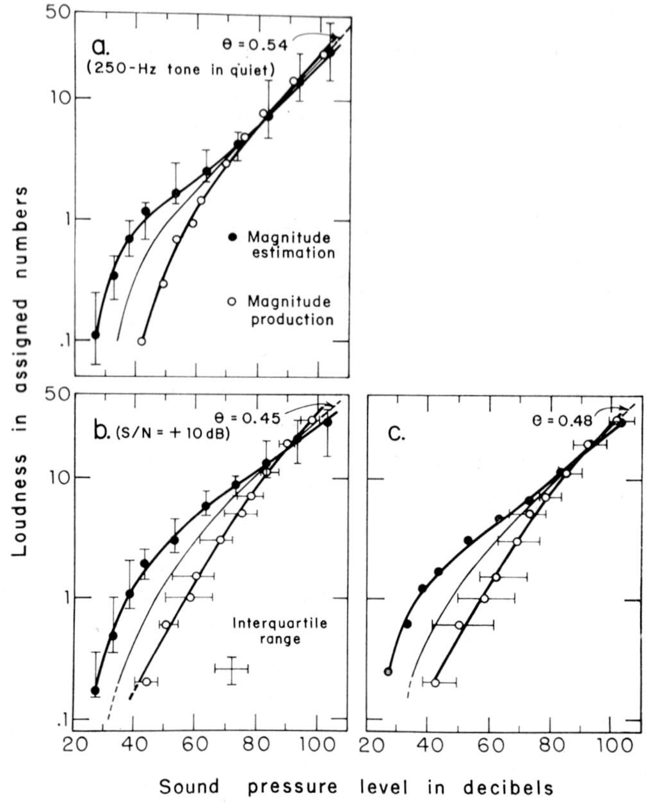

Fig. 1. (*a*) Loudness of a 250-Hz tone as a function of SPL. Filled and unfilled circles represent group geometric means obtained by magnitude estimation and production, respectively. Vertical bars show the interquartile range of judgments based on magnitude estimation. The middle curve is the magnitude-balance function. (*b*) Same as (*a*) except that the 250-Hz tone was masked by a noise band with cut off frequences at 390 and 2400 Hz. The signal-to-noise ratio was constant at + 10 dB. Vertical and horizontal bars represent interquartile ranges of magnitude estimation and production data, respectively. (*c*) Same as (*b*) except that the 250 Hz tone and the noise band were heard in alternation. Horizontal bars represent interquartile ranges of magnitude production data.

of magnitude balance agrees well with a 250-Hz function determined earlier by Hellman & Zwislocki (1968). Near threshold, loudness is proportional to sound intensity. Over the middle range of SPLs the 250-Hz curve is steeper than the 1000-Hz function in quiet, but at SPLs above 70 dB it is as steep as the 1000-Hz function. In this instance, the curve above about 70 dB SPL obeys a power function of sound pressure with an exponent of 0.54. Although 0.54 is somewhat smaller than the accepted ISO standard of 0.60, it falls well within the distribution of exponents that is characteristic of the loudness function (Stevens, 1969).

The effect on loudness of introducing a 390–2400-Hz noise band at a constant signal-to-noise ratio of + 10 dB is shown in Figure 1b. The curve of magnitude balance differs from the one in quiet only at high SPLs where the exponent decreases from

0.54 to 0.45. However, not all of the reduction in exponent can be ascribed to the masking effect of the noise; some of the reduction may be due to non-masking effects of the noise (Hellman & Zwislocki, 1964).

Figure 1c indicates the magnitude of the non-masking effect in the present study. The same noise and tone intensities were used as in Figure 1b except that the tone and noise were presented, not together but in alternation. This change alone reduced the exponent at high intensities from 0.54 to 0.48. Hence, the actual masking effect of the noise presented at a signal-to-noise ratio of +10 dB is quite small. It reduces the exponent at high intensities from 0.48 to 0.45.

The loudness functions shown in Figure 1 are consistent with the results of loudness matching. Figure 2 presents group geometric means of loudness matches by six to seven listeners for signal-to-noise ratios of +10 and 0 dB. The triangles mean the listeners adjusted the loudness of the unmasked tone, and the circles that they adjusted the loudness of the masked tone. The two signal-to-noise ratios produce essentially the same result. Consequently, one curve serves for both the filled and unfilled triangles, and another curve for both the filled and unfilled circles. The overall average curve (thin line) has a slope of 1.0 at low intensities, and a somewhat smaller slope of 0.95 at high intensities. In agreement with Figure 1, the slope of 1.0 implies that the loudness functions in noise and in quiet are equally steep at low intensities, whereas the slope of 0.95 implies that the noise reduces the loudness exponent slightly at high intensities. The matching data are also consistent with measurements of mutual masking between equally loud, widely spaced tones (Howes, 1950). Those results show that, at low and moderate loudness levels, there is no interference in the ear between

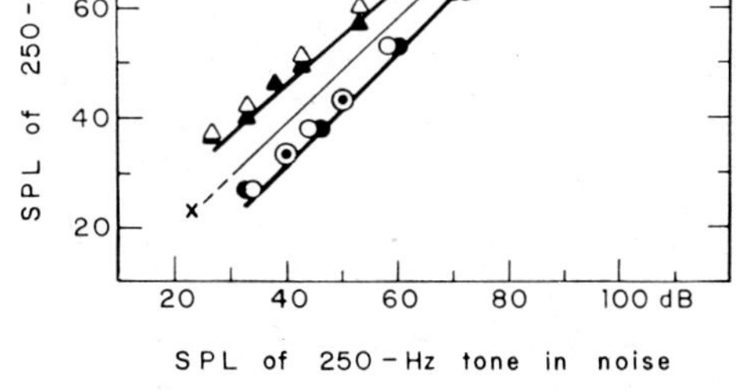

Fig. 2. Loudness matches obtained between a 250-Hz tone in quiet and a 250-Hz tone in noise. Group geometric means are shown for two signal-to-noise ratios, +10 and 0 dB. Filled and unfilled triangles are group means of six to seven listeners who varied the loudness of the unmasked tone. Filled and unfilled circles are group means of six to seven listeners who varied the loudness of the masked tone. The cross designates the threshold of audibility.

the component frequencies and thus, no loudness reduction of one tone by another. At loudness levels above 60 dB, where the excitation patterns of the components overlap, the loudness of the low-frequency tone is negligibly altered by the masking effect of the adjacent high-frequency tone.

Effect of Signal-to-Noise Ratio of —10 dB

The preceding section dealt with the effect on loudness of partially masking the high-frequency excitation produced in the ear by the 250-Hz tone. This section deals with the effect of more completely masking this high-frequency tail. The signal-to-noise ratio was constant at −10 dB, while the low-frequency cutoff of the noise was varied. The data obtained by loudness matching are shown in Figure 3. As in Figure 2, each point is the geometric mean of 12 to 14 loudness judgments by six to seven listeners. The triangles mean the loudness of the unmasked tone was adjusted, and the circles that the loudness of the masked tone was adjusted.

Figure 3a compares the masking effect of two noises with different lower cutoff frequencies. The unfilled points are for a 390–2400-Hz band and the filled points are for a 345–2400-Hz band. Both bands produce nearly identical results and can be represented by a single function. The average curve has a slope of 1.0 at low intensities. In the vicinity of 60 dB SPL the slope decreases smoothly to a value of 0.80 which remains constant above 70 dB SPL. Thus, the main effect of the noise is a 20% reduction in the slope (exponent) of the 250-Hz loudness function above 70 dB SPL. However, despite this reduction in slope and therefore in loudness, the tone continues to grow louder over a stimulus range of nearly 100 dB. The results of loudness matching

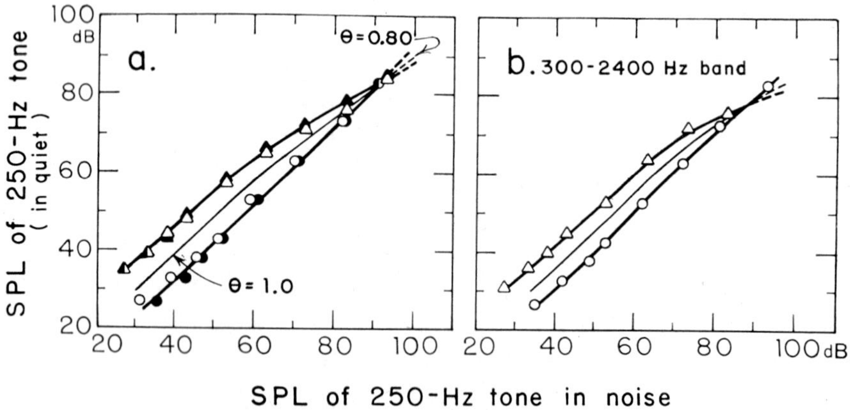

Fig. 3. (*a*) Masking effect of a 390–2400-Hz noise band (unfilled symbols) compared to the effect of a 345–2400 noise band (filled symbols). The signal-to-noise ratio was constant at −10 dB. Triangles and circles represent group geometric means of six to seven listeners who varied the loudness of the unmasked and masked tones, respectively. (*b*) Loudness-balance data obtained with a 300–2400-Hz noise band. Plot similar to that in 3*a*.

concur with those of magnitude estimation and magnitude production (Hellman, 1973).

When the signal-to-noise ratio is −10 dB, the curve of magnitude balance below about 60 dB SPL is as steep in noise as in quiet. At and above 60 dB SPL, the loudness function in noise has a constant exponent of 0.40. Above 70 dB SPL this exponent relative to the exponent of 0.48 obtained during alternate presentation of tone and noise (Figure 1c) yields an exponent ratio that closely approximates the slope (exponent) of 0.80 obtained by loudness matching (see Figure 3a).

It is evident that in the present experiments the listeners disregarded the loudness of the noise, for the matching results in Figures 2 and 3a are contrary to the results obtained when listeners are asked to judge the overall loudness of a combination of tone and noise (see Fishken, 1971). The combination tends to be louder, especially at low SPLs of noise than the tone alone. These last data also showed that judging the overall loudness of noise plus tone does not alter the slope of the loudness function at high intensities.

Finally, Figure 3b shows the effect on loudness of the noise with its low-frequency cutoff decreased to 300 Hz. Up to about 70 dB SPL, the average curves in Figures 3a and 3b appear the same. Above 70 dB the 300–2400 Hz band produces a function that bends somewhat, which suggests, as do the listeners' spontaneous comments, that the loudness of the 250-Hz tone approaches saturation. Presumably, when the frequency difference between the 250-Hz test tone and the low-frequency cutoff of the noise is only 50 Hz, the noise encroaches on the tone itself, cutting into both the height and the spread of the tone's excitation pattern at high intensities (see Zwicker, 1958).

The present findings are consistent with earlier results which showed that, when a 1000-Hz tone is centered in a band of noise, reducing the noise bandwidth but maintaining constant the spectrum level tends to steepen the masked loudness function (Hellman, 1970). More direct evidence is provided by the loudness-balance data of Zwicker (1958) for a tone at 3200 Hz masked by an adjacent high-pass noise at a constant signal-to-noise ratio of −6 dB. Those data accord with the assumption that the exponent for the *specific* loudness function at SPLs above 30 dB is about 20% lower than the exponent of the subjectively measured loudness function (Zwicker, 1963). The present results also agree with earlier measures of the partial masking of tones at 690 and 830 Hz by an adjacent narrow-band noise with very steep skirts (Scharf, 1964). The agreement between Scharf's data and those of the present study, in which the noise had rather flat skirts, indicates that the sharpness of the filter cutoff is not a critical variable.

Conclusions

The results suggest the following conclusions:

(1) Masking the high-frequency tail produced in the ear by a 250-Hz tone does not reduce the range over which loudness increases with stimulus intensity. Loudness continues to grow, but at a slower rate, over a range of nearly 100 dB.

(2) Regardless of sound frequency, the spread of excitation toward high frequencies

contributes to loudness primarily by increasing the exponent of the loudness function. Stevens' power law remains essentially intact even when the frequency distribution of excitation is confined to a relatively narrow band.

(3) Consistent with the evidence accumulated by Zwislocki (1965, 1969, 1972), the loudness function for a 250-Hz tone, like the function for a 1000-Hz tone, shows that near threshold, loudness is directly proportional to sound intensity.

The implications of these conclusions are directly relevant to the current search for a neurophysiological basis for the loudness function (Goldstein, 1974; Kiang, 1968; Stevens, 1970; Zwislocki, 1965, 1969, 1972). Physiological measurements reveal that the discharge rate of eighth-nerve fibers, as well as those in the cochlear nucleus, reaches saturation within 40 dB above threshold (e.g., Galambos & Davis, 1943; Greenwood & Goldberg, 1970; Kiang, 1965). Kiang (1968) has further demonstrated that the range of thresholds acıoss fibers responding maximally to a narrow band of frequencies is less than 30 dB. If indeed loudness increases with stimulus intensity over a 100-dB range, despite complete masking of the excitation produced at frequencies above the test or characteristic frequency, one more restriction has been added to the possible interpretation of the mechanism for loudness coding.

References

Fishken, D. Loudness summation between tones and noise. Unpublished doctoral dissertation, Northeastern University, 1971.

Fletcher, H., & Munson, W. A. Relation between loudness and masking. *Journal of the Acoustical Society of America*, 1937, **9**, 1–10.

Galambos, R. & Davis, H. The response of single auditory nerve fibers to acoustic stimulation. *Journal of Neurophysiology*, 1943, **6**, 39–57.

Goldstein, J. L. Is the power law simply related to the driven spike response rate from the whole auditory nerve? In this volume, p. 223–229.

Greenwood, D. Aural combination tones and auditory masking. *Journal of the Acoustical Society of America*, 1971, **50**, 502–543.

Greenwood, D. & Goldberg, J. Response of neurons in the cochlear nuclei to variations in noise bandwidth and to tone noise combinations. *Journal of the Acoustical Society of America*, 1970, **47**, 1022–1040.

Hawkins, J. E. Jr., & Stevens, S. S. Masking of pure tones and speech by white noise. *Journal of the Acoustical Society of America*, 1950, **22**, 6–13.

Hellman, R. P. Effect of noise bandwidth on the loudness of a 1000-Hz tone. *Journal of the Acoustical Society of America*, 1970, **48**, 500–504.

Hellman, R. P. Effect of high-frequency tail on the loudness of a 250-Hz tone. *Journal of the Acoustical Society of America*, 1973, **54**, 337. (Abstract)

Hellman, R. P. & Zwislocki, J. J. Monaural loudness function at 1000 cps and interaural summation. *Journal of the Acoustical Society of America*, 1963, **35**, 856–865.

Hellman, R. P. & Zwislocki, J. Loudness function of a 1000-cps tone in the presence of a masking noise. *Journal of the Acoustical Society of America*, 1964, **36**, 1618–1627.

Hellman, R. P. & Zwislocki, J. J. Loudness determination at low frequencies. *Journal of the Acoustical Society of America*, 1968, **43**, 60–64.

Howes, D. H. The loudness of multi-component tones. *American Journal of Psychology*, 1950, **63**, 1–30.

Kiang, N. Y.-S. Discharge patterns of single fibers in the cat's auditory nerve. Research Monograph 35. Cambridge Mass.: M.I.T. Press, 1965.

Kiang, N. Y.-S. A survey of recent developments in the study of auditory physiology. *Annals of Otology, Rhinology, and Laryngology*, 1968, **77**, 1–20.

Kiang, N. Y.-S., Pfeiffer, R. R., Warr, W. B., & Backus, A. S. N. Stimulus coding in the cochlear nucleus. *Annals of Otology, Rhinology, and Laryngology*, 1965, **74**, 463–486.

Kiang, N. Y.-S., Sachs, M. B., & Peake, W. T. Shapes of tuning curves for single auditory nerve fibers. *Journal of the Acoustical Society of America*, 1967, **42**, 1341–1342.

Luscher, E. & Zwislocki, J. Adaptation of the ear to sound stimuli. *Journal of the Acoustical Society of America*, 1949, **21**, 135–139.

Munson, W. A. & Gardner, M. B. Loudness patterns – A new approach. *Journal of the Acoustical Society of America*, 1950, **22**, 177–190.

Scharf, B. Partial masking. *Acustica*, 1964, **14**, 16–23.

Scharf, B. Fundamentals of auditory masking. *Audiology*, 1971, **10**, 30–40.

Shaw, E. A. G. Earcanal pressure generated by circumaural and supra-aural earphones. *Journal of the Acoustical Society of America*, 1966, **39**, 471–479.

Stevens, S. S. The measurement of loudness. *Journal of the Acoustical Society of America*, 1955, **27**, 815–829.

Stevens, S. S. Problems and methods of psychophysics. *Psychological Bulletin*, 1958, **54**, 177–196.

Stevens, S. S. Cross-modality validation of subjective scales for loudness, vibration and electric shock. *Journal of Experimental Psychology*, 1959, **57**, 201–209.

Stevens, S. S. On Predicting Exponents for cross-modality matches. *Perception and Psychophysics*, 1969, **6**, 251–256.

Stevens, S. S. Neural events and the psychophysical law. *Science*, 1970, 170, 1043–1050.

Stevens, S. S. & Greenbaum, H. Regression effect in psychophysical judgment. *Perception and Psychophysics*, 1966, **1**, 439–446.

Stevens, S. S. & Guirao, M. Loudness functions under inhibition. *Perception and Psychophysics*, 1967, **2**, 459–465.

Wegel, R. L. & Lane, C. E. The auditory masking of one sound by another and its probable relation to the dynamics of the inner ear. *Physical Review*, 1924, **23**, 266–285.

Zwicker, E. Ueber Psychologische und Methodische grundlagen der Lautheit. *Acustica*, 1958, **8**, 237–258.

Zwicker, E. Ueber die Lautheit von ungedrosselten und gedrosselten Schallen. *Acustica*, 1963, **13**, 194–211.

Zwicker, E., Flottorp, G. & Stevens, S. S. Critical bandwidth in loudness summation. *Journal of the Acoustical Society of America*, 1957, **29**, 548–557.

Zwislocki, J. J. Analysis of some auditory characteristics. In R. D. Luce, R. R. Bush, & E. Galanter (Eds.), *Handbook of Mathematical Psychology*. New York: John Wiley & Sons, Inc., 1965, pp. 1–97.

Zwislocki, J. J. Temporal summation of loudness: An analysis. *Journal of the Acoustical Society of America*, 1969, **46**, 431–441.

Zwislocki, J. J. Central masking and neural activity in the cochlear nucleus. *Audiology*, 1971, **10**, 48–59.

Zwislocki, J. J. A theory of central auditory masking and its partial validation. *Journal of the Acoustical Society of America*, 1972, **52**, 644–659.

Zwislocki, J. J., Buining, E. & Glantz, J. Frequency distribution of central masking. *Journal of the Acoustical Society of America*, 1968, **43**, 1267–1271.

TEMPORAL ORDER AND AUDITORY PERCEPTION[1]

IRA J. HIRSH

Washington University and Central Institute for the Deaf

Abstract. Varying the onset times of two or more acoustic events, which comprise *temporal sequences*, results in a variety of perceptual phenomena, depending in part on the range of time intervals used. Onset-time differences from 1 to 20 msec give rise to qualities that are interpretable on relatively peripheral physiological grounds, and may be associated with unitary or fused, non-successive perceptions. Time differences between 20 and 100 msec encompass a range of phenomena that are best interpreted by invoking figure properties of sequences. These need not involve separate verbal reports of "order," as is more typical of a third range, well beyond 100 msec. While various filter models may be applied to the shortest range and its discrimination responses, and while decision models may be applied to the longest range and its judgments of successive, separated events, the intermediate range requires Gestalt-like rules for adequate interpretation.

The patterns of auditory perception have several 'form qualities': the spectrum or harmonic arrangement, the sequential form, and a variety of speech-related aspects that may involve other than auditory properties. The subject of the present essay is the acoustic sequence, a temporal string of acoustic events. While sequences may differ from each other in several ways, the focus here will be the order in which the events occur in the sequence. One would have hoped that the recent increase in the number of experimental studies on the perception of temporal order would have provided a single, whole account of this aspect of perception, but unfortunately the wider the range of time intervals, of different tasks, and of the training of subjects, the more disparate appear to be the results, and the more numerous the possible theoretical approaches. The present purpose is to re-examine these results within a structure that offers some simple rules for categorization of phenomena.

Typically, a listener is asked to recognize the order of events within a sequence either by identifying the sequence, by reproducing the sequence, by reporting the temporal position of one item, or by discriminating between two sequences that are identical except with respect to the order of their component events. In addition to these variations in the listener's task, other sources of disparity are the level of training of the listeners, the number of events in the sequence, the kinds of sounds represented in such events, and the manner of presentation of the sequences, whether as single stimulus patterns, or as continuously recycled pattern series, with or without breaks between successive sequences. Then, there is also wide variation in interpretation of results depending upon the verbal report of a listener.

One framework for delineating the different phenomena utilizes the range of times or time differences in the stimulus pattern (Hirsh, 1959). Thus, it was suggested that very small time changes would give rise to changes in the quality of fused events, that

[1] Preparation of this paper was supported by Public Health Service grant NS 03856 from the National Institute of Neurological Diseases and Stroke to the Central Institute for the Deaf.

H. R. Moskowitz et al. (eds.), Sensation and Measurement. 251–258. *All Rights Reserved.*

is, events whose components would not be reported as successive by the listener (one as opposed to two or more). Somewhat larger time differences would give rise to changes in the figural or Gestalt properties of a sequence whose components could be judged to be distinct and successive, but changes in stimulus order would be responsible only for changes in those figural aspects. The order of individual stimulus events in such circumstances would not, for example, be imitated (e.g., tapping) nor even labelled "order" by untrained listeners. Finally, a range of time values was suggested in which the sequential order of separated events could be identified through an item-by-item analysis of the pattern, with correct imitation or repetition of the parts. Under this scheme there is not a single psychological scale that corresponds to a scale of temporal grain, but rather different ranges within which performance increases with time for each of several different kinds of judgment.

Now it appears that the time range alone will not suffice to delineate these different sets of phenomena or judgments. There appears to be an interaction between such judgments and the types of sounds that are employed in the sequences. The concepts of "channel" and "stream" enter here as mediators for grouping, and suggest that the rules for the perception of event order are not the same within a channel as they are between channels. Indeed, if we broaden our concern beyond the auditory system, then the notion of channel becomes even clearer, as does the interaction. One of the aims of this essay is to suggest that the listener's performance with respect to perceived order may help to clarify what is meant by a "channel," and also how much overlap lies between "channels" and "streams."

Two Events

The simplest case where the question of order can arise is one in which two events, *A* and *B*, are presented monaurally or diotically, and the subject is asked to distinguish between *AB* and *BA*. The question may also be put in terms of which event came first or which started the two-event sequence. For hearing, a variety of sound pairs was used to establish the minimum time required between the onsets of the two events for the order to be reported correctly 75% of the time (Hirsh, 1959). In general this minimum time appeared to be about 18 msec with relatively little variation attributed to the different kinds or levels of sounds used. Listeners in that experiment were highly trained and furthermore could listen to the pairs over and over again until they reached a decision.

The lack of dependence of this minimum time on the particular sounds used led to a further study in which the same time value was found to describe the ability of observers to report correctly on the order of two auditory events, two visual events (separated in space), and two tactile stimuli, as well as pairs of events that were comprised of one stimulus in each of two of these three sensory modalities (Hirsh & Sherrick, 1961). Here again the observers were well trained and could inspect the pairs over and over again until a decision was reached.

Subsequently, a single stimulus pair, namely a light and a sound, was used to ascertain the role of training and repetition in the temporal-order judgment. In untrained subjects, who had the opportunity on each trial to observe only a single pair, correct identification of order required a difference of 60 msec when a sound preceded the light, and about 100 msec when the light preceded the sound (Hirsh & Fraisse, 1964). (Such asymmetry was not found in the earlier results with well-trained subjects.) Studying repeated presentation and training, Gengel & Hirsh (1970) found a clear difference of about 15 msec between single and repeated presentations and, similarly, a more marked improvement with training for single presentations than for repeated presentations. Thus even the earliest trials for repeated presentations yielded 75% correct thresholds of about 25 msec, which then decreased to 17 or 18 msec after ten trials, whereas single presentations showed thresholds almost as high as those reported by Hirsh & Fraisse (1964) of about 45 msec, which decreased to 25–30 msec after about ten test sessions.

In the simple, two-event case, these different phenomena can be categorized according to the time ranges involved and the interaction between such times and both tasks and training (Hirsh, 1959). When the time differences between the onsets of two events are even smaller, from 1 to 15 msec, listeners can discriminate (*AB* vs *BA*) changes, since they give rise to different onset characteristics, phase relations or predominance of different frequencies in the start or termination of an event complex (Efron, 1973; Patterson & Green, 1970). From the middle of this range to 20 or 30 msec, highly trained observers can learn to respond with words that are ordinarily used to designate order or direction of change, e.g., "*A* came first," or "pitch moved upward." In the range 60 to 100 msec, even untrained listeners can thus report correctly the order of events.

The two-event sequence is a barely adequate example of perceptual-figure properties (of which "upward moving pitch" is one). Such properties do not emerge in a compelling way simply because other features are salient and provide simpler cues. One has only to notice a characteristic end or start to discriminate *AB* from *BA*, even across sensory modalities. At very short times, only such cues are available (Efron, 1973). They cannot be delimited, however, by the time range alone. For example, Sternberg & Knoll (1973) set aside such peripheral "special cues" from their theory of temporal-order decisions, but use the 20-msec thresholds from earlier experiments (Hirsh, 1959) as proper examples of decision processes. Yet, Broadbent & Ladefoged (1959) argued that that same time resulted in a quality change rather than order perception.

Three or More Events

The judgment of the order of two events represents the simplest case. As we increase the number of components in a sequence beyond two, not only is the mere number increased but the complexity of the task and the description of the complexity are increased. In the case of two events, the observer has only to recognize the characteristics of one of the two in the initial or terminal position or, where this is impossible, to fabricate some sort of a figural "construction" as Neisser & Hirst (1973) put it.

In the case of three events, at the very least one must recognize properties of those stimuli that are both initial and terminal in order to identify order of components within a sequence. Such recognition is further subject to rules of pattern organization which have been made evident, if not clear, in a variety of studies.

Divenyi & Hirsh (1973) constructed three-tone sequences or melodies consisting of temporally contiguous pure tones in the region of 1 kHz. The task of the listener was to identify which of six possible melodic forms had been played after each single presentation. Analysis of the results, particularly by means of confusion matrices, permitted a report not only on the correctness of overall responses but also on the correctness of parts or features of these temporal patterns. Melodies in which the frequencies jumped in a unidirectional manner were easier to recognize than those with inflections or changes in direction. Furthermore the appearance of the highest of the three frequencies in the terminal position turned out to be a strong identifying feature. In general, however, it appeared that the listeners' performance remained relatively good even with tonal durations down to only a few milliseconds.

It has been difficult to relate such a result to the earlier results of Warren, Obusek, Farmer, & Warren (1969), who reported that contiguous sounds, each lasting 200 msec, could not be reliably identified with respect to order when either three or four such sounds comprise the sequence. There were several differences in the two studies. Here, no listener had the opportunity to be trained in the experiment. Instead, each sequence was presented to each listener only once. Thus the listeners were naive in the experiment, but also their previous experience relevant to the task, for example training in music, was unknown. Another difference was that there was no terminal or final component; instead the sequence was continuously repeated without breaks. A third important difference was that Warren *et al.* used sounds very different from each other, i.e., not all members of a particular sound group, consisting as they did of a buzz, a hiss, one or two different tones, or a vowel. This early report of Warren *et al.* and a subsequent one by Warren & Obusek (1972) suggested that durations longer than a half second were required to get naive listeners to order correctly such contiguous sounds.

In the meantime Thomas, Hill, Carroll, & Garcia (1971) as well as Warren & Obusek (1972) showed that considerably less duration was required if all the sounds were vowels of American English. Thomas *et al.* showed a sharp increase in the recognition of the order of such sounds as the duration was increased from a range below 100 msec to one greather than 100 msec. Furthermore Bregman & Campbell (1971) have reported that only 100 msec per stimulus is required when sequences of six tones are presented to listeners for order identification. This time is not different from that for order identification of two events by naive observers (Hirsh & Fraisse, 1964).

In the same report Bregman & Campbell introduced the notion of "auditory streaming," following on an older concept of Miller & Heise (1950) that concerned separation of groups of elements according to their proximity in frequency. Thus it was that in the Bregman & Campbell study the reported order of three of the six tones that were either high or low in frequency was more correct than was the order across frequency groups. These subsequent studies appear to emphasize dependence of judgment of order on the membership of sequence components in a single perceptual channel, perceptual class or stream, or simply into a whole figure by virtue of some aspect of "belongingness."

Pattern Perception

As stated at the outset, temporal order of events is a feature of auditory patterns, or auditory figures. It will be useful to speculate through some of the Gestalt laws of visual perception to define what would be a good figure (Julesz & Hirsh, 1972). A good figure involves a circumscribed *area*, and in auditory terms this may mean a circumscribed range of frequencies as well as a restricted range of time. The patterns of Miller & Heise (1950) and Heise & Miller (1951), and the streams of Bregman & Campbell exemplify the frequency dimension. As for maximum time, there is simply very little information about how spread out in time elements can be before they lose their relatedness.

Good continuation is manifest in the identification study of Divenyi & Hirsh (1973), where simple, unidirectional pitch changes in three-tone melodies define the easiest patterns to identify. Another example (Bregman & Dannenbring, 1973) involves connecting remote parts (but see below).

One other characteristic of elements that appear to belong together, with respect to comprising a figure over time, is not an aspect that one will find among the Gestalt laws. It concerns the repeated occurrence of such elements with each other in the past experience of the observer. Think of the learned units of specialists in bird calls, sonar operators and musicians. Either this associationistic view or perhaps a more modern view, involving 'listening in the speech mode,' must be invoked to suggest how a series of speech sounds comprises a temporal figure even though they may occupy very different bandwidths, frequencies, etc.

Streams and Channels

A stream flows in already established channels; and channels are formed by the flowing of streams. It is suggested that both of these observations from nature are evidenced in auditory perception. Let us remind ourselves of the difficulty in which the airport control-tower operator finds himself when he must monitor the speech of several talkers (pilots) simultaneously. Much of the early literature on this multi-channel listening has been reviewed by Broadbent (1958). The ability of such listeners to monitor several sources of speech simultaneously is enhanced by whatever means are available to give the several voices separate identities. Thus, they may be separated spatially in different loudspeakers, may be processed through different filters so that they have different qualities, or they may, in the case of only two, be delivered to separate ears. These are all examples of stream segregation, some depending on the utilization of channels already established in the listener, and others depending on features characteristic of the streams themselves.

The segregation of different groups of tones that depends upon regions of frequency (Bregman & Campbell, 1971; Miller and Heise, 1950) is a relative grouping depending on the relations of the tones to each other. In addition, however, there appears to be evidence for established channels in the auditory system that make such streaming easier. The separation of frequencies more different than about 15% (Miller and Heise, 1950) does correspond, with the frequencies used, to a critical bandwidth. The critical band is also a crude approximation to the limits of frequency grouping in the study by Bregman & Campbell. The identification of three-tone melodies (Divenyi & Hirsh, 1973) appears to be optimum when the range of frequencies lies between one and two critical bands.

A more direct approach to this question is provided by Nabelek, Nabelek, & Hirsh (1970) who presented tone bursts containing a rapid frequency change to listeners and found that the pitch assigned such complex tone bursts was sometimes a single, fused pitch, and in other circumstances was divided or separated and assigned to both the initial and the terminal portions of the bursts. Although the critical region separating fusion from separation was a complex product of the frequency change and the time for which the change occurred, the critical band seemed again to be implicated.

One can bring two temporal figures or streams more closely into relation with another, thus comprising a single as opposed to separate figures by, so to speak, drawing connecting lines. Thus, if one puts in frequency transitions, either complete or incomplete, between those frequencies that are segregated into separate streams, there is less segregation (Bregman & Dannenbring, 1973). Similarly one can more easily obtain pitch fusion for complex tone bursts (Nabelek, Nabelek, & Hirsh, 1973) with frequency glides or transitions between initial and terminal tones than when a burst consists only of initial and final tones without any transition.

Recapitulation

When events *A* and *B* are separated by brief times, from 1 to 20 msec, and when listeners discriminate *AB* from *BA*, almost any waveform or spectrum features that change with this separation time can subserve the discrimination. Such "quality" discriminations may, with sufficient training, be evidenced also by labelling responses like "*A* came first." These brief time intervals may also play a role in discrimination or identification of longer patterns, like *ABC*, especially when a salient cue appears at the end of a pattern.

In the range from 20 to 100 msec, event order gives unique form to sequences, even those of only two events. But in the simple two-event case there is an overlap with the time range for more easily available quality cues. The order property of such sequence patterns requires, however, that the individual events belong to a *common group* by virtue of sensory channel (intramodal), of figure-relations among the elements, or of special code-common features like speech or the melodic phrases of music.

The ordering of several events that are unrelated by such properties requires decision processes related to the outputs of different channels and possibly mechanisms for the switching of attention. Thus the times required for such order judgments are quite long, of the order of a half second, until particular elements develop strong learning. The exceptions are strings of only two events, where 'first' or 'second' perceptions need not be related in storage over time.

The elegant analytic treatment of models of temporal order judgment, by Sternberg & Knoll (1973) does not encompass all these examples of perceived order. It is restricted in two respects. First, it deals only with decisions concerning first arrival in a pair of arrivals or compounds of such pairs. Second, its insistence on independent channels necessarily excludes from its scope those very cases that are here considered as aspects of the perception of auditory figures.

It is not likely that any single theoretical account of the auditory perception of temporal order can encompass the entire range of time intervals, phenomena, or perceptual tasks. There appear, instead, to be three distinct categories, which can be identified by a combination of time intervals, tasks and the features that seem to be most important for perceived order.

References

Bregman, A. S., & Campbell, J. Primary auditory stream segregation and perception of order in rapid sequences of tones. *Journal of Experimental Psychology*, 1971, **89**, 244–249.

Bregman, A. S., & Dannenbring, G. L. The effect of continuity on auditory stream segregation. *Perception and Psychophysics*, 1973, **13**, 308–312.

Broadbent, D. E. *Perception and communication.* New York: Pergamon, 1958, pp. 15–35.

Broadbent, D. E., & Ladefoged, P. Auditory perception and temporal order. *Journal of the Acoustical Society of America*, 1959, **31**, 1539–1540.

Divenyi, P. L., & Hirsh, I. J. Identification of the temporal order of three tones. *Journal of the Acoustical Society of America*, 1973, **54**, 315–316 (Abstract).

Efron, R. Conservation of temporal information by perceptual systems. *Perception and Psychophysics*, 1973, **14**, 518–530.

Heise, G. A., & Miller, G. A. An experimental study of auditory patterns. *American Journal of Psychology*, 1951, **64**, 68–77.

Hirsh, I. J. Auditory perception of temporal order. *Journal of the Acoustical Society of America*, 1959, **31**, 759–767.

Hirsh, I. J., & Sherrick, C. E. Perceived order in different sense modalities. *Journal of Experimental Psychology*, 1961, **62**, 423–432.

Julesz, B., & Hirsh, I. J. Visual and Auditory Perception: An Essay of Comparison. In E. E. David, Jr. & P. B. Denes (Eds.). *Human communication: A unified view.* New York: McGraw-Hill, 1972, pp. 283–340.

Miller, G. A., & Heise, G. A. The trill threshold. *Journal of the Acoustical Society of America*, 1950, **22**, 637–638.

Nabelek, I. V., Nabelek, A. K., & Hirsh, I. J. Pitch of tone bursts changing frequency. *Journal of the Acoustical Society of America*, 1970, **48**, 536–553.

Nabelek, I. V., Nabelek, A. K., & Hirsh, I. J. Pitch of sound bursts with continuous or discontinuous change of frequency. *Journal of the Acoustical Society of America*, 1973, **53**, 1305–1312.

Neisser, U., & Hirst, W. Effect of practice on the identification of auditory sequences. *Perception and Psychophysics*, 1973, **15**, 391–398.

Patterson, J. H., & Green, D. M. Discrimination of transient signals having identical energy spectra. *Journal of the Acoustical Society of America*, 1970, **48**, 894–905.

Sternberg, S., & Knoll, R. L. The perception of temporal order. In S. Kornblum (Ed.) *Attention and performance*, vol. IV. New York: Academic Press, 1973, pp. 629–685.

Thomas, I. B., Hill, P. B., Carroll, F. S., & Garcia, B. Temporal order in the perception of vowels. *Journal of the Acoustical Society of America*, 1970, **48**, 1010–1013.

Warren, R. M., & Obusek, C. J. Identification of temporal order within auditory sequences. *Perception and Psychophysics*, 1972, **12**, 86–90.

Warren, R. M., Obusek, C. J., Farmer, R. M., & Warren, R. P. Auditory sequence: Confusion of patterns other than speech and music. *Science*, 1969, **164**, 586–587.

THE LINK BETWEEN SPEECH PRODUCTION AND SPEECH PERCEPTION

DAVIS H. HOWES

Boston University School of Medicine and Boston Veterans Administration Hospital

Abstract. The invariance governing the distribution of word frequencies in samples of spoken discourse is utilized to measure the number of words in a speaker's vocabulary, defined as all words with non-zero probabilities of occurrence. The calculated number of words with non-zero probabilities is found to increase systematically with sample size, showing that most words are totally unavailable during the production of discourse. This finding suggests that the permanent vocabulary is stored in a protected mode, making it totally unavailable for use. In discourse, the cognition the speaker wishes to express releases temporarily a small subset of related words from protected storage, and the word actually spoken is selected from this semantic field. When applied to speech perception, this model suggests a new interpretation of experiments on the facilitation of word perception by context or familiarity and of some recent studies on the perception of speech sounds.

The influence of Smitty Stevens on those who studied with him, especially in those exciting days when the Psycho-Acoustical Laboratory was at full strength, had a depth and breadth that those who knew him only through his publications could scarcely appreciate. In audition it would have been hard to do an experiment that did not in one way or another bear the imprint of his thinking. But he also had an intense interest in the craftsmanship of science that led him far and wide over the whole spectrum of research. Unlike most academic discussions of scientific method, which are apt to be vague and supererogatory, his were invariably trenchant and rooted in the solid earth of the investigator's practical contest with a stubborn nature. Many of his arguments have found their way into his articles on operationism and measurement, but cold print cannot convey that special quality of illumination that Smitty imparted to a favorite point through the forcefulness of his personality and the rich embroidery he would weave about the theme. Lessons learned from these spontaneous expositions were not soon forgotten. Though he sometimes disparaged the role, Smitty was in fact a superb teacher to those who served their apprenticeship with him.

The material I wish to present here, while only indirectly related to Smitty's own researches, bears his imprint through these lessons on the scientific process. One of his theses that impressed me most vividly was the importance of pursuing invariances, in contrast with the emphasis then so prevalent in psychology of searching for significant differences. The doctrine went far beyond his published accounts (e.g., Stevens, 1951) and was intertwined with the importance of reducing problems to fundamental measurement and with the dictum that theories are needed only when the proper measurements can't be carried out. The argument as he developed it spontaneously was overwhelming; I was left with the conviction that it was almost a moral obligation to exploit an invariance when one came your way. Thus when I resumed my study of central mechanisms of language and speech I felt compelled to take another look at

H. R. Moskowitz et al. (eds.), Sensation and Measurement. 259–269. All Rights Reserved.

what appeared to be that field's most remarkable invariance, Zipf's law, although I had previously shared the general opinion of the day that it was little more than a curiosity or artifact. This problem has occupied me, off and on, ever since. The results of this investigation and some of its implications for the storage of verbal information and the perception of speech, form the topic of this paper.

Zipf (1932, 1935) had shown that the number of different words used 1, 2, 3... times in any sizable sample of spontaneous discourse follows the same distribution regardless of the language and the subject or form of discourse. Originally he had proposed that this invariance obeys an inverse square law,

$$v(x) = a/x^2, \tag{1}$$

where $v(x)$ is the number of words occurring x times and $a = v(1)$, but later (Zipf, 1949) he treated the data in a disguised form of the integral of (1),

$$x = a/r(x), \tag{2}$$

where $r(x)$ denotes the rank of a word occurring x times in order of frequency. In this latter form he presented graphical tests of an astonishing array of verbal materials, including samples from languages with diverse structures and histories such as English, German, Chinese, and the American Indian languages Nootka, Dakota, and Plains Cree. Having no experience with quantitative data, Zipf failed to recognize this equation as, at best, a rough rule of thumb. The deviations from Equation 2 in Zipf's innumerable graphs of linguistic data follow such a regular course, however, that his work did establish that some kind of invariance governs word-frequency data.

This invariance can be exploited in two directions. One is to derive it from an explanatory theory or model of the underlying linguistic processes. Zipf himself attempted to account for Equation 2 by a pseudo-mathematical appeal to a general principle of least effort, an argument that stimulated Benoit Mandelbrot (1953) to formulate the problem as one of coding information with minimum cost. Mandelbrot showed that the generalized Pareto distribution, of which Zipf's equation is a special case, offers a better description of the data and can be derived from very general postulates about the cost of coding information in linguistic form. Other, less successful, models for deriving the Zipf law were proposed by Simon (1955), Good (1953), and others.

A second way of exploiting this invariance, and one more in accord with Stevens' scientific philosophy, is to utilize its potential for measuring fundamental quantities. An obvious candidate is the size of an individual's vocabulary. The extraordinary dimension of the storage and retrieval problem presented by the vocabulary has received scant attention in recent years, owing to the intense interest in syntax aroused by the theories of Chomsky and Miller and in the acoustic aspects of speech perception by the discoveries of the Haskins Laboratories, K. Stevens, Fant, and others. By even the most conservative estimates the brain of any literate person must store tens of thousands of words. Every time a speaker utters a word this vast permanent memory must be searched in order for the appropriate word to be retrieved. To understand the mechanism by which the brain accomplishes this remarkable feat we must first be able to measure the size of the memory store involved.

Carroll (1938) first attempted to use the Zipf invariance for this purpose, deriving an expression for the number of words in the vocabulary from Equation 2. The results were unsatisfactory, however, and Carroll rightly concluded that Equation 2 does not satisfactorily represent the invariance underlying Zipf's law. The English statistician Yule (1944) suggested a more general approach to the problem, using the frequency distributions in the form of Equation 1 instead of the rank distributions of Equation 2. Drawing on his experience with accident statistics, Yule pointed out that the frequency distribution obtained from any sample of discourse is incomplete, inasmuch as an unspecified number of words not appearing in the same were nevertheless 'at risk' during its production. These should appear in the sample distribution as words occurring 0 times. Hence W, the number of words in the speaker's vocabulary, can be represented by the sum $R+v(0)$, where $v(0)$ is the unknown number of words at risk but unused and $R=\sum v(x)$, $x=1, 2, \ldots, N$ is the number of different words appearing one or more times in the sample. Given a satisfactory expression for $v(x)$, the number of words occurring one or more times, the unknown quantity $v(0)$ may be inferred to give an estimate of vocabulary size. Yule was unable to find a satisfactory expression, however, and did not pursue his argument further, having rejected Zipf's inverse square law on the dual grounds that it failed to describe the data adequately and implied a vocabulary of unlimited size.

Another suggestion of Yule's led to my first venture into the field. One method of minimizing the problem presented by the unknown number of words with zero sample frequencies is to consider the number of occurrences of all words occurring exactly **x** times in the sample, $n(x)=x\cdot v(x)$, since for $x=0$, $n(x)=0$. By serendipity I found that word-frequency data in this form are very well represented by the lognormal distribution function. Certain difficulties persisted, however. If $n(x)$ is lognormal, it is easily proved that the distribution of word frequencies $v(x)=n(x)/x$ should also be lognormal. Unfortunately, my attempts to obtain satisfactory fits to the data in this form were unsuccessful. Furthermore, study of the parameters derived from the lognormal $n(x)$ distributions led to the puzzling conclusion that an individual's vocabulary, even if he is aphasic, is unlimited in size (Howes, 1964).

These persistent failures to derive an estimate of vocabulary size from the Zipf invariance led me to formulate more carefully the concept of the vocabulary as it relates to the word frequency distribution. In spontaneous discourse a speaker typically gives verbal form to ideas, memories, perceptions, and so forth that he wishes to express; he transforms meanings or cognitions into a sequence of phonemes. The verbal system is a kind of transducer, converting information stored in cognitive or pre-verbal form into linguistic events. The smallest unit by which this transducing system can operate is the word (morpheme), inasmuch as smaller units such as the phoneme or syllable have no cognitive significance. The sequence of phonemes a speaker produces at any given time therefore is determined by which word (or larger unit) the transducing system has selected on the basis of the cognitive information to be expressed. The vocabulary of a speaker is defined by the set of all possible selections the transducing system can make. Each element of the vocabulary may be represented by a point connected (*a*) to one or more input pathways that can be excited by cognitions or meanings and (*b*) to a single output pathway leading to a neural template that specifies the sequence of phonemes constituting the spoken word. Every word a person can utter meaningfully thus corresponds to a point in his vocabulary.

Several limitations on the interpretation of vocabulary measurements follow from these definitions. (*a*) The measurements relate exclusively to the number of elements in the active, or output, vocabulary. (*b*) Certain word strings may be selected as units (e.g., *thank you*) and thus have independent representation in the vocabulary. Since the component words can also be used separately, measurements of vocabulary based on word statistics represent a minimum bound on the size of the actual store. (*c*) The vocabulary includes only words used propositionally, in the sense of Hughlings Jackson (1931); nonsense words or imitations of arbitrary speech sounds may utilize the same motor mechanisms as words produced through the vocabulary, but their production bypasses the vocabulary mechanism itself. (*d*) In the adult, the size of the vocabulary is effectively a constant during any time period measured in hours or days. New elements may be added to the adult's vocabulary from time to time, but at a rate that is negligible relative to the number already in storage.

With these considerations in mind we can define a measure of vocabulary size as follows. Each vocabulary element is by definition a possible event, capable of excitation via at least one input pathway; it therefore has a probability greater than zero. More precisely, since the probability, θ, of any given word can be expected to vary in time, it is the expectation or average value of θ that is greater than zero. The size of the vocabulary is accordingly the number of elements for which $\theta > 0$. If there are M such elements, their mean probability is

$$\bar{\theta} = \frac{1}{M} \sum_{i=1}^{i=M} \theta_i . \tag{3}$$

Since every possible outcome of a verbal selection is included, the sum of the M elements with non-zero probabilities is unity,

$$\sum_{i=1}^{i=M} \theta_i = 1 . \tag{4}$$

It follows that the total number of words in the vocabulary is the reciprocal of the mean probability of its elements,

$$M = 1/\bar{\theta} . \tag{5}$$

At this point we introduce the invariance of Zipf in the following general form. We assume that the probabilities of all M words in any person's vocabulary are distributed according to some probability law $f(\theta)$ whose mean $\bar{\theta}$ exists. Since the probability that any given word will occur $x=0, 1, 2, \ldots$ times in a random sample of N selections from the vocabulary is given by the binomial distribution, the expected number of words occurring exactly x times in N selections from a vocabulary is

$$v(x, N) = M \int_0^1 B(x; \theta, N) f(\theta) \, \mathrm{d}\theta, \quad x = 0, 1, 2, \ldots, N, \tag{6}$$

where $B(x; \theta, N)$ is the binomial of x for probability θ and the sample size N. For large samples, the binomial will be approximated under fairly general conditions of sampling, and thus Equation 6 is not limited to sampling with Bernoulli trials.

Equations 5 and 6 together provide a method of determining the number of words in the vocabulary of a speaker from samples of his discourse. Given any hypothetical expression for the probability law $f(\theta)$, we test its validity by comparing the observed number of words occurring 1, 2, 3,... times in samples of N words with the expected number $v(x, N)$ for all $x>0$. Then from the mean of the function $f(\theta)$ the number of words in the vocabulary, M, is calculated by Equation 5. Obviously the calculated values of M will depend critically on the expression chosen for $f(\theta)$, since a large proportion of the vocabulary will consist of words with very small probabilities and expected frequencies less than 1. The correspondence between the expected frequencies $v(x, N)$ and the empirical word frequency distribution therefore must be evaluated with great care.

Following my previous experience with occurrence distributions I have examined the specific hypothesis that the function $f(\theta)$ is lognormal (see Howes, 1971, for the mathematical development of this assumption). The lognormal is determined by two parameters, the mean μ and variance σ^2 of the transformed variate $y=\log_e \theta$. These two parameters can be evaluated from the incomplete observed word-frequency distributions by a method based on Fisher's solution to the maximum-likelihood equations for the parameters of a truncated normal distribution (Hald, 1952). From the moments of the lognormal it is easily shown that on this hypothesis the vocabulary size is

$$M = e^{-\mu - \frac{1}{2}\sigma^2}, \tag{7}$$

and numerical integration of Equation 6 shows that the function $v(x, N)$ is given approximately by the discrete form of the lognormal,

$$v(x, N) = M \int_{x-\frac{1}{2}}^{x+\frac{1}{2}} \mathrm{d}\Lambda(x), \tag{8}$$

where $\Lambda(x)$ is the lognormal distribution for $x=N\theta$.

Extensive tests of Equation 8 have been made using the data from my corpus of spoken English, which comprises more than 250000 words transcribed from interviews with 41 individuals varying widely in age, education, and occupational level (Howes, 1966). The interviews were conducted in an open-ended manner, the subject being

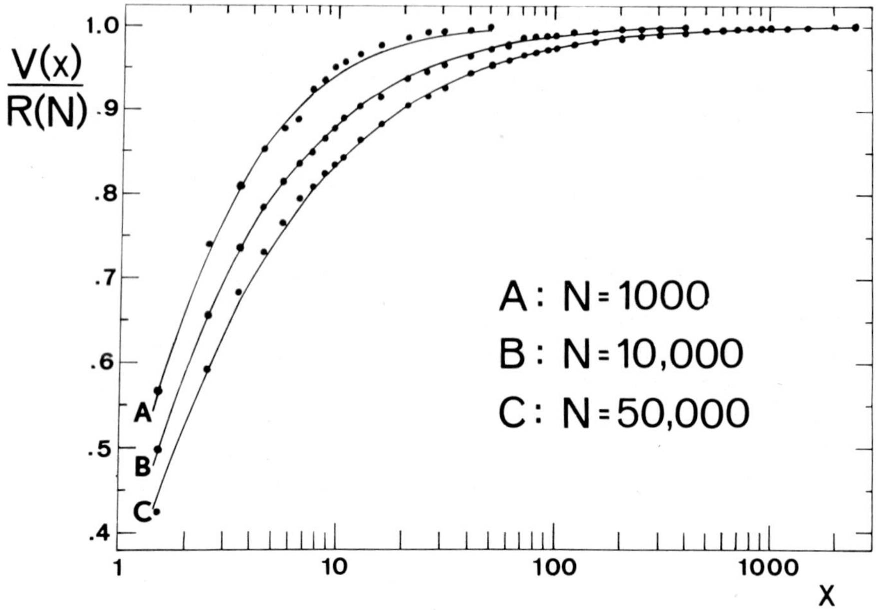

Fig. 1. Word-frequency distributions for samples of different size from the same speaker. The ordinate shows the cumulative proportion of words (types) occurring one or more times. The theoretical lines represent lognormal distributions truncated at the point $x=\frac{1}{2}$.

asked to talk freely and the interviewer intervening only to introduce new topics whenever the subject seemed to be running out of conversation. This procedure was used in order to obtain a complete record, as far as possible, of the words generated by the subject during a given interval. Samples of writing, where the subject may edit his output before writing it down, are for this reason a less reliable source of data.

Figure 1 shows the word-frequency distributions, plotted cumulatively on a logarithmic frequency scale, for samples of 1000, 10000, and 50000 words from one subject who was interviewed for more than 6 h. The smooth lines represent theoretical values of $v(x, N)$ calculated from the lognormal hypothesis by Equation 8. Visually, these curves fit the 3 sets of data well.

For more exact tests the χ^2 test of goodness of fit was applied to the distributions for 40 independent samples of 5000 words from 36 different speakers, including 5 independent samples from the subject whose data appear in Figure 1. The data were grouped to give an expected number of at least 5 words per frequency class; the number of classes ranged from 19 to 21 for different subjects. The values of χ^2 exceeded the 0.05 level of significance for only 2 of the 40 samples, exactly the number expected if the observed points represent random samples from the theoretical values. The sum of the 40 χ^2 values was 832.5 with 783 degrees of freedom ($p>0.20$). Since the power of the χ^2 test is great for such large numbers of observations (Cohen, 1969), this result indicates that the lognormal gives nearly perfect fits to the observed word-frequency distributions. Similar results were obtained with samples of 1000 words from the same individuals.

In view of these results, calculations of vocabulary size by Equation 7 can be accepted as based on tested assumptions. For the subject who gave more than 50000 words, M was calculated from the parameters μ and σ^2 estimated from samples ranging in size from 1000 to 65000. These calculated values are shown by the solid circles in Figure 2. The value of M clearly increases with sample size; an exponential function of the form

$$M = W(1 - e^{-aN}), \tag{9}$$

indicated by the smooth line in the figure, gives a good representation of this relationship. Here W is a constant representing the limit of M as $N \to \infty$ and is approximately 20000 for this individual. Comparable increases in M are found in the data from all 36 subjects, although data are available for the others only in the range from $N = 1000$ to $N = 5000$.

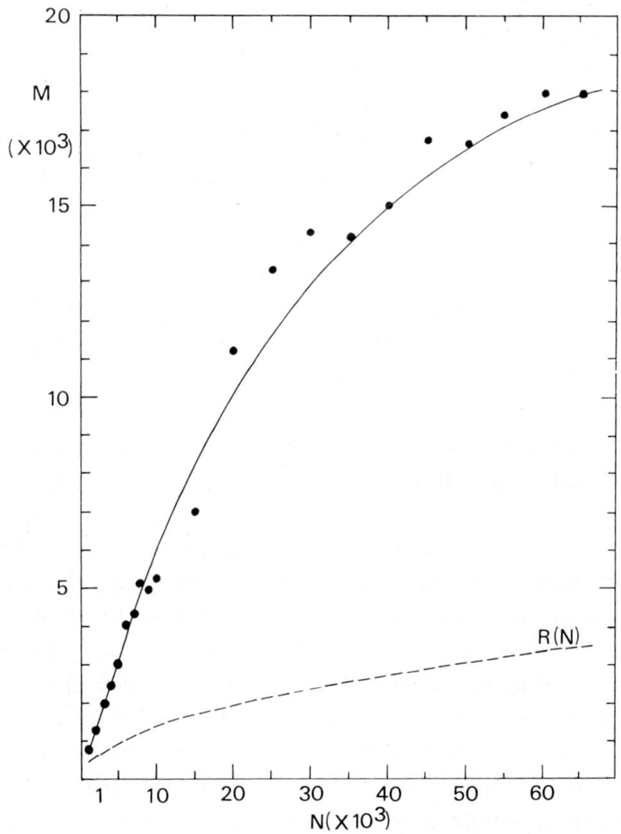

Fig. 2. The number of words with non-zero probabilities, M, calculated from samples of varying size from the same speaker. The solid line represents Equation 9 with $W=20000$. The dashed line labelled $R(N)$ shows the number of words appearing at least once in each sample.

The dashed line in Figure 2 represents the observed number of different words in each sample, i.e., those occurring one or more times. Thus the vertical distance between each point and the dashed line below it indicates the number of words with non-zero probabilities but zero sample frequencies, $v(0)$; these are the words assumed to be available for selection but not actually used. It can be seen that the proportion of such words is generally greater than half, and that it systematically increases with sample size over the range available.

These measurements clearly show that the vocabulary, as we have defined it, is not the ensemble from which selections of words are made in discourse. For the vocabulary, as an essentially permanent memory store, cannot possibly increase at the rapid rate indicated by the points in Figure 2, nor could it be limited to the relatively small number of words (3200 or less) indicated by the values of M calculated from samples of 1000 to 5000 words. If selections were made directly from the vocabulary, we would expect M to be independent of sample size and thus to describe an essentially horizontal line in Figure 2. And $v(0)$, the number of words with zero frequency, would have to decrease with N.

The results, although unexpected, nevertheless are not actually inconsistent with our previous definitions. We defined the vocabulary as the set of all words whose probabilities have *non-zero expected values*, recognizing that the probability of any given word may vary in time. Let us suppose that at some point in time a word in the vocabulary becomes totally unavailable and has a probability of zero. If it remains in that state throughout an interval of time (t_0, t_1) its average probability over that interval will be zero. But if during a subsequent interval (t_1, t_2) the word temporarily becomes available and attains a probability greater than zero its average probability over the interval (t_0, t_2) will be greater than zero. Then we have $M_2 > M_1$, where M_1 is the number of words with non-zero average probabilities in the interval (t_0, t_1) and M_2 the number in the larger interval (t_0, t_2). As the time interval is extended indefinitely, moreover, M will approach a limiting value W, representing the total number of elements in permanent storage. By allowing words to pass in and out of a temporary state of zero probability we can account for the major features of the data shown in Figure 2.

The vocabulary exists, then, in a kind of protected mode of storage, to which the neural mechanism that determines the actual word produced at a given time has no direct access. Instead, the vocabulary is scanned by a separate mechanism that releases a relatively small subset of vocabulary elements from the protected mode. The selection mechanism scans only this smaller set of elements to determine the word that is produced. After a selection has been made, all vocabulary elements revert to the protected mode. The only vocabulary elements ever scanned by the selection mechanism therefore are those that appear at least once in open mode; these elements constitute the verbal ensemble to which the invariance of Zipf applies.

The mathematical results give no indication of the criteria by which the scanning mechanism determines which words are released from protected mode at a given time. Inasmuch as the inputs to the vocabulary represent cognitive or semantic information, the temporary ensemble presumably consists of words related to the semantic aspects of the cognition that is being expressed. Accordingly, we assume that only semantically related words exist in open mode at the same time.

Although other models of the selection process can be suggested, the fundamental distinction between one mechanism that scans the vocabulary to specify a small temporarily available ensemble of words, and a second mechanism that selects the word to be produced, appears to be required by the data. A two-tiered process of this kind makes good sense when the engineering aspects of processing information are taken into consideration. Even for the subject whose data appear in Figure 2, who was a milkman of modest verbal skills, a vocabulary of 20000 words is indicated; and this figure is derived from the calculated values of M, which must be considered a lower bound on the actual number of stored elements. The data from the initial segments of the curves for subjects of greater verbal ability indicate vocabularies numbering well over 100000 words. A mechanism for scanning such a memory in order to select the appropriate alternative each time a word is produced, whether by some kind of semantic feature analysis or in a frequency-dependent search, staggers the imagination, especially in view of the relatively slow time constants of neural elements and the rapid rate at which words can be produced propositionally. Nor is it evident that any great economies could be achieved by parallel processing, as some have suggested. A two-tiered search has the advantage that the initial scan need only be very rough and therefore can be performed rapidly, whereas the ultimate choice of a word, which to be accurate requires scanning a relatively rich store of information, requires a selection from only a few alternatives. In this way the remarkable flexibility of human language, whereby the system is capable of finding any one of a vast number of possible words in response to an appropriate stimulus, can be achieved both rapidly and accurately.

So far we have been concerned exclusively with the role of the vocabulary in the production of discourse. Let us now turn to the part it plays in the perception and comprehension of speech. Here the verbal system acts as a transducer in the reverse direction, accepting as its input a sequence of phonemes and evoking congitions or meanings as its output. The phonemic input sequence must be matched with the neural template corresponding to the correct vocabulary element for a word to be recognized and understood. Some process therefore must be postulated by which the listener's entire vocabulary can be searched to find the right template.

It is this search process that is of interest here. Given the enormous number of words a person can understand, it is difficult to imagine that a neural mechanism simply scans templates and compares each one with the input sequence until a match is found. It seems unlikely, moreover, in view of the vast amounts of information involved, that separate vocabularies are established for the production and perception of speech. We have just seen that a two-tiered search of the vocabulary is indicated for production of discourse. Let us consider briefly how this model might operate to reduce the scanning requirements for the perception of speech.

As before, we assume that the vocabulary itself is stored in a protected mode that renders it totally inaccessible to the scanning mechanism. At any given time a relatively small set of vocabulary elements is temporarily released from the protected mode by excitation from whatever cognitions are then active in the listener. The phonemic templates of only this small subset of words are scanned and compared with the input sequence. If a match is achieved, the cognitions connected to the selected vocabulary element are activated and the word is perceived and understood. If not, the vocabulary elements that have been scanned revert to protected storage, and new semantic fields are successively released until a match is achieved. Rapid search of the entire vocabulary is possible because cognitive information is utilized in addition to the phonemic input.

The listener thus plays an active role in speech perception. In continuous dialogue the sequence of cognitions evoked in the listener must correspond roughly to the sequence of cognitions that led the speaker to his selection of words. Since a word must be in an activated semantic field in order to be perceived, the cognitive information supplied by the context will greatly facilitate speech perception in continuous discourse. Telling the subject the semantic category to which a word belongs (such as animal names), or showing him a list containing the word, would have a similar facilitative effect on its recognition. When no other cognitive information is available to the listener, on the other hand, the words most likely to be in an activated semantic field will be those he most frequently uses. Consequently, the threshold of a word presented in isolation should be inversely related to its frequency of usage. Since this last effect depends on random sampling of semantic fields, moreover, it should be quantitatively smaller than the effects produced by factors, such as context, directly influencing the listener's semantic fields. Thus many of the cognitive effects on speech perception that have been established experimentally (cf. Neisser, 1967) follow directly from the assumption of a two-tiered model of vocabulary search.

A peripheral mechanism must be postulated for constructing the phonemic input to the vocabulary out of the acoustic record provided by the auditory system. The properties required of this mechanism account for some well-established results of experiments with speech sounds. The perceptual significance of the phoneme, according to the present model, resides in its function as an element of the neural templates associated with vocabulary elements, not as an element of the acoustic record of speech. Phonemes therefore are not segmented in the acoustic record, but in the output of the peripheral mechanism, where they must be registered (and thus perceived) as discrete elements to permit comparison with the stored templates of the vocabulary. Since the same neural templates are used in both the production and perception of speech, moreover, parallels between the two peripheral systems for entering the vocabulary are to be expected. Thus the principal conclusions of the Haskins Laboratories, based on their experiments with synthetic speech sounds (Liberman, Cooper, Shankweiler, & Studdert-Kennedy, 1967), can be explained without appealing to their motor theory of speech perception. Moreover, the absence of distinctive acoustic cues for the boundaries between words, which the Haskins analysis does not account for, can be explained by the present theory as a consequence of the discrete changes between successive semantic fields.

By pursuing the invariance represented by Zipf's law to its logical conclusion, then, we arrive at a new conception of the vocabulary as a link between speech perception and speech production. Both processes utilize the same mechanism for generating temporary semantic fields to reduce the scanning requirements for searching the entire permanent vocabulary. What distinguishes them is the type of information used for scanning the vocabulary elements in those fields. Thus in the rapid interchange between speaking and listening that is the hallmark of good conversation we can perhaps find the reflection of a basic principle underlying the way in which we process verbal information.

References

Carroll, J. B. Diversity of vocabulary and the harmonic series law of word-frequency distribution. *Psychological Record*, 1938, **2**, 379–386.

Cohen, J. *Statistical power analysis for the behavioral sciences.* New York: Academic Press, 1969.

Good, I. J. The population frequencies of species and the estimation of population parameters. *Biometrika*, 1953, **40**, 237.

Hald, A. *Statistical theory with engineering applications.* New York: Wiley, 1952.

Howes, D. Application of the word-frequency concept to aphasia. In A. V. S. de Reuck & M. O'Connor (Eds.), *Disorders of language.* London: Churchill, 1964, pp. 47–75.

Howes, D. Vocabulary size estimated from the distribution of word frequencies. In H. Myklebust (Ed.), *Progress in learning disabilities*, vol. 2. New York: Grune & Stratton, 1971, pp. 94–110.

Jackson, J. H. In James Taylor (Ed.), *Selected writings of John Hughlings Jackson.* London: Hodder & Stoughton, 1931.

Liberman, A. M., Cooper, F. S., Shankweiler, D. P., & Studdert-Kennedy, M. Perception of the speech code. *Psychological Review*, 1967, **74**, 431–461.

Mandelbrot, B. Contribution à la théorie mathématique des jeux de communication. *Publications de L'Institut de Statistique de L'Université de Paris*, 1953, **2**, 1–124.

Neisser, U. *Cognitive psychology.* New York: Appleton-Century-Crofts, 1967.

Simon, H. A. On a class of skew distribution functions. *Biometrika*, 1955, **42**, 425–440.

Stevens, S. S. Mathematics, measurement, and psychophysics. In S. S. Stevens (Ed.), *Handbook of experimental psychology*, New York: Wiley, 1951, pp. 1–49.

Yule, G. U. *The statistical study of literary vocabulary.* Cambridge: The University Press, 1944.

Zipf, G. K. *Selected studies of the principle of relative frequency in language.* Cambridge: Harvard University Press, 1932.

Zipf, G. K. *The psycho-biology of language.* Boston: Houghton Mifflin, 1935.

Zipf, G. K. *Human behavior and the principle of least effort.* Cambridge: Addison-Wesley Press, 1949.

MATCHING LOUDNESS AND VOCAL LEVEL: AN EXPERIMENT REQUIRING NO APPARATUS[1]

ROBERT J. IRWIN
University of Auckland
and
A. WILLIAM MILLS
Tufts University

Abstract. Both the loudness of a sound and the apparent magnitude of a self-produced vocal response (autophonic response) can be described as power functions of sound pressure, although with different exponents. Two scales, one of loudness, the other of autophonic level, can therefore be specified as a function of the same sound pressures. Under these circumstances theory predicts that loudness should be proportional to the square root of apparent autophonic level. Two separate but similar classroom experiments were performed, in each of which one person made autophonic responses of six different magnitudes whose loudnesses were judged by the members of the class. The obtained exponents between the two scales so erected was 0.52 in one demonstration and 0.53 in the other, thus confirming the prediction. The experiments used no apparatus since the only specification of the stimulus required was that the sound pressure produced by one subject should be the same as that judged by another.

Experiments on cross-modal matching (Stevens, 1959) require that subjects judge when two stimuli, sensed by different modalities, are equal in apparent magnitude. By this means pairs of stimuli of apparently equal magnitudes are determined. If the subjective magnitude of each stimulus bears a known relation (as specified by some psychophysical function) to its physical magnitude then it follows that pairs of stimuli corresponding to apparently equal magnitudes must bear a predictable relation to each other. For example, if the sensation of two different stimulus-dimensions are power functions of their respective stimuli, then it can be shown that such stimuli, matched in subjective magnitude, should also be related by a power function, but with an exponent equal to the ratio of the exponents of each dimension. This deduction, which is due to Stevens, therefore provides a check on the validity of the separate scales of apparent magnitude – a check which is, however, a necessary consequence but not a sufficient proof of their validity, because other functions (such as a logarithmic one) lead to the same deduction.

A special case of cross-modal matching has been reported by Lane, Catania, & Stevens (1961). They asked subjects to match the apparent magnitude of the vocal response (autophonic response, as the authors called it) to the loudness of a white noise. From independent experiments (e.g. Stevens, 1955) the loudness of white noise, when judged by one of the direct methods such as the method of magnitude estimation, is proportional to the 0.6 power of the sound pressure. The apparent level of a subject's autophonic response, as measured by the method of production, is

[1] Reprinted from *British Journal of Psychology*, 1965, **56**, 2 and 3, pp. 143–146.

H. R. Moskowitz et al. (eds.), Sensation and Measurement. 271–274.

proportional to about the 1.17 power of the sound pressure produced (Lane *et al.*, 1961). It follows that if a subject adjusts the loudness of a noise to seem similar in magnitude to one which he himself is producing, the sound pressure of the vocal response should be the 0.6/1.17 power of the sound pressure of the equated noise. This prediction was confirmed by Lane *et al.* for the autophonic response of the vowel [ɑ], and the loudness of white noise.

Lane's experiment is a special case of cross-modal matching because the two modalities (speech and hearing) are both described as functions of the same physical dimension, namely, sound pressure. For this reason it affords an opportunity of performing the converse experiment: instead of measuring pairs of stimuli corresponding to equal sensations, one can measure pairs of sensations corresponding to equal stimuli. The magnitude of the stimuli need not be known, so long as for any pair of judgements they are the same.

Thus given the following psychophysical functions (and ignoring constants which govern the size of units),

$$L = P^{0.6} \quad \text{and} \quad A = P^{1.17}, \tag{1}$$

where L is loudness, A is apparent magnitude of autophonic response, and P is sound pressure; then, if L and A are found for identical values of P,

$$L^{1.17} = A^{0.6} \tag{2}$$

or

$$\log L = 0.6/1.17 \log A\,; \tag{3}$$

$\log L$ should then be a linear function of $\log A$, with a constant of proportionality of 0.51. Note that physical magnitudes do not appear in Equation 3.

This function provides the basis for an instructive demonstration of cross-modal matching that can be performed in the classroom. Two such demonstrations are now described.

Method

Each author carried out an independent but procedurally similar experiment. In one experiment the subjects were nineteen students of a second-year psychology class at the University of Auckland, and in the other they were twenty-five students of a first-year course at Tufts University. The subjects were read instructions which asked them to estimate the loudness of the vowel [ɑ] which would be said by the teacher. The first vowel emitted was to be the standard stimulus, and was assigned a loudness of ten; other vocal productions were to be given numerical estimates proportional to their loudnesses, bearing in mind that the first one had a loudness of ten. (This is the method of magnitude estimation.) The teacher then produced six different autophonic levels whose magnitudes bore a specified relation to the magnitude of the standard: these relations were one-fifth, one-half, once, twice, three times, and ten times. The standard was presented first, and each of the five remaining magnitudes was presented twice in a predetermined and random order. (This is the method of magnitude production.) The modulus of the autophonic scale was set by producing the standard at what was deemed to be a conversational level.

Results

The results of the two experiments are shown separately in Figure 1. The experi-

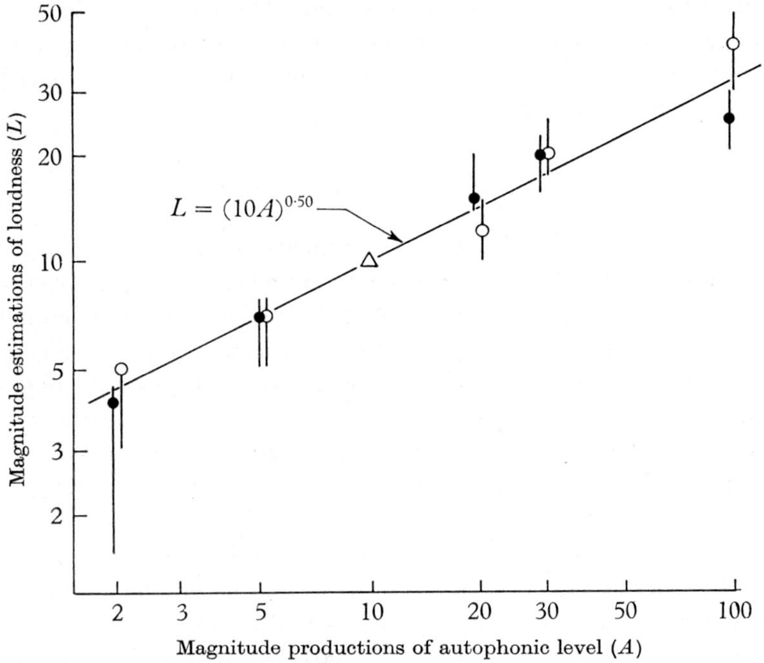

Fig. 1. Estimates of the loudness of a vocal response plotted as a function of its apparent autophonic level. The filled and open circles are independent estimates from different experiments. The filled circles have been displaced slightly to the left of the open circles for the sake of clarity. The triangle represents the standards which were arbitrarily assigned to that point on both scales. The vertical lines extend $\pm$ one quartile from the medians. The straight line is the theoretical outcome predicted from the separate psychophysical equations which specify each subjective scale as a function of sound pressure.

mental points represent the median estimations of the loudness of each of the vocal levels produced. The filled circles are the medians of 38 judgements from 19 subjects, and the open circles are those of 50 judgements from 25 subjects. Each point represents two sets of judgements described as a function of the same stimuli: one set of judgements about loudness, and the other about autophonic level. The triangle at the co-ordinates (10, 10) represents the standards which were arbitrarily assigned to that position on both scales. The vertical lines around each point extend plus and minus one quartile from the medians.

The solid line is the theoretical outcome predicted from the separate psychophysical functions of equation 1. The constant 10 in the equation that describes the line merely reflects the choice of units. The method of least squares was used to determine what power function fitted the medians best. The best-fitting exponent for the filled circles is 0.52, and that for the open circles is 0.53; the theoretical equation thus represents the data well. The data may therefore be described by saying that the judgements of loudness were approximately proportional to the square-root of the apparent magnitude of the autophonic response. The largest discrepancy between theory and experiment is shown by the most right-hand points, where one of the obtained medians underestimates the theoretical outcome of 31.62 by 6.62 units, and the other overestimates it by 8.38 units.

Discussion

Three characteristics distinguish these experiments from the usual one on cross-modal matching. First, instead of determining the locus of stimuli corresponding to equal sensory magnitudes, they determined the locus of sensory magnitudes corresponding to equal stimuli. Secondly, whereas the same subject usually makes the judgements of both stimuli, here the person who produced the autophonic responses was not the one who estimated their loudness, or, at any rate, their loudness unconfounded by the effects of producing them. Thirdly, both sensory modalities were scaled on the same physical dimension, not different ones. But since the sense of hearing is the only one capable of transducing small sound pressures, the psychophysical equation for the autophonic response may be somewhat misleading. Its exponent cannot reflect, as is claimed for other exponents (Stevens, 1961), the operating characteristic of its transducer, for the ear is the transducer of sound pressure, and its exponent is 0.6. Although it may be possible to specify both loudness and autophonic level as a function of sound pressure, the judgements must be made of different stimuli, otherwise loudness could not be proportional to the square root of autophonic level when both are described as functions of the same stimuli. Warren (1962), on the other hand, suggested that judgements of both loudness and vocal level are based on estimates of distance: a sound twice as loud as another has a sound pressure of one twice as near, and a vocal level twice another is one whose sound pressure is projected twice as far. This explanation must therefore invoke additional hypotheses to account for the non-linear relation between loudness and vocal level reported by Lane *et al.* (1961), and also found in the present experiments.

Despite these differences from the customary experiment on cross-modal matching, or perhaps because of them, we believe these experiments illustrate a feasible and instructive demonstration which can be performed in the classroom without any apparatus.

References

Lane, H. L., Catania, A. C., & Stevens, S. S. Voice level: autophonic scale, perceived loudness, and effects of sidetone. *Journal of the Acoustical Society of America*, 1961, **33**, 160–167.

Stevens, S. S. The measurement of loudness. *Journal of the Acoustical Society of America*, 1955, **27**, 815–819.

Stevens, S. S. Cross-modality validation of subjective scales of loudness, vibration, and electric shock. *Journal of Experimental Psychology*, 1959, **57**, 201–209.

Stevens, S. S. Psychophysics of sensory function. In W. A. Rosenblith (Ed.), *Sensory communication.* New York: M.I.T. and Wiley, 1961.

Warren, R. M. Are 'autophonic' judgements based on loudness? *American Journal of Psychology*, 1962, **75**, 452–456.

PREDICTION OF PAIRED-COMPARISON AND MAGNITUDE-ESTIMATION JUDGMENTS OF NOISINESS[1]

KARL D. KRYTER

Stanford Research Institute, Menlo Park, Calif.

Abstract. Paired comparisons and magnitude estimations of the subjective noisiness or unacceptability of noises that differed with respect to both spectral and temporal characteristics were obtained from some 72 subjects. In the present tests, subjects making repetitive judgments of noises that vary simultaneously with respect to several physical dimensions appear to base their judgments primarily on the peak levels reached by each noise. The results indicate that subjective noisiness of complex sounds can be better predicted by the physical measures that have been designated as PNdBM and dBD_2 than by dBA or by the recently proposed units, PLdB and dBE. The method of magnitude estimation is a much more efficient and effective procedure, for present purposes, than the method of paired comparisons.

Inasmuch as the development of standardized procedures for the measurement and evaluation of environmental noise depends to a large extent upon psychological tests conducted in the laboratory, it is of practical as well as theoretical importance to continue to test and improve, if possible, the efficiency and reliability of these tests. Accordingly, a series of paired-comparison and magnitude-estimation judgment tests were conducted of the subjective annoyance of noises (primarily aircraft) that differed widely with respect to both spectral complexity and duration. Also, the relative accuracy with which various older and two new (Stevens, 1972) physical units of sound measurement predict the perceived noisiness of such sounds, as judged in these two test methods, was investigated. Perceived noisiness (PN) and perceived noise level (PNL) are subjective quantities either judged or calculated.

Procedure

ACOUSTIC ENVIRONMENT

All tests were conducted in an anechoic chamber. Stimuli were presented via loudspeakers. Physical measures of the noises were computed from 24 one-third octave bands, from 50 to 10000 Hz, whose sound pressure levels were sampled and averaged over half-second time intervals at the position of the listeners' ears. From these measures the so-called maximum level (PNL) and effective level (EPNL) of the noises were calculated in various units of physical measurement. These units and related frequency weightings and calculation procedures are given in detail in Anon (1961), Kryter (1970), and Stevens (1972) and are summarized in Table 1 and Figure 1.

NOISE STIMULI

The various noise stimuli used are described in Table 2. All the noises were recorded

[1] This paper is based on work done by the author under Contract NAS1-11602 with the National Aeronautics and Space Administration, Langley Research Center, Virginia.

H. R. Moskowitz et al. (eds.), Sensation and Measurement. 275–283. *All Rights Reserved.*

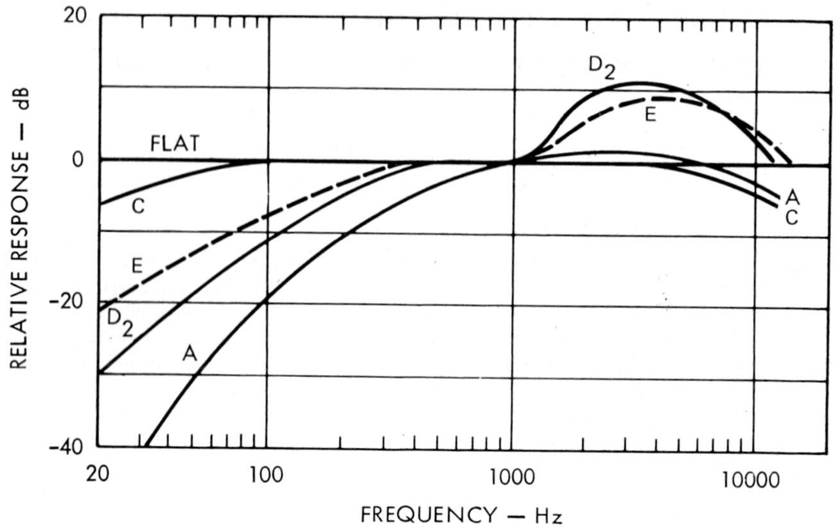

Fig. 1. Frequency weightings applied to overall sound level measurements (Flat, *A*, *C* from Anon, 1961; D_2 from Kryter, 1970; *E* from Stevens, 1972).

TABLE 1

Units of physical noise measurement

I dBA, dBD_2, dBC, and dBE are read from a sound level meter, with specified weightings (see Figuse 1) and meter action set on "slow."
PndB and PNdBM with and without pure-tone corrections (t_1 and t_2) are defined by Kryter (1970). PLdB is defined by Stevens (1972).

II PNL is the level for each of the above units, present in each successive half-second interval of a noise occurrence.
Max PNL is the maximum level reached on a sound level meter over all weighted frequencies or the maximum PNdB, PNdBM (t_1) (t_2) and PLdB level reached during successive half-second intervals of a noise occurrence.

III EPNL is taken as the integration on a $10 \log_{10}$ basis of the half-second PNL values present between the 10-dB downpoints from the half-second interval in which the max PNL occurred.

on magnetic tape. The tape recordings were re-recorded onto master tapes in which the levels and sequences were appropriately varied to provide the test material.

PAIRED-COMPARISON TEST

The aircraft and air-conditioner noises were paired with each of two standard noises on a test tape. The noises were recorded with a 4-s pause between pairs and about a 1-s pause within a pair. The subjects judged which in each pair they considered "the more unacceptable, bothersome or annoying, considering each noise in its entirety." The standard noise (the output of an electronic random noise generator shaped to have a low-frequency roll-off below 63 Hz of 3 dB oct^{-1} and a high-frequency

TABLE 2

Noises used in paired-comparison and magnitude-estimation tests

Noise		Nominal max level	Duration to 10-dB downpoints
Standard 1 (S1)		80 dBA	4 s
Standard 2 (S2)		73 dBA	9 s
Comparison noises		Presented in 5 steps, 4 dB apart	
"VSTOL" 1 (V1)[a]	737 Takeoff at ½ speed recording	72–88 dBA	8.7 s
"VSTOL" 2 (V2)[a]	737 Landing at ½ speed recording	70–86 dBA	6.0 s
"VSTOL" 3 (V3)[a]	737 Flyby at ½ speed recording	72–88 dBA	16.8 s
"VSTOL" 4 (V4)[a]	Vertol simulation recording	70–86 dBA	15.4 s
"VSTOL" 5 (V5)[a]	Vertol simulation recording	70–86 dBA	18.8 s
F1	737 Takeoff	72–88 dBA	5.2 s
F2[b]	737 Landing	70–86 dBA	3.4 s
F3	737 Flyby	72–88 dBA	16.9 s
F4	747 Takeoff	72–88 dBA	6.2 s
F5	747 Landing	70–86 dBA	7.2 s
F6	DC-8 Landing (nacelle treated)	72–88 dBA	9.6 s
F7	DC-8 Landing (nacelle untreated)	66–82 dBA	6.7 s
AC	Recording of room air conditioner	70–86 dBA	9.3 s

Note 1. S1 and S2 shaped at rate of 20 dB 0.5 s^{-1} below max level; at max level for 1.5 s.
Note 2. All noises "faded" at rate of 30 dB 0.5 s^{-1} when level reaches 15 dB below max dBA level.
[a] Recordings furnished by NASA Langley Research Center.
[b] The F2 noise had atypical "skirts" that caused difficulties in making certain physical measurements and was omitted for this reason from further data analysis.

roll-off above 500 Hz of 6 dB oct^{-1}) and the comparison noises were presented at the levels indicated in Table 2. The sequence of comparison noises and levels was random on the test tapes which contained a total of 240 pairs of noises.

The percentage of subjects who judged unacceptable each comparison noise at each of its levels was plotted against the sound pressure level of the comparison noise. The values for the two orders of presentation (when the comparison preceded and when it followed the standard noise in a pair) were averaged. An example of a paired-comparison test function for aircraft noise F1 is given in the upper graph of Figure 2.

Magnitude-estimation test

Each noise at each of the levels used in the paired-comparison test was re-recorded in a random order onto a master test tape with about 3 s between noises, and with 81 noises on a given tape. The first noise on each test tape was the standard noise S1 presented at a maximum level of 80 dBA. The subjects were instructed to ascribe the number 10 to the magnitude of relative unacceptableness of that first noise. They were then to judge each succeeding noise in relation to the standard, assigning each one an appropriate number, e.g. if the second sound appeared to be twice as noisy or un-

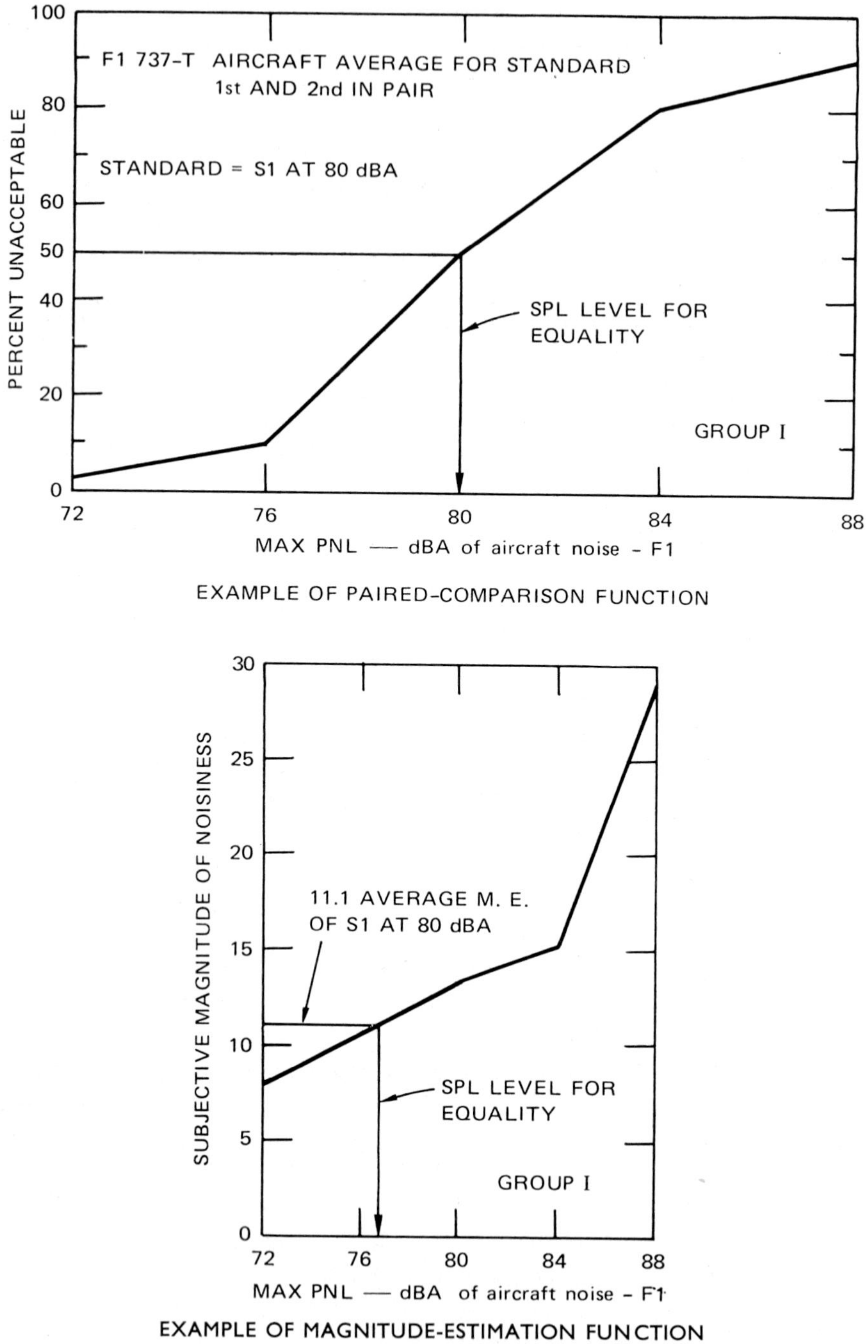

Fig. 2. Examples of graphs developed from the results of paired comparisons (upper) and magnitude estimations (lower).

acceptable it was to be called 20. (The standard noise was presented, without being identified in any way, an additional five times during the course of one test tape of 81 noises.)

The average of all subjects' judgments of a given noise was plotted against the level, as measured by a particular unit of physical noise measurement, at which the noise was presented. The average number assigned the standard, on its five unidentified presentations, was first noted. The graphs prepared for each of the other noises was then entered to determine the physical noise levels required to achieve the same numerical magnitude of subjective noisiness. An example of how the magnitude-estimation data were interpreted is given in the lower graph of Figure 2.

SUBJECTS

Three groups of 24 adult subjects each were selected. Group I was given the paired-comparison test first and the magnitude-estimation test about two weeks later. Group II received the magnitude-estimation test first and the paired-comparison test second about one week later. Group III received the paired-comparison test first and the magnitude-estimation test two days later.

Results

MAGNITUDE ESTIMATION

The results, in standard-deviation units, are shown in Table 3. These standard deviations are calculated by taking the square root of the average of the sum of the squared differences between: (*a*) the average level, as measured by a given physical unit, at which the noises were judged to have the same subjective magnitude; and (*b*) the level of each individual noise when judged to have the same magnitude. If

TABLE 3

Magnitude estimation

Standard deviations of differences between physical levels of the noises and the mean of the distribution of the levels that elicit an equal subjective magnitude of acceptability

	Group					Group			
Max PNL	I	II	III	Average	EPNL	I	II	III	Average
dBC	5.51	5.42	5.41	5.45	EdBC	5.73	6.00	5.60	5.78
dBA	2.21	2.02	2.20	2.14	EdBA	2.65	3.01	3.01	2.89
dBD_2	2.20	1.53	2.03	1.92	$EdBD_2$	1.89	2.09	2.26	2.08
dBE	2.71	2.11	2.39	2.40	EdBE	3.26	3.13	3.08	3.16
PLdB	2.45	1.73	2.15	2.11	EPLdB	2.68	2.69	2.68	2.68
PNdB	2.21	1.48	1187	1.85	EPNdB	2.47	2.48	2.39	2.45
PNdBM	2.22	1.40	2.08	1.90	EPNdBM	2.30	2.12	2.39	2.27
$PNdBM_{t1}$	2.81	2.26	2.49	2.52	$EPNdBM_{t1}$	1.80	1.72	1.86	1.79
$PNdBM_{t2}$	2.80	1.50	1.63	1.89	$EPNdBM_{t2}$	1.80	1.75	1.98	1.84
$PNdB_{t2}$	1.98	1.58	1.74	1.77	$EPNdB_{t2}$	1.85	2.00	1.75	1.87
Average	2.71	2.10	2.40	2.40	Average	2.64	2.70	2.70	2.68

TABLE 4

Paired-comparison test

Standard deviations of differences between the physical level of a standard noise and of comparison noises that are found to be subjectively equal in acceptability according to paired-comparison tests

Standard 2						Standard 2					
Group						Group					
Max PNL	I	II	III	Average	Aver. of S1 and S2	EPNL	I	II	III	Average	Aver. of S1 an dS2
dBC	5.29	7.32	7.31	6.64	6.13	EdBC	5.86	7.41	6.71	6.66	6.60
dBA	2.23	3.84	2.81	2.96	2.69	EdBA	2.73	3.60	2.78	3.04	3.14
dBD_2	1.68	3.25	1.99	2.31	1.98	$EdBD_2$	1.81	2.84	2.93	2.53	2.50
dBE	2.00	3.41	2.46	2.62	2.52	EdBE	2.95	3.85	2.59	3.46	3.47
PLdB	1.83	3.48	2.24	2.52	2.28	EPLdB	2.56	3.65	3.41	3.21	3.07
PNdB	1.83	3.58	2.04	2.48	2.12	EPNdB	2.23	3.49	2.79	2.84	2.81
PNdBM	1.62	3.37	2.00	2.33	2.03	EPNdBM	1.92	3.35	2.41	2.56	2.57
$PNdBM_{t1}$	2.68	3.11	2.73	2.84	2.43	$EPNdBM_{t1}$	2.05	2.83	2.02	2.30	2.19
$PNdBM_{t2}$	2.17	3.84	2.52	2.84	2.33	$EPNdBM_{t2}$	2.57	3.96	2.88	3.14	2.78
$PNdB_{t2}$	2.32	3.54	2.56	2.81	2.28	$EPNdB_{t2}$	2.99	2.80	3.03	2.94	2.80
Average	2.37	3.87	2.87	3.04	2.68	Average	2.77	3.78	3.26	3.27	3.19

there were perfect agreement between the physical unit of measurement and the subjective judgments, the physical levels would be identical and the distribution of differences from the average would be zero.

PAIRED-COMPARISON TEST

Table 4 gives the standard deviations of the distribution of differences between the level of standard S2 and the level of each of the comparison noises when judged equally unacceptable and when measured in terms of the various physical units. As with the magnitude-estimation tests, the Max PNL units exhibit average standard deviations or errors of prediction that are at least as small as those for EPNL. The last two columns of each section of Table 4 permits a comparison of the results with S2 and the average of the results with S1 and S2. The results with the 9-s standard noise S2 hardly differ from those with the 4-s standard S1; i.e. the results for S1 and S2 averaged are little different from the results for S2 only.

Table 4 indicates that the paired-comparison judgments made by Group II were generally more variable than those made by Groups I and III. Since the three groups performed about equally well in their magnitude estimations, it may be that the paired-comparison test is adversely influenced by previous experience with a magnitude-estimation test, but that the reverse is not true.

COMPARISON OF MAX PNL WITH EPNL

One of the surprising things revealed in both Tables 3 and 4 is that the Max PNL units of physical measurement predict so well the subjective judgments of noises that varied so much in duration–sounds lasting from 4 s to over 18 s. Some laboratory tests and some field tests with actual aircraft flyovers have demonstrated noises of longer duration are less acceptable than the same noises when of shorter duration (Kryter, 1973).

TABLE 5

Rank ordering of average standard deviations for combined magnitude-estimation and paired-comparison results and for the three groups of subjects combined

Max PNL			EPNL			Aver. PNL and EPNL		
Rank	Unit	Stand. Dev.	Rank	Unit	Stand. Dev.	Rank	Unit	Stand. Dev.
1	dBD_2	1.95	1	$PNdBM_{t1}$	1.99	1	dBD_2	2.12
2	PNdBM	1.97	2	dBD_2	2.29	2	$PNdB_{t2}$	2.19
3	PNdB	1.99	3	$PNdBM_{t2}$	2.31	3	PNdBM	2.20
4	$PNdB_{t2}$	2.03	4	$PNdB_{t2}$	2.34	4	$PNdBM_{t2}$	2.23
5	$PNdBM_{t2}$	2.14	5	PNdBM	2.42	5	$PNdBM_{t1}$	2.24
6	PLdB	2.20	6	PNdB	2.63	6	PNdB	2.31
7	dBA	2.42	7	PLdB	2.88	7	PLdB	2.54
8	dBE	2.46	8	dBA	3.07	8	dBA	2.71
9	$PNdBM_{t1}$	2.48	9	dBE	3.32	9	dBE	2.89
10	dBC	5.79	10	dBC	6.60	10	dBC	5.99

We have no explanation of why the Max PNL and EPNL units predicted the present results in such a similar fashion. Perhaps in spite of the instructions to judge a noise in its entirety the subjects placed heavier weight upon the "peak" levels of the noises as being, under the laboratory circumstances, the most obvious aspect of the various noises that could readily and reliably be comparatively judged and subjectively quantified.

RANK ORDER OF PHYSICAL UNITS

Table 5 is a summary of how well, in terms of the standard deviation, the various physical units of measurement predicted the results of the subjective tests. These deviations range from near 2 dB for the best units to over 6 dB for the worst units.

The results in Table 5 are in substantial agreement with previous experiments; the D_2 overall frequency weighting and the PNdBM third-octave band means of frequency weighting give, in general, better predictions of the subjective judgments than do the other units of physical measurement. Also, the tone corrections, t_1 and t_2, improve the predictions but, as usual in such complex experiments, only slightly (Kryter, 1973).

MAGNITUDE SCALE OF PERCEIVED NOISINESS

A special feature of magnitude estimation is that a ratio scale of the subjective quantity (noisiness or unacceptability) is obtained from the numerical values ascribed to the

TABLE 6

Ratios between the magnitude estimates given to different levels of same noise

	dB Diff. between two levels of same noise		
	8 dB	10 dB	16 dB
Group I	1.85	2.4	4.1
Group II	1.78	1.79	3.01
Group III	1.80	2.12	3.27
Average	1.81	2.10	3.46

noises by the subjects. It has typically been found that when judging non-impulsive noises, at least in the mid-to-high range of intensities, a 10-dB increase in the sound pressure level of the noise doubles its subjective loudness or noisiness. Table 6 shows that the same rule applies to the present results.

Conclusions

It is concluded that:

1. The standard deviations with which the various units of physical noise measurement predicted the subjective judgments of perceived noisiness or unwantedness were

approximately the same for both the methods of magnitude estimation and paired comparison.

2. As appeared in an earlier study (Clarke & Kryter, 1972), the paired-comparison procedure (which required the presentation of some 240 pairs of noises to the listeners) is about one-sixth as efficient as the method of magnitude estimation (which required the presentation of but 81 noises) in the determination of the point of subjective equality. In addition, the magnitude estimates provided a scale factor, over the intensity range tested, of perceived noisiness.

3. The results suggest that subjects faced with judging noises that vary in several physical-temporal aspects tend to choose the maximum level reached by each noise as the primary basis for making their judgments.

4. Frequency weightings D_2 and PNdBM were consistently better by a small but practically significant amount (about 3.5 dB over a range of ± 3 standard deviations) than the overall frequency weightings of A and E and the one-third octave band procedure of PLdB.

5. The scale of perceived noisiness as determined by magnitude estimation was consistent with that typically found for both loudness and perceived noisiness, namely, a doubling of perceived magnitude followed each increase of 10 dB in intensity.

References

Anonymous. *American standard specification for general purpose sound level meters.* ASAS1.4-1961, New York: American National Standards Institute, 1961.

Clarke, F., & Kryter, K. D. *The methods of paired comparisons and magnitude estimation in judging the noisiness of aircraft.* NASA CR-2107. Washington, D.C.: National Aeronautics and Space Administration, 1972.

Kryter, K. D. *The effects of noise on man.* New York: Academic Press, 1970.

Kryter, K. D. A note on the quantity (effective) perceived noisiness and units of perceived noise level. *Journal of Sound and Vibration*, 1973, **25**, 383–393.

Stevens, S. S. Perceived level of noise by Mark VIII and decibels (E). *Journal of the Acoustical Society of America*, 1972, **51**, 573–601.

VOICE SPECTRUM AND SIDETONE SPECTRUM

HARLAN LANE

Institut d'Etudes Linguistiques et Phonétiques, Université de Paris III

and

A. P. VAN TESLAAR

New York University in France

When a speaker hears his own voice fed back to him with altered intensity or timing, he adjusts the properties of his speech to compensate for the apparent distortion of his message. These adjustments appear to be designed to provide the listener with intelligible messages rather than to provide the speaker with some acoustic feedback required for elaborating speech. When it comes to a third type of sidetone distortion, changes in spectral properties or timbre, much is claimed but little is known. On the one hand, the speaker might modify the source spectrum or the vocal tract transfer function so as to compensate for changes in the apparent timbre of his voice, pre-emphasizing high frequencies under low-pass sidetone filtering, and conversely. On the other hand, reductions in regions of the sidetone spectrum have been claimed to yield corresponding reductions in the voice spectrum. In fact the present experiment found no appreciable changes in the long-term spectra of sentences read by four speakers under seven conditions of sidetone filtering, once fluctuations in sidetone level were controlled. The speakers proved to be more intelligible, however, when they heard their voices filtered while speaking than when they did not.

When a speaker hears his own voice fed back to him with altered intensity or timing, he adjusts the properties of his speech to compensate for these distortions. The substantial experimental literature on voice changes induced by sidetone distortion is reviewed by Lane and Tranel (1971), who conclude that such changes are designed to provide the listener with intelligible messages rather than to provide the speaker with some acoustic feedback required for elaborating speech. Reductions in sidetone level, or increases in ambient noise level, cause systematic increases in voice level that are half as large in decibel units (Lane, Tranel, & Sisson, 1970). This is just what would be predicted on the hypothesis that the speaker matches perceived decreases in signal level, or increases in noise level, so as to preserve the signal-to-noise ratio and hence his intelligibility. Figure 1 shows the changes in voice level of a group of subjects who were instructed to match noise levels, to communicate in noise, and to communicate with altered sidetone. The three tasks are functionally the same and all of them validate the pair of underlying sensory scales which tell us that loudness grows about half as fast as autophonic level.

With regard to temporal distortion, increased sidetone delay leads systematically to a slower rate of speaking (Huggins, 1968), among other voice modifications (Chase, Sutton, & First 1959).

With regard to spectral distortion of sidetone, much is claimed but little is known. On the one hand, the speaker might modify the source spectrum or the vocal tract transfer function so as to compensate for changes in the apparent timbre of his voice,

H. R. Moskowitz et al. (eds.), Sensation and Measurement. 285–294. *All Rights Reserved.*

pre-emphasizing high frequencies when the sidetone is low-pass filtered and pre-emphasizing low frequencies when the sidetone is high-pass filtered. On the other hand, a reduction in some region of the sidetone spectrum might yield a corresponding reduction in the voice spectrum as Tomatis (1956, 1960) contends. Of

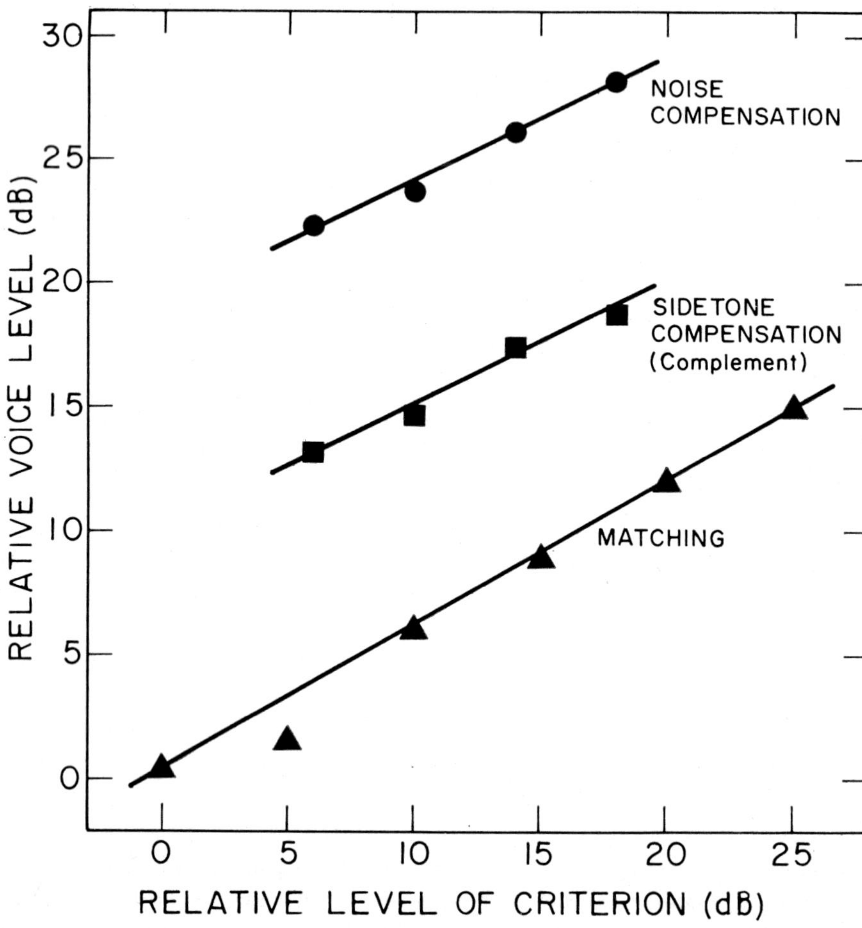

Fig. 1. Effect on voice level of (1) changes in the level of a sound that speakers were instructed to match, (2) changes in sidetone amplification during communication over an interphone, and (3) changes in noise level during communication over an interphone. (From Lane & Tranel, 1971)

course, the voice spectrum might show no significant effect of changes in sidetone spectrum.

We have found only a single study of changes in voice spectrum under distortion of sidetone spectrum. Zachman (1966) had 20 speakers utter the vowel [u] with normal and filtered sidetone, and found that filtering led indiscriminately to increases in the frequencies of formants one and two. However, Zachman did not report sidetone and voice levels whereas the results summarized above suggest that filtering sidetone with the attendant reduction in its level, would have increased voice level. Greater voice level is accompanied, in turn, by a shift toward higher frequencies, both in the energy distribution of the source spectrum (Fant, 1959) and in the resonant properties of the vocal tract. For the vowel [u], Sundberg (1971) found that a 10-dB increase in the level of the sung vowel ($F_0 = 130$ Hz) led F1 to increase from 287 to 300 Hz and F2 from 650 to 686 Hz.

The purpose of the present study, then, was to examine the effects on voice spectrum of changes in sidetone spectrum while controlling for indirect effects due to changes in voice level. Accordingly, before reading the sentences whose long-term spectra were measured, our speakers always increased the level of the filtered sidetone so as to restore its original loudness.

Method

Subjects. Three female and one male student at the University of Paris, with no known history of speech or hearing disorders, were employed individually in sessions lasting approximately one hour. Under each of seven sidetone filtering conditions, *S* read two test sentences twice, then a phonetically balanced list of 27 French monosyllables, and finally the two test sentences again, twice each. The sentences were chosen to differ substantially in their long-term spectra; they were: (A) "Cécile solicite la Sicile" and (B) "Les murmures monotones des moutons."

Apparatus. The *S* was seated in an audiometric room and instructed to remain about one foot from a dynamic microphone (Beyer M-260). Her speech was recorded on one channel of a tape recorder (Revox A-77) which supplied two variable bandpass filters (Krohn-Hite 310-C) arranged in cascade (nominal attenuation 48 dB oct^{-1}). The filtered signal was returned to the other channel of the tape recorder. The *S* could monitor either her normal or filtered sidetone with a headset (Hosiden DH-03-S) connected through a variable attenuator and switching network (Grason-Stadler audiometer 162) to the outputs of the tape recorder outside the room. The cutoff frequencies for filtering were chosen to fall approximately midway (log scale) between the center frequencies of adjacent octave bands in the spectral measurements. The low-frequency cutoffs were 350, 700, 1400, and 2800 Hz; the high-frequency cutoffs, 700 and 1400 Hz. The seventh condition was wideband: 60 to 20000 Hz.

Sidetone matching. In matching the loudness of the filtered to the normal sidetone, prior to the experiment proper, *S* was encouraged to talk spontaneously while switching back and forth between the two ouputs of the tape recorder, each time adjusting the level of the filtered sidetone with the variable attenuator, so as to zero in on the loudness of the unfiltered sidetone. When *S* was satisfied with the loudness match, *E* noted the decibel gain or drop *S* had introduced, and then adjusted the filters to provide the next condition of sidetone filtering. A different, arbitrary order of conditions was used for each *S*. When *E* exposed *S* again to the filtered sidetone conditions during the experiment, he reintroduced the corresponding decibel gains, so as to hold sidetone loudness and hence *S*'s voice level approximately constant.

Spectral measurement. The final reading of each of the sentences under each filtering condition was selected for spectral measurement. (A preliminary check with the data from one *S* revealed no discernible change in the long-term spectrum from the first to the fourth reading.) The recorded sentence was played repeatedly through a frequency analyser tuned successively to each of the eight octave bands from 125 to 16000 Hz (Bruel & Kjaer 2107 and 1612). The frequency analyser supplied a graphic level recorder (B & K 2305; writing speed 500 mm s^{-1}), which provided for each sentence a recording of its instantaneous log rms level in each octave band. To average the level of the sentence in each band over its entire duration, the graphic records were traced with a planimeter and the average level read directly to an accuracy of 0.25 dB. The average level per cycle was calculated for each octave band and expressed relative to that of the entire spectrum (computed from the sum of the band levels).

Results

The average sidetone gains introduced by the *S*s (top, Figure 2) offset the substantial sidetone losses due to filtering (bottom), leaving voice level relatively constant over the seven filtering conditions (center) for both sentences A and B. The median fluctuation in voice level was 1 dB, and all fluctuations greater than 3 dB were due to one of the two sentences produced by a single speaker. Fant (1959) found that a 10-dB increase in voice level was associated with a 3-dB per octave high-frequency emphasis in the output spectra of vowels. For at least seven of the eight speaker-sentences in the present experiment, then, we can consider that such slight fluctuations in level as did occur would have negligible effects on the slope of the speech spectra.

Average spectra for three female speakers reading with wideband sidetone are shown in Figure 3. Although the slope of the spectral envelope is generally not very sensitive to the choice of text, by using short passages with selected vowels and consonants it was possible to vary the slope in order to detect differential effects of sidetone filtering, if any. The high-frequency emphasis of sentence A (top) compared to B (bottom) is largely due to its many fricative segments and high front vowels. For comparison, the average spectrum reported by Dunn & White (1940; five female speakers reading for 2.5 min) has been replotted in the coordinates of Figure 3 (middle) alongside the combined average spectrum of our sentences A and B. Long-term average spectra reported by several other investigators fit quite well with these (Benson & Hirsh, 1953; Blomberg & Elenius, 1971; Fant, 1959; French & Steinberg, 1947).

The effect of sidetone filtering on the speech spectrum – or, rather, the absence of any such effect – is apparent from Figure 4, which shows the spectra obtained in each of the seven filtering conditions from a representative speaker (sentence A).

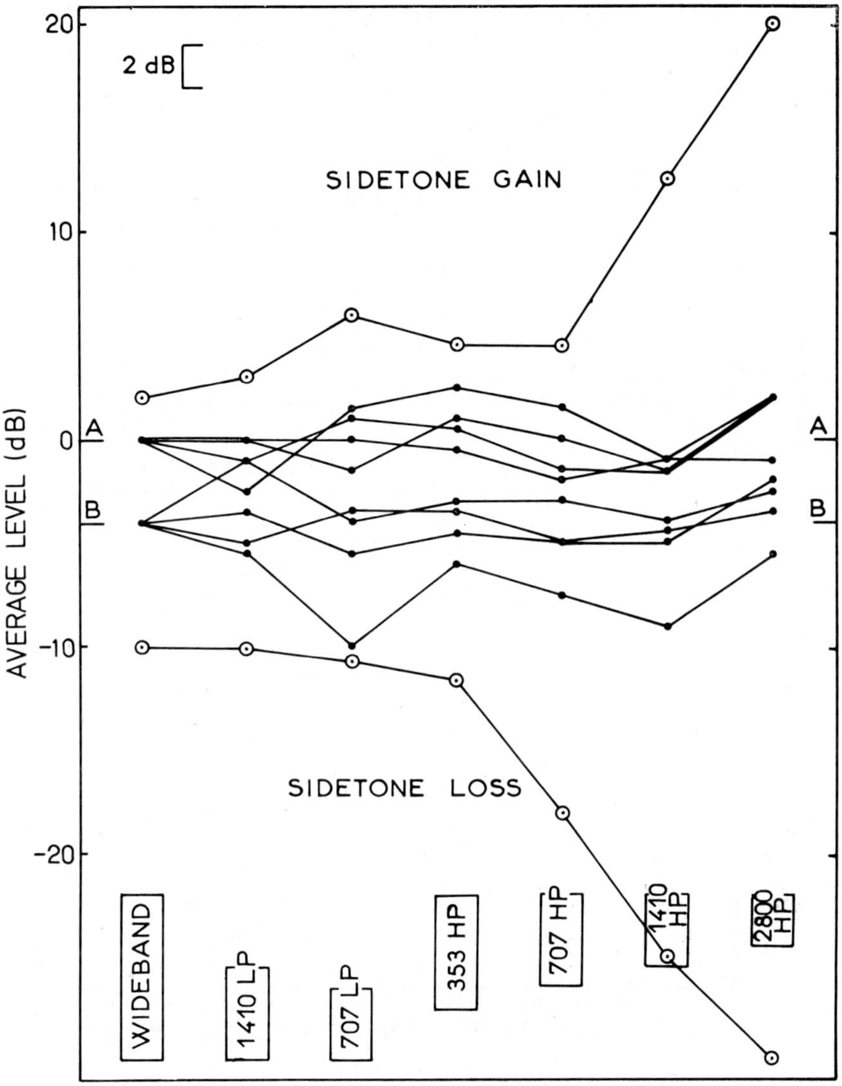

Fig. 2. When speakers compensate for sidetone losses due to filtering by introducing sidetone gain, their voice levels remain approximately constant. Each value of sidetone gain is the mean of four determinations. Voice levels shown for each speaker in each filtering condition are expressed in decibels relative to the level in the wideband condition (sentences A and B). Sidetone losses in each of the six filtering conditions were calculated from data reported by Dunn & White (1940).

The seven spectra are almost perfectly congruent. Such slight fluctuations as may be discerned seem unrelated to the filtering condition.

In order to examine the relation between speech spectrum and sidetone spectrum for all eight speaker-sentences, Figure 5 gives the slopes of the corresponding spectral envelopes, obtained under each of the seven sidetone filtering conditions. (The slopes

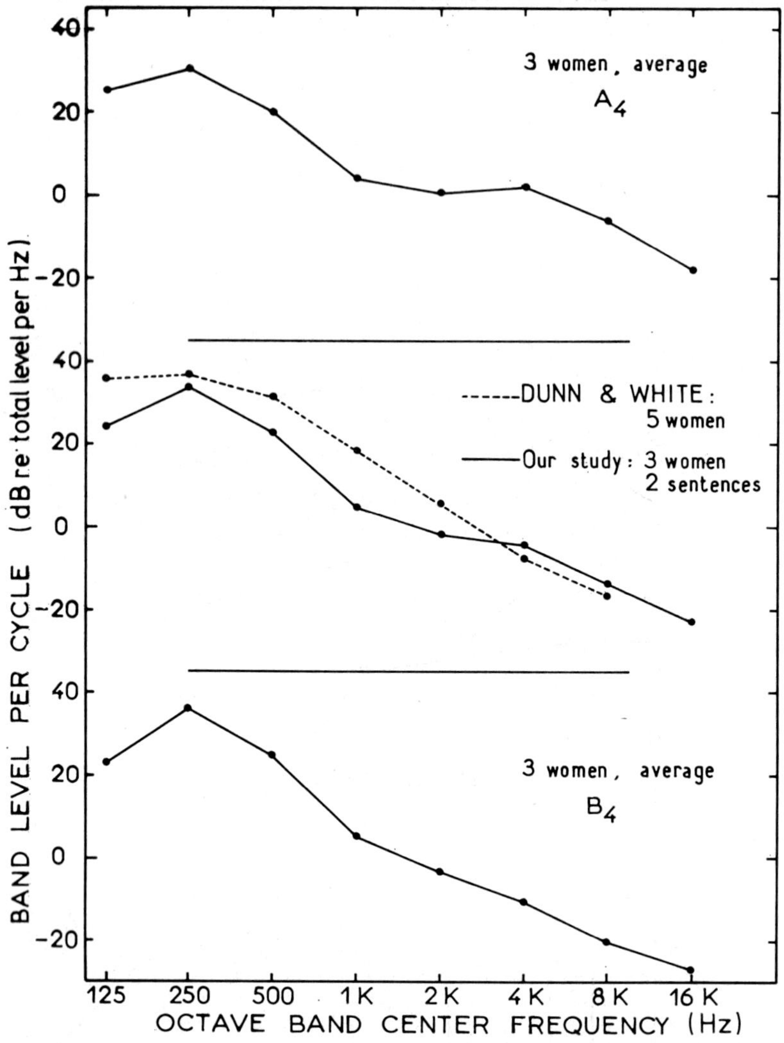

Fig. 3. Average voice spectra of three female speakers are shown for test sentences A and B (wide-band sidetone). The combined spectrum is then compared with that reported by Dunn and White for five women reading English passages.

were fit by the method of least squares to the band levels between 250 and 8000 or 16000 Hz.) It is evident that the eight utterances show little and nonsystematic variation in spectral slope over the sidetone conditions. The largest fluctuation in slope is less than 2 dB per octave. Both the compensation and matching hypotheses of sidetone filtering effects fail to find support in these data. Spectral slopes do not flatten under low-pass sidetone filtering and do not steepen under high-pass filtering. Nor is the converse true. A test for differences among regression slopes (Quenouille, 1966) showed the variations among the slopes to be nonsignificant in each of the eight cases.

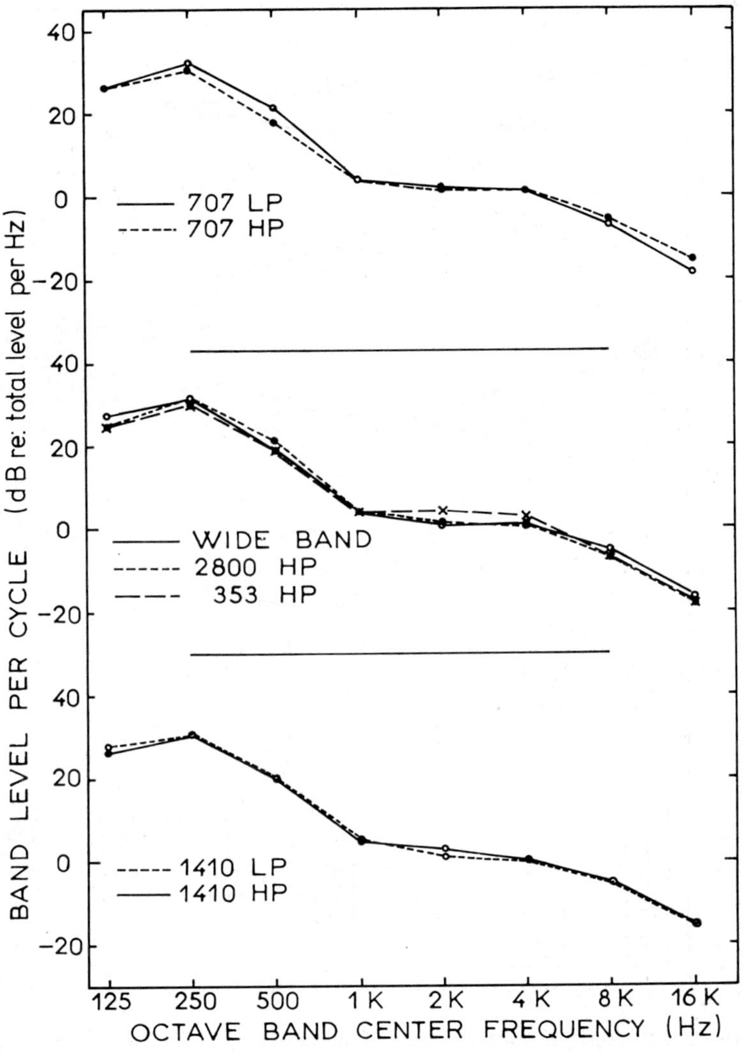

Fig. 4. Voice spectra of a typical female speaker under seven conditions of sidetone filtering (sentence A).

The weakest indication of a systematic effect of sidetone filtering on voice spectrum, which places no requirement on the size or direction of the effect, would be to find significant agreement among the speakers in the rank ordering of their spectral slopes across the seven sidetone conditions. The Kendall Coefficient of Concordance (Siegel, 1956) was small and nonsignificant for both sentences ($W_A = 0.17$; $W_B = 0.15$), showing that the variations in slope over the seven sidetone conditions were unrelated from one speaker to the next. There are, however, wide differences in slope associated with the nature of the sentence, as discussed earlier, and, secondarily, with the speaker.

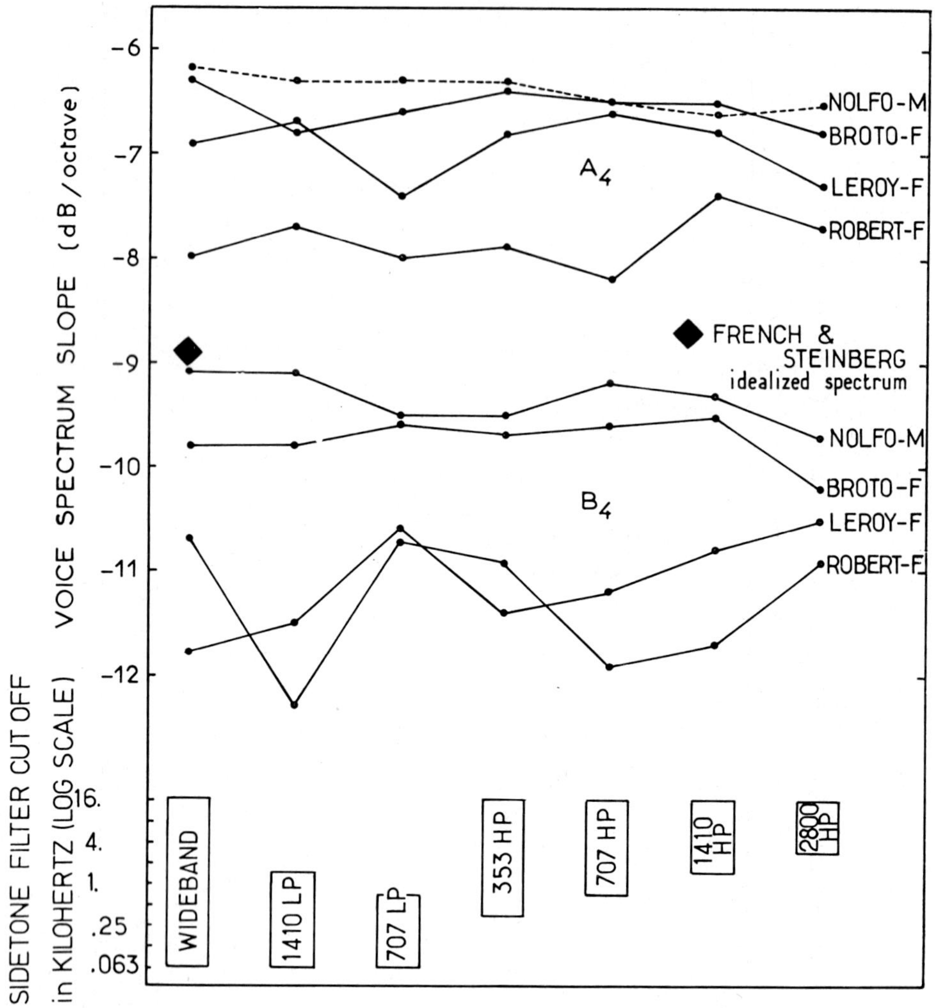

Fig. 5. Least-squares slopes of voice spectra of four speakers reading two sentences under seven conditions of sidetone filtering.

The male *S* in this sample had flatter spectral slopes than the females. The general picture that emerges from Figure 5 is that each speaker has a characteristic spectral slope which varies substantially and predictably as a function of the construction of the short sentences but insignificantly as a function of the sidetone filtering while the sentences were read.

Discussion

Etienne Lombard (1911) was probably the first to study systematically the effects of sidetone distortion on voice. He exposed his patients to noise in various ways while they were speaking, and attributed the observed increases in voice level to an ear-voice reflex. Further research showing that perturbations in sidetone level and timing perturb speech (Fletcher, Raff, & Parmley 1918; Lee, 1950) led to the widely-accepted but largely false servomechanism model (Fairbanks, 1954), according to which speaking is regulated at its every moment by its auditory feedback. In this tradition, Tomatis (1960) claimed that sidetone spectrum as well as level and timing regulates speaking and, more stringently, that "the voice of a subject contains only those harmonics that he can hear" (p. 197). Accordingly, he constructed an "appareil à effet Tomatis" – an electronic circuit for filtering sidetone – whose use has been claimed to speed foreign-language learning (Vettier, 1960) and speech therapy (Le Gall, 1961). The present study finds, on the contrary, no systematic effect of sidetone spectrum on voice spectrum, once voice level is held constant. It is simply untrue that "there is a precise and complete correspondance between the frequencies ... of sounds heard and emitted" (Le Gall, 1961, p. 22).

If we suppose that the speaker compensates for distorted listening conditions not to hear himself better but in order to be heard better, then diverse experimental findings fall into line for the first time. Among the most striking findings are that a speaker raises his level as much to match a noise as he does to communicate in one, and that reducing the premium on effective communication correspondingly reduces the change in voice level. This "intelligibility hypothesis" (Lane & Tranel, 1971) would likewise predict that if a speaker's message is filtered to the point of reducing his intelligibility, he will introduce compensatory changes. Peters (1955) found in fact that 600-Hz low-pass filtering of sidetone leads speakers to read word lists more intelligibly. He recorded the lists in both normal and filtered sidetone conditions, and then played them to listeners in ambient noise intense enough to reduce the intelligibility of the control lists to an average of 60%; the lists recorded under filtered sidetone were significantly more intelligible by 5%. To see if similar results would be obtained with other values of sidetone filtering and speakers of a different language, we asked four French college students to transcribe the seven recorded word-lists of one of our female speakers while we adjusted the ambient noise level to yield an average intelligibility of 60%. We then played the lists recorded by a different female speaker and by the male speaker. The 2 speakers, 6 filtering conditions, and 4 listeners permitted 48 comparisons, in 36 of which the speaker proved to be more intelligible when he had spoken with filtered sidetone. (In three cases, there was no difference.) The average increase in intelligibility was 6.4% for the female speaker (Mann-Whitney, $U=19.5$, $p=0.03$) and 10.3% for the male speaker ($U=25$, $p=0.07$). Since this enhanced intelligibility apparently cannot be traced to changes in the average long-term spectrum or the level of the utterance, it is probably due to small changes at the segmental level which vary with the particular vowel or consonant articulated.

References

Benson, R. W. & Hirsh, I. J. Some variables in audio spectrometry. *Journal of the Acoustical Society of America*, 1953, **25**, 499–505.

Blomberg, M. & Elenius, K. Statistical analysis of speech signals. Unpublished report QPSR 4/1970, Speech Trans. Lab., Stockholm, 1971, pp. 1–8.

Chase, R. A., Sutton S., & First, D. Bibliography: Delayed auditory feedback. *Journal of Speech and Hearing Research*, 1959, **2**, 193–200.

Dunn, H. K. & White, S. D. Statistical measurements on conversational speech. *Journal of the Acoustical Society of America*, 1940, **11**, 278–288.

Fairbanks, G. A. Systematic research in experimental phonetics. I: A theory of the speech mechanism as a servosystem. *Journal of Speech and Hearing Disorders*, 1954, **19**, 133–139.

Fant, C. G. M. Acoustic analysis and synthesis of speech with applications to Swedish. *Ericsson Technics*, 1959, **1**, 1–108.

Fletcher, H., Raff, G. M., & Parmley, F. Study of the effects of different amounts of sidetone in the telephone set. Western Electric Company, Report 19412, Case 120622. Murray Hill, New Jersey, 1918.

French, N. R. & Steinberg, J. C. Factors governing the intelligibility of speech sounds. *Journal of the Acoustical Society of America*, 1947, **19**, 90–119.

Huggins, A. W. F. Delayed auditory feedback and the temporal properties of the speech material. *Zeitschrift für Phonetik*, 1968, **21**, 53–60.

Lane, H. & Tranel, B. The Lombard sign and the role of hearing in speech. *Journal of Speech and Hearing Research*, 1971, **14**, 677–709.

Lane, H. L., Tranel, B., & Sisson, C. Regulation of voice communication by sensory dynamics. *Journal of the Acoustical Society of America*, 1970, **47**, 618–624.

Lee, B. S. Effects of delayed speech feedback, *Journal of the Acoustical Society of America*, 1950, **22**, 824–826.

Le Gall, A. *Le redressement de certaines déficiences psychologiques et psycho-pédagogiques par l'appareil à effet Tomatis*. Paris: Centre du Langage, 1961.

Lombard, E. Le signe de l'élévation de la voix. *Annales des Maladies de l'Oreille et du Larynx*, 1911, **37**, 101–119.

Peters, R. W. The effect of filtering of sidetone on intelligibility. *Journal of Speech and Hearing Disorders*, 1955, **20**, 371–375.

Quenouille, M. *Introductory statistics*. New York: Pergamon, 1966.

Siegel, S. *Nonparametric statistics for the behavioral sciences*. New York: McGraw Hill, 1956.

Sundberg, J. The level of the "singing formant" and the source spectra of professional bass singers. Unpublished report QPSR 4/1970, Speech Trans. Lab., Stockholm, 1971, pp. 21–39.

Tomatis, A. Relations entre l'audition et la phonation. *Annales de Télécommication* 1956, **2**, 3–8.

Tomatis, A. Conditionnement audio-vocal. *Bulletin de l'Academie Nationale de Médecine*, **144**, 197–200.

Vettier, R. *l'Appareil électronique à effet Tomatis et l'etude des langues*. Paris: Ste. Aurel, 1960.

Zachman, T. A. The effects of bandpassed filtered sidetone upon vocal production of the vowel [u]. *Journal of Auditory Research*, 1966, **6**, 441–443.

THE SLOPE OF THE LOUDNESS FUNCTION: A PUZZLE[1,2]

WILLIAM J. McGILL
Columbia University

Abstract This paper deals with the slope of the loudness function considered as a sensory parameter. Shapes of individual loudness functions are examined in a measurement situation in which loudness is estimated by marking a point on a line. It is shown that such personalized loudness functions can be converted to power functions by computing zero points differing widely from listener to listener. The slopes of the computed loudness functions also differ markedly.

It is then shown that the slopes and zero points are closely related. All are simple transformations of a single loudness function with a slope of 0.30. The transformation is that of an elastic scale with a fixed unit system stretched between the righthand margin (maximum loudness) and the estimated zero point. This interpretation seems to be consistent with a single (sensory) loudness function reported through an elastic transformation (judgmental anchoring) reflecting the range of loudnesses the listener expects to hear.

The author begins by arguing with Stevens's conclusions on the slope of the loudness function, ends by conceding reluctantly that Stevens was correct, and rediscovers the anchoring phenomenon along the way.

In a series of papers Stevens (cf. 1956) has shown that loudness can be measured by instructing *S* to make numerical responses. The responses are then plotted against sound intensities to form a relation that is known as the loudness function.

Whatever else they are, the responses are *not* numbers. They are responses. Stevens' procedure capitalizes on our lifetime of commerce with quantification and estimation. It assumes that a normal subject can use his skill in estimation in order to evaluate an internal event quantitatively. Consequently, when the measurement is free of bias, the numbers are thought to represent loudnesses more or less accurately.

But perhaps normal subjects seldom respond to the intensity of sound in all the ways that numbers suggest. The responses may look or sound numerical, and they can often be plotted, but some sort of demonstration is demanded if we are to believe that they also have quantitative significance. On the other hand, even an obstinate critic would agree that magnitude estimations of loudness behave a bit like numbers. The thing that is not clear is how much real quantification is achieved. Conceivably magnitude estimations also involve processes allied to learning, set, and concept formation. There seems to be good evidence (Garner, 1954a; Garner, 1954b) that the latter distort the numbering system but we do not know what form these distortions take and how serious they are in ordinary loudness measurements.

The substance of this paper is that it attempts to show that certain loudness

[1] Reprinted from Messick, S. & Gulliksen, H. (Eds.), *Psychological scaling*, New York: Wiley, 1960. Abstract to this article added by the author.

[2] This research was supported by The United States Air Force under Contract No. AF 41(657)-126, monitored by Aero Medical Laboratory, Directorate of Research, Wright Air Development Center, Wright-Patterson Air Force Base, Ohio.

The assistance of J. Howett and G. Yonemura in carrying out this study is gratefully acknowledged.

H. R. Moskowitz et al. (eds.), Sensation and Measurement. 295–307.

functions are "personal equations." They reveal a good deal about the process of estimation in the individual but not very much about loudness, at least in their raw form. However, with some effort they can be brought into correspondence with Stevens' loudness function, and hence made to reveal something of the process of distortion.

Apparatus and Method

The loudness functions were obtained with 1000-Hz tones at various sound pressure levels. The tones were generated by a Hewlett-Packard 200AB oscillator and controlled in intensity by two 110 dB attenuators calibrated in 1 dB steps. Stimuli were presented to the subject via a Grason-Stadler electronic switch and interval timer that turned tones on and off in the regular sequences described below. Listening was binaural. The earphones used were Telephonics type TDH-39 dynamic receivers. Sound pressure levels were determined in a 6 cm^3 standard coupler.

Subjects estimated loudness by making a pencil mark on a line six inches long. The line was an absolute rating scale whose left-hand end symbolized "the weakest tone you could possibly hear," while the right-hand end was supposed to be the "loudest tone you could possibly hear." Each tone was rated on a separate line and prior ratings were covered from sight. The lines were numbered in sequence from 1 to 100 on successive sheets of paper. The tone was picked off as it was turned on by the electronic switch, amplified and then rectified so as to actuate two automatic counters. The *S* used one counter to keep his place on the rating sheet, while *E* used the other to program the attenuator. Loudness ratings are reported as the distance (in 1/64ths of an inch) from the left-hand end of the line to the pencil mark. Two rating methods were used.

Method 1. Stimuli were chosen in 10 dB steps from 30 dB to 100 dB. The *E* ran through the eight tones in the series in ascending order while *S* listened. During this preview the tones were 1.5 s in duration and spaced 2 s apart. Then *E* presented the same eight intensities in random order now spaced 6 s apart and *S* rated each one. The entire procedure was repeated 10 times.

Method 2. Sixty stimuli were chosen in 1 dB steps from 41 dB to 100 dB sound pressure level. The sequence was presented five times, each time in a different random order. No previews of any kind were given. All tones were 1.5 s in duration spaced 6 s apart.

Reproducibility of the Loudness Function

Loudness functions obtained from different individuals using Method 1 (described in the previous section) are clearly different, although this is not surprising since the judgments themselves are variable. The basic question is whether the differences between individuals are simply reflections of the "noise level" of the loudness judgments, or whether they are reproducible parametric differences.

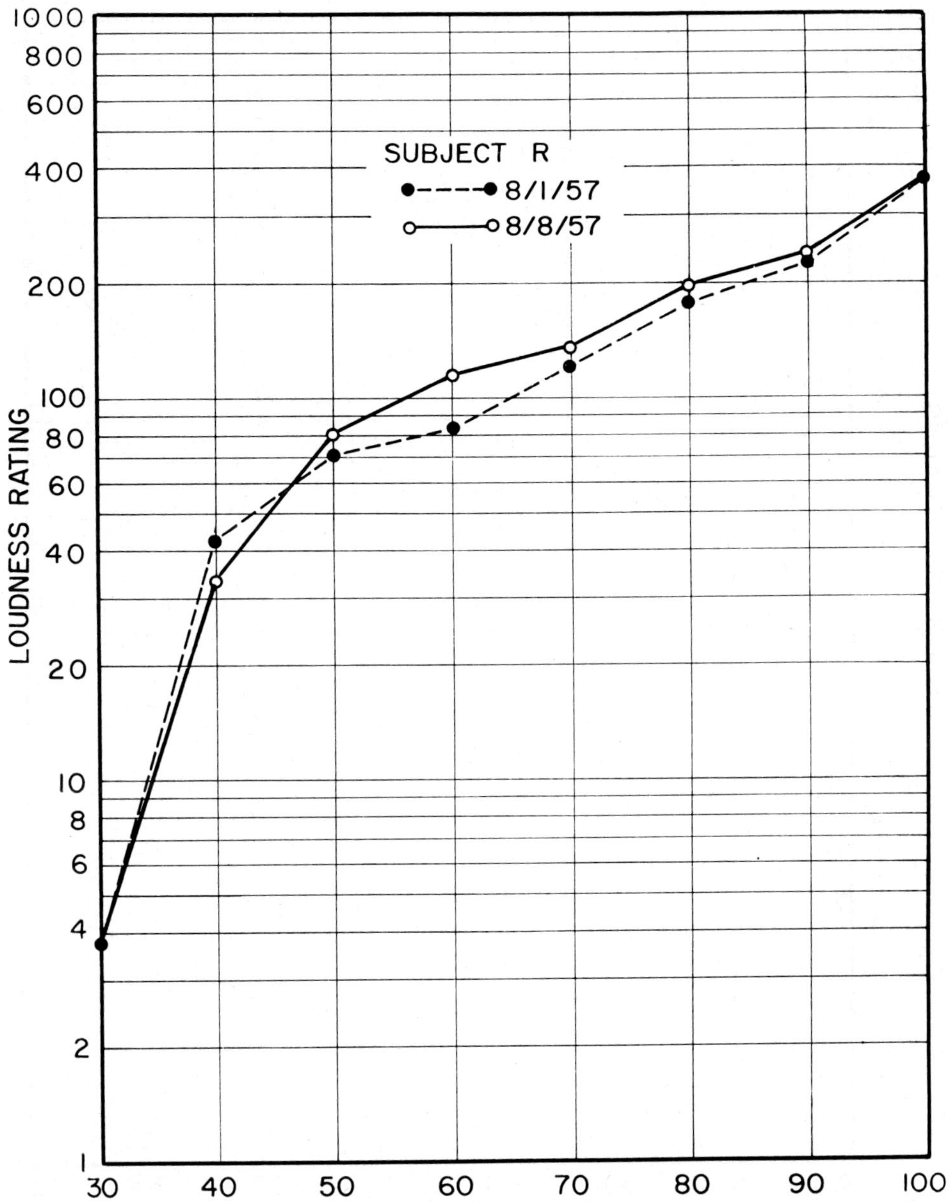

Fig. 1. Individual loudness functions redetermined after an interval of approximately one week (Subject R).

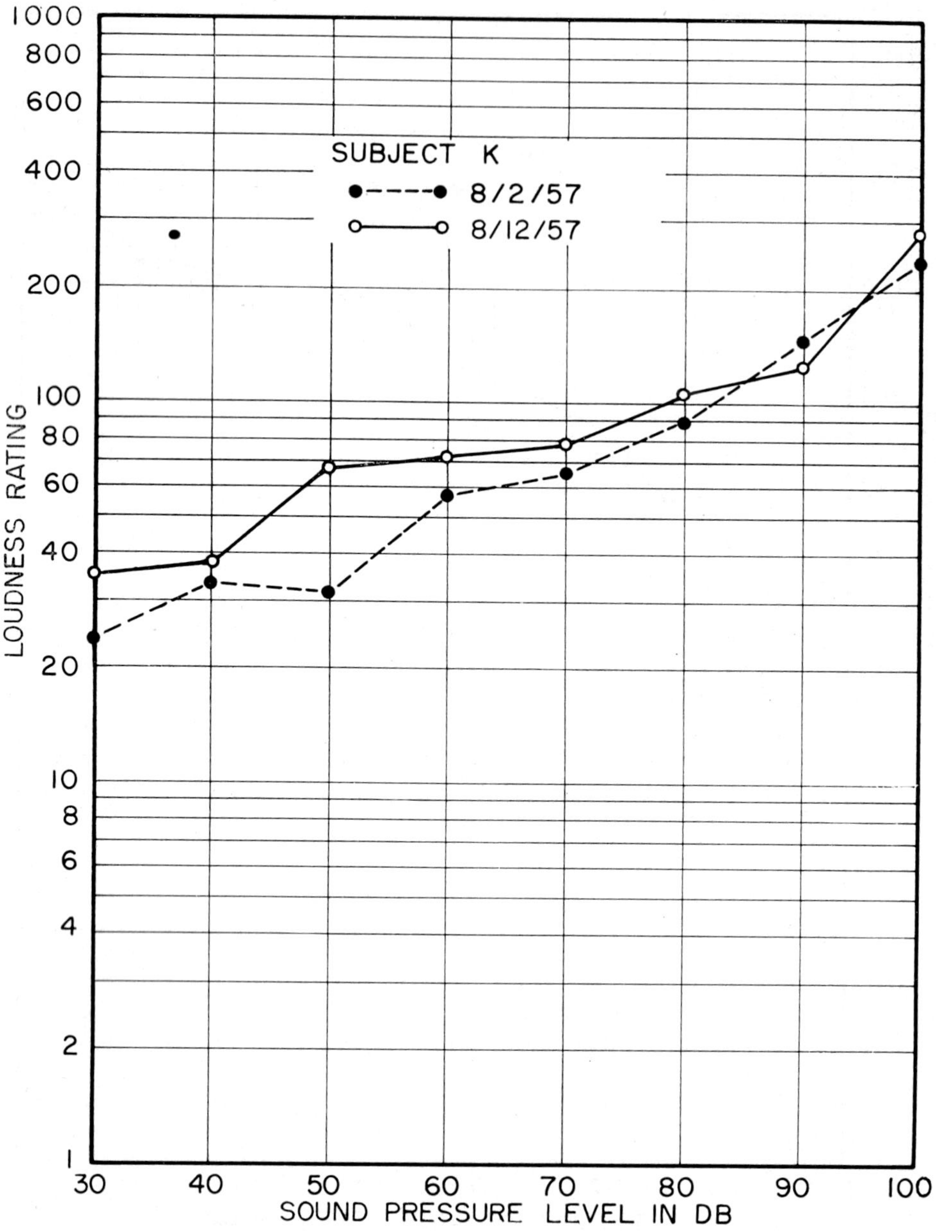

Fig. 2. Individual loudness functions redetermined after an interval of approximately one week (Subject K).

Figures 1 and 2 illustrate our findings on this point. They show two individual loudness functions and redeterminations of the same functions after an interval of approximately one week. The points on each curve are averages of 10 ratings at each intensity. The reproducibility of these loudness functions seven days or so after the original determination is hardly perfect, but it is not discouraging either. On the other hand, the individual loudness functions seem to be quite different, at least in the intensity range from 30 to 60 dB. Accordingly we can infer that the principal differences between subjects are not random but reflect stable parameters.

The two loudness functions illustrated are taken from 12 cases in which we have tried this sort of reproduction. The complete data follow the pattern just described. The functions are highly stylized but reproducible. The differences are most evident at low intensities. They are a little bit like a signature or a thumbprint in helping us to identify the subject.

Statistical Properties of Loudness Ratings

It is by no means surprising to find stable differences between subjects in situations where they make estimates of magnitude. Free judgments are notoriously mobile. Garner (1954a) has shown that it is easy to condition such differences systematically. When subjects show us the phenomenon spontaneously, it suggests that they have been differentially conditioned before we ever get them into earphones. But even though we can suggest how the differences between the loudness functions might occur, we are still unable to explain or to eliminate them. Averaging over subjects simply exacerbates the problem because the individual loudness functions do not exhibit similar curvature. Hence an analysis of the conditions producing the individual differences is practically mandatory before we can decide which loudness function to pick as typical. Specifically we are after an additional insight that will help us to convert all individual functions to the same general form.

With this in mind we undertook a more detailed study of loudness ratings using Method 2 in which all 1 dB steps from 41 to 100 dB are given in random order. The intervals between tones were silent and no stimuli other than those to be judged were ever presented. Ten subjects were run through this procedure with the outcome shown in Figure 3. Intensities are grouped together in 5 dB intervals. Consequently each data point in Figure 3 is an average taken over 25 judgments of intensities spread uniformly through the interval. The disagreements are again most prominent at low intensities. This effect is certainly related to the log transform on the loudness axis, and might lead us to look for some other manipulation, if it were not for the pattern of variability associated with the loudness estimates.

Figure 4 shows one of the 10 loudness functions plotted on an arithmetic loudness coordinate. Boundary regions covering one standard deviation above and below the average rating are also indicated by the dashed-line envelope around the curve. The judgmental variability evidently depends on intensity, increasing as intensity increases. Estimation is most reliable at low intensities and most erratic at high in-

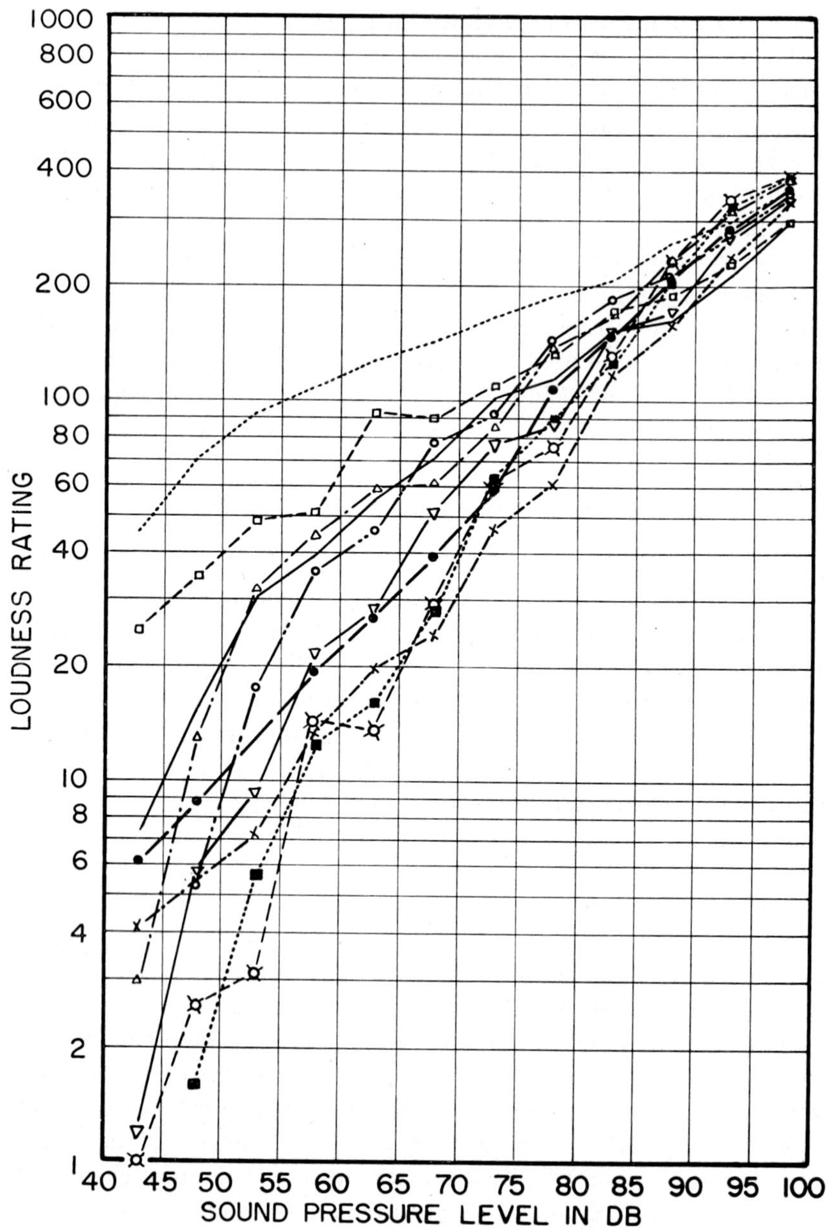

Fig. 3. Absolute ratings of the loudness of brief 1000-Hz tones obtained from 10 different individuals under constant conditions.

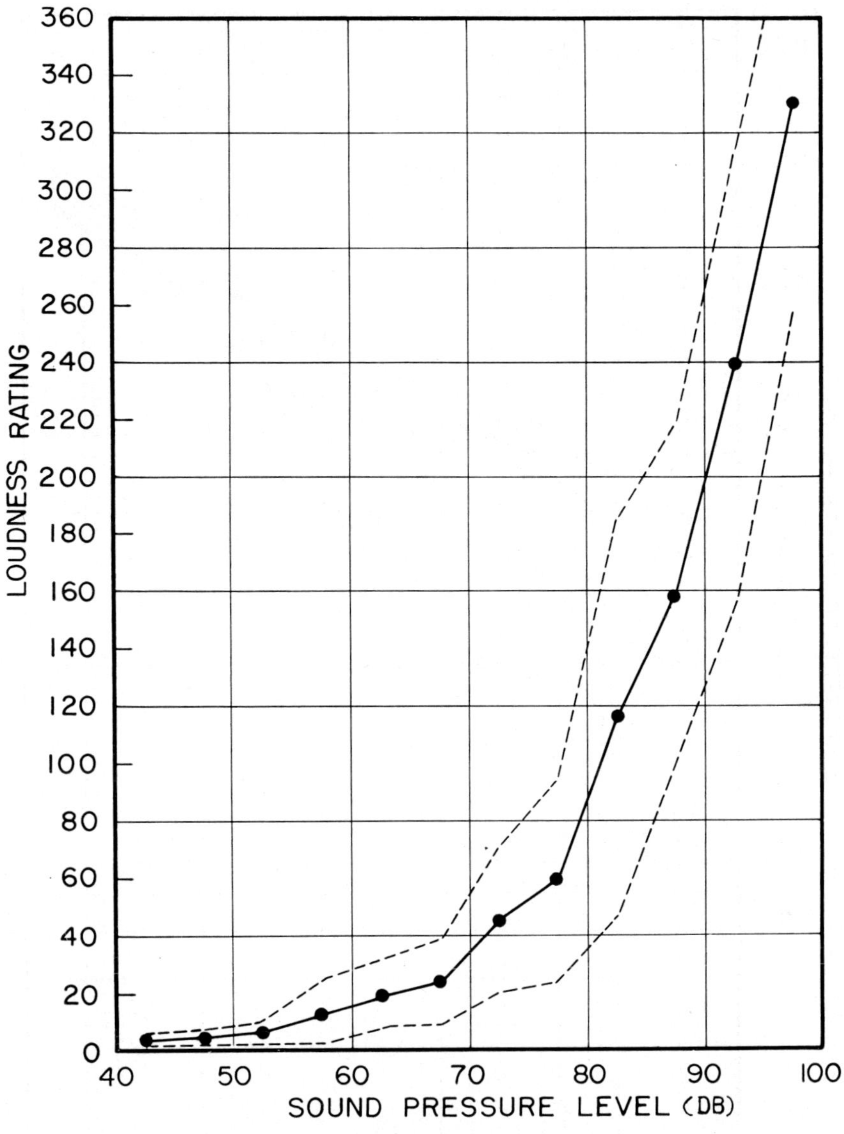

Fig. 4. One of the loudness functions shown in Figure 3, replotted on an arithmetic loudness scale. The dotted envelope is the region enclosing plus or minus one standard deviation around the mean rating.

tensities. This relation is observed for all 10 loudness functions with the single qualification that as the loudness function becomes flatter, the relation between intensity and variability is weaker. Hence it seems that variability of loudness ratings is related to loudness rather than to intensity.

The foregoing seems to indicate that log loudness will show uniform variability. The transformation, however, is not quite adequate in most cases. On log loudness

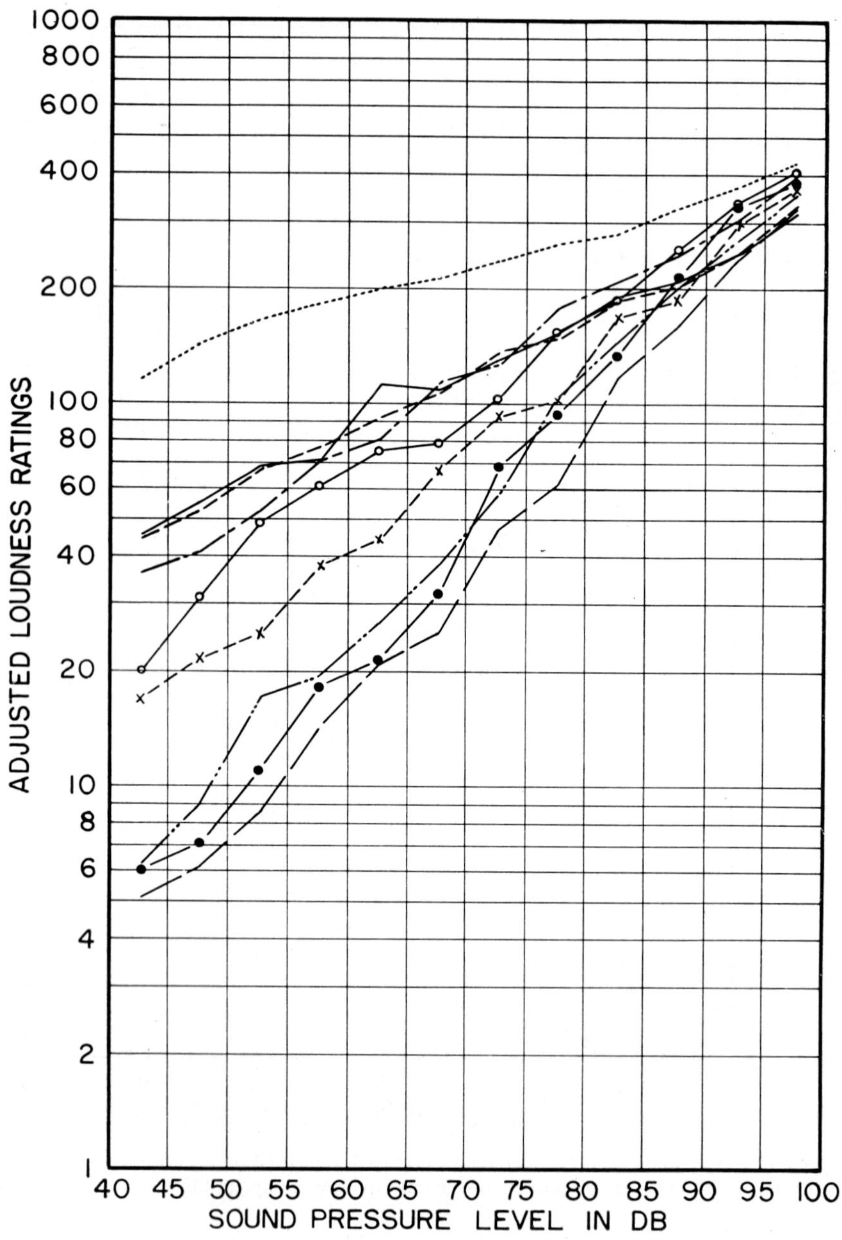

Fig. 5. Individual loudness functions adjusted for differences in zero point. A constant is added to all ratings of each individual in order to approximate linearity.

coordinates the scatter of the judgments at the low intensities seems to expand; just the reverse of the condition seen on the arithmetic plot. The few cases that are made linear by the log transform have uniform variability in log loudness.

These observations taken together suggest that whatever produces linearity on the log-log plot of the individual functions also produces uniform variability. It happens that both conditions can be corrected simultaneously by adding a constant to the ratings given by an individual with a curved loudness function, i.e., by treating the loudness functions as interval scales.

Hence our method of loudness estimation seems to have produced interval judgments. The loudness functions, compensated for differences in "zero point," are given in Figure 5, and the individual curves are now seen to be linear. The computed constants represent the displacement of each S's reference point to the left of our reference point. The adjustments are designed to produce linearity if the loudness functions are power functions. Our method is crude but it leads to a unique adjustment for each S, and the constant does straighten out the individual loudness functions. The idea is that a power function will produce equal loudness ratios corresponding to equal decibel differences. For example,

$$\frac{L_{43} + L_0}{L_{68} + L_0} = \frac{L_{73} + L_0}{L_{98} + L_0},$$

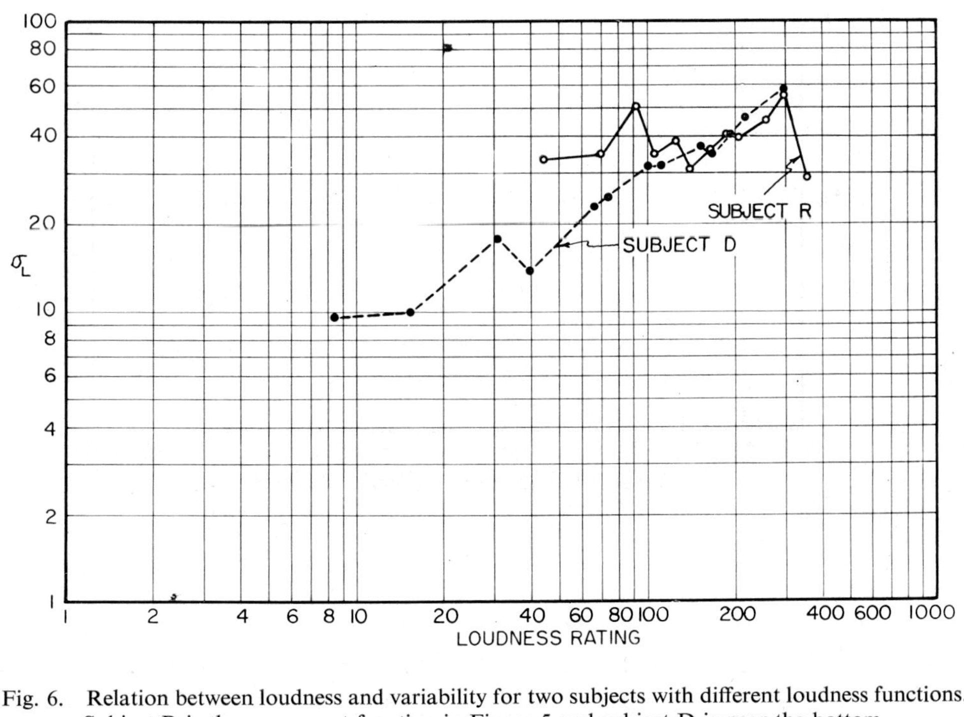

Fig. 6. Relation between loudness and variability for two subjects with different loudness functions. Subject R is the uppermost function in Figure 5 and subject D is near the bottom.

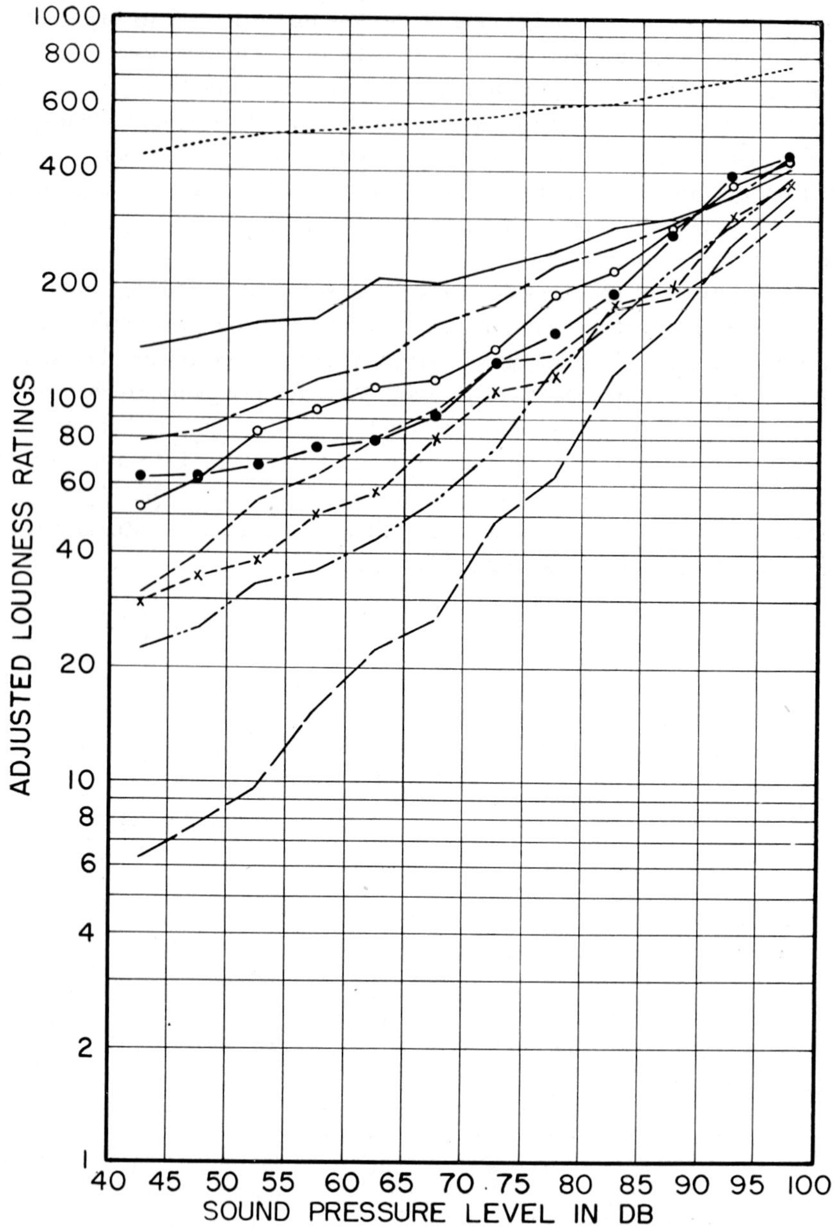

Fig. 7. Individual loudness functions adjusted for differences in zero point. A constant is added to all ratings in order to approximate uniform variability.

where L_0 is the displacement of the reference point, L_{43} is the loudness rating corresponding to 43 dB and the other terms are defined analogously. The constant is estimated from

$$L_0 = \frac{L_{68}L_{78} - L_{43}L_{98}}{L_{43} + L_{93} - L_{68} - L_{73}}.$$

This quantity is computed for each S and added to the ratings shown in Figure 3 in order to produce the adjusted ratings plotted in Figure 5.

Alternatively, a variation of Thurstone's criterion (Thurstone, 1928) may be used to find the individual reference points. Thurstone defined the zero point as the scale value for which variability disappears. His procedure requires a relation between loudness and variability similar to that observed in the present experiment and illustrated in Figure 6 for two Ss with very different loudness functions. To find the reference point, a linear equation is set up between L and σ_L. Then σ_L is made arbitrarily small and the equation is solved for the corresponding value of L. By experimentation we have found that a value of $\sigma_L = 6$ produces constants similar to those computed from the linearity criterion (Figure 5). The loudness functions adjusted by Thurstone's criterion are shown in Figure 7. Incidentally, Thurstone's criterion applied literally leads to a reversal in the curvature of the loudness function, i.e., it "over-corrects." The approximate correspondence of the two criteria is the basis for our statement that the adjustments required for linearity and for uniform variability are essentially the same.

Slopes and Anchors

In outline the previous section suggests that our individual loudness functions are interval judgments and can be converted into power functions by estimating a zero point. However, the slopes of these adjusted functions are different and this is a puzzle. It is hard to believe that the sensory process changes so radically from person to person. Apparently something else is involved. This "something" seems to transform the sensory process, and the transformation affects both the slope of the function and the location of the reference point. In Figure 8 the nature of the transformation is shown more clearly. The estimated displacement of the "zero point" is plotted as a function of the slope of the resulting loudness function. The constants in Figure 8 are derived from the Thurstone criterion but this is not critical. The linearity criterion produces a similar relation. In any case the function in Figure 8 strongly indicates that the transformation of the loudness function involves an evaluative mechanism that has similar properties for all subjects. It behaves like a ruler that can be stretched. As it stretches, the units spread out. The sensory event is held up against this ruler and read off in terms of its rubbery units. Our data indicate that most Ss agree on where to put the right-hand edge of the ruler but they disagree about its length.

The rubber-scale phenomenon was first described by Rogers (1941) and McGarvey (1943), who showed that it is produced by an anchoring stimulus. McGarvey de-

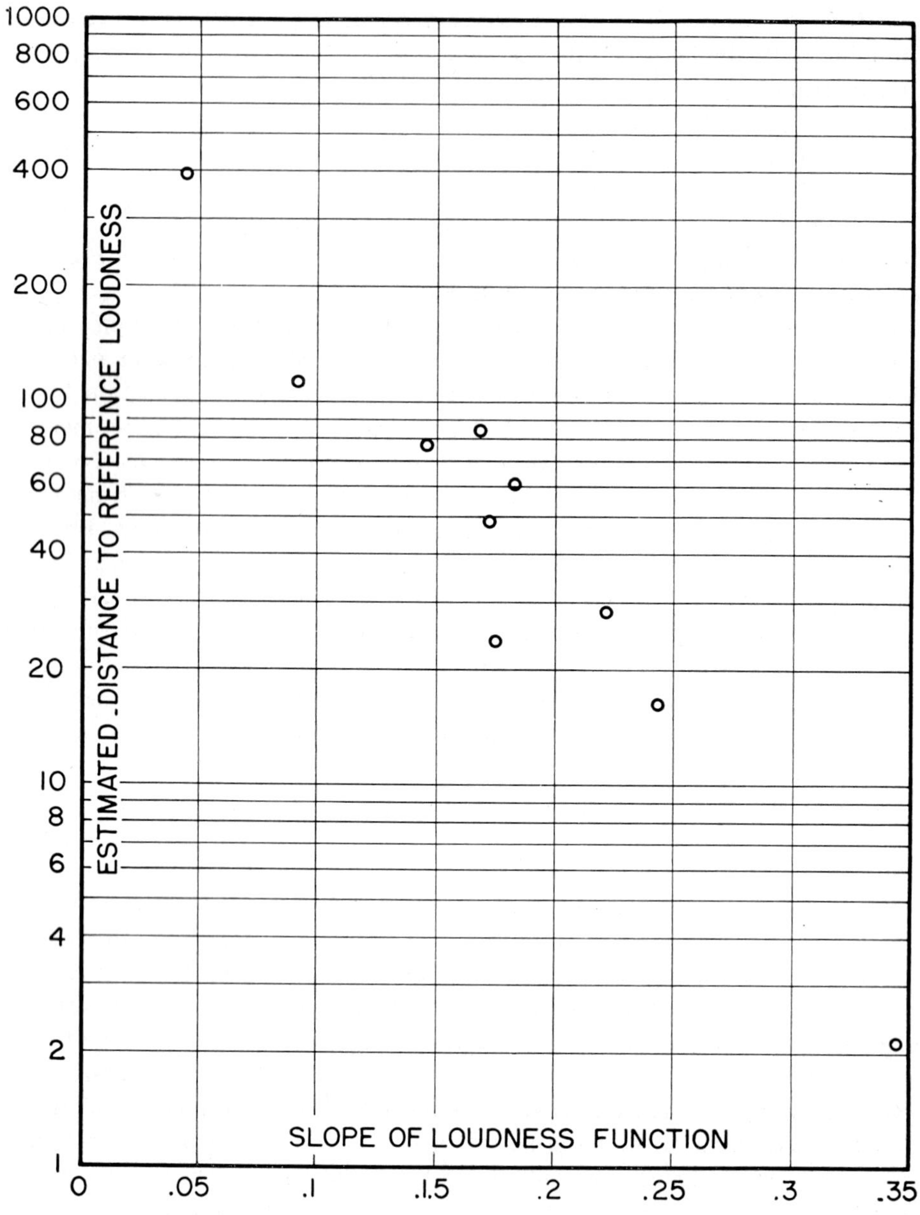

Fig. 8. Empirical relation between two parameters of individual loudness functions. The estimated distance to the reference (zero) point is plotted against the slope of the resulting loudness function (variability criterion). Each point represents one individual.

monstrated that the subjective evaluation scale stretches to accommodate the anchoring stimulus and that the scale units spread out as the scale expands.

There is no explicit analogue of the anchoring stimulus in the present experiment, unless it is the silent interval. But the data seem to indicate that the differential conditioning we find may be due to differential anchoring.

Stevens (1955; 1956; Stevens & Galanter, 1957) has reviewed a large body of evidence and has added a good deal more of his own work to show that the loudness function follows a cube root law. According to Stevens, the slope of the function is 0.30 on the log-log coordinates. This loudness function emerges as an asymptote of the present experiment. When *S*'s reference point corresponds with the reference point used for evaluating his ratings, the slope of his loudness function is found to be approximately 0.30, as Stevens maintains.

References

Garner, W. R. Context effects and the validity of loudness scales. *Journal of Experimental Psychology*, 1954, **48**, 218–224. (a)

Garner, W. R. A technique and a scale for loudness measurement. *Journal of the Acoustical Society of America*, 1954, **26**, 73–88. (b)

McGarvey, H. Anchoring effects in the absolute judgment of verbal materials. *Archives of Psychology* 1943, Vol. 39 (86, Whole No. 281). (Abstract)

Rogers, S. The anchoring of absolute judgments. *Archives of Psychology*, 1941, Vol. 37 (42, Whole No. 261).

Stevens, S. S. The measurement of loudness. *Journal of the Acoustical Society of America,* 1955 **27**, 815–829.

Stevens, S. S. The direct estimation of sensory magnitudes: Loudness. *American Journal of Psychology*, 1956, **69**, 1–25.

Stevens, S. S., & Galanter, E. H. Ratio scales and category scales for a dozen perceptual continua. *Journal of Experimental Psychology*, 1957, **54**, 377–411.

Thurstone, L. L. The absolute zero in intelligence measurement. *Psychological Review*, 1928, **35**, 175–197.

LOCALIZATION OF UNLIKE TONES FROM TWO LOUDSPEAKERS[1]

BERTRAM SCHARF

Northeastern University, Boston

Abstract. Listeners judged the location of a pair of tones presented separately from two loudspeakers in an anechoic room. Both speakers were 3 m from the listener's head, one 45° to the left and the other 45° to the right. When the tones in the two speakers were at the same frequency, a single fused sound was heard coming from the side of the speaker that was energized between 2 and 60 msec sooner than the other speaker. Known as the *precedence* or *Haas* effect, the dominance of the leading tone was also observed when the two tones differed in frequency. As the frequency difference widened, however, the effect weakened, but was still measurable for tones differing by 1900 Hz. At all frequency separations, the effect was clearest when the lower-frequency tone was turned on first.

Although Smitty Stevens coined the term, anechoic room, he didn't have such a room available in the 1930s when he wanted to measure the localization of pure tones. So he and Ed Newman set up a tall swivel-chair on the roof of one of Harvard's buildings in order to find out how well a listener can localize pure tones in space. Out in the open, there were no walls and ceilings to reflect sounds and complicate the sound field. The tones were presented from a single loudspeaker located on a circular frame, with the listener in the center. From those measurements came Stevens' & Newman's (1936) classic paper on auditory localization which showed, among other things, that we are a good deal poorer in localizing tones around 3000 Hz than at lower and higher frequencies.

Stevens doesn't seem to have returned to the problem of auditory localization until much later as advisor for Mills' thesis on the minimum audible angle, a project carried out in the anechoic room next to Smitty's office in Memorial Hall (Mills, 1958). Meanwhile, Newman joined with Wallach & Rosenzweig (1949) to show that a click, music, or speech presented from two separated speakers is heard to come from only the speaker which is energized first, provided the onset time difference is not less than 1 msec nor more than 50 msec. They called this dominance of the leading sound source the *precedence* effect. In Europe it is better known as the *Haas* effect, after the German engineer who published useful data on the optimal time and intensity differences that yielded the best-sounding speech coming from two separated loudspeakers (Haas, 1951). All the published measurements of the precedence effect have been on complex sounds like speech and clicks, and the literature implies that the effect doesn't work well for pure tones. Defying that warning, I went ahead and measured the precedence

[1] I wish to thank Professor J. Jauhiainen and Dr E. Lampio for making available the anechoic room and the necessary equipment at the Acoustics Laboratory of the Helsinki University of Technology. I also thank J. Toivanen and M. Pulakka for their assistance, and J. C. Armington, B. Gottschalk, A. W. Mills, and E. B. Newman for criticisms of an earlier draft of this manuscript. Supported by PHS grant 5 R01 NS 07270-04.

H. R. Moskowitz et al. (eds.), Sensation and Measurement. 309–314.

effect not only with pure tones but with pure tones at a different frequency in each loudspeaker.

Method

Measurements were made in a 4 m by 4 m anechoic room. Two double-cone loudspeakers were placed 3 m from the listener's head, one 45° to the left and the other 45° to the right of the median plane. Each loudspeaker was energized from a separate tone generator through a one-third-octave bandpass filter. (The rise/fall time varied from 1 to 2 msec, depending on frequency.) Tones were set equally loud and presented for 500 msec (and in some series for 6 msec) approximately every two seconds until the subject had marked the position or positions of the sound or sounds relative to his head on polar coordinates. The onset time difference, ΔT, between the two speakers was measured on an oscilloscope from the half-power points, and was varied from 0 to 500 msec; in half the trials the left speaker came on first.

The first series of measurements was made with the same frequency in both loudspeakers. Frequency was set at 500, 2000, or 5000 Hz. In the second and more extensive series, the frequency separation, ΔF, between the tone in the left speaker and the tone in the right speaker was varied from 0 to 4200 Hz around a geometric center frequency of 2000 Hz. In half the sessions, the lower frequency was in the left speaker, and in the other half in the right speaker. In both the single-frequency and double-frequency series, tones were presented at loudness levels of approximately 45, 65, and 85 phons. Three men, including the author, and one woman served as *O*s. The *O* sat in one corner of the room with his head on a chin rest.

No attempt was made to blindfold the *O* or screen the loudspeakers because preliminary trials showed that the visual clues had almost no effect on the judgments. For example, *O*s often reported the sound was in back of them although they knew that only the walls of the room were there.

Results and Discussion

Figure 1 shows that the precedence effect holds quite nicely for two separated loudspeakers energized by 500-msec sinusoids. When the left speaker was turned on first (negative values on the abscissa) a single tone was heard as coming from the left, and when the right speaker was turned on first the tone was heard from the right. Each point is based on at least six judgments for which the *O* reported a single sound locus; split judgments are excluded. (At ΔTs longer than 60 msec, the tones were always split.) Judgments were scored left or right when they were more than 15° to the left or right of the median plane, whether in front or back of the listener. Percentages on the abscissa of Figure 1 often do not sum to 100 because center judgments are not included. Only the data for 45 and 65 phons are shown; the 85-phon data were similar to those at 65 phons.

Generally, localization was better (i.e. was toward the leading speaker) at 65 and 85 phons than at 45 phons, and was better for 6-msec tones than for the 500-msec

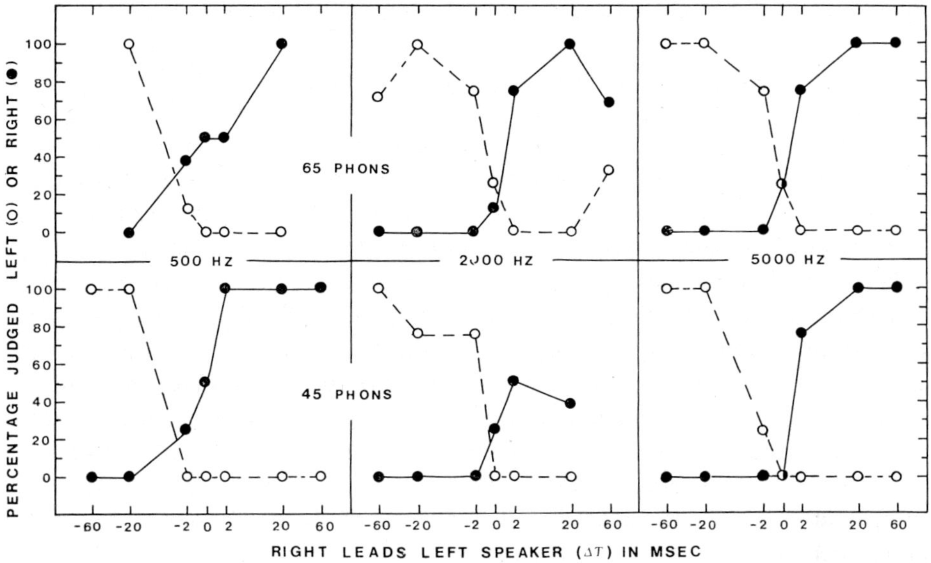

Fig. 1. Localization of a pair of tones, presented at the same frequency from two separated loudspeakers, as a function of onset time difference. (The tones were presented at three different frequencies and two loudness levels.)

tones shown in the figure. Although the sound usually seemed to come from the same side as the leading loudspeaker, the 500-Hz and 2000-Hz tones were heard in back 40% of the time, the 5000-Hz tones almost never. Stevens & Newman (1936) reported a very similar distribution of front-back confusions for pure tones from a single speaker. Their *O*s made front-back errors nearly 40% of the time for tones at 500 and 2000 Hz, and less than 20% of the time for tones at 5000 Hz.

When the same frequency went to both speakers, a single fused sound was heard until the temporal separation became greater than 20 to 60 msec. When a different frequency went to each speaker, then a single sound was heard only at small frequency and time separations. Nevertheless, although two distinct pitches could be heard the auditory image often appeared to be in a single place. For the purpose of the present analysis, sounds are classified as fused so long as they shared a common locus, whether or not they had a single pitch. (Tones must be much closer in frequency to yield a single pitch than to yield a single position. See Thurlow & Bernstein, 1957.)

At a ΔT of 0 msec, listeners usually heard the two simultaneous tones as a single sound located in front of them between the two speakers or at a corresponding position in back. A single image was reported ninety percent of the time even when the two tones differed as much as 900 Hz (one tone, 1600 Hz, the other, 2500 Hz). When ΔT was larger than 0 msec, the tones split up at narrower ΔFs; how much narrower depended on loudness level. At 45 phons, fused images were still reported more than seventy percent of the time when ΔF was 600 Hz and ΔT was about 40 msec; at 65 phons, seventy-percent fusion persisted until ΔF reached 400 Hz and ΔT reached about 30 msec; at 85 phons, fusion persisted until ΔF was again 400 Hz but ΔT could not exceed 20 msec.

Fused judgments were combined and scored left, center (within 15° of the median plane), or right. A striking dominance was noted for the fused sound to be judged toward the side from which the lower-frequency tone originated. Overall, sounds were judged nearly twice as often toward the low-frequency side than toward the high-frequency side. This ratio was larger at the wider ΔFs than at the narrower ΔFs. Since the low-frequency tone was just as often in the left speaker as in the right speaker, this low-frequency bias is not tied to a position bias. In fact, right and left seemed to be treated equally, as also suggested in Figure 1. Given this low-frequency bias, it seemed appropriate to score the judgments according to whether the sound was localized toward the low-frequency side or toward the high-frequency side.

Figure 2 plots the percentage of fused sounds that were judged either toward the low-frequency side (unfilled circles) or toward the high-frequency side (filled circles) as a function of ΔT. These data were collected at 65 phons with 500-msec tones. The time separation is the difference between the onsets of the low-frequency tone and the high-frequency tone, regardless of whether the leading tone was in the left or right speaker. A negative value means the high-frequency tone was turned on first. The percentage of judgments to the center is not shown, but can be calculated at a given ΔT by subtracting the sum of the percentages of judgments toward one side or the other. Although each stimulus combination was judged sixteen times (eight with the low frequency in the left speaker and eight with the low frequency in the right) by the four *O*s, not all combinations were fused so that many of the data points in Figure 2 are based on fewer than sixteen judgments, but never on fewer than six. Owing to the small numbers involved and variability among the four *O*s, only general trends in these data are noteworthy.

The precedence effect is demonstrated in Figure 2 when the filled circles (sound locus judged toward the high-frequency side) are associated with high percentages at *negative* ΔTs (which means the high-frequency speaker was turned on first), and the unfilled circles are associated with high percentages at *positive* ΔTs. At the two narrower ΔFs of 160 Hz and 400 Hz, the precedence effect comes through clearly, and the sound is localized toward the leading side. The low-frequency bias is shown by the higher percentages for the unfilled than for the filled circles, which means that *O*s localized more often toward the low-frequency than toward the high-frequency side. The same bias is seen at the two wider ΔFs, and the precedence effect is still evident but weak. The reason for the low-frequency bias is not clear. A strong low-frequency dominance in the lateralization of sounds presented through earphones has also been reported (Scharf, 1972; Yost, Wightman, & Green, 1971).

Similar but less extensive results were obtained with tones lasting 6 msec instead of 500 msec. The major difference was that at the shorter duration, fusion did not persist much beyond a ΔT of 20 msec.

Summarizing Figures 1 and 2, we see that the precedence or Haas effect applies to pure tones of the same frequency and also of different frequencies. However, it must

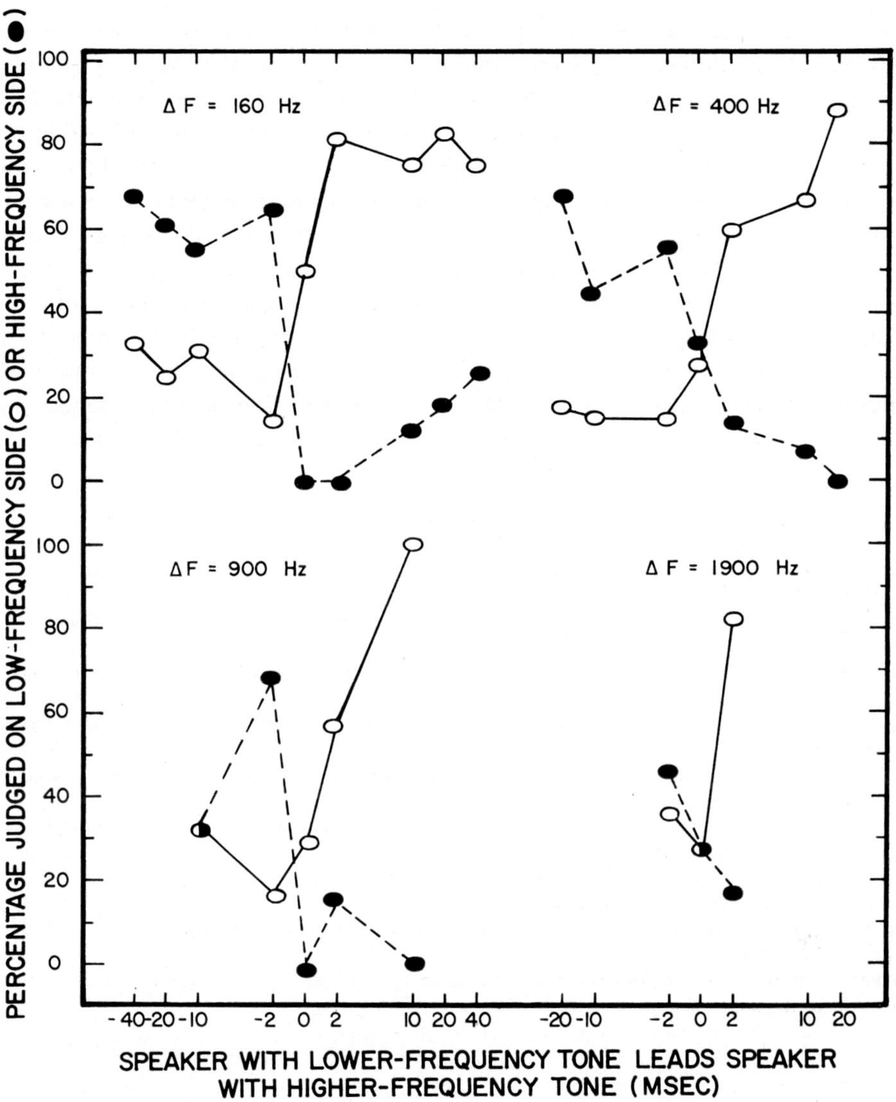

Fig. 2. Localization of a pair of tones, presented at different frequencies from two separated loudspeakers, as a function of onset time difference. (The frequency difference, ΔF, between the two tones, whose geometric mean was 2000 Hz, is the parameter. Loudness level was 65 phons. Half the time the lower-frequency tone was in the loudspeaker on *O*'s left and the other half in the speaker on the right.)

be emphasized that the greater the difference in frequency the smaller the time difference at which the effect disappears and two separate sound images are heard. Sounds too different in both spectral composition and temporal features are heard as separate. (The precise limits for this splitting seem to vary widely from *O* to *O*.)

Although listeners report a single sound from the side of the leading loudspeaker, they hear more than just the leading sound. Usually the fused sound seems like two tones played simultaneously in the same place. Moreover, the loudness of the two tones is greater than either alone. A large number of loudness measurements showed that the loudness of the two tones, whether fused or not, increased with ΔF in much the same way as two tones presented through a single earphone provided ΔT was under 20 msec (Scharf, 1974). As in earphone listening, loudness first began to increase with ΔF when the two tones were separated by more than a critical band (Zwicker, Flottorp, & Stevens, 1957). The loudness level of two simultaneous tones separated by 4200 Hz was as much as 10 phons greater than the level of either tone presented alone.

Although the experimental results were gathered in an anechoic room, the precedence effect with unlike tones is easily demonstrated in normal reverberant rooms. Consequently, in auditoria the optimal fusion or integration time may depend upon the difference in spectral composition between direct and reflected sounds.

References

Haas, H. v. Über den Einfluss eines Einfachechos auf die Hörsamkeit von Sprache. *Acustica*, 1951, **1**, 49–58.

Mills, A. W. On the minimum audible angle. *Journal of the Acoustical Society of America*, 1958, **30**, 237–246.

Scharf, B. Frequency selectivity and sound localization. Paper presented at the Symposium on Hearing Theory, Eindhoven, The Netherlands, June, 1972.

Scharf, B. Loudness summation between tones from two loudspeakers. *Journal of the Acoustical Society of America*, 1974, in press.

Stevens, S. S., & Newman, E. B. The localization of actual sources of sound. *American Journal of Psychology*, 1936, **48**, 297–306.

Thurlow, W. R., & Bernstein, S. Simultaneous two-tone pitch discrimination. *Journal of the Acoustical Society of America*, 1957, **29**, 515–519.

Wallach, H., Newman, E. B., & Rosenzweig, M. R. The precedence effect in sound localization. *American Journal of Psychology*, 1949, **62**, 315–336.

Yost, W. A., Wightman, F. L., & Green, D. M. Lateralization of filtered clicks. *Journal of the Acoustical Society of America*, 1971, **50**, 1526–1532.

Zwicker, E., Flottorp, G., & Stevens, S. S. Critical band width in loudness summation. *Journal of the Acoustical Society of America*, 1957, **29**, 548–557.

PSYCHOPHYSICAL CORRELATES OF MIDDLE-EAR-MUSCLE ACTION

W. DIXON WARD

Hearing Research Laboratory, University of Minnesota, Minneapolis

Abstract. The psychophysical correlates of middle-ear muscle activity are anything but clear. The acoustic reflex (AR) reduces TTS at and from low frequencies, and it reduces the TTS caused by impulse noise. A shift in absolute threshold at low frequencies is observed in people who can do *something* that may be a voluntary contraction of the muscles, but not in people whose reflex is presumably aroused by external stimuli. As for changes in the loudness of suprathreshold stimuli, the evidence is contradictory: Some evidence suggests that the loudness of a low-frequency test tone is reduced when the AR is aroused by a contralateral stimulus only when the test tone is very loud; other evidence suggests that the loudness level is reduced the same number of phons no matter what the tone's intensity; still other evidence suggests that loudness is not reduced at all, but rather enhanced, particularly at high intensities. Thus the precise manner in which the AR, separated from central interactive influences, has an effect on psychophysical judgments, demands further investigation.

When this volume was originally planned, I had intended to write an essay comparing the use of subjective musical intervals vs numerical relations in the scaling of pitch, a topic over which Professor Stevens and I had had numerous fairly heated discussions while I was his student, in the hope that this might induce him to re-examine his position on this matter. However, when the book became a memorial volume instead of a Festschrift, a less controversial article seemed more appropriate. Accordingly, I have attempted to review the action of the middle-ear muscles on psychoacoustic phenomena at high intensities, a topic in which opinion plays a less salient role than in scaling of pitch.

A loud sound presented to the normal intact auditory system causes the muscles of the middle ear – the stapedius and the tensor tympani – to contract. These two antagonistic muscles pull on their respective attachments, stiffening the middle-ear transmission system and thereby reducing the level of the sound that reaches the cochlea. Consequently, the action of the middle-ear muscles (MEM) should affect the absolute threshold, judgments of loudness, the threshold for discomfort and pain, and temporary threshold shifts (TTSs) produced by intense stimuli. Furthermore, these effects should be time-dependent, since the muscles need time to attain equilibrium, and soon thereafter begin to relax even in the presence of a sustained arousal stimulus. Clearly, then, the effect of the MEM on perception can be expected to be complicated. In this paper, I review the psychophysical aspects of MEM-arousal in an attempt to show that linearity of perceptual processes at high intensities should not be assumed, and indeed does not occur.

Voluntary Contraction

The first psychophysical demonstrations of the protection afforded by the MEM were

H. R. Moskowitz et al. (eds.), Sensation and Measurement. 315–324.

carried out on persons who believed themselves able to contract these muscles voluntarily (Smith, 1943). On the basis of data from such individuals, collected over many years, Reger (1960) showed that the threshold shift associated with this voluntary action can be more than 30 dB at frequencies below 1000 Hz but then drops to 0 dB at 2000 Hz and above. Possibly, however, a part of this threshold shift could be attributed to masking by noise produced by the contracting muscles.

To assess that possibility, Reger (1960) determined how the MEM affected the loudness of a low-frequency tone. Owing to loudness recruitment, a constant muscle noise that might raise the absolute threshold would not affect the loudness of a tone well above the masked threshold. Reger's *O*s adjusted the level of one 125-Hz, 1-s tone to match in loudness a second 125-Hz tone presented 200 msec later to the same ear. The second tone was accompanied by a 500-Hz tone, also in the same ear, at an intensity great enough to arouse the MEM reflex (a reflex-arousal stimulus or RAS). Figure 1 shows the sensation level at which the first, unaccompanied tone was judged to be as loud as the second, accompanied tone. The results imply that the auditory reflex (AR) activated by the RAS reduced the loudness of the second tone, and that the more intense the RAS was, the more it reduced loudness. Moreover, the effect is like that of a true attenuator, the reduction in decibels being independent of the level of the 125-Hz tone.

Since Békésy (1941) had reported that a low-frequency tone decreased in loudness when an intense high-frequency tone was presented to the opposite ear, Reger (1960)

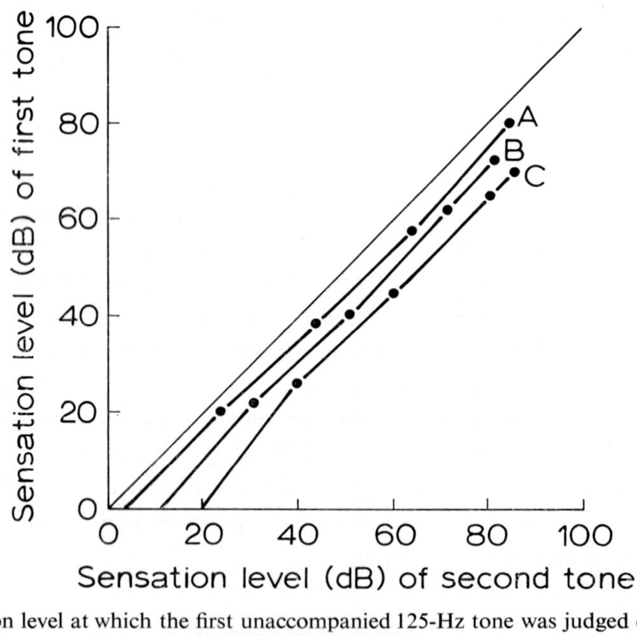

Fig. 1. Sensation level at which the first unaccompanied 125-Hz tone was judged equal in loudness to a second 125-Hz tone which was accompanied by a 500-Hz arousal tone. All tones were presented to the same ear. The sensation level of the arousal tone was 80 dB (A), 100 dB (B), or 110 dB (C). From Reger (1960).

repeated the experiment with the RAS (the 500-Hz tone) in the opposite ear. Having attributed Békésy's finding to the consensual nature of the MEM reflex, Reger expected and found the same kind of constant attenuation of the 125-Hz tone in the dichotic as in the monotic presentation. However, the attenuation was less, being only about 10 dB in the case of the 110-dB RAS, in comparison to 18 dB in the monotic situation. This reduced effect is consistent with Møller's (1961) deduction from impedance measurements that an ipsilateral RAS produces a stronger contraction than a contralateral RAS.

All these results seemed reasonable and straightforward: the contraction of the muscles increases with the intensity of the RAS, thus attenuating any low-frequency tone, whether of low, moderate, or high intensity. One should be able to use Reger's paradigm to study the relative effectiveness of noise vs tones and high vs low frequencies. Also, by varying the temporal relation between the RAS and brief test stimuli, one could study the growth and recovery of the loudness reduction as the MEM swiftly contracts and slowly relaxes.

Reduction of TTS

If an RAS reduces the energy reaching the cochlea by X dB, then one would expect that in order to produce a given TTS, X dB greater energy would have to be delivered to the earphone in the presence of the RAS than in its absence. In one application of this procedure, I determined the effective attenuation of short impulses (similar to gunfire) produced by a 250-msec 1000-Hz RAS at 100 dB SPL presented to the other ear at various times before the impulses (Ward, 1962b). In this case, 2-min exposures were given to pulses presented at the rate of 25 per minute at successively higher levels. The TTS at 4 kHz 30 s after exposure at one level was measured, and if a criterion TTS of 20 dB had not been produced, then a 2-min exposure at the next higher level was given, and so on until the criterion was reached. On subsequent days, this process was repeated but with the RAS presented 25, 62, 100 or 150 msec before each pulse. Figure 2 shows both some straightforward results (e.g., MK and KA) and some peculiar ones (YT). As in Figure 1, the effective attenuation is equal to the horizontal distance separating the curves. VA-R represents an ear that was later found to have no reflex as measured by the impedance bridge. Here the presence of the contralateral RAS had no effect whatsoever.

In another experiment, the action of the MEM in reducing the TTS produced by the RAS itself was investigated (Ward, 1962a). A 5-min monaural exposure to a 700-Hz pure tone at 125 dB SPL produced a TTS 15 s after exposure of about 30 dB that decreased to about 20 dB at 2 min post-exposure (short-dashed line in Figure 3). On the other hand, a narrow-band noise of the same SPL and center frequency produced only 17 dB of TTS immediately after exposure, dropping to 10 dB by 2 min (solid curve). When the tone and noise were given simultaneously but separately to each ear, the TTS produced by the tone (long-dashed curve) was no greater than that produced by the noise alone. A similar effect was found for 1400-Hz stimuli, but the

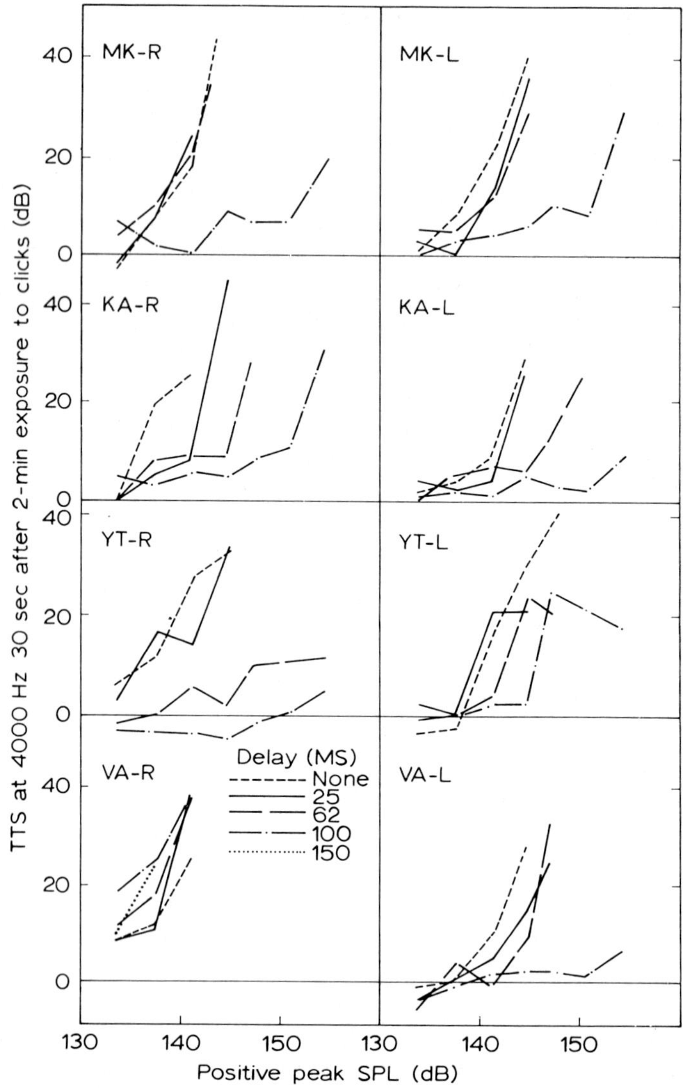

Fig. 2. Examples of the growth of $TTS_{0.5}$ at 4000 Hz as the level of successive 2-min exposures to 25 pulses per min is raised from 133 dB SPL to a level sufficient to produce 20 dB or more of TTS. The short-dashed line shows the TTS produced with no reflex-arousal stimulus. The other curves show the changes that occur when a 1000-Hz arousal tone at 100 dB SPL is presented to the contralateral ear. The parameter is the delay, in milliseconds, between onset of the arousal tone and presentation of the pulse. From Ward (1962a).

difference was much smaller, and the TTS from a 2000-Hz tone was unaffected by the simultaneous presentation of the corresponding narrow band of noise to the contralateral ear. These results are consonant with the effective attenuation implied by Reger's original results. It also appears that a noise, presumably because of its time varying property, is able to maintain contraction of the muscles better than a pure tone.

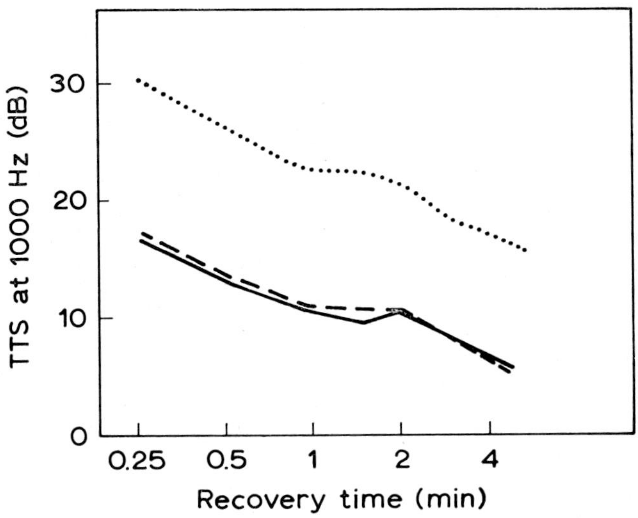

Fig. 3. Course of recovery from TTS at 1000 Hz following a 5-min exposure at 125 dB SPL to: (a) a 700-Hz pure tone (dotted curve); (b) a narrow band of noise centered at 700 Hz (solid curve); (c) a 700-Hz tone, but with the noise simultaneously presented to the other ear (dashed curve). From Ward (1962b).

Contralateral Remote Masking

Interpretation of data from contralateral remote masking (CRM), however, is not so straightforward. The basic procedure in measuring CRM and other types of masking is illustrated in Figure 4 (Ward, 1961). The ordinate here is in all cases the change in threshold of a pulsed 500-Hz test tone in the left ear associated with presentation of a steady noise whose intensity is given by the abscissa and whose spectral composition is the parameter. If one puts a 300–600-Hz band of noise into the LE, then ordinary direct masking results; a 10-dB increase in masker level will produce a 10-dB increase in the masking, and the MEM have nothing to do with this function, because any action of the muscles will affect both the noise and the test tone equally. The same unity slope is seen when the 300–600-Hz noise is in the other ear, but the curve is shifted by the 60 dB that corresponds to transcranial attenuation; the 3–4 dB of threshold shift produced by 60- or 70-dB SPL 300–600-Hz contralateral noise is classical "central masking."

The effects of a high-frequency octave band of noise are more complicated. When a 2400–4800-Hz noise is presented to the same ear, then the observed shift in threshold will be due partly to the "remote masking" caused by the generation of low-frequency distortion products within the cochlea, and partly to the attenuation produced by the reflex. As can be seen, a curvilinear growth function is found, with a 10-dB increase in the high-frequency noise producing as much as a 20-dB rise in threshold.

A naive view of the action of the 2400–4800-Hz noise presented to the contralateral ear (the rightmost curve) might be that here only the effect of the reflex will be in-

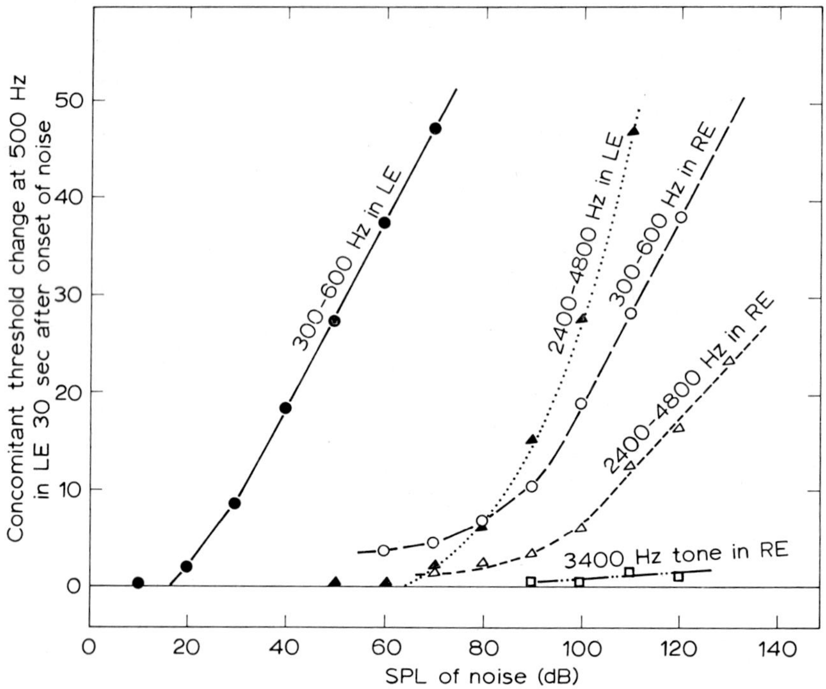

Fig. 4. Masking of a 500-Hz tone by high- and low-frequency bands of noise in the same and in the opposite ear. From Ward (1961).

volved; even with a 130-dB noise in the RE, the effective level in the LE due to transcranial conduction would be only 70 dB SPL (130 dB–60 dB), which would produce only about 2 dB of threshold shift by remote masking, so that 21 of the 23 dB of shift actually observed could be attributed to the reflex.

However, such an assumption neglects the fact that the 130-dB high-frequency noise is producing very intense distortion products in the RE, so that considerable central masking of the 500-Hz test tone might well be expected. For example, it can be seen that 110 dB of high-frequency noise produces nearly 50 dB of shift in the same ear; 130 dB would be apt to generate as much as 100 dB or more of shift. If this were so, surely the massive neural discharge along the ipsilateral pathways would be expected to produce considerable central interference, quite apart from any action of the MEM.

The test of this hypothesis involves the study of persons known to have missing or inoperative MEM. In patients with Bell's palsy (Ward, 1967), in those in whom the stapedius had been cut during stapedectomy (Fletcher & King, 1963), and in those in whom the MEM had been paralyzed by curare (Smith, Loeb, Fletcher, & Thomas, 1966), CRM was nearly as great as in normal ears.

Also, the threshold shift is just as great for a 50-msec tone pip whose onset coincides with that of the contralateral masker as one which begins 100 msec later (Ward, 1967), even though the impulse-noise study (Figure 2) indicated that as much as 150 msec is needed before the full protective effect is reached. Apparently contralateral remote masking is not a good indicator of the attenuation produced by arousal of the reflex, because this attenuation is overshadowed by central effects.

Central Effects (Loudness Enhancement)

Indeed, the experiments of Prather (1961) indicate that under some conditions, the judged loudness of a tone can be *enhanced* by simultaneous presentation of a white noise to the contralateral ear. This increase in loudness was confirmed by Vigran (1965) who used a narrow-band noise instead of white noise, in order to minimize the direct-masking effect of transcranially-conducted sound. So it is clear that with simultaneous presentation of arousal and test stimuli, two opposing factors are always involved: the attenuation produced by the MEM, and the loudness enhancement associated with simultaneity.

A recent attempt to minimize central effects has been reported by Gjaevenes, Gran, & Rollag (1969). Instead of presenting the 45-msec maskee simultaneously with a 540-msec masker (a 2000-Hz tone at 105-dB SPL), they inserted an interval of 35 msec between the end of the masker and the onset of the test tone. Since the muscles do not fully relax for an appreciable fraction of a second after removal of the arousal stimulus, there should still exist considerable effective attenuation through the period concerned (80 msec after cessation). And indeed they found a shift at 500 Hz of about 10 dB, slightly less at lower frequencies, and considerably less at higher frequencies. Unfortunately for a simple explanation, however, a listener with known inoperative MEM, as shown by impedance measurements, displayed as much threshold shift as normals, so that even "residual CRM" seems to depend more on central factors than on the reflex. This conclusion was supported by the fact that the magnitude of the impedance change was calculated by Gjaevenes *et al.* to predict at most only a 2- or 3-dB threshold shift even in the normal ears.

On the other hand, despite the failure of our attempts to confirm, using threshold shifts, the attenuation values implied by Reger's voluntary contractors, there is no doubt that the MEM somehow do protect the ear. Mills & Lilly (1970) recently confirmed the implication of my earlier finding, i.e. that the difference between the traumatizing power of a pure tone and a band of noise is ascribable to the action of the MEM. Six stapedectomized ears and 6 normals were exposed to both a 710-Hz pure tone and a narrow band of noise (cutoff frequencies at 660 and 710 Hz), each at 110 dB SPL. Whereas the TTS produced by the tone in the normals was twice as great as that produced by the noise, the stapedectomized patients showed the same TTS for both conditions.

The implication of these results is that the action of the MEM is non-linear – that high-intensity stimuli are attenuated more than low-intensity ones, a conclusion reached by Loeb & Riopelle (1960). They found only slight contralateral threshold shifts associated with a high-frequency tone at 100 or 105 dB SPL. But by balancing for loudness a tone heard alone against one accompanied by the arouser, they showed that as the intensity of the accompanied tone increased, the intensity disparity required for equal loudness also increased. That is, a given arousal tone seemed to have more effect on an intense low-frequency tone than on a weak one, which implies some sort of a peak-limiting mechanism. Measurements in cadaver ears of the attenuation produced by known tensions induced in the MEM tend to confirm this nonlinearity (Neergaard, Andersen, Hansen, & Jepsen, 1964).

Over-Recruitment and Pain

Lack of a reflex should – other things being equal – lead to "over-recruitment" in the affected ear for low-frequency sounds, since the self-limiting action normally found is absent. This was already observed in 1938 by Perlman, on a patient with Bell's palsy, and the lowering of the "discomfort" level has since been amply confirmed (Hansen, 1965; Tato, 1960). It must be pointed out, however, that Jepsen (1955) found that only slightly more than half of his palsy cases showed any change in the *pain* threshold. Although according to absolute judgments the sounds were louder, they were not necessarily more painful. This agrees with our observation (Ward, Selters, & Glorig, 1961) that presentation of a reflex-arousal tone has no influence on the painfulness of a given high-intensity click. That is, although the RAS may eliminate the TTS produced by a 150-dB click, it has no effect on the painfulness of each click. This probably means that the pain arises from extreme movement of the eardrum.

MEM Impedance Changes

If the protection afforded by the MEM depends on the impedance change produced, then one would expect a negative correlation between the degree of impedance change produced by a low-frequency noise and the subsequent TTS. (Many experiments have shown that there is no relation between CRM and TTS, but in view of the fact that CRM is at best only partly dependent on MEM activity, this is hardly surprising.) Johansson, Kylin, & Langfy (1967) report that when they selected, on the basis of impedance measurements, two persons with a short reflex latency and fast rise time, and two with a long latency and slow rise time, the former showed much less TTS at 500 and 1000 Hz after a 15-min exposure to 300–1200-Hz noise at 110 dB SPL. This implies that a short latency and swift rise time are correlated with a more sustained and powerful contraction, but in view of the questionable selection process, the problem demands closer scrutiny. In fact, the latest study of the relation between the AR and susceptibility to TTS (Brasher, Coles, Elwood, & Ferres, 1969) has given negative results. Sixteen young men were exposed for 25 min to octave-band noise centered on 1000 Hz (105 dB SPL), to noise centered on 4000 Hz for the same time at the same level, and to impulse noise. There were no significant correlations between any of the resultant TTSs and any measure of the AR including the reflex threshold, its relative strength at onset, and its strength after 2 min of exposure. One problem here is how to compare the reflex strengths of two individuals. Using the Madsen apparatus, as both Johansson *et al.* and Brasher *et al.* did, one cannot even be sure that a given deflection from the null position means the same *relative* change in impedance in two different ears, much less the same absolute change.

Conditioning the MEM

Finally, consider the conditionability of the reflex. Years ago, I conducted some unpublished experiments in which I compared the TTS produced by pulses delivered at a regular rate with the TTS produced by the same number of pulses delivered randomly in time. No difference was found, implying that the reflex could not be conditioned. On the other hand, after participating in a long series of studies of TTS from impulses, 6 of the 14 subjects claimed that they could voluntarily reduce the loudness of a low-frequency noise. Therefore, these six listeners were given two series of exposures to pulses delivered at regular intervals; in one series the subject was asked to anticipate each click with a MEM contraction, and in the other he was asked not to do so (Fleer, 1963). The resulting TTSs implied that this voluntary contraction produced about 10 dB of effective protection. Also, Brasher *et al.* (1969) report that in many persons a large impedance change can be observed when, during an exposure to gunfire in which the subject himself pulls the trigger, a deliberate misfire is introduced by the experimenter (unknown to the subject). If such strong reactions can result from anticipation, it is hard to see why my listeners did not gradually develop an anticipatory response quite involuntarily during exposure at regular intervals. Possibly the important difference here is that the subject is active in the one situation, but passive in the other.

Bibliography

Békésy, G. von. Über die Messung der Schwingungsamplitude der Gehörknöchelchen mittels einer kapazitiven Sonde. *Akustische Zeitschrift*, 1941, **6**, 1–16.

Brasher, P. F., Coles, R. R. A., Elwood, M. A., & Ferres, H. M. Middle-ear muscle activity and temporary threshold shift. *International Audiology*, 1969, **8**, 579–584.

Fleer, R. Protection afforded against impulsive noise by voluntary contraction of the middle ear muscles. In *Middle Ear Function Seminar*, Report No. 576, J. L. Fletcher, Ed. U.S. Army Medical Research Laboratory, 1963, pp. 196–200.

Fletcher, J. L. & King, W. P. Susceptibility of stapedectomized patients to noise induced temporary threshold shifts. *Annals of Otology, Rhinology and Laryngology*, 1963, **71**, 900–907.

Gjaevenes, K., Gran, S. & Rollag, Ö. Contralateral remote masking and the aural reflex. *Journal of the Acoustical Society of America*, 1969, **46**, 918–923.

Hansen, S. Phonophobia evaluated with Bekesy audiometry. *International Audiology*, 1965, **4**, 53–55.

Jepsen, O. Studies on the acoustic stapedius reflex in man. Thesis, Aarhus Univ., Denmark, 1955.

Johansson, B., Kylin, B. & Langfy, M. Acoustic reflex as a test of individual susceptibility to nosei: a preliminary report. *Acta Oto-laryngologica*, 1967, **64**, 256–262.

Loeb, M. & Riopelle, A. J. Influence of loud contralateral stimulation on the threshold and perceived loudness of low-frequency tones. *Journal of the Acoustical Society of America*, 1960, **32**, 602–610.

Mills, J. H. & Lilly, D. J. Temporary threshold shift produced by pure tones and by noise in the absence of an acoustic reflex. *Journal of the Acoustical Society of America*, 1970, **50**, 1556–1558.

Møller, A. Bilateral contraction of the tympanic muscles in man. Report No. 18, Speech Transmission Lab., Royal Institute of Technology, Stockholm, Feb. 1961.

Neergaard, E. B., Andersen, H. C., Hansen, C. C., & Jepsen, O. Experimental studies on sound transmission in the human ear. III: Influence of the stapedius and tensor tympani muscles. *Acta Otolaryngologica*, 1964, Suppl. **188**, 280–286.

Perlman, H. B. Hyperacusis. *Annals of Otology, Rhinology and Laryngology*, 1938, **47**, 947–953.

Prather, W. F. Shift in loudness of pure tones associated with contralateral noise stimulation. *Journal of Speech and Hearing Research*, 1961, **4**, 182–193.

Reger, S. N. Effect of middle ear muscle action on certain psycho-physical measurements. *Annals of Otology, Rhinology and Laryngology*, 1960, **69**, 1179–1198.

Smith, H. D. Audiometric effects of voluntary contraction of the tensor tympany muscle. *A.M.A. Archives of Otolaryngology*, 1943, **38**, 369–372.

Smith, R. P., Loeb, M., Fletcher, J. L., & Thomas, D. M. The effect of moderate doses of curare on certain auditory functions. *Acta Oto-laryngologica*, 1966, **62**, 101–108.

Tato, J. M. Personal communication, 1960.

Vigran, E. Loudness change of pure tones with contralateral noise stimulation. *Journal of the Acoustical Society of America*, 1965, **37**, 1134–1138.

Ward, W. D. Studies on the aural reflex. I: Contralateral remote masking as an indicator of reflex activity. *Journal of the Acoustical Society of America*, 1961, **33**, 1034–1045.

Ward, W. D. Studies on the aural reflex. III: Reflex latency as inferred from reduction of temporary threshold shift from impulses. *Journal of the Acoustical Society of America*, 1962, **34**, 1132–1137. (a)

Ward, W D. Damage-risk criteria for line spectra. *Journal of the Acoustical Society of America* 1962, **34**, 1610–1619. (b)

Ward, W. D. Further observations on contralateral remote masking and related phenomena. *Journal of the Acoustical Society of America*, 1967, **42**, 593–600.

Ward, W. D., Selters, W., & Glorig, A. Exploratory studies on temporary threshold shift from impulses. *Journal of the Acoustical Society of America*, 1961, **33**, 781–793.

LOUDNESS AND EXCITATION PATTERNS OF STRONGLY FREQUENCY MODULATED TONES

EBERHARD ZWICKER

Institut für Elektroakustik, Technische Universität München

Abstract. The loudness level of sinusoidal frequency-modulated tones (1500 Hz ± 700 Hz) was measured as a function of their frequency of modulation and sound pressure level. The purpose was to find out how loudness depends on the time structure of the spectrum while the level is kept constant. The results indicate that loudness remains constant up to frequencies of modulation of 16 Hz, then rises and reaches a new constant value between 64 Hz and 128 Hz. This partly unexpected effect is compared with values calculated on the basis of incompletely known excitation patterns for such frequency-modulated tones. The first direct estimations of such excitation patterns are given.

The loudness of steady-state sounds is an important subject of investigation. Stevens (1955, 1957, 1961) was one of the first authors to point out how knowledge about loudness could be used to calculate its value from the physical parameters of a sound. Several other authors (Bauch, 1956; Brittain, 1939; Fletcher & Munson, 1933; Zwicker, 1958; Zwicker & Feldtkeller, 1955; Zwicker, Flottorp, & Stevens, 1957) published similar or related results. Thus, our present understanding of the formation of the loudness of steady-state sounds including the influence of critical bands (Zwicker *et al.*, 1957) and psychoacoustical excitation (Zwicker, 1958; Zwicker & Feldtkeller, 1967) seems to be almost complete, at least for the basic effects.

The formation of the loudness of sounds with strong temporal patterns, on the other hand, remains more or less unclear. Existing approximations designed for technical use employ the sound intensity weighted with an RC-network having a time constant τ of 25 msec (Niese, 1965) or 100 msec (Zwicker, 1969). Nevertheless, the way in which the loudness of such sounds is formed really remains mostly unexplored. Some investigations have been started and a model for the formation of the loudness of sounds with strong temporal patterns has been proposed (Zwicker, 1968), but more research is necessary.

The investigation described in this article is part of this research, but – in contrast to classic experiments – frequency was changed drastically as a function of time, while amplitude was kept constant. The loudness of sinusoidally, frequency modulated tones, whose instantaneous frequency $f=f_0 \pm \Delta f$, was measured. For $f_0=1500$ Hz and $\Delta f=700$ Hz the frequency of the tone varied between 800 Hz and 2200 Hz. The important parameter, the frequency of modulation f_{mod}, was changed drastically. Since it is generally accepted that loudness is formed by integration over time, two quasi steady-state conditions can be expected: (A) for very slow changes in frequency, i.e. for very small f_{mod}, the ear should respond the same way as to steady pure tones (no integration); (B) for very rapid changes in frequency, i.e. for very large f_{mod}, the ear integrates totally over the period of modulation and again reaches a steady-state

H. R. Moskowitz et al. (eds.), Sensation and Measurement. 325–335.

condition. The reaction of the ear for f_{mod} between these two quasi steady-state conditions can not be predicted and has to be measured.

Physical Description of the FM Tones

For condition A, small f_{mod}, the sound is best described by plotting the actual frequency as a function of time as in Figure 1. Since the frequency f_{mod} of the sinuisoidal modulation is varied over a wide range during these experiments, it is convenient to use a relative measure of time. Accordingly, time is expressed on the abscissa of Figure 1 in eight parts of one full period of f_{mod}. The left-hand ordinate gives the instantaneous frequency, f, and the right-hand ordinate the corresponding value on the critical-band scale. When $f_{mod} = 1$ Hz, the duration of the period is 1 s and condition A holds. When $f_{mod} = 500$ Hz, the period is only 2 msec and condition B is reached. The sound should then be described by its spectrum in order to comply with the response characteristics of the ear.

The sound pressure $p(t)$ of a frequency modulated tone follows the equation

$$p(t) = \hat{p} \cos\left(\omega_0 t + \frac{\Delta\omega}{\omega_{mod}} \cos \omega_{mod}\, t\right).$$

The term within the brackets corresponds to the time-dependent frequency shown in

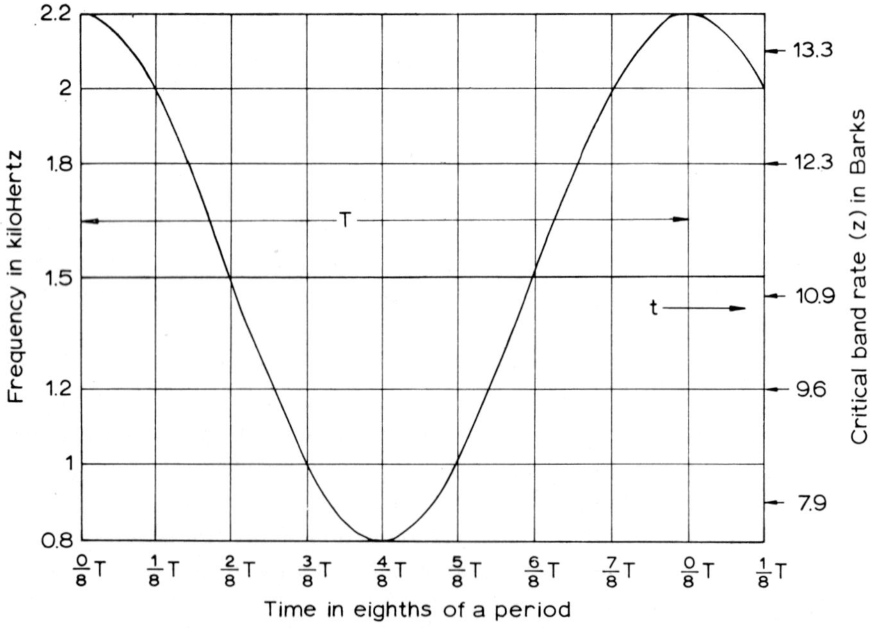

Fig. 1. Change in frequency of a strongly frequency modulated tone as function of time. The time scale is divided into eights of the period $T = 1/f_{mod}$. The arrows on the right indicate frequencies converted to critical band rates at which masked thresholds were measured.

Figure 1. In this equation, the separate frequency components are not obvious. However, certain Bessel-function identities can be applied directly to yield the equation

$$p(t) = \hat{p} \sum_{n=-\infty}^{+\infty} J_n \frac{\Delta\omega}{\omega_{\text{mod}}} \cos\left[\omega_0 t + n \cdot \omega_{\text{mod}}\, t + \frac{n\pi}{2}\right].$$

From this equation, the sound-pressure level, L, of the spectral lines can be calculated with the aid of the tables of Jahnke, Emde, & Lösch (1966). Figure 2 gives two examples of the calculated spectra. The upper plot is for an f_{mod} of about 32 Hz which corresponds to the characteristic value

$$\frac{\Delta\omega}{\omega_{\text{mod}}} = \frac{\Delta f}{f_{\text{mod}}} = 22.$$

The density of the lines, spaced symmetrically at distances of f_{mod} around the center frequency, indicates that in this case the ear may be unable to resolve all the components because so many fall within the same critical band.

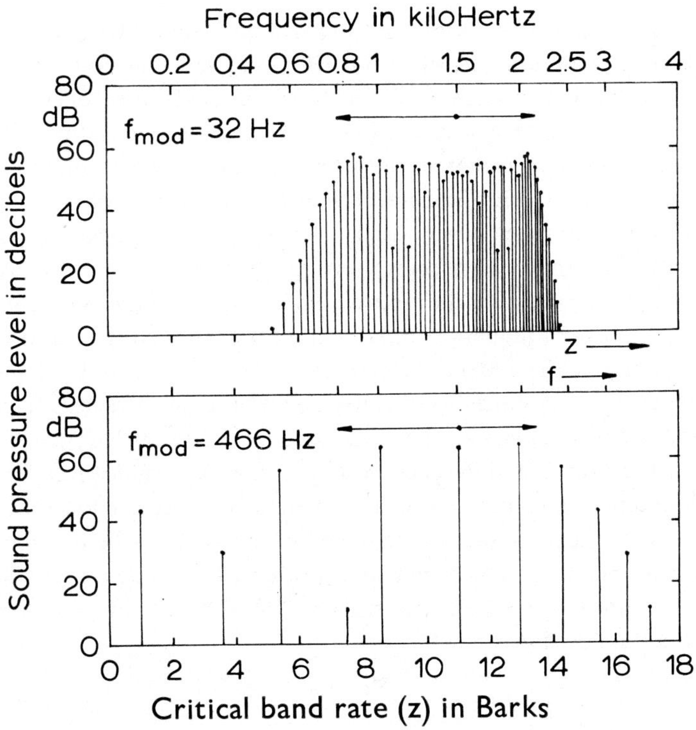

Fig. 2. Bessel spectra of sinusoidally frequency modulated tones for modulation frequencies, f_{mod}, of 32 Hz and 466 Hz. The level of the spectral lines is plotted against a linear critical-band rate scale. At the top is given the corresponding nonlinear frequency scale. Double arrows indicate the frequency range covered by the modulated tone.

The spectrum for $f_{mod}=466$ Hz, which approximates $\Delta f/f_{mod}=1.5$, shows only five important lines plus some additional ones more than 20 dB down. In this case the ear may be able to separate most of the lines as indicated by the fact that such a signal has no audible time structure, but sounds like a complex of tones. The spectra in Figure 2 are plotted on a linear critical-band rate scale, z, while the frequency, f, is indicated on the upper nonlinear scale. This configuration shows that the lower-frequency spectral lines can be resolved more easily by the ear, since in the higher frequency range more lines fall within a given critical band. Moreover, Figure 2 makes evident that the spectrum is wider than the range over which frequency is varied ($2\Delta f$), indicated by the double arrow. The difference between spectral width and $2\Delta f$ is small at a low f_{mod}, and relatively large at 466 Hz. The level of the FM-tones, with spectra as plotted in Figure 2, is 70 dB SPL. The level L of the corresponding spectral lines indicates that for smaller f_{mod} *more lines* but with *lower levels* are produced. This is so because the total intensity and thereby the overall level must be constant regardless of the number of lines.

Apparatus and Method

A Wavetec AM-FM generator produced the stimuli. The center frequency, 1.5 kHz, and the frequency deviation, Δf, of ± 700 Hz were kept constant, while f_{mod} varied between 1 Hz and 512 Hz in steps by a factor of 2. These 10 FM tones plus pure tones at 1 kHz, 1.5 kHz, and 2 kHz were compared in loudness with a narrow-band noise one critical band wide and centered at 1 kHz. Sounds were presented at four sound pressure levels, 30 dB, 50 dB, 70 dB, and 90 dB. The method of tracking combined with the method of adjustment was used. The observer was asked to track at least five times up and five times down before setting the motor-driven attenuator (Kaiser, 1952) to the position that gave the impression of equal loudness. Eight normal observers took part in the loudness comparisons. First, the narrow-band noise (NBN) was kept constant and the FM or the pure tones were varied in level; in the second part of the experiment the tones were constant and the noise varied. Each of the 832 data points represents the mean of the final adjustment and the average of the tracking trace. Most of the time, the difference between these two values was less than 3 dB. When the difference exceeded 6 dB, the match was repeated. No characteristic difference between the two sets of data could be found, whether individually or averaged. The sounds to be compared were presented 1 s each, separated by a silent period of 0.4 s through a single ear phone (DT 48) with an equalizing network (Zwicker & Feldtkeller, 1967).

Results

The loudness matches of all observers are plotted with the level of the narrow band noise on the ordinate and the level of the frequency modulated tones or pure tones on the abscissa. Figure 3 shows the average values and the interquartile ranges for modulation frequencies of 1 Hz, 8 Hz, 64 Hz, and 512 Hz. The four data sets are

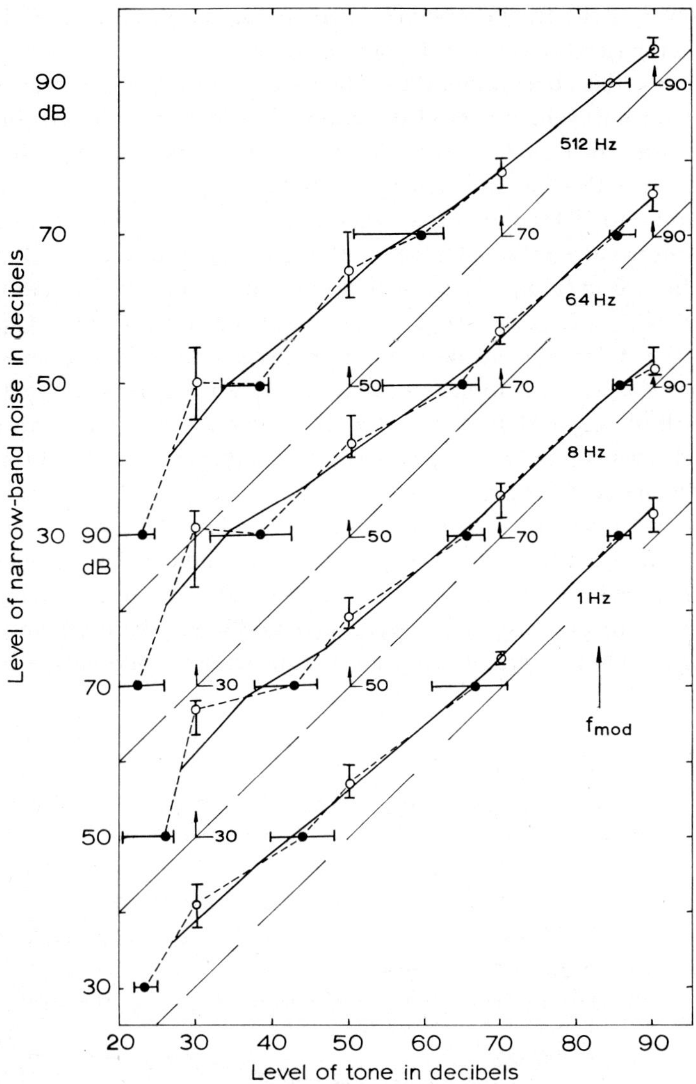

Fig. 3. Results of loudness comparisons between FM tones and a critical band of noise centered on 1 kHz at four different frequencies of modulation, f_{mod}. Unfilled circles are the means obtained when the noise was varied, filled circles when the tone was varied. Vertical and horizontal lines drawn through the data are the corresponding interquartile ranges. Solid curves represent the averages of all the data. Curves are separated by 20dB relative to the ordinate; the true ordinate values are on the 45° lines.

separated by 20 dB each to avoid confusion. The lower scale on the ordinate belongs to a modulation frequency of 1 Hz, the upper scale to 512 Hz. The appropriate scales for $f_{mod} = 8$ Hz and 64 Hz are indicated on the 45-degree lines.

The unfilled circles with vertical bars in Figure 3 were obtained by varying the level of the narrow-band noise. The filled circles with horizontal bars were obtained by varying the level of the frequency-modulated tones. As observed and described by Stevens (1955) the *varied* level is set higher at low levels and lower at very high levels. At medium levels this effect diminishes. The two sets of data have been averaged by connecting (solid lines) the points of bisection of the straight (dotted) lines between the filled and the open circles. Near the highest level, 90 dB, the solid lines were extrapolated 1 or 2 dB so as to reach $L_{FM}=90$ dB.

The solid curve for 1 Hz shows that when L_{FM} was 30 dB, the level of the narrow-band noise centered at 1 kHz had to be 39 dB for the noise to sound as loud as a tone at 30 dB modulated in frequency between 800 Hz and 2200 Hz once per second. The difference, $\Delta L = L_{NBN} - L_{FM}$, is 9 dB at $L_{FM}=30$ dB, but only 4 dB at $L_{FM}=90$ dB as indicated by the difference on the ordinate between the solid line and the dashed 45-degree line. For a modulation frequency of 512 Hz ΔL becomes 15 dB at $L_{FM}=$ 30 dB and 5 dB at $L_{FM}=90$ dB. The value ΔL required for equal loudness is always positive, which means that at the same level the frequency modulated tone is always louder than the narrow-band noise.

Plots like those in Figure 3 have been drawn for all ten frequencies of modulation and for the 1-kHz, 1.5–kHz, and 2-kHz pure tones. As indicated above, the differences $\Delta L = L_{NBN} - L_{FM}$ and $\Delta L = L_{NBN} - L_{Tone}$ are the most interesting data. Figure 4 presents ΔL as a function of f_{mod} at levels $L_{FM}=30$ dB, 50 dB, 70 dB, and 90 dB. The difference, ΔL, tends to increase from low frequencies of modulation to high ones

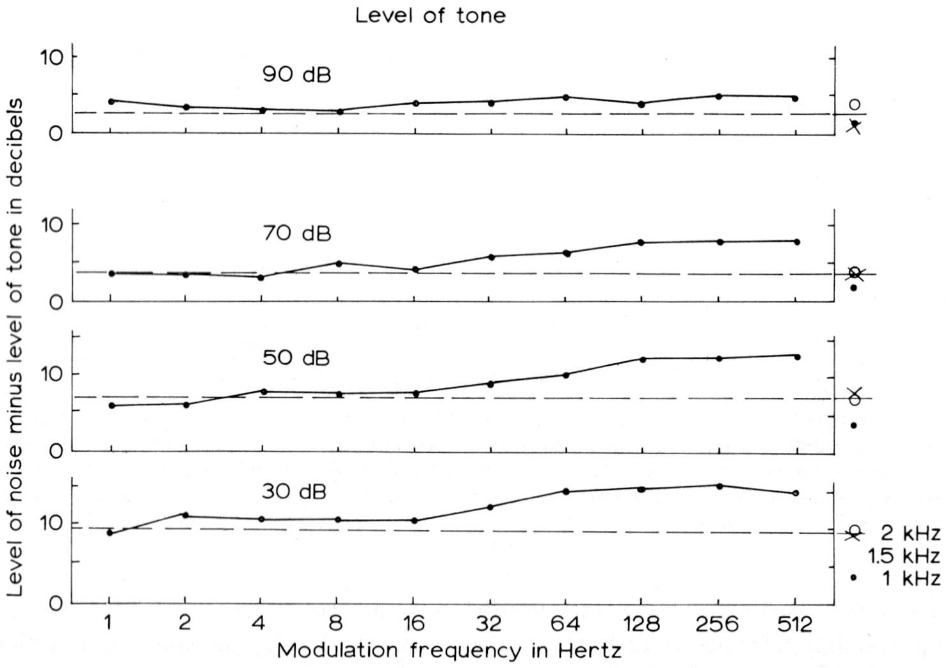

Fig. 4. Difference between the level of the narrow-band noise and the FM tone needed for equal loudness plotted as a function of the frequency of modulation. Parameter is the level of the tone. Symbols at the right indicate the level difference between the noise and a pure tone.

(especially at lower levels) as it varies between 3 dB and 16 dB. Since the comparison noise (one critical band widc) is centered at 1 kHz while the frequency modulated sounds are spread over a wide range of frequencies (between at least 800 Hz and 2.2 kHz), it seems reasonable that the FM tones are louder than the noise. However, it cannot be assumed that the equal-loudness contours are totally horizontal over the whole range of stimulating frequencies. The results of the loudness comparisons between the 1-kHz, 1.5-kHz, and 2-kHz tones and the narrow-band noise are used in place of the usual equal-loudness contours. The data were averaged in the way shown in Figure 3 and are plotted as dots (1 kHz), crosses (1.5 kHz), and open circles (2 kHz) on the right ordinate of Figure 3. On the assumption that the loudness of the FM tone varies most of the time between the two loudest tones, the horizontal dashed lines in Figure 4 indicate the average between the two highest values of $\Delta L = L_{\mathrm{NBN}} - L_{\mathrm{Tone}}$. Taking this effect into account and using the dashed horizontal lines as a kind of reference value, we can discuss the results in Figure 4.

At low frequencies of modulation the loudness of the FM tone is close to the averaged loudness level of the two loudest pure tones. At high frequencies of modulation, however, the loudness is clearly larger. The increment starts at modulation frequencies of 16 Hz to 32 Hz and reaches its asymptotic value between 64 Hz and 128 Hz. The effect is largest at lower and medium levels and less pronounced at the highest level used (90 dB). Since the model of loudness summation, based on the pattern of psychoacoustical excitation (see Zwicker & Scharf, 1965), describes most of the measured facts very well in the steady-state condition, it may be interesting to know the excitation-critical band rate-time patterns produced by the frequency modulated tones.

Related Excitation Patterns

Psychoacoustical excitation is based on the masking of pure tones by the sound in question. For steady-state conditions the just masked tone has a duration no shorter than 200 msec. To measure the temporal pattern of the excitation, the signal has to be as short as possible, i.e., as short as the smallest critical band allows. In a preliminary sequence of measurements the signals were 5-msec tone impulses with a Gaussian shaped envelope (rise time of 2 msec) sent through a third-octave band filter centered on the frequency of the tone impulse. The masker, a frequency modulated tone, was set at 50 dB or 70 dB SPL, while the frequency of modulation was varied between 0.5 Hz and 128 Hz. The masked thresholds of two observers were measured monaurally by the method of tracking. The 5-msec signal was presented every second at a time corresponding to one of the eighths of a period as depicted in Figure 1. The frequencies of the signal were chosen in such a way that they spread almost equally over the frequency range of interest. Furthermore, they were far enough from both the masker frequency occurring at the eighths of the period and the frequencies produced by the Bessel-spectra at high f_{mod} so as to avoid disturbing beats. Eight frequencies, five inside and three outside the frequency range of the FM tone, were used: 700 Hz, 900 Hz, 1200 Hz, 1450 Hz, 1800 Hz, 2100 Hz, 2400 Hz, and 3000 Hz.

In Figure 1, the corresponding critical-band rates are indicated by small arrows on the right.

From many preliminary results, three examples, at modulation frequencies of 0.5 Hz, 8 Hz, and 128 Hz and at a masker level of 70 dB, are shown in Figure 5. The sound-pressure level of the 5-msec signal at threshold is plotted as a function of critical-band rate. (The level of the 5-msec impulse is that of the original pure tone out of which the impulse is cut.) Parameter on the individual curves, as coded in the figure legend, is the time of signal presentation in eighths of a period. To avoid a confusing figure, only four of the eight times are presented.

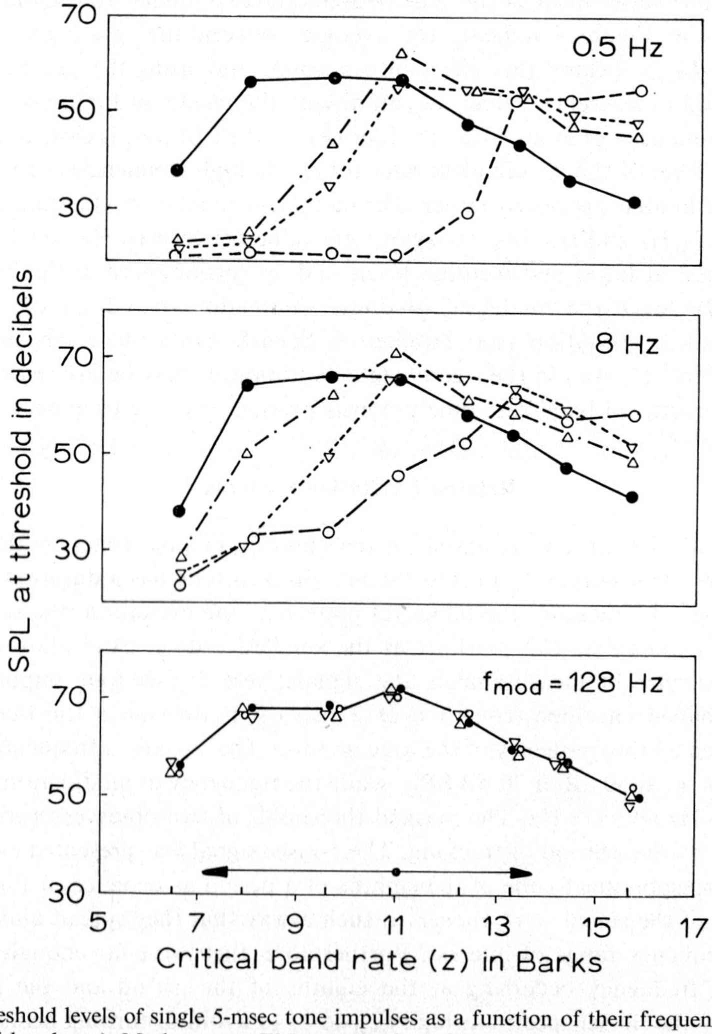

Fig. 5. Threshold levels of single 5-msec tone impulses as a function of their frequency (expressed as the critical-band rate). Maskers were FM tones at three different frequencies of modulation, f_{mod}, 0.5 Hz, 8 Hz, and 128 Hz. Thresholds were measured at four different moments of the modulation period, T (circles: 0/8 T; triangles: 2/8 T; dots: 4/8 T; inverted triangles: 6/8 T).

At a modulation frequency of 0.5 Hz the ear reacts as in a steady-state condition. The dots (4/8 period), for example, give the threshold at the moment that the masking FM tone reaches its lowest frequency, 800 Hz, which corresponds to a critical-band rate of 7.2 Bark. The data represent, in effect, samples from a masking curve produced by an 800-Hz tone. Although the peak of the curve, where masking is greatest, was not measured and difference tones produced in the ear may have influenced the absolute value of the threshold at 7.9 Bark and 9.6 Bark, the curve is similar to that produced by a masking 800-Hz tone at a level of 70 dB. The other three curves in the top section of Figure 5 are also similar to their corresponding steady-state frequencies, namely, 1500 Hz (∇ and Δ) and 2200 Hz (○). For a frequency of modulation of 0.5 Hz the ear reacts almost exactly as in the steady-state condition.

At $f_{mod} = 8$ Hz the threshold pattern, and so also the excitation pattern, still resembles the pattern at 0.5 Hz. However, careful inspection indicates some changes: (*a*) The threshold in quiet is never reached between 7.9 Bark and 10.9 Bark for 0/8 period (○); (*b*) most of the thresholds are higher; (*c*) the 2/8-period curve (Δ) and the 6/8-period curve (∇) deviate from each other in a regular manner although the actual masking frequency (1500 Hz) is the same in both cases (the difference between forward and backward masking becomes effective); (*d*) threshold differences among the four curves are smaller.

At $f_{mod} = 128$ Hz the thresholds measured on four different phases of the period lie so close together that they can all be summarized by a single curve. The masked threshold curve and thereby the excitation pattern show no temporal effects; they have again reached a quasi steady-state condition.

Together with other data from this preliminary experiment, these findings may be generalized as follows: (*a*) at modulation frequencies around 1 Hz, the excitation pattern can be thought of as being determined by the actual frequency and level of the stumulus; (*b*) at modulation frequencies of 128 Hz and higher, the excitation pattern can be regarded as determined by the Bessel-spectrum of the stimulus; (*c*) the transition between the two conditions starts at $f_{mod} = 8$ Hz and ends at 128 Hz.

Conclusions

On the basis of the model of loudness summation (Zwicker & Scharf, 1965) the two quasi steady-state conditions reached, one at very low frequencies of modulation and the other at very high frequencies of modulation, were expected. Loudness calculated by means of the model agrees quite well with the data. In these calculations, the average loudness of the two loudest tones (dashed lines in Figure 4) was used at low frequencies, and the Bessel-spectrum levels were converted to critical-band levels for use at high frequencies of modulation.

The effects at medium frequencies, however, were unexpected. In the relevant literature (Niese, 1961; Port, 1963; Reichardt, 1970; Zwicker, 1969; see also IEC-impulse sound-level meter) it is agreed that the loudness of impulses is achieved by integrating sound intensity (square of sound pressure) over a certain time, τ, where the value of τ varies between 25 msec and 100 msec. In sound level meters or loudness analyzers with a time constant of 100 msec, the intensities in each critical band are averaged at f_{mod} higher than 1.5 Hz (from $f=1/2\pi\tau$); for a time constant of 25 msec, the intensities are averaged at f_{mod} higher than 6 Hz. At modulation frequencies above these limits imposed by the time constant, not just one single critical band is covered during the frequency sweep, but almost all critical bands are excited at the same time. A situation similar to increasing the bandwidth – while total intensity is kept constant – is then reached, and loudness should increase. Loudness meters like Pfeiffers' (1966) and the Hewlett-Packard loudness analyser clearly show this increment. The results presented in Figure 4, however, indicate that the measured loudness first begins to increase at higher frequencies of modulation (around 32 Hz).

This unexpected effect points out that a model of loudness incorporating a *single* time constant for sound intensity is too simple. Models similar to one described earlier (Zwicker, 1968), containing not only linear but also nonlinear networks, may be able to account for this effect.

The combined excitation critical-band rate and time pattern, however, is the basic pattern from which most hearing sensations are derived (Zwicker, 1970). It seems also to play an important role in the formation of the loudness of frequency modulated tones. Further research is necessary to investigate this complex pattern as carefully and as accurately as possible, while taking into account the numerous parameters involved. Such data may make possible a more accurate model not only of the spatial summation but also of the temporal summation of loudness.

References

Bauch, H. Die Bedeutung der Frequenzgruppe für die Lautheit von Klängen. *Acustica*, 1956, **6**, 40–45.

Brittain, F. H. The loudness of continuous spectrum noise and its application to loudness measurements. *Journal of the Acoustical Society of America*, 1939, **11**, 113–116.

Fletcher, H., & Munson, W. A. Loudness, its definition, measurement and calculation. *Journal of the Acoustical Society of America*, 1933, **9**, 82–108.

Fletcher, H., & Munson, W. A. Relation between loudness and masking. *Journal of the Acoustical Society of America*, 1939, **9**, 1–10.

Jahnke, E., Edme, F., & Lösch, F. *Tafeln höherer Funktionen* (7th ed.). Stuttgart: Teubner Verlag, 1966.

Kaiser, W. Das Békésy-Audiometer der Technischen Hochschule Stuttgart. *Acustica*, 1952, **2** (Beiheft 4), 235–238.

Niese, H. Das Zusammenwirken der Einflüsse von Geräuschbandbreite und Geräuschzeitfunktion auf die Lautstärke. *Hochfrequenztechnik und Elektroakustik*, 1961, **70**, 79–91.

Niese, H. Eine Methode zur Bestimmung der Lautstärke beliebiger Geräusche. *Acustica*, 1965, **15**, 117–126.

Pfeiffer, Th. Ein Lautstärke-Messgerät für breitbandige und impulshaltige Schalle. *Acustica*, 1966, **17**, 322–334.

Port, E. Zur Lautstärkeempfindung und Lautstärkemessung von pulsierenden Geräuschen. *Acustica* 1963, **13** (Beiheft 1), 224–233.

Reihardt, W. Subjective and objective measurement of the loudness level of single and repeated impulses. *Journal of the Acoustical Society of America*, 1970, **47**, 1557–1562.

Stevens, S. S. The measurement of loudness. *Journal of the Acoustical Society of America*, 1955, **27**, 815–829.

Stevens, S. S. On the psychological law. *Psychological Review*, 1957, **64**, 153–181.

Stevens, S. S. Procedure for calculating loudness, Mark VI. *Journal of the Acoustical Society of America*, 1961, **33**, 1577–1585.

Zwicker, E. Über psychologische und methodische Grundlagen der Lautheit. *Acustica*, 1958, **8** (Beiheft 1) 237–258.

Zwicker, E. A model describing temporal effects in loudness and threshold. *Reports of the VI International Congress on Acoustics, Tokyo*, 1968, S.A21–A24.

Zwicker, E. Der Einfluss der zeitlichen Struktur von Tönen auf die Addition von Teillautheiten *Acustica*, 1969, **21**, 16–25.

Zwicker, E. Masking and psychological excitation, as consequences of the ear's frequency analysis. In R. Plomp, & G. F. Smoorenburg (Eds.), *Frequency analysis and periodicity detection in hearing*. Leiden, The Netherlands: A. W. Sijthoff 1970, pp. 376–394.

Zwicker, E., & Feldtkeller, R. Über die Lautstärke von gleichförmigen Geräuschen. *Acustica*, 1955, **5**, 304–316.

Zwicker, E., & Feldtkeller, R. *Das Ohr als Nachrichtenempfänger* (2nd ed.), Stuttgart: Hirzel Verlag, 1967.

Zwicker, E., Flottorp, G., & Stevens, S. S. Critical band width in loudness summation. *Journal of the Acoustical Society of America*, 1957, **29**, 548–557.

Zwicker, E., & Scharf, B. A model of loudness summation. *Psychological Review*, 1965, **72**, 3–26.

PART III

VISION, TASTE, WARMTH

THE EFFECTS OF CAFFEINE ON TERMINAL DARK ADAPTATION[1]

A. LEONARD DIAMOND
Simon Fraser University

and

ESTHER M. SMITH
University of Hawaii

Abstract. The lower liminal threshold for light in the fovea was observed under the administration of: (*a*) 6 g of caffeine and (*b*) 9 g of calcium lactate placebo. The time-response relationship of the drug effect was observed for 80 min after dosage. The results showed that caffeine produced a highly significant reduction in the luminance necessary for terminal threshold perception. The course of the drug induced change was a decline in threshold luminance during the first 40 to 60 min. The maximum effect for four subjects averaged 0.23 logmL. The drop in threshold was maintained (except for fluctuations) for the remainder of the 80 min test session. Cyclical fluctuations in the response occurred in both control and caffeine conditions. Caffeine also counteracted a decrement in sensitivity which occurred during the latter part of placebo sessions.

Dark adaptation refers to the increase in the brightness sensitivity of the eye as a function of time in the dark. A psychophysical measurement of the sensitivity increase is obtained from judgments of least luminance perceptible at given points in time after cessation of light exposure. Thus, as sensitivity increases, threshold (least) luminance decreases. The initial portion of the dark adaptation function drops off rapidly and levels off in 6–10 min for foveal threshold (Diamond & Gilinsky, 1955; Johannsen, McBride, & Wulfeck, 1956). The latter part of the function determines the terminal threshold, at the portion of the curve where adaptation is essentially complete.

Characteristics of the dark adaptation function have been found to be dependent upon (*a*) stimulus conditions (Hillman, 1958; Hansen, Anderson, & Winterberg, 1960); (*b*) the adaptation of the eye (Hecht, Haig, & Chase, 1937; Mote & Riopelle, 1951; and Wolf, Zigler, & Cowen-Solomons, 1960); and (*c*) the physiological state of the individual (Hecht & Mandelbaum, 1939; McFarland, Roughton, Halperin, & Niven, (1944); Hecht, Hendley, Frank, & Haig, 1946). In the three latter experiments, visual threshold was employed as the dependent variable in studies designed to determine the effects on the organism of respiratory variables and drugs. Drugs have also been used in dark adaptation studies (Mandelbaum, 1941; Diamond & Cole, 1970) to test aspects of theories concerning photochemical processes and neural mechanisms underlying the visual response.

The use of drugs, including caffeine, as modifying agents of the physiological processes related to dark adaptation has a history of conflicting experimental results. Mandelbaum (1941) cites a comprehensive review by Adams (1929) of studies con-

[1] This work was supported by research grant NSF G9588 from the National Science Foundation.

H. R. Moskowitz et al. (eds.), Sensation and Measurement. 339–349. *All Rights Reserved.*

cerned with neurotropic drug effects on dark adaptation. Mandelbaum's evaluation of experimental methods employed indicates that the results of early research are not conclusive due to incomplete control of variables relevant to visual phenomena. In his own experiment, with appropriate visual controls, he studied the effects of caffeine on dark adaptation after exposure of the eye to a bright light (1500 mL for 3 min). No caffeine effect was observed in the entire function, obtained during 30 min of dark adaptation. The same results were found in a similar study by Rose & Schmidt (1947).

In contrast to the above results, Ditchburn & Power Steele (1941) found that caffeine increased the rate of dark adaptation during the first minute. Also, in a study by Diamond & Cole (1971) it was found that foveal terminal threshold (after 10 min of dark adaptation) was lower with caffeine than with placebo for the entire range of nine test-field areas. A double dose of caffeine, moreover, decreased threshold further.

The above contradictory findings suggest the possibility that conditions relevant to the phenomena being observed have not been controlled at times, thus preventing the isolation and measurement of the caffeine effect on visual threshold. Of the many controls that are necessary in visual threshold experiments (Hecht & Schlaer, 1938; McDonald, 1940; Mandelbaum, 1941), the studies described above meet the needed *visual* requirements. Evaluation in terms of controls pertinent to pharmacological effects is difficult since few are specified.

General factors cited as influencing the outcome of studies of drug effects are: the situational variables of behavior measurement, pharmacological variables, and characteristics of the organism (*Psychopharmacology Service Bulletin*, 1961). The latter factor (condition of the subject) is one which has particularly been left unspecified in the above dark adaptation studies. The condition of the individual includes state of health, age, body weight, prior and present activity, and the time relationship of dosage to food intake. In addition, other aspects of the subject to be considered are tolerance for caffeine (Winsor & Strongin, 1933; Womack & Cole, 1934), individual differences in reactivity (Kornetsky, Humphries, & Evarts, 1957), and the effects of suggestion and of the route of drug administration (Wolf, 1950). Wolf found that both drugs and placebo produced identical responses when administered by injection due to an adrenal reaction to the mode of administration. However, oral administration of drugs, where taste was controlled, produced differential effects for drug and placebo conditions. Mandelbaum (1941) and Rose & Schmidt (1947) used injections with no mention of a pre-test of subject reactions.

Ditchburn & Power Steele (1941) demonstrated the importance of control of tolerance for caffeine. They found no caffeine effect on dark adaptation for individuals who drank coffee frequently when given a dose as large as 8 g. However, the moderate coffee drinker showed a defiinite though small increase in the rate of dark adaptation when given doses of 6 to 10 g of caffeine.

Another variable which appeared relevant was proximity of food intake to drug administration. McFarland & Forbes (1941) found that food increased sensitivity to light in normal subjects tested before and after a meal, an effect in the same direction as that found for caffeine (Diamond & Cole, 1970).

In view of the above findings, reported in the literature, it was decided to study the effects of caffeine (as compared to a placebo condition) on the foveal threshold response at terminal threshold, with control of some relevant variables; namely, physical condition, tolerance for caffeine, food intake, route of drug administration and dose size. In addition, appropriate controls for visual and other pharmacological variables were included in the apparatus and in the design of the experiment.

To control for the many sources of variation in absolute threshold which occur from day to day (Wertheimer, 1955), dark adaptation curves were obtained in each session for 20 min prior to drug administration. This procedure established a daily base response to permit adjustment of the curves for day to day differences in response level, similar to the procedure used by McFarland & Evans (1939).

Method

Apparatus. The components of the apparatus were (*a*) the luminance sources and optical devices to vary the luminance of the test field as it appeared to the subject (see Figure 1) and (*b*) the adapting and test fields as seen by the subject.

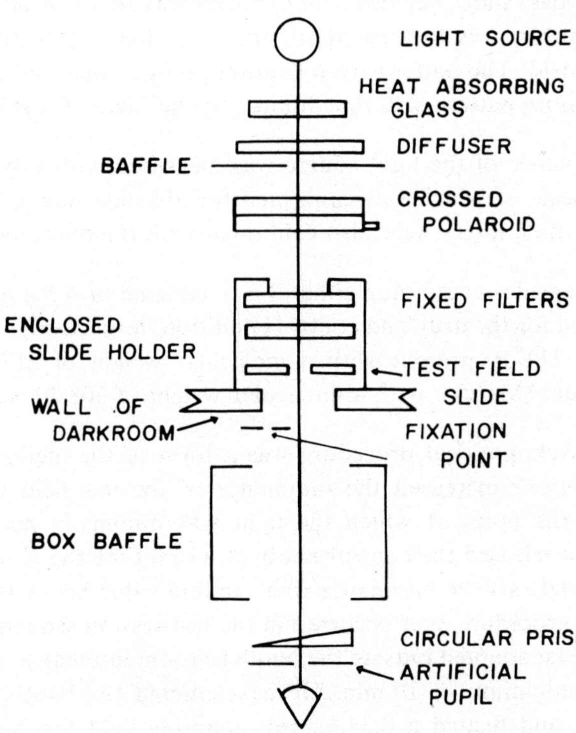

Fig. 1. Apparatus schematic.

Luminance controls. The luminance source for the test field was a 150 W projection lamp operated at 115 V and 1.3 A ac. The light path, in sequence from the lamp to the test field, included a section of heat-absorbing glass, a milk-white plastic diffuser, neutral density crossed-polaroids, and finally, neutral density Wratten filters. The polarizers, operated by the experimenter (*E*) or subject (*S*) reduced the luminance of the test field continuously over a calibrated range of 0.5 log units. The Wratten filters, inserted between the polarizers and the test field, changed test luminance in discrete steps over a range of 4.0 log units. The maximum luminance available at the test field was 2.97 log mL.

The experimental room was a blackened, light-tight booth. The box baffle (see Figure 1) prevented the possibility of any extraneous light reaching the eye. A chin rest, arm rest, and an adjustable chair permitted the *S* to maintain a steady comfortable position.

Pupil size was held constant by a 3 mm artificial pupil mounted in optical trial frames worn by the *S* during testing. All *S*s used only the right eye, the left was occluded.

Adapting and test fields. The light adapting field, located 2 ft to the *S*'s left, was $11° \times 14°$ of visual angle and had a luminance of 0.34 log mL. The circular test field 122 cm in front of the *S*'s eye, was defined by a hole punched in black paper which was mounted in a glass slide. The test-field diameter was 14′ of visual angle. A fixation point 1.0′ in diameter, was located 31′ in the nasal horizontal direction from the center of the test field. The pattern from fixation point to outer edge of the test field covered 40′, the entire pattern was thus limited to the fovea (Polyak, 1941).

Calibration. Luminance of the light source was measured with a Welch Densichron photometer, the scale of which was calibrated for absolute luminance. The crossed polarizers and Wratten filters were also calibrated with the photometer.

Drugs. Identical capsules containing either 3 g of caffeine or 4.5 g of calcium lactate (placebo) were used for the drug and control condition, respectively. Caffeine alkaloid (Merck), hydrous U.S.P. powder with a molecular weight of 212.21 and calcium lactate, N.F. powder (Merck), with a molecular weight of 308.30 were used.

Procedure. The psychophysical procedure was a form of the method of adjustment (Stevens, 1951). The *S* increased the luminance of the test field from well below threshold just to the point at which the light was minimally perceived. He then signalled the *E* and released the control knob, at which time the *E* read the polarizer scale and immediately set the luminance to a random value below threshold.

The adaptation procedure as it occurred in the test-session sequence of events was as follows: The *S* first adapted outside the booth to room luminance of approximately 1.0 log mL for a minimum of 10 min. He next entered the booth, sat down, then turned to his left, and fixated a 0.34 log mL adapting field for 2 min. During this light adaptation time the *S* adjusted his trial frames in which the artificial pupil was mounted. The adapting light was turned off and the *S* began making judgments immediately. From two to six responses a min were made during 7-min test periods, with a rest of 3 min between each period. Judgments were recorded for 100 min after the end of light adaptation. In each session two capsules of caffeine (6 g) or calcium lactate (9 g) were administered 20 min after the light adaptation.

In pre-experimental training, *S*s were instructed to hold their visual fixation constant, except for necessary blinking, to turn the polarizer control slowly to avoid overshooting the point where light was first visible, and to maintain the same criteria for the threshold response in terms of amount of light responded to. Judgments where overshooting had occurred were not signalled; the *S* reduced the luminance and made another judgment. Overshooting rarely occurred after the training sessions. Practice continued until the standard deviation (SD) of the responses became consistent for this procedure at about 0.06 log mL.

Pharmacological controls. Conditions of drug administration were stabilized as follows. A single blind technique was used to control effects of suggestion in that the drug and placebo were not identifiable by the *S* and he was not informed, and a cross-over design was used in which each *S* served as his own control to give validity to individual comparisons. Drugs were given orally with 5 oz of water. Only one condition (drug or placebo) was observed on each day. Conditions were assigned randomly over days. A base measure of threshold was obtained each day in the first 20 min of the test sessions, prior to the introduction of drugs or placebo conditions to permit adjustment of the data for day-to-day differences in the response level, independently of the drug effect.

The condition of the *S* was controlled with regard to the following factors: fatigue, lack of sleep, anxiety, illness, medication, and use of dietary items containing xanthines. The *S* was instructed to avoid or report occurrences of these factors, and data obtained under such conditions were eliminated. Test sessions were scheduled a minimum of 2 h after the last meal. *S* KVE was given caffeine 2.5 h after lunch, the other *S*s were tested 3 h or longer after the previous meal. Two *S*s, KVE and RS, rarely used xanthine-containing dietary items; EG normally had 2 cups of coffee a day, AE usually drank 5 cups a day. All *S*s omitted such items from their diet for 12 h prior to testing.

Results

Figure 2 shows the course of dark adaptation in the fovea for each *S* under two conditions, caffeine and placebo (non-caffeine) administration, as a function of time. The ordinates of the points on the graphs represent the minimum luminance of the test field necessary for perception of the stimulus. Along the abscissa is plotted time after cessation of the adapting light. The time at which the drug condition was introduced is indicated by an ordinate at the 20-min point. Each point on a curve represents the average of data collected during successive 5-min intervals and is a mean of 10 to 30 separate determinations of threshold.

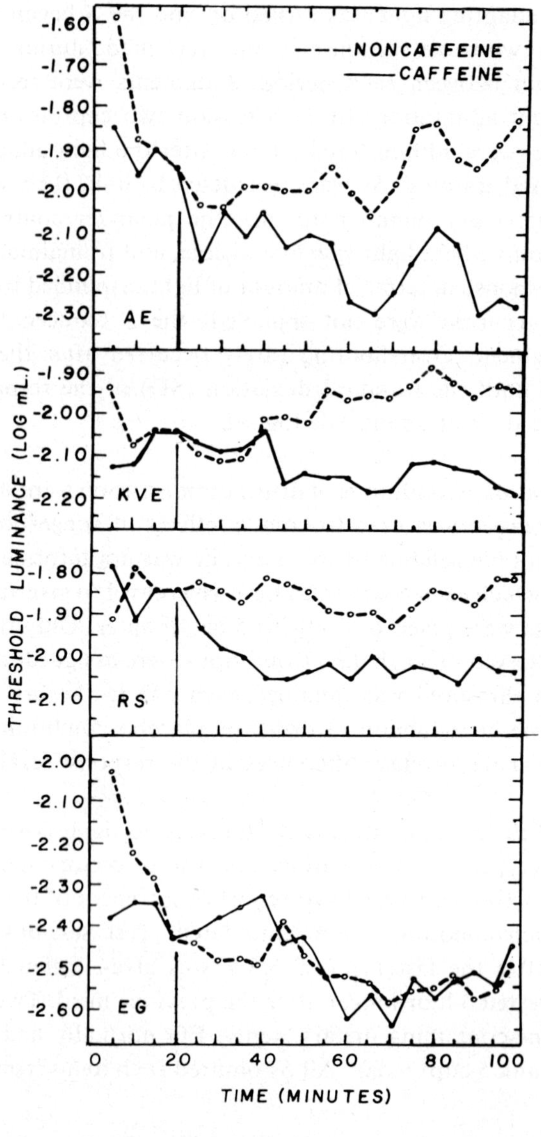

Fig. 2. The effect of caffeine on threshold luminance as a function of time for each *S*.

The entire caffeine and non-caffeine curves were shifted to superimpose the pre-drug threshold points obtained at 20 min of dark adaptation so as to adjust curves for day to day differences in absolute threshold.

The major features of the threshold functions are: (*a*) the separation of the caffeine and non-caffeine curves which occur as early as 5 min after administration for AE and RS, at 25 min after dosage for KVE, indicating an increase in sensitivity to light following administration of caffeine; (*b*) the increasing separation of the caffeine

TABLE 1

Mean threshold luminances for caffeine (C) and noncaffeine (NC) conditions

	Subjects									
	AE		KVE		RS		TG		Average	
	C	NC	C	NC	C	NC	C	NC	C	NC
Min	Log mL									
5	−3.65	−3.39	−3.91	−3.72	−3.70	−3.57	−4.16	−3.81	−3.85	−3.74
10	−3.77	−3.68	−3.89	−3.85	−3.58	−3.70	−4.13	−4.01	−3.84	−3.81
15	−3.71	−3.71	−3.85	−3.82	−3.63	−3.63	−4.14	−4.08	−3.82	−3.81
20	−3.75	−3.75	−3.81	−3.81	−3.63	−3.63	−4.22	−4.22	−3.84	−3.84
25	−3.97	−3.84	−3.85	−3.86	−3.72	−3.61	−4.20	−4.23	−3.89	−3.87
30	−3.84	−3.83	−3.87	−3.88	−3.77	−3.63	−4.17	−5.27	−3.88	−3.89
35	−3.91	−3.79	−3.86	−3.88	−3.79	−3.66	−4.15	−4.27	−3.90	−3.87
40	−3.85	−3.79	−3.80	−3.78	−3.84	−3.60	−4.12	−4.28	−3.86	−3.84
45	−3.93	−3.80	−3.94	−3.78	−3.84	−3.62	−4.24	−4.18	−3.96	−3.83
50	−3.90	−3.80	−3.92	−3.79	−3.83	−3.64	−4.22	−4.27	−3.93	−3.85
55	−3.92	−3.74	−3.93	−3.71	−3.81	−3.68	−4.31	−4.31	−3.96	−3.82
60	−4.06	−3.80	−3.93	−3.74	−3.84	−3.69	−4.41	−4.30	−4.01	−3.85
65	−4.09	−3.86	−3.96	−3.73	−3.79	−3.69	−4.35	−4.33	−4.00	−3.86
70	−4.04	−3.78	−3.95	−3.73	−3.73	−3.84	−3.71	−4.42	−4.38	−4.02
75	−3.97	−3.64	−3.88	−3.71	−3.82	−3.67	−4.31	−4.31	−3.93	−3.81
80	−3.88	−3.63	−3.88	−3.67	−3.83	−3.63	−4.34	−4.33	−3.94	−3.78
85	−3.92	−3.72	−3.89	−3.70	−3.70	−3.85	−3.64	−4.31	−3.95	−3.80
90	−4.09	−3.74	−3.90	−3.73	−3.79	−3.66	−4.30	−4.36	−3.95	−3.84
95	−4.05	−3.68	−3.94	−3.70	−3.82	−3.60	−4.33	−4.34	−3.99	−3.80
100	−4.06	−3.62	−3.96	−3.70	−3.82	−3.60	−4.24	−4.27	−3.95	−3.78

Note: Caffeine administered at 20 min. Differences between caffeine and non-caffeine means larger than 0.09 logmL are significant beyond the 0.01 level of confidence.

and non-caffeine curves for AE, KVE and RS due both to a continued decline of the caffeine curve and to a rise in the placebo curves, and (*c*) a 20- to 30-min cycling effect, appearing in both the control and caffeine curves after 45 min of dark adaptation.

The separation of the paired functions is significant at the 0.01 level of significance at 5 min after administration of caffeine for AE and RS and at 25 min after dosage for KVE. All differences between drug and placebo curves of 0.09 log units or larger were found to be significant beyond the 0.01 level of probability using Student's one-tailed t test (Edwards, 1960). Table 1 presents the means for each S at 5-min intervals.

The data for EG differ from that for the first three Ss in two respects: (*a*) the placebo curves for EG are similar to the caffeine curves in that the threshold continues to drop over time and to almost the same extent as in the drug condition and (*b*) the caffeine curve drops below the control curve only between 60 and 70 min, and the separation at these points is not significant. There was no consistent change in

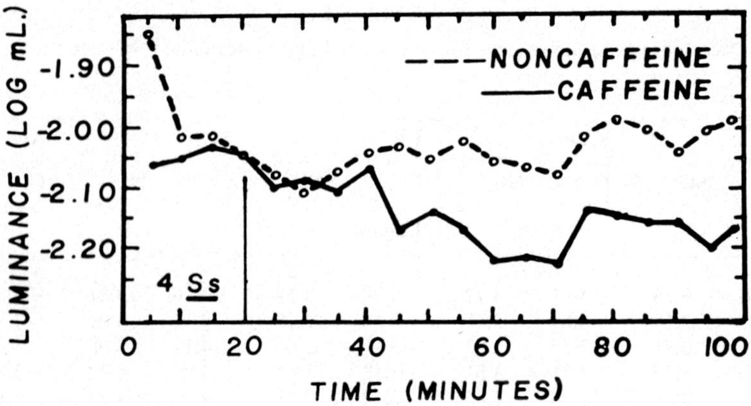

Fig. 3. The effect of caffeine on threshold luminance as a function of time. Average curve over 4 *S*s.

variability associated with the use of caffeine or duration of the test session for any of the *S*s.

In Figure 3 are shown the average curves for 4 *S*s. Corresponding values are given in Table 1. The complete absence of overlap between the caffeine and non-caffeine curves, after the drug action occurs, indicates a highly significant difference between the two functions (beyond the 0.01 level of confidence).

Discussion

The present experiment was carried out to test further the effect of caffeine on terminal visual threshold, particularly with respect to time after the administration of the drug.

The results show first that Mandelbaum's generalization that caffeine does not affect the dark adaptation curve does not hold in all situations. Not only is the early part of the curve affected by caffeine as found in the Ditchburn *et al.* study, but it significantly affects the terminal portion of the curve as shown in the present experiment. Why Mandelbaum did not get a caffeine effect and why our experiment did might be explained in terms of the individual differences obvious in our own results in Figure 2. That is, not all *S*s showed a separation between drug and placebo curves. In other words, Mandelbaum, who used only two *S*s, could easily have selected ones who were not susceptible to caffeine, or for whom the experimental situation involved some form of increased activation with lowering of threshold during the placebo condition as well as during the caffeine condition.

What the variables are that might make for these individual differences are not clearly evident at this time, although one pertinent variable is suggested by the present data. That is, the results seem to show that the sooner caffeine administration follows eating, the more the effect is delayed. In Figure 4 are plotted data from a pilot study combined with data from the present experiment. The latency of the caffeine effect (time of threshold drop after drug administration) is plotted as a function of time

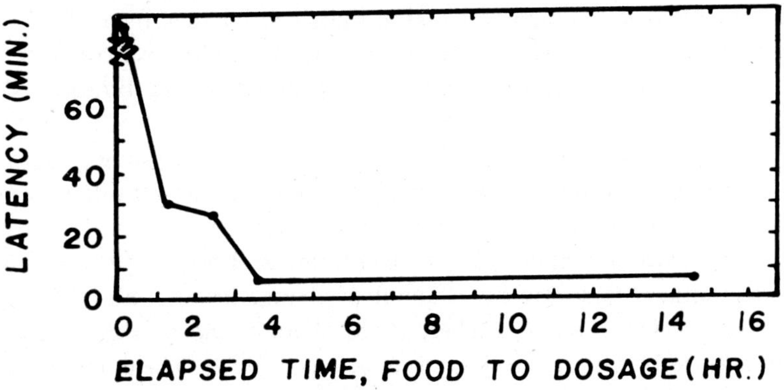

Fig. 4. Latency of threshold drop as a function of time after eating. Average curve over 4 *S*s.

after eating. It appears that latency decreases as time after eating increases. Since all points on the curve are not taken from the same *S*, this experiment will have to be repeated, but it does suggest that proximity of food intake to drug administration might change caffeine effectiveness.

Other factors that might account for inter-subject variability are the individual differences in drug reaction such as (*a*) the large differences found to occur in the rate of absorption and elimination of caffeine (Axelrod & Reichenthal, 1953), (*b*) the presence of a conditioned mode of response set up prior to the use of placebo conditions such that no difference between drug and control results is obtained and (*c*) the existence of a state of stress, anxiety or other excitation which prevents the detection of a drug reaction in the same direction (Wolf, 1941).

Other interesting phenomena seen in our data include (*a*) a rise in the control curves after 40 to 60 min of adaptation and (*b*) the cycling of threshold in the terminal portion of both the control and caffeine curves.

The rise in the control curves found for three *S*s was also found in Wertheimer's (1955) data. A study by Domey, McFarland, & Chadwick (1960) shows a rise in threshold near the end of a 40-min function to be a characteristic only of the curves for a 20 to 29 yr age group. All other groups (from 10 to 90 yr of age) showed level or gradually declining curve terminals.

The cycling frequently occurs after about 45 min of repeated threshold judgments and is shown as 20- to 30-min fluctuations superimposed on the general trend of each function. These cycles did not appear to be eliminated by caffeine. They did not always occur at a constant time in the daily curves and tend to be averaged out somewhat in the curves presented but are reliable effects for each *S*. Subjective reports suggest that periods of sleepiness and wakefulness might account for these fluctuations.

All of the fluctuations in threshold found in the above cited experiments and in the present experiment seemed to indicate a necessity for comparing the effect of caffeine at any given time in a test session with a placebo threshold response obtained at the same time in a similar session rather than with a threshold obtained prior to administration of the drug. Actually, a highly significant change from the 20-min pre-drug threshold occurred in the caffeine curves for all *S*s. However, the time-response curves also serve to demonstrate time of onset, peak effect and duration of the drug reaction and *S* differences in reactivity.

The use of calcium lactate as a placebo had no effect on threshold. Control curves obtained in a pilot study in which no capsules were given did not differ from placebo curves. The 5 oz of water given, likewise had no effect.

The extent of the caffeine-induced change at terminal threshold (0.10 to 0.33 log mL below control data) is less than the amount of change brought about by age, a rise of 0.40 log units (McFarland & Fisher, 1955). Anoxia and insulin raised threshold 0.50 log units (Wald, Harper, Goodman, & Krieger, 1942). The comparative magnitude and direction of the caffeine change indicate that, with the dose used, while a highly significant increase in sensitivity is obtained, the extent of the effect is not indicative of an extreme shift in physiological balance or neural functioning.

References

Adams, D. Dark adaption (a review of the literature). *Medical Research Council, Special Report Series*. 1929, No. 127.

Axelrod, J., & Reichenthal, J. The fate of caffeine in man and a method for its estimation in biological material. *Journal of Pharmacology and Experimental Therapeutics*, 1953, **107**, 519–523.

Diamond, A. L. & Cole, R. E. Visual threshold as a function of test area and coffeine administration, *Psychonomic Science*, 1970, **20**, 109–111.

Diamond, A. L., & Gilinsky, A. S. Dark-adaptation luminance thresholds for the resolution of detail following different durations of light adaptation. *Journal of Experimental Psychology*, 1955, **50** 134–143.

Ditchburn, R. W., & Power Steele, E. J. Effect of caffeine and bromide on dark adaption. *Nature*, 1941, **147**, 745–746.

Domey, R. G., McFarland, R. A., & Chadwick, E. Dark adaptation as a function of age and time: II. A derivation. *Journal of Gerontology*, 1960, **15**, 267–282.

Edwards, A. L. *Experimental design in psychological research*. New York: Rinehart, 1960.

Hansen, J. A., Anderson, E. M. S., & Winterberg, R. P. Studies on dark adaption. V: Effect of various sizes of centrally fixated pre-exposure fields on foveal and peripheral dark adaptation. *Journal of the Optical Society of America*, 1960, **50**, 895–899.

Hecht, S., Haig, C., & Chase, A. M. The influence of light adaptation on subsequent dark adaptation of the eye. *Journal of General Physiology*, 1937, **20**, 831–850.

Hecht, S., Hendley, C. D., Frank, S. R., & Haig, C. Anoxia and brightness discrimination. *Journal of General Physiology*, 1946, **29**, 335–351.

Hecht, S., & Mandelbaum, J. The relation between vitamin A and dark adaptation. *Journal of the Americal Medical Association*, 1939, **112**, 1910–1916.

Hecht, S., & Schlaer, S. An adaptometer for measuring human dark adaptation. *Journal of the Optical Society of America*, 1938, **28**, 269–275.

Hillman, B. M. Relationship between stimulus size and threshold intensity in the fovea measured at four exposure times, *Journal of the Optical Society of America*, 1958, **48**, 422–428.

Johannsen, D. E., McBride, P. I., & Wulfeck, J. W. Studies on dark adaptation. I: The pre-exposure tolerance of the dark-adapted fovea. *Journal of the Optical Society of America*, 1956, **46**, 67–71. (a)

Johannsen, D. E., McBride, P. I., & Wulfeck, J. W. Studies on dark adaptation. II: The pre-exposure tolerance of the human fovea adapted to different brightness levels. *Journal of the Optical Society of America*, 1956, **46**, 266–269. (b)

Kornetsky, C., Humphries, O., & Evarts, E. V. Comparison of psychological effects of certain centrally acting drugs in man. *Archives of Neurology and Psychiatry*, 1957, **77**, 318–323.

Mandelbaum, J. Dark adaptation: Some physiologic and clinical considerations. *Archives of Opthalmology*, 1941, **26**, 203–239.

McDonald, R. Some basic principles of dark adaptation. *Archives of Opthalmology*, 1940, **23**, 841–851.

McFarland, R. A., & Evans, J. N. Alterations in dark adaptation under reduced oxygen tensions. *American Journal of Physiology*, 1939, **127**, 37–50.

McFarland, R. A., & Fisher, M. B. Alterations in dark adaptation as a function of age. *Journal of Gerontology*, 1955, **10**, 424–428.

McFarland, R. A., & Forbes, W. H. The effects of variations in the concentration of oxygen and of glucose on dark adaptation. *Journal of General Physiology*, 1940, **24**, 69–98.

McFarland, R. A., Roughton, F. J. W., Halperin, M. H., & Niven, J. I. The effects of carbon monoxide and altitude on visual thresholds. *Journal of Aviation Medicine*, 1944, **15**, 381–394.

Mote, F. A., & Riopelle, A. J. The effect of varying the intensity and the duration of pre-exposure upon foveal dark adaptation in the human eye. *Journal of General Physiology*, 1951, **34**, 657–674.

National Institute of Health, *Psychopharmacology Service Center Bulletin*, 1961.

Polyak, S. L. *The retina*. Chicago: University of Chicago Press, 1941.

Rose, H. W., & Schmidt, I. Factors affecting dark adaptation. *Journal of Aviation Medicine*, 1947, **18**, 218–230.

Stevens, S. S. *Handbook of experimental psychology*. New York: John Wiley, 1951.

Wald, G., Harper, P. V., Goodman, H. C., & Krieger, H. P. Respiratory effects upon the visual threshold. *Journal of General Physiology*, 1942, **25**, 891–904.

Wertheimer, M. The variability of auditory and visual absolute thresholds in time. *Journal of General Psychology*, 1955, **52**, 111–147.

Winsor, A. L., & Strongin, E. I. A study of the development of tolerance for caffeinated beverages *Journal of Experimental Psychology*, 1933, **16**, 725–734.

Wolf, E., Zigler, M. J., & Cowen-Solomons, H. B. Variability of dark adaptation. *Journal of the Optical Society of America*, 1960, **50**, 961–965.

Wolf, S. Effects of suggestion and conditioning on the action of chemical agents in human subjects – The pharmacology of placebos. *Journal of Clinical Investigation*, 1950, **29**, 100–109.

Womack, N. A., & Cole, W. H. Effect of caffeine on basal metabolism. *Proceedings of the Society for Experimental Biology and Medicine*, 1934, **31**, 1248–1250.

SCALING OF SATURATION AND HUE SHIFT: SUMMARY OF RESULTS AND IMPLICATIONS

TAROW INDOW

Keio University, Tokyo, Japan

Abstract. The results were reviewed of experiments in which a difference scale ψ_D, based upon equisection, and a magnitude scale ψ_M, based upon ratio judgments, were constructed for saturation of various hues as well as for hue shift between two adjacent primary hues of aperture colors. The same nonlinearity between ψ_D and ψ_M as in prothetic continua was found for the saturation and the hue shift; this seems to suggest that saturation is a quantitative change of balance between two components, chromatic and achromatic, and that the hue shift is between the two primary hue components. A number of anomalous results were observed with yellow. The implications of these results for opponent color theory are discussed.

Two Kinds of Scales: φ_M and φ_D

The following empirical fact has been made indisputably clear by the late S. S. Stevens. For the sensory attribute corresponding to a stimulus continuum φ, we have to distinguish different types of scales $\psi(\varphi)$[1] according to what kind of judgment we wish to predict from $\psi(\varphi)$, because one $\psi(\varphi)$ is in general not linearly related to another $\psi(\varphi)$. In the present article, two types of unidimensional scales are discussed in relation to saturation and hue of colors.

Difference scale $\psi_D(\varphi)$: Whenever $[\psi_D(\varphi_i)-\psi_D(\varphi_j)]\geqslant[\psi_D(\varphi_k)-\psi_D(\varphi_l)]$, we would expect the perceptual difference between φ_i and φ_j to be judged larger than, or equal to, the perceptual difference between φ_k and φ_l.

Magnitude scale $\psi_M(\varphi)$: Whenever $\psi_M(\varphi_i)/\psi_M(\varphi_j)=r\,(r>0)$, we would expect the perceptual ratio of φ_i to φ_j to be judged equal to r.

According to the well-known classification of scales in terms of admissible transformation, which was also introduced by Stevens (1946, 1951), ψ_D must be regarded as an interval scale (I) and ψ_M as a ratio scale (R). Somewhat contrary to common expectation, however, abundant experimental evidence has been accumulated by Stevens to show that ψ_M and ψ_D are in general not linearly related, and when ψ_D is plotted against ψ_M, the relationship is convex upward. Stevens also found the same nonlinearity between ψ_D and ψ_M with nonsensory continua such as the seriousness of crime (Stevens, 1966). The situation is different with the pitch of tones (Stevens & Volkmann, 1940). Stevens coined the term *metathetic* to describe continua on which ψ_D is found to be linearly related to ψ_M, and he once conjectured that qualitative sensory attributes such as saturation of color would belong to that group (Stevens & Volkmann, 1940). However, in later articles, he carefully omitted reference to satura-

[1] The notation favored by Stevens, φ for a physical process and ψ for a psychological process, is used in the present article.

H. R. Moskowitz et al. (eds.), Sensation and Measurement. 351–362. *All Rights Reserved.*

tion when he listed examples of metathetic continua (e.g., Stevens, 1957; Stevens & Galanter, 1957), and in later experiments a similar nonlinearity between ψ_D and ψ_M was observed for saturation (Indow, 1967; Indow & Stevens, 1966; Panek & Stevens, 1966) as well as for hue (Indow & Stevens, 1966). From the standpoint of admissible transformations, ratio scales R must be included as a special case of interval scales I, and hence the relationship among the four types of scales can be schematized as in Figure 1. Remember that R vs I and ψ_M vs ψ_D are distinctions in terms of two entirely different principles.

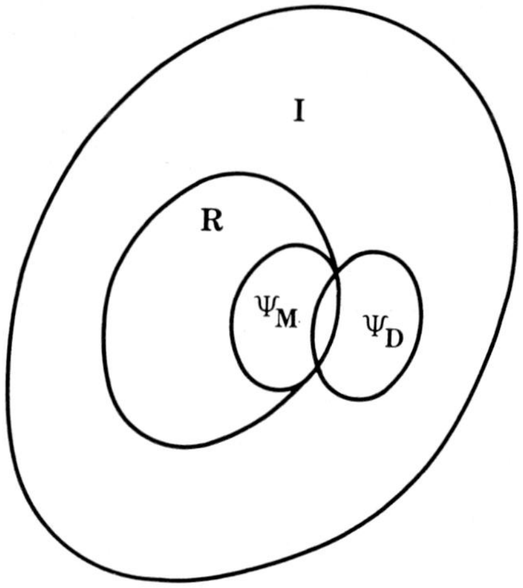

Fig. 1. Relationship among interval (I), ratio (R), magnitude (ψ_M) and difference (ψ_D) scales.

In the domain of colorimetry and color science, interest has been exclusively focussed upon $\psi_D(\varphi)$. A number of formulas for color difference have been developed to predict the perceptual difference between two given colors (e.g., Vos, Friele, & Walraven, 1972; Wyszecki & Stiles, 1967). The color samples of the Munsell system are based on the principle that two neighboring samples along a given dimension differ perceptually by the same amount (Newhall, 1940; Newhall, Nickerson, & Judd, 1943). That circumstance presumably results because the impression of difference is a natural consequence of viewing two object colors simultaneously or in succession. In fact, it is impossible to define a simple ratio when two colors differ in more than one attribute. On the other hand, a ratio judgment is not impossible between two colors that differ with respect to one attribute only. The impression of ratio is especially natural and vivid when the brightness of the illumination or of the aperture color is changed from one level to another, and many investigators have undertaken the ratio scaling of brightness (for example, Bartleson & Breneman, 1967, 1973; Hanes, 1949a, b; Onley, 1960; J. C. Stevens & S. S. Stevens, 1963). Similarly, $\psi_M(\varphi)$ of saturation has been investigated with aperture colors by Galifret (1959), Indow (1967 and in preparation), Indow & Stevens (1966), Onley (1963), Panek & Stevens (1966), and with object colors by Mattiello & Guirao (1973) and Ohsumi (1968).

For the continuous shift of hue between two adjacent primary hues both $\psi_D(\varphi)$ and $\psi_M(\varphi)$ were also obtained by Indow & Stevens (1966) and Indow (in preparation). For example, when an aperture color changes from red to yellow through orange while the brightness is kept constant, ψ may represent either the redness or the yellowness in the intermediate hue. In the section to follow, some of the results obtained by the author in the above-mentioned studies will be reviewed.[2] In the scaling of saturation the dominant wavelength (λ_d) and the luminance[3] (Y) of the color stimulus were kept constant, and φ represents the colorimetric purity P_c unless otherwise stated. In the scaling of hue shift, two color stimuli corresponding to the adjacent primary hues were mixed, both of which were very close to 100% in P_c and had the same value of Y. In this case, φ represents the mixture ratio of the stimulus corresponding to the primary hue that is represented by ψ. According to the mixture ratio, the hue of the color shifts along the spectrum locus while Y is held constant. The scaling of the two continua, saturation and hue shift, is parallel in effect because ψ represents a change to a highly saturated color of a given hue, either from the achromatic color or from the adjacent hue, and φ represents the mixture ratio of the color stimulus, either with white light or with the other color stimulus.

Scales of Saturation and Hue Shift

1. For both saturation and hue shift, $\psi_M(\varphi)$ is approximated quite well by a power function of φ, no matter what method is employed to obtain ψ_M. Hereafter the exponent of $\psi_M(\varphi)$ is denoted by β. In order to give some idea about the data of individual *S*s, three examples of data, for both saturation and hue shift, are shown in Figure 2. Each sample represents a different degree of goodness of fit. These data were obtained with aperture color by the method in which the *S* freely varied φ and assigned numbers proportional to the impression at issue (Marks & J. C. Stevens, 1966; J. C. Stevens & Guirao, 1964). Examples for object colors are given in Figure 3, where φ represents Munsell chroma C. Though C is said to be approximately proportional to P_c, with a constant that varies according to λ_d and Y (Judd & Nickerson, 1967), at least for each of these colors, C is approximated by a power function of P_c with an exponent whose value is not unity. Hence, $\psi_M(\varphi)$ for P_c is also a power function, but with an exponent of different value, as shown in Figure 3. The following facts are noteworthy.

1.1. The absolute threshold φ_0 is fairly high for saturation and hue shift, so that the points in the lower left corner of the plots of Figure 2 are very close to the level of φ_0. Nevertheless, since the $\log \psi_M$ was throughout linearly related to $\log \varphi$, it was not necessary to make any "threshold correction" (e.g., subtract φ_0 from φ) to establish

[2] Through the courtesy of Professor Stevens, the author had an opportunity to carry out an additional experiment in the Laboratory of Psychophysics in June 1972, which will be reported elsewhere in the near future under the title, Scaling of saturation and hue in the extraspectral region.

[3] As suggested by Stevens, Y is denoted in dB re 10^{-10} L, and hence 70 dB corresponds to 1 mL.

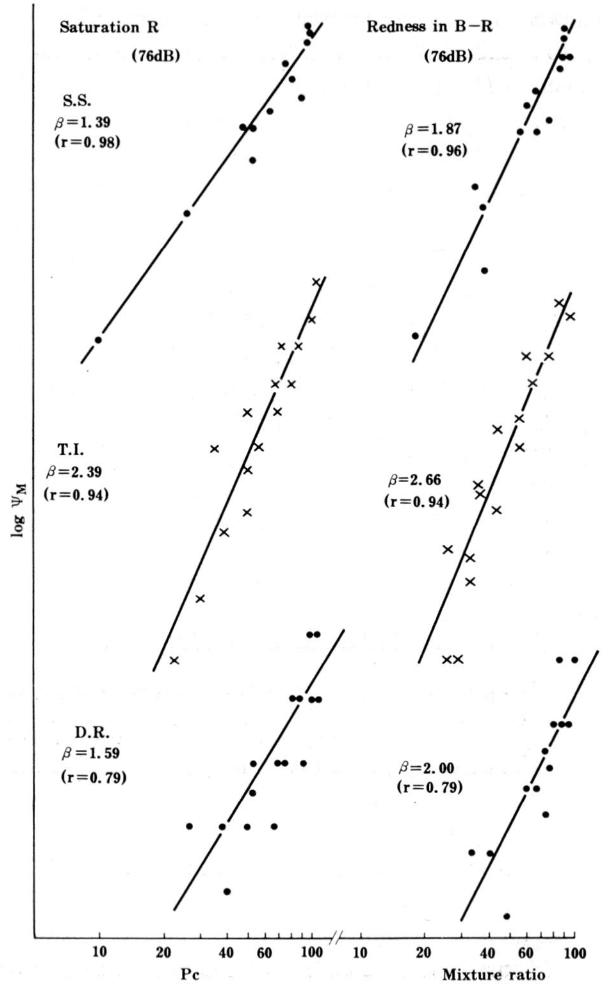

Fig. 2. Examples of individual power functions $\psi_M(\varphi)$ where φ represents colorimetric purity for the saturation of red or the mixture ratio of a red stimulus ($\lambda_d = 632$ nm) for a hue shift from blue to red (Indow, in preparation). The value of the exponent β of $\psi_M(\varphi)$ is given in each case. Goodness of fit is given in terms of the correlation coefficient r between log ψ_M and logφ. The examples represent three levels of fit of all the data obtained: good, medium, and poor.

the power relation. (For some continua such a correction is apparently necessary, but not here.)

1.2. That $\psi_M(\varphi)$ is a power function of P_c holds for saturation not only of primary hues but also of intermediate hues such as magenta and violet.

1.3. That $\psi_M(\varphi)$ is a power function of the mixture ratio holds for hue shift, not only

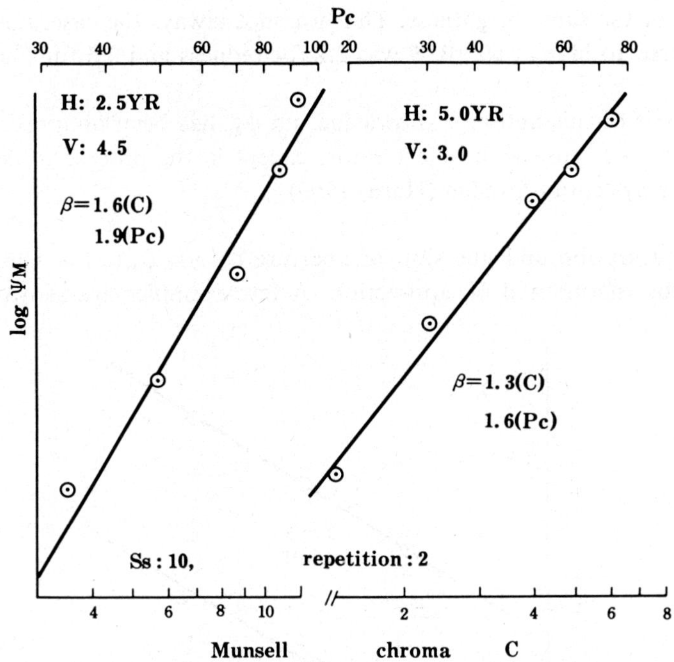

Fig. 3. Saturation $\psi_M(\varphi)$ of object colors obtained by magnitude estimation, where the abscissa φ represents Munsell chroma C (Ohsumi, 1968). The relation between C and colorimetric purity P_c is also shown. As C is approximated by a power function of P_c, $\log \psi_M$ is still linear to $\log P_c$, but the exponent β changes when plotted against $\log P_c$. Both values of β are given.

along the spectral locus but also in the extra spectral region from red to blue through magenta and violet.

1.4. The value of β for saturation varies systematically according to λ_d and Y, and the value for hue shift varies according to the pair of adjacent primary hues and Y. It goes without saying that the value of β could not be completely free of the experimental procedure used to obtain $\psi_M(\varphi)$, and individual differences were also fairly large, as is clear from the examples in Figure 2. However, it has invariably been found true with the colors used in the experiments that $\beta > 1$, which implies that the dynamic range of the stimulus is expanded in these sense modalities. For the saturation of yellow, β even reaches as high as 5, and it is not rare for other hues that $\beta > 2$. Compared with β of the more than 20 power functions that Stevens has reported for other sense modalities (1960, 1961, 1962, 1967), the situation is extraordinary. Note that β is dimensionless and therefore directly comparable across different modalities.

1.5. For hue shift, the values of β for the two primary hue components were almost the same in some cases. For example, β was 2.0 for redness and 1.9 for yellowness in an orange of 81 dB. Moreover, those values were very close to the 1.8 for the saturation of a red of the same brightness. That was not always the case, however. In the change from red to blue at 69 dB, β was 2.2 for redness and 3.3 for blueness.

1.6. To the best of this author's knowledge, no ψ_M has been obtained for hue shift in the above-stated sense with object colors except in the process of developing the Natural Color System in Sweden (Hard, 1969).

2. For both saturation and hue shift of aperture colors, $\psi_D(\varphi)$ is a linear function when scaled by the method of equisection. A few examples are shown in Figure 4

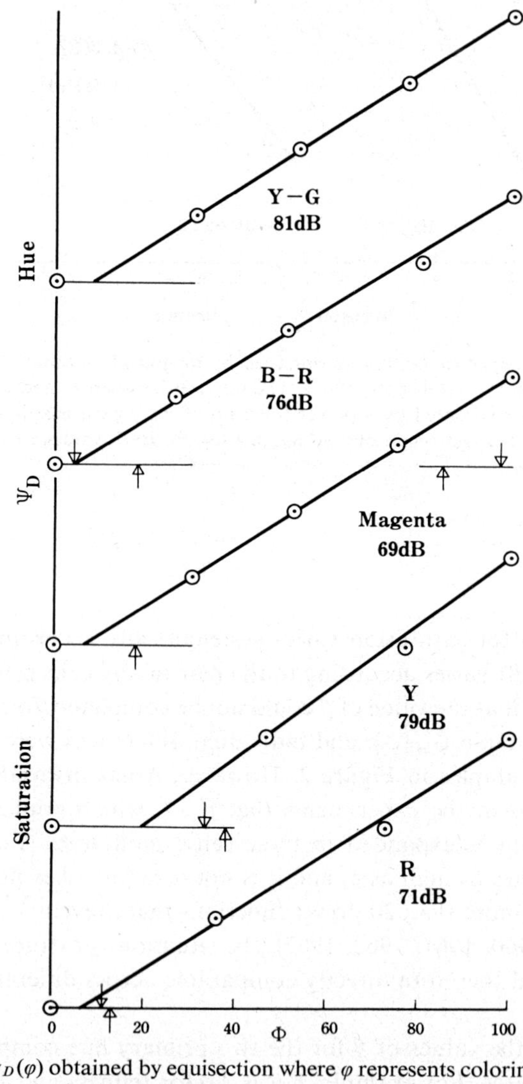

Fig. 4. Examples of $\psi_D(\varphi)$ obtained by equisection where φ represents colorimetric purity for saturation and the mixture ratio for hue shift (Indow in preparation; Indow and Stevens, 1966). The arrows represent absolute thresholds by the method of limits.

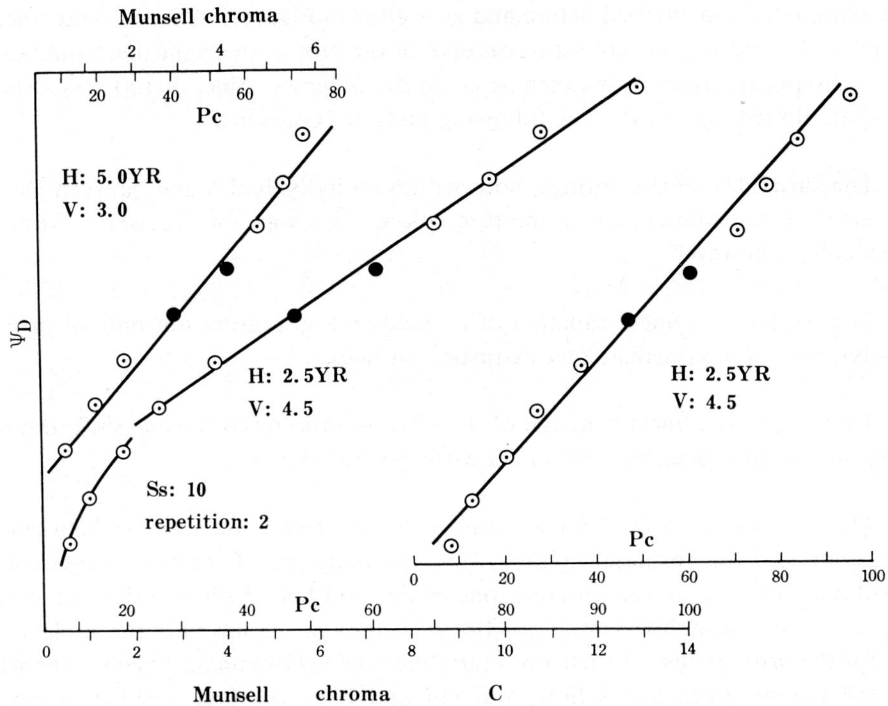

Fig. 5. Saturation $\psi_D(\varphi)$ of object colors where φ represents Munsell chroma C at the left and colorimetric purity P_c at the right (Ohsumi, 1968). The nonlinearity of 2.5 YR in the left-hand plot almost vanishes in the right-hand plot. Two colors shown by circles, were fixed and $\psi_D(\varphi)$ was obtained by extrapolations on both sides.

from results obtained when the stimuli at the two ends were set at 0 and 100 in P_c or in the mixture ratio. The spatial order was counterbalanced by setting 100 once at the left and once at the right. As there was no substantial difference in results between the two spatial orders, only averages are shown in Figure 4. Absolute thresholds determined by the method of limits are shown by arrows, pointing down for the descending series and up for the ascending series. Since the Munsell hue steps in the chromaticity diagram are fairly uniform between two adjacent primary hues, the linearity between ψ_D and φ for hue shift appears to hold for object colors. Since two series of colored papers happened to be available, in which C changed with extremely fine gradations and H and V were practically constant, a modified form of equisection was applied to obtain ψ_D for saturation, and the results are shown in Figure 5. Instead of fixing colors at both ends, a pair of colors denoted by the filled circles in the center of Figure 5 served as the standards, and the colors were selected so as to form a perceptually uniform series as a whole. The number of colors to be placed on both sides of the standard pair was at the subject's (S) disposal. In other words, the series was constructed through extrapolation rather than interpolation. Except for the region of very desaturated colors as in the example shown at the left, ψ_D is linear against

C as expected. As mentioned before and as is clear in Figure 5, C is not quite linearly related to P_c, and it is of interest to observe in the plot at the right that nonlinearity almost disappears when P_c is taken as φ. In the other example, $\psi_D(\varphi)$ was also linear when plotted against P_c. The following facts are noteworthy.

2.1. The variability of the settings, both within an individual S and between Ss, was very small in the equisection of aperture colors. This was not necessarily true with object colors, however.

2.2. That $\psi_D(\varphi)$ is a linear function of P_c holds for saturation not only of primary hues but also of intermediate and extraspectral hues.

2.3. That $\psi_D(\varphi)$ is a linear function of the mixture ratio holds for hue shift, not only along the spectral locus but also in the extraspectral region.

2.4. The straight line $\psi_D(\varphi)$ for aperture color intersects the abscissa between the point $\varphi=0$ and the absolute threshold, i.e., the midpoint of the two arrows. In the case of hue shift, that is true with only one component hue. With the other component hue, ψ_D passes through the point $\varphi=100$ even though the absolute threshold is not zero for the primary hue. If such a primary hue is called dominant, then for the pairs, red and yellow, green and yellow, and red and blue, the first member is always, dominant. The dominant hue seems to be analogous to the spectral color in saturation whereas the subordinate hue is analogous to the achromatic color.

2.5. As with the value of β (1.4), yellow behaves differently from the other colors. Its absolute threshold is extraordinarily high. Nevertheless the linearity of $\psi_D(\varphi)$ still holds.

2.6. Except for yellow, the slope of the straight line $\psi_D(\varphi)$ in terms of P_c does not vary much with λ_d and Y.

3. As stated in Sections 1.4 and 2, for both saturation and hue shift, each $\psi_M(\varphi)$ is an accelerated function of φ, whereas $\psi_D(\varphi)$ is a linear function of φ. Consequently, $\psi_M(\varphi)$ is convex downward when plotted against $\psi_D(\varphi)$, as shown by the examples in Figure 6. The upper plot of Figure 6 follows the conventional pattern in which all curves were plotted so as to meet at two fixed end points corresponding to φ_L and φ_U (filled circles). Since the range of φ over which $\psi_M(\varphi)$ and $\psi_D(\varphi)$ are compared is defined somewhat arbitrarily, φ_U was put at 100 in P_c and φ_L was determined as follows. In a previous study (Indow & Stevens, 1966), families of saturation scales $\psi_M(\varphi)$ for the four primary hues at various levels of Y were constructed on a common unit. The unit was named by Stevens a *crome*, according to which, for a red of 71 dB, $\psi_M(100)=100$ with an exponent β of 1.7. Then φ_L was defined as the value of P_c that satisfies the condition $\psi_M(\varphi_L)=\psi_M(\varphi_0)+0.02\,[\psi_M(100)-\psi_M(\varphi_0)]$ where

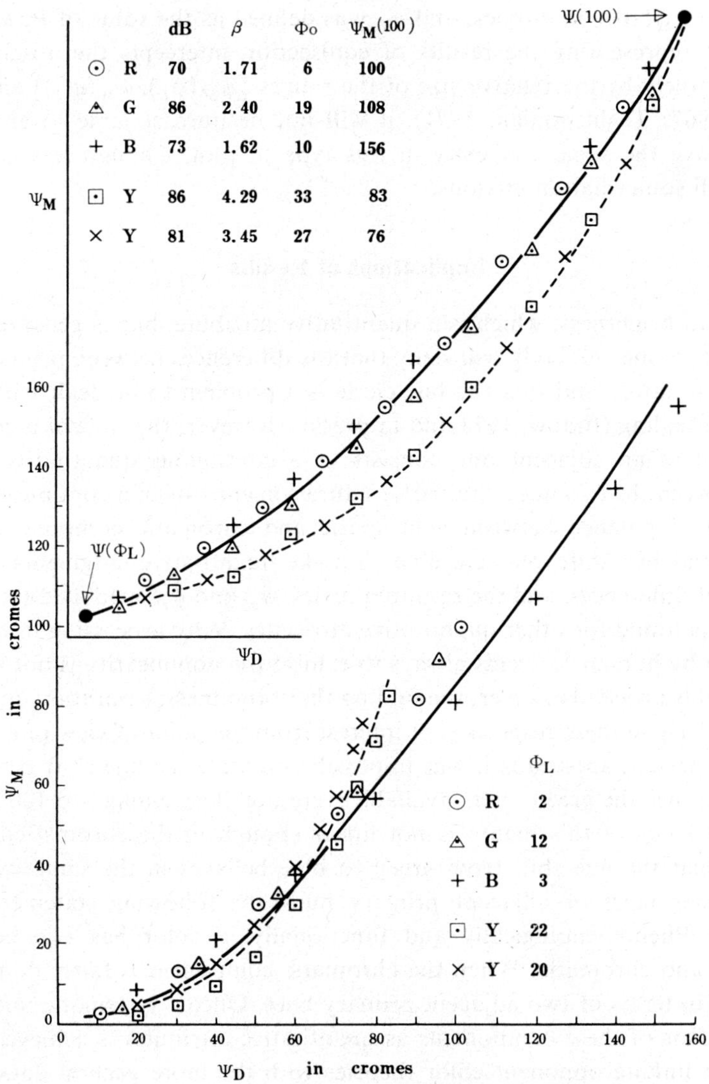

Fig. 6. Examples of nonlinearity between ψ_M and ψ_D in saturation (Indow & Stevens, 1966). For details, see the text.

$\psi_M(\varphi)$ is given in cromes and φ_0 represents the absolute threshold. Note that $\psi_M(\varphi_0)$ is obtained only by extrapolation, whereas $\psi_M(\varphi_L)$ is meaningful as a scale value to predict ratio judgments, and $\psi_D(\varphi)$ can be safely assumed to be linear over the range from φ_L to φ_U. The convexity in this plot is determined solely by the range (φ_L, φ_U) and the exponent β of $\psi_M(\varphi)$. As will be clear from Figure 6, yellow is anomalous because the range (φ_L, φ_U) is not small enough to compensate for the anomalous large value of β for yellow. In the lower plot of Figure 6, $\psi_M(\varphi)$ in cromes was simply plotted against $\psi_D(\varphi)$, where $\psi_D(\varphi)$ was defined as increasing linearly from $\psi_D(\varphi_L)=0$

to $\psi_D(100)=\psi_M(100)$ in cromes, and φ_L was defined as the value of P_c at which the straight line representing the results of equisection intercepts the abscissa. If β is determined solely by the relative size of the ranges $[\psi_M(\varphi_L), \psi_M(\varphi_U)]$ and $[\varphi_L, \varphi_U]$ (Poulton, 1967; Teghtsoonian, 1971), it will not be unreasonable to expect all the curves to have the same convexity in this type of plot. Though less conspicuous, yellow is still somewhat anomalous.

Implications of Results

In contrast to brightness, which is a quantitative attribute, hue is generally regarded as a qualitative one. Nobody will deny that the differences between primary hues are qualitative in nature and that the hue cicrle is a problem to be dealt with by multidimensional scaling (Indow, 1973 and in press). However, the shift of a color from a primary hue to an adjacent one consists of a continuous quantitative change of balance between the two hues. Similarly, saturation consists of a continuous quantitative change of balance between achromatic and chromatic components. In both saturation and hue shift, *S*s were able to make quantitative judgments in terms of ratios and of differences, and the resulting scales, ψ_M and ψ_D, exhibited the same nonlinearity as is found for other quantitative attributes. Why processing of quantitative information by human *S*s seems always to exhibit the nonlinearity is not the primary concern in this article. However, the finding that brightness, saturation, and hue shift behave similarly in these respects is of interest from the point of view of color theory.

With the present apparatus it was impossible to scale the hue shift between green and blue because the green filters available were not close enough to 100% in P_c and the spectral locus of this region is not linear enough in the chromaticity diagram. Assuming that the hue shift from green to blue behaves in the same way as those between other pairs of adjacent primary hues, the following statement could be formulated. Phenomenologically and functionally, a color has two components, achromatic and chromatic. When the chromatic component is fairly dominant, it is describable in terms of two adjacent primary hues. Once a systematic understanding of the behavior of these components as quantitative attributes is achieved, it should be useful in linking opponent color theories with the more general data concerned with color appearance. No matter at what stage or zone two sets of chromatic opponent response processes and one achromatic process are assumed, predictions from the opponent theories have been tested mainly by threshold data or data obtained by simple matching (e.g., Hurvich & Jameson, 1955, 1957; Walraven, 1973). Sooner or later, an experimental test of the theories should be extended to scales of saturation and hue shift, and even to scales of color difference. Among the results described here, two findings seem to be of special interest in this context: the linearity of $\psi_D(\varphi)$ and the anomalous behavior of yellow. The former is suggestive of the mechanism by which a perceptual color difference is generated, and the latter accords with the special position of yellow in opponent color theories. There are three different receptors in the retina: red (R), green (G), and blue (B). Yellow (Y), as the opponent of blue, is usually assumed to be synthesized at a later stage. It will be interesting, for example, to relate β_Y to β_R and β_G for the purpose of explaining the anomalous large value of β_Y. However, quantitative discussion of this kind needs more systematic data concerned with color appearance and color differences.

References

Bartleson, C. J., & Breneman, E. J. Brightness perception in complex fields. *Journal of the Optical Society of America*, 1967, **57**, 593–597.

Bartleson, C. J., & Breneman, E. J. Differences among responses of observers in scaling brightness. Paper presented at the second congress of the International Colour Association, York, July, 1973.

Galifret, Y. Les psychophysiques de la saturation chromatique. *L'Année Psychologique*, 1959, **59**, 35–46.

Hanes, R. M. A scale of subjective brightness. *Journal of Experimental Psychology*, 1949, **39**, 438–452. (a)

Hanes, R. M. The construction of a brightness scale from fractionation data: A validation. *Journal of Experimental Psychology*, 1949, **39**, 719–728. (b)

Hard, A. Quality attributes of colour perception. Survey lecture presented at the AIC International Colour Congress, Stockholm, June, 1969.

Hurvich, L. M., & Jameson, D. Some quantitative aspects of an opponent colors theory. II: Brightness saturation, and hue in normal and dichromatic vision. *Journal of the Optical Society of America* 1955, **45**, 602–616.

Indow, T. Saturation scales for red. *Vision Research*, 1967, **7**, 481–495.

Indow, T. Colour atlases and colour scaling. Survey lecture presented at the second congress of the the International Colour Association, York, July, 1973.

Indow, T. Applications of multidimensional scaling in perception. In E. C. Carterette & M. P. Friedman (Eds.), *Handbook of perception*. Vol. 2. New York: Academic Press, in press.

Indow, T., & Stevens, S. S. Scaling of saturation and hue. *Perception and Psychophysics*, 1966, **1**, 253–271.

Judd, D. B., & Nickerson, D. One set of Munsell re-notations. National Bureau of Standards Report 192693, *U.S. Department of Commerce*, 1967.

Marks, L. E., & Stevens, J. C. Individual brightness functions. *Perception and Psychophysics*, 1966, **1**, 17–24.

Mattiello, M. L. F., & Guirao, M. Lightness and saturation for surface colours. Paper presented at the second congress of the International Association of Colour, York, July, 1973.

Newhall, S. M. Preliminary report of the O.S.A. subcommittee on the spacing of the Munsell colors. *Journal of the Optical Society of America*, 1940, **30**, 617–645.

Newhall, S. M., Nickerson, D., & Judd, D. B. Final report of the O.S.A. subcommittee on the spacing of the Munsell colors. *Journal of the Optical Society of America*, 1943, **33**, 385–418.

Onley, J. W. Brightness scaling of white and colored stimuli. *Science*, 1960, **132**, 1668–1670.

Onley, J. W., Klingberg, C. L., Dainoff, M. J., & Rollman, G. B. Quantitative estimates of saturation. *Journal of the Optical Society of America*, 1963, **53**, 487–493.

Ohsumi, K. Scaling of continuous changes of object color. Unpublished graduation thesis, Keio University, 1968.

Panek, D. W., & Stevens, S. S. Saturation of red: A prothetic continuum. *Perception and Psychophysics*, 1966, **1**, 39–66.

Poulton, E. C. Population norms of top sensory magnitudes and S. S. Stevens' exponents. *Perception and Psychophysics* 1967, **2**, 312–316.

Stevens, J. C., & Guirao. M. Individual loudness functions. *Journal of the Acoustical Society of America*, 1964, **36**, 2210–2213.

Stevens, J. C., & Stevens, S. S. Brightness function: Effects of adaptation. *Journal of the Optical Society of America*, 1963, **53**, 375–385.

Stevens, S. S. On the theory of scales of measurement. *Science*, 1946, **103**, 677–680.

Stevens, S. S. Mathematics, measurement, and psychophysics. In S. S. Stevens (Ed.), *Handbook of experimental psychology*. New York: John Wiley, 1951, pp. 1–49.

Stevens, S. S. On the psychophysical law. *Phychological Review*, 1957, **64**, 153–181.

Stevens, S. S. On the new psychophysics. *Scandinavian Journal of Psychology*, 1960, **1**, 27–35.

Stevens, S. S. The psychophysics of sensory function. In W. A. Rosenblith (Ed.), *Sensory communication*. Cambridge, Mass.: The MIT Press, 1961, pp. 1–33.

Stevens, S. S. In pursuit of the sensory law. Second Public Klopsteg Lecture. Northwestern University, 1962.

Stevens, S. S. A metric for the social consensus. *Science*, 1966, **151**, 530–541.

Stevens, S. S. Intensity functions in sensory systems. *International Journal of Neurology*, 1967, **6**, 202–209.

Stevens, S. S., & Galanter, E. H. Ratio scales and category scales for a dozen perceptual continua. *Journal of Experimental Psychology*, 1957, **54**, 377–411.

Stevens, S. S., & Volkmann, J. The relation of pitch to frequency: A revised scale. *American Journal of Psychology*, 1940, **53**, 329–353.

Teghtsoonian, R. On the exponents in Stevens' law and the constant in Ekman's law. *Psychological Review*, 1971, **78**, 71–80.

Vos, J. J., Friele, L. F. C., & Walraven, P. L. (Eds.), *Color metrics*. Soesterberg: AIC/Holland c/o Institute for Perception TNO, 1972.

Wyszecki, G., & Stiles, W. S. *Color science: Concepts and methods, quantitative data and formulas*. New York: John Wiley, 1967.

SMITTY STEVENS' TEST OF RETINEX THEORY

EDWIN H. LAND[1]

Research Laboratories, Polaroid Corporation, Cambridge, Mass.

Abstract. This paper describes an experiment that Smitty performed while I was giving the William James lectures at Harvard. It was a modification of Craik's and Cornsweet's experiments using mixtures of red and blue instead of black and white. Smitty's experiment tested whether the colors produced were the colors one would expect from the predictions of Retinex theory. This paper describes the experiment, the predictions, and the results.

In 1966 and 1967 I had the priviledge of giving the William James lectures and working with Smitty, who was my host from the Harvard faculty. Early in the lectures I showed experiments which demonstrated that color sensations did not depend upon the relative amount of long-, middle-, and short-wave light falling at a point on the retina (Land, 1962; Land, 1964; Land & McCann, 1971). The experiments that led to this conclusion also led me to propose that the visual system acted as if all the receptors of one type associated with each other to form an image of the entire field of view. The image thus formed from one set of receptors is independent of the images formed from the other sets. This meant that all the long-wave cone receptors, for example, might associate with each other to form an image that assimilated all the information carried to the eye from the long-wave portion of the light. Similarly, images would be constructed from the middle-wave information and also from the short-wave information. In the Young-Maxwell approach the interaction is between a member of one set of receptors and a member of a second set and a member of a third set, the three members being at one point on the retina. Retinex theory requires no interaction between any member of the first set and any member of the second set and any member of the third set. The only interactions required are within a set; the members of a given set interact with each other.

With each of the separate sets generating separate images, the comparison area by area of the three separate images in super-position becomes the basis of color. The comparison could occur in the retina or it could occur in the cortex. Experiments in visual physiology cannot as yet define the location of the interactions that must be occurring. Therefore, I coined the word Retinex (made of "retina" and "cortex") to designate the physiological mechanisms that generate these images.

> We do think that, in a mathematically functional sense, these images exist independently. We are not urging that the retinal elements with the same peak sensitivity have to be *directly* connected to each other, but rather that, in the retinal-cerebral liaison, those elements with the same peak sensitivity cooperate to form a mechanism that has the capacity to establish an image [Land, 1964, p. 248].

[1] I wish to thank my colleagues Jeanne Benton and John McCann for their assistance in repeating Smitty's experiments and their assistance in writing the manuscript. In addition, I would like to thank Jay Scarpetti for making the reproductions of the experiments shown in the figures, Tom Taylor and Steve Auerbach for finding the best film-filter combination and Marie Watson for preparing the drafts of this manuscript.

H. R. Moskowitz et al. (eds.), Sensation and Measurement. 363–368. *All Rights Reserved.*

I turned then to the description of the image that is generated by a Retinex. When the members of a given set interact with each other, there comes into being a scale of lightnesses produced by that set. Every area in a scene will be characterized by three lightnesses; and the color experience in viewing an area is determined by these three lightnesses.

The spectral sensitivities of the sets of cone receptors in the retina overlap. Therefore in spite of their operational independence, no set can respond by itself to a single band of wavelengths. Even the use of a single wavelength will not isolate a single set of cone receptors. However, an image can be produced on the rod Retinex without producing an image on the other Retinexes. By dropping the level of illumination below the threshold of vision for the cone Retinexes while still well above the threshold of vision for the rod Retinex, we can examine and describe the characteristics of an image produced by the interactions within a single set of receptors. What we then see with the rod Retinex is a black, gray and white image. I have referred to the image we see with this single Retinex as an image made up of lightnesses.

Our use of the word lightness is in some respects similar and in other respects different from its previous use in the literature. LeGrand (1968, p. 225) defines lightness as the psychological attribute corresponding to a reflectance factor. Evans (1948, p. 159) describes lightness as the mental perception of reflectance and distinguishes it from brightness, which he describes as the mental perception of luminance. The reason we chose lightness rather than brightness is that in complex images and real-life situations sensations correspond well with the reflectance of objects and poorly with the amount of light coming from them (Land, 1964). There are other definitions of lightness referring to colored objects in a way that is irrelevant to Retinex theory. The Optical Society of America (1953) defines lightness as the "perception by which white objects are distinguished from gray and light from dark colored objects [p. 373]." In this sense, lightness is defined as Value in the Munsell system. In Retinex theory, three independent lightnesses are combined to generate color. Each color, whether it is a dark gray or light red, is determined by the long-, middle-, and short-wave lightnesses. This is different from the Munsell Value, which describes only how light or dark the color is.

Smitty felt that we were imposing on the word lightness a set of properties somewhat different from those it had had in the past. Our position would be clearer if we coined a new word that was defined in our own terms. He proceeded to coin a new word *grexity* and gave our definition of lightness to it. He derived it from the Greek word γϱηύς meaning gray woman and the German word *greckse* meaning to groan and grumble.

> Grexity is not dependent upon illumination. Grexity is not reflectance. In order to see grexity one has to be only on the rods – or have the same grexity on all three Retinexes. Grexity is an experience [Stevens, personal communication, 1967].

Whether one uses lightness or grexity as a name, the next problem is how one evaluates a colored image to determine the lightnesses or grexities of each part of it. A rough approximation of the long-, middle-, and short-wave lightnesses of an object can be made by holding an appropriate color separation flilter to the eye. If only long-wave light reaches the retina, the image we see is made up of the approximate lightnesses of the long-wave retinex. A reddish wash covers the entire image, but there is little or no variation in redness and the red is not nearly as saturated as a bright red object in a multicolored image. Similarly, we can look through narrow band green and blue filters and see approximate lightness images of the middle- and short-wave Retinexes.

Smitty became interested in the Craik-Cornsweet effect as a test of Retinex theory. His interest in this effect was aroused because the lightnesses of two areas do not correspond with either the reflectances or luminances of the discs. Craik's experiment (1966) used a spinning disc made of black and white papers. When a disc is spun, the reflectances of all the points at any given distance from the center are averaged. The reflectance is constant for any radial distance and proportional to the ratio of white to black papers at that radial distance. In Craik's experiments, there was the same ratio of white to black papers at the center and at the outside. In between these areas of uniform average reflectance was an abrupt increase and gradual decrease in the amount of black paper. Craik's disc is very similar to Cornsweet's except that it contains only one of these changes, whereas Cornsweet's contains two. To visualize Craik's disc look at Cornsweet's in Figure 1a and imagine a disc with only one cusp.

For simplicity of this and later discussions we will refer to the areas that are uniform in reflectance and equal to each other as the "center" and the "outside ring." The exciting realization is that the center does not appear the same lightness as the outside ring even though the same energy is coming from all the points in both.

Cornsweet's experiment (1970) is essentially the same as Craik's using a *pair* of opposed gradients separated by an abrupt edge (Figure 1a). The center of the stationary disc is half white and half black. At about a third of the way along the radius, starting at the outside rim, the amount of white paper gradually increases, abruptly decreases to less than half, and then gradually increases back to half white and half black at two-thirds the distance along the radius. When this disc is spun, the two uniform areas which have the same reflectance are seen as different. The inner area appears darker than the outer area and the gradients tend to vanish.

Figure 1b shows a second Cornsweet disc in which the cusps have been reversed. This time the cusp nearer the outside rim gradually increases the amount of black paper whereas in disc la it increased the amount of white paper. Again the center and outside ring have identical quantities of black and white papers. Only the direction of the *gradual change – abrupt edge – and gradual change* have been reversed. In the spinning part of this figure, the center looks lighter than the outer ring.

Smitty created a colored version of the Craik-Cornsweet effect to test whether the color sensations produced by the disc were those predicted by Retinex theory. The important property of this disc is that the image in long-wave light is the inverse of the image in short-wave light. In long-wave light the red paper is very light and the blue paper is very dark. If Figure 1c is viewed with a red filter it will appear the same as the stationary part of Figure 1a. In short-wave light the opposite is true; the red paper is dark and the blue paper is light. Consequently, the direction of the cusp is reversed. If Figure 1c is viewed through a blue filter it will appear the same as the stationary part of Figure 1b. This inverse relationship causes the effect of the *gradual change – abrupt edge – gradual change* to reverse. In long-wave light the Craik-Cornsweet effect makes the whole inner area look darker (see spinning part of Figure 1a). In short-wave light the Craik-Cornsweet effect makes the whole inner area look lighter (see spinning part of Figure 1b). The light coming from the center of the disc is identical in composition to that coming from the outside ring. Nevertheless, Smitty argued, the center and outside ring should be differently colored if Retinex theory is correct. The center should look bluer since it looks lighter in the short-wave light and darker in the long-wave light. The outside ring should look redder since it looks lighter in long-wave light and darker in short-wave light.

Figure 1c is a color photograph of a disc made of red and blue papers. If this disc is viewed through a red filter the red paper appears light and the blue paper appears dark. If the same disc is viewed through a blue filter, the blue paper appears light and the red paper appears dark. (If the disc is viewed with a green filter both red and blue papers appear dark and the same lightness.)

Figures 2a, 2b, 2c are a set of photographs of the spinning disc taken with standard color separation filters. The center and outside ring both sent to the eye or camera the same energy at each wavelength. Nevertheless, the center was darker than the outside in long-wave light and the center was lighter than the outside in short-wave light. On the basis of these photographs one would expect from Retinex theory that the center of the colored disc should look bluer and the outside look redder even though they have the same wavelength-energy distribution. Figure 1d of the spinning disc shows that indeed the center is seen as bluer and the outside as redder.

The colors of the spinning disc are those that we would expect and predict from Retinex theory. To photograph this experiment we used color separation filters whose spectral sensitivities were much narrower than the pigments in the eye. A better way to analyze the lightnesses that the receptors generate would be to make a photographic image with a black and white film that has the same spectral sensitivity as the receptor in question. Three such photographs, one for each cone spectral sensitivity, would be a record of the information sent to each set of receptors.

We prepared such a set of photographs, which we call Retinex records, by first measuring the spectral response of a commercial negative film (Polaroid type 55 P/N). We then calculated, with the aid of a computer, the spectral response of the film when combined with a variety of different filters. Each film-filter combination was compared to the absorption curves of the pigments in the human retina. We used a set of curves that was the average of a number of measurements made by Paul Brown (personal communication, 1973). These measurements were made using the difference-spectra technique described by Brown & Wald (1963). These long-, middle-, and short-wave absorption curves were multiplied by the transmission of the eye and the absorption of the macular pigment to estimate the resultant net sensitivity of the pigments in the intact eye (Wyszecki & Stiles, 1967). The results are shown in Figure 3. The best fit for the long-wave pigment was provided by the combination

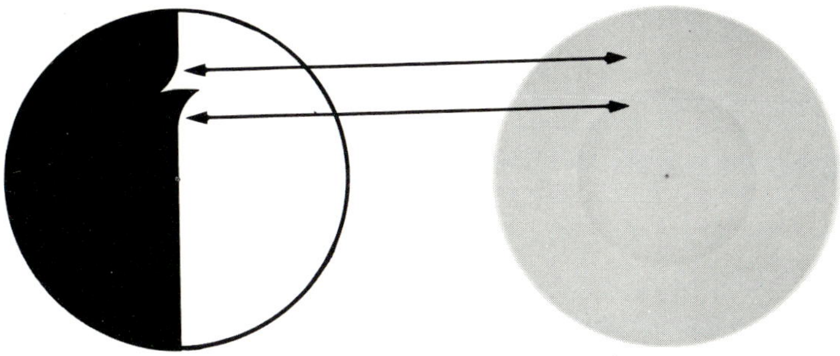

Fig. 1a. Photographs of Cornsweet's disc.

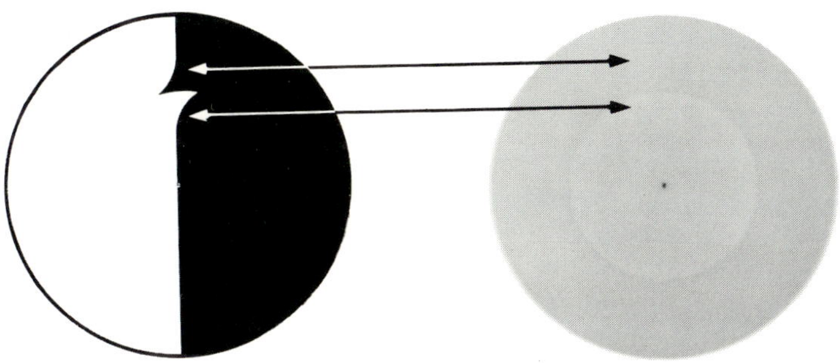

Fig. 1b. Photographs of above disc with cusps reversed.

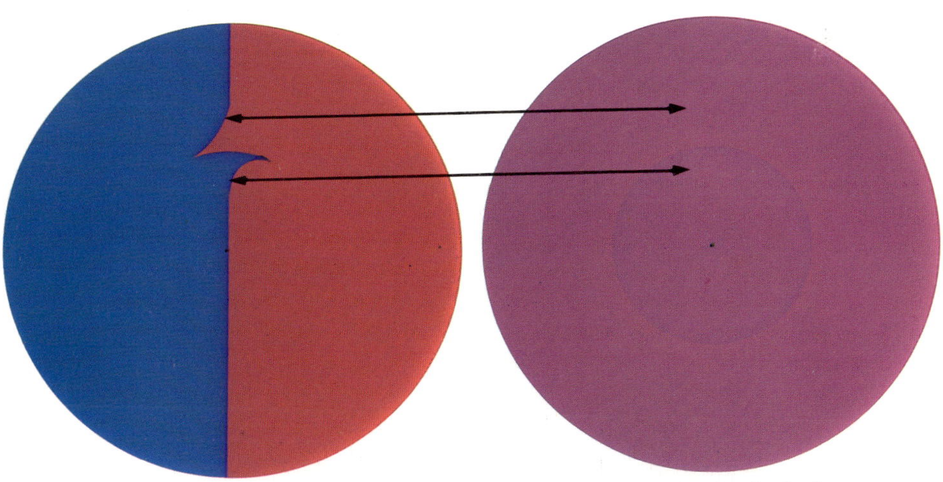

Fig. 1c. Photograph of stationary colored disc.

Fig. 1d. Photograph of spinning colored disc.

Fig. 2a. Long-wave Wratten #25 record.

Fig. 2d. Long-wave Retinex record.

Fig. 2b. Middle-wave Wratten #58 record.

Fig. 2e. Middle-wave Retinex record.

Fig. 2c. Short-wave Wratten #47B record.

Fig. 2f. Short-wave Retinex record.

Fig. 2. Six color separation photographs of the spinning disc shown in Fig. 1d. The left hand column has photographs taken with standard color separation filters: Top (2a) Wratten #25 (long-wave), center (2b) Wratten #58 (middle-wave), bottom (2c) Wratten 47B (short-wave). The right hand column has photographs taken with broad band filters that match the sensitivity of the pigments in the retina. Top (2d) Polaroid type 55 P/N film with Wratten #9 and CC 20C filters, center (2e) type 55 P/N film with Wratten 8, 13 and CC 20C filters, bottom (2f) type 55 P/N film with Wratten #47 and 86A filters. Each disc was photographed with a series of neutral gray papers beside it. The negative was developed and prints were made so that the reflectances of the gray papers in the print reproduced the reflectance of the original gray papers. This insured that the photographic process did not introduce larger differences in reflectance than those in the original target.

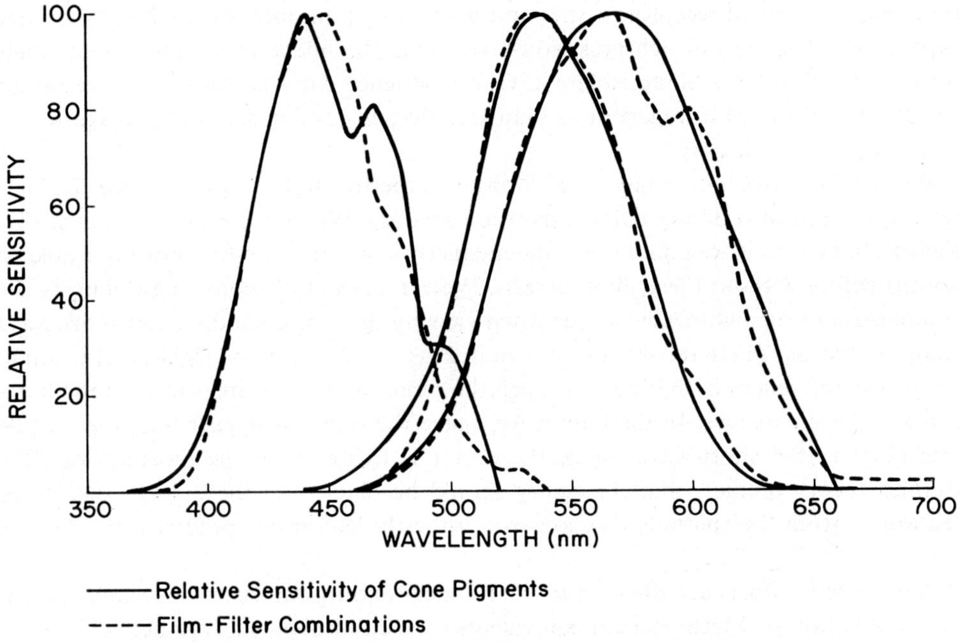

Fig. 3. The normalized spectral sensitivity of the three film-filter combinations used to match the spectral sensitivities of the three pigments in the retina. The film-filter combinations are shown with the dotted lines. The data from P. Brown's normalized measurements multiplied by the transmission of the eye and macular pigment are shown by the dotted lines.

of the above mentioned film and Wratten 9 and CC 20C filters. The middle-wave pigment was matched by the film and Wratten 8, 13, and CC 20C filters. The short-wave pigment was matched by the film combined with Wratten 47 and 86A filters.

As we see from Brown's curves in Figure 3 the spectral sensitivities of the visual pigments overlap broadly. If we illuminated a scene with the entire range of wavelengths to which a single pigment is sensitive, then we would see a large variety of colors because more than one Retinex would respond. The photographic intermediates enable us to isolate lightnesses that would ordinarily be combined into color sensation. This photographic technique performs two functions: First, the system provides spectral sensitivities which are the same as those of the visual pigments. Second, it generates black and white silver pictures for a human observer to examine. It is the human visual system which converts the photographic pattern in silver into lightness. Ideally we would like our observer to examine the black and white pattern with only one set of cones, reporting the lightnesses appropriate to that cone set. However, at any point in the silver pattern the reflectance is essentially the same throughout the visible spectrum. Therefore, with a black and white photograph we stimulate all the receptors with the same information, in this case the energies absorbed by a single visual pigment. If we assume that all the Retinexes process the information in an identical manner, then we can propose that sending this identical information to several sets of receptors is the same as sending it to only one, and that the three superimposed images in lightness would resemble the image in lightness on a single Retinex if it were possible to isolate it. Our experience with the isolated image on the rod Retinex leads us to regard it as plausible that any isolated Retinex image would be black, white and gray.

We can improve our analysis of Smitty's experiment by making three Retinex records instead of ordinary color separation records. We now can see the image that each Retinex sees if we could see it independetly – whereas we had not been able to do this before without these photographs. We can predict the color sensations by the comparison of the lightnesses we see when viewing the long-, middle-, and short-wave Retinex records. These records are shown in Figs. 2d, 2e, 2f in the right hand column. There are differences in lightness between the center and outer areas in both the long- and short-wave images. In the long-wave image the center is darker than the outside ring (2d); in the short-wave image the center is lighter than the outside ring (2f). Retinex theory predicts that the center should be bluer than the outside. The color sensations from the spinning disc are seen to be the sensations predicted by Retinex theory.

Our present efforts are directed toward understanding the visual mechanisms that generate lightness. Mathematical equivalents of such mechanisms are necessary for a complete model that uses the light on the retina as the input, lightnesses as the intermediates, and compared lightnesses, namely color sensations, as the outputs. One should realize the importance of the Retinex record in ascertaining the lightness of each area and the importance of lightnesses in determining the color of each area. In experiments shown at the William James lectures, in experiments Smitty performed, in experiments with rod-cone interactions (McCann & Benton, 1969), as well as in many others, the multiple lightnesses of each area predicted the color sensations. We have not yet found a situation in which lightnesses have not been able to predict color sensations accurately.

References

Brown, P. K., & Wald, G. Visual pigments in human and monkey retinas. *Nature*, 1963, **200**, 37–43.

Cornsweet, T. N. *Visual perception*. New York and London: Academic Press, 1970.

Craik, K. J. W. *The nature of psychology*. Cambridge, England: The University Press, 1966.

Evans, R. M. *An introduction to color*. New York: Wiley, 1948.

Land, E. H. Colour in the natural image. *Proceedings of the Royal Institution*, 1962, **39**, 1–15.

Land, E. H. The Retinex. *American Scientist*, 1964, **52**, 247–264.

Land, E. H., & McCann, J. J. Lightness and retinex theory. *Journal of the Optical Society of America*, 1971, **61**, 1–11.

LeGrand, Y. *Light, color and vision*. (2nd ed.) London: Chapman and Hall, 1968.

McCann, J. J., & Benton, J. L. Interaction of the long-wave cones and the rods to produce color sensations. *The Journal of the Optical Society of America*, 1969, **59**, 103–107.

Optical Society of America, Committee on Colorimetry. *The science of color*. New York: Cromwell, 1953.

Wyszecki, G., & Stiles, W. S. *Color science*. New York, London, and Sydney: John Wiley & Sons, 1967.

SPATIAL SUMMATION IN THE WARMTH SENSE[1]

LAWRENCE E. MARKS

John B. Pierce Foundation Laboratory and Yale University

Abstract. The warmth sense is characterized by generous spatial summation: perceived strength of warmth sensation increases with increasing areal extent of stimulation as well as with increasing stimulus intensity. When intensity is low, area exerts its greatest effect, in that warmth depends on the product of stimulus area and intensity – i.e., on total power in watts. Response to integrated heat input at low intensity enables the warmth sense to help maintain constant body temperature. As stimulus intensity increases, area's relative influence on warmth diminishes until the pain threshold is reached, whereupon spatial summation vanishes. Lack of summation at high intensity enables the warmth sense to help protect the skin from potentially damaging heat. The level-dependence of spatial summation is reflected in the way stimulus size influences the psychophysical power functions that relate warmth sensation to stimulus intensity: the larger the areal extent of the stimulus, the smaller the exponent of the power function.

There has been a tradition in the study of the senses whereby vision and hearing dominate interest and concern. The psychophysical properties of those two senses are highly adapted to complex processing of spatial and temporal information. But deserving of greater attention than has usually been paid to them are, among others, the thermal senses: warmth and cold. As compared to vision and hearing, the thermal senses are less "informational," more "motivational." Whereas vision and hearing provide the organism with information about the external world, the thermal senses to a large extent provide the organism with information about its own body. Warmth and cold help to mediate two important biological functions, namely the maintenance of constant internal body temperature and the protection of the body from potentially damaging extremes of environmental heat and cold. The present paper reviews recent studies of the warmth sense that explain how the psychophysical property of spatial summation serves to mediate these two functions.

Especially suitable to the psychophysical study of the thermal senses are the direct scaling procedures devised and developed by S. S. Stevens. Foremost among these is the method of magnitude estimation (Stevens, 1956). Magnitude estimation is a rapid, convenient, and comprehensive means to evaluate the way that sensory intensity depends on the intensity, composition, spatial extent, duration, etc., of stimulation [for a survey, see Marks (1974)]. It is an ideal procedure for study of warmth sensations: because time is needed for the skin to dissipate the heat absorbed from each stimulation, warmth stimuli can be presented only at a relatively slow rate, e.g., one stimulation every 30–45 s. Given such a slow rate, direct matching becomes prohibitively long and tedious. Magnitude estimation, on the other hand, is a much more efficient procedure, in that a judgment is obtained upon every presentation of a stimulus: thus it becomes possible, in a single experimental session to map out the

[1] This paper was supported by United States Public Health Service Grant ES-00354.

H. R. Moskowitz et al. (eds.), Sensation and Measurement. 369–378. *All Rights Reserved.*

effects on sensation of several stimulus variables. Furthermore, matching functions can be derived readily from results of magnitude estimation. Examples are given below in the discussion of area-intensity reciprocity (Figures 5 and 6).

Summation at Absolute Threshold

A prominent aspect of warmth sensation is that it displays generous spatial summation over large regions of the body. When stimulus intensity is low, there is almost a perfect trading between stimulus intensity and areal extent of stimulation. Measurements of absolute threshold by Hardy & Oppel (1937) and by Kenshalo, Decker, & Hamilton (1967) have shown that one stimulus of intensity φ and area $10A$, and another of intensity 10φ and area A will be about equally effective in arousing a minimal sensation of warmth. That is, at threshold the trading relation between area and intensity is expressed approximately as

$$A\varphi = \text{constant}. \tag{1}$$

Suprathreshold Summation of Warmth

But absolute threshold is only one end-point – the bottom – of the warmth continuum. The other end-point – the upper terminus of warmth sensation – is marked by the

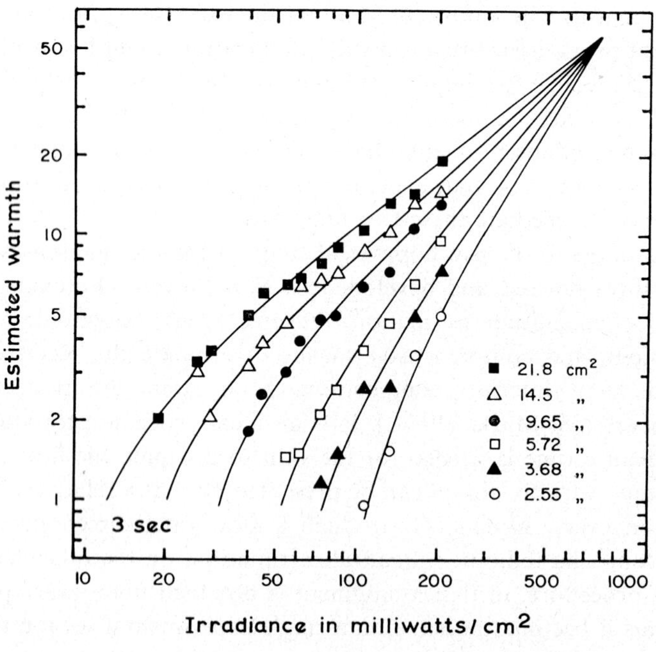

Fig. 1. Magnitude estimation of warmth as a function of stimulus irradiance. The parameter is areal extent of stimulation of the forehead (3-s exposures).

absolute threshold for pain. Studies by Greene & Hardy (1958) and by Murgatroyd (1964) have demonstrated that at the pain threshold there is virtually no spatial summation.

An interesting and important feature of spatial summation in the warmth sense is the way summation changes from full (complete reciprocity) near the warmth threshold to zero (no summation) near the pain threshold. Degree of spatial summation declines progressively as stimulus intensity is augmented. Figure 1 displays, in double-logarithmic coordinates, magnitude estimates of the warmth aroused by 3-s exposures of the forehead to radiant stimulation (J. C. Stevens & Marks, 1971). Each set of data points represents the results obtained for a different stimulus size.

Each curve fitted to the data points is a power function of the form

$$\psi = k(\varphi - \varphi_0)^{\beta}, \tag{2}$$

where ψ represents estimated warmth, φ represents irradiance, and φ_0 is a constant related to the absolute threshold of warmth. Thus all of the functions obey S. S. Stevens' (1957) general power law. The value of φ_0 is, for warmth, inversely proportional to areal extent, thereby reflecting the complete reciprocity between area and intensity near threshold that is expressed by Equation 1. Of special interest is the systematic influence that area exerts on the value of the exponent β (slope of the func-

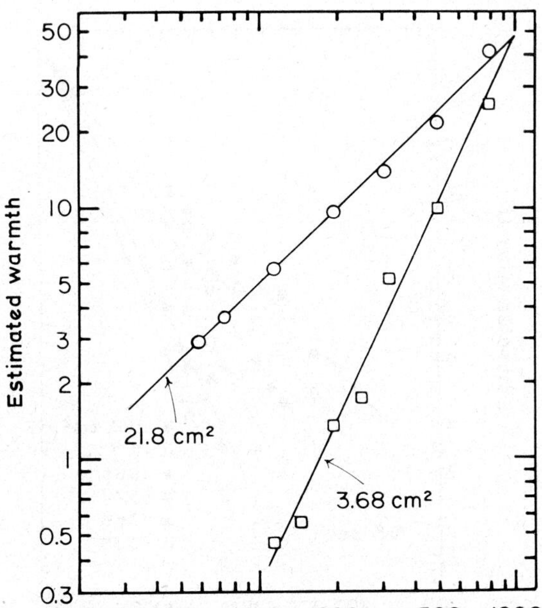

Fig. 2. Magnitude estimation of warmth as a function of stimulus irradiance. Three-sec exposures of 3.68 and 21.8 cm² of the forehead.

tion in log-log coordinates). The size of β indicates how warmth grows with irradiance, and, as Figure 1 depicts, as area increases the slope (size of β) decreases.

From the fact that β varies with area, it follows that degree of spatial reciprocity depends on level of stimulus irradiance. The power functions in Figure 1 show that at any level of irradiance, the larger the size of the stimulus, the greater the warmth. But as irradiance grows stronger, the relative effect of area diminishes, until, the extrapolated portions of the curves predict, at some high irradiance, all of the functions converge. [For a description of the procedure whereby the convergence point was determined, see J. C. Stevens' (1974) paper in this volume, p. 157.] Presumably, if the subjects were stimulated at such a high level, the warmth aroused would have been the same given any areal extent of stimulation. At the point of convergence, where spatial summation is no longer evident, irradiance equalled about 800 milliwatts cm^{-2} (mW cm^{-2}), a level that falls close to the absolute threshold for pain produced by 3-s stimulation with radiant heat (Adair, J. C. Stevens, & Marks, 1968).

A subsequent experiment helped confirm what the extrapolated functions in Figure 1 predicted, namely that psychophysical functions for warmth obtained with different stimulus sizes do converge at or near the pain threshold (Marks & J. C. Stevens, 1973). In that experiment, the forehead was stimulated with 3-s exposures to irradiances that ranged all the way up to 800 mW cm^{-2}. As Figure 2 shows, the psychophysical functions appear to converge just a little above that level, at about 1000 mW cm^{-2}.

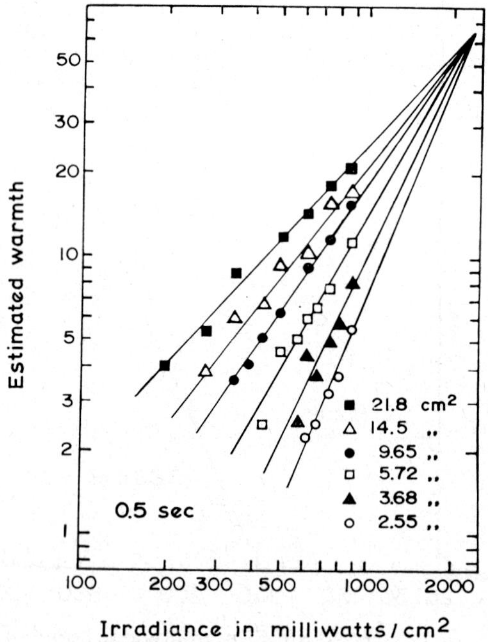

Fig. 3. Magnitude estimation of warmth as a function of stimulus irradiance. The parameter is areal extent of stimulation of the forehead (0.5-s exposures).

Summation as a Function of Stimulus Duration

The pain threshold is not a constant value, at least not when it is expressed in terms of stimulus irradiance. Though pain does not display much, if any, spatial summation, it displays considerable temporal summation (Hardy, 1956). If the hypothesis that warmth functions converge at pain threshold is correct, then the point of convergence, like threshold per se, must depend on duration.

When the skin is heated over only a short duration, warmth still displays spatial summation (Marks & J. C. Stevens, 1973). Figure 3 displays psychophysical functions obtained by irradiating several areal extents of the forehead for 0.5 s, instead of 3 s. Again the functions appear to converge on a single point, but this time at a much higher level of irradiance, about 2300 mW cm^{-2}. This increase in the irradiance at convergence is reasonably consistent with the way pain threshold increases when duration is shortened. The results therefore support the hypothesis that the disappearance of spatial summation at high intensity corresponds to the appearance of thermal pain.

Spatial Summation on Different Regions of the Body

Families of power functions obtained with different stimulus sizes, like those displayed in Figures 1 and 3, have been obtained on several regions of the body besides the forehead. These include the back (J. C. Stevens & Marks, 1971), the cheek, the forearm, and the calf (the last three as yet unpublished). The picture that emerges is, in every case the same: Given 3 s of radiant stimulation, the warmth increases in accordance with S. S. Stevens' power law, and the power functions obtained with different stimulus sizes appear to converge at an irradiance of 800–1000 mW cm^{-2}, i.e., at or near the pain threshold. It is a general feature of the warmth sense that, whatever the region of skin surface stimulated, spatial summation is a level-dependent phenonemon. Area exerts a larger effect when stimulus intensity is low than when it is high.

Neural Locus of Summation

Evidence that the warmth sense can sum the neural effects of stimulation over large areal extents may be construed as suggesting that summation takes place at least in part somewhere in the central, rather than peripheral, nervous system. An experiment by Hardy & Oppel (1937) helps bolster that view. They found the absolute threshold for warmth to be about 30% lower when two hands instead of one were stimulated. Neural signals from the two hands are, of course, carried over separate spinal nerves, so inputs from the two hands can combine only at a central locus.

Suprathreshold warmth also displays summation of neural signals that are carried by separate peripheral nerves (Marks & J. C. Stevens, 1973). Figure 4 shows average magnitude estimates of the warmth aroused by radiant stimulation (3 s) of the forehead using three stimulus configurations: a small field presented to one side of the midline (neural signals carried by one nerve), a field twice as large presented to one

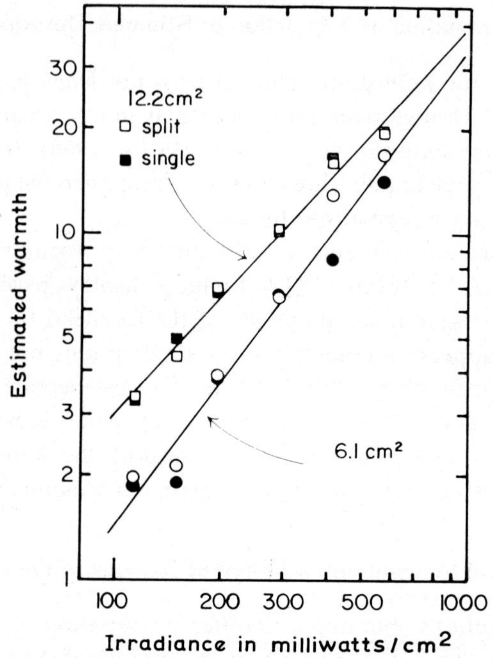

Fig. 4. Magnitude estimation of warmth as a function of stimulus irradiance (3-s exposures). Circles: small, single field. Squares: large field, unitary (filled) and split (unfilled).

side of the midline (again, neural signals carried over one nerve), and a field of the same total area as the larger field, but split half to the left, half to the right of midline (half of the signals carried by one nerve, half by the other). As Figure 4 makes clear, the warmth aroused by the large field was just about the same regardless of whether the signals were carried by one (filled symbols) or by two (unfilled symbols) peripheral nerves. That is to say, spatial summation of warmth crosses dermatome boundaries. A significant portion of warmth summation must, therefore, take place somewhere in the central nervous system. A similar conclusion may be drawn for vibratory touch, which also displays spatial summation across widely disparate regions of the body (Craig, 1966).

Reciprocity between Area and Irradiance

Families of psychophysical functions like those shown in Figures 1, 3, and 4 contain sufficient information to calculate how irradiance and areal extent must covary in order to preserve a constant level of warmth sensation. This calculation may be accomplished by making horizontal cuts at various levels of warmth through each family of functions and reading off the combinations of area and irradiance. Figure 5 gives contours of constant warmth derived from the psychophysical functions in Figure 1 (3-s stimulation of the forehead). Around the absolute threshold the area-irradiance reciprocity is nearly perfect. A line of slope equal to -1 implies complete

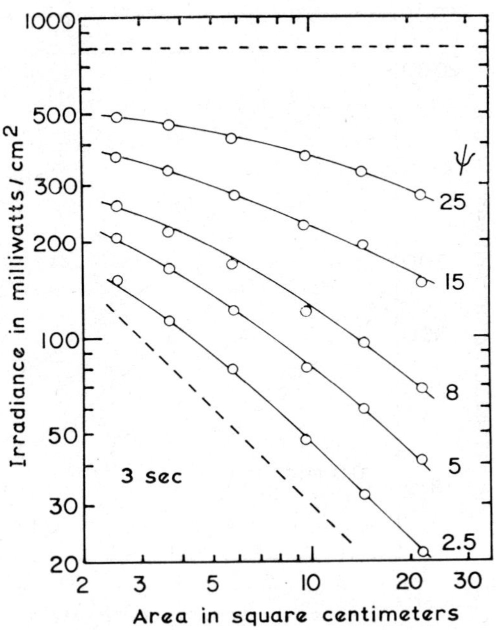

Fig. 5. Equal-warmth contours, showing how irradiance and areal extent of stimulation must convary to maintain constant warmth. The parameter is the level of estimated warmth ψ. The points were determined by making horizontal cuts in the psychophysical functions in Figure 1 (3-s stimulation).

spatial reciprocity of the form given by Equation 1. At higher and higher stimulus levels, however, area becomes relatively less and less effective a determinant of warmth, and degree of spatial summation diminishes. This is shown by the way the curves get flatter and flatter. Finally, at a high enough level, summation is totally absent, as the dashed, horizontal line indicates. This level – 800 mW cm^{-2} – corresponds approximately to the absolute threshold for pain.

The shapes of these constant-warmth contours are of some interest. Nearly all of them have a concave downward form. These shapes appear time and again, in contours constructed from all of the families of warmth functions. They are also apparent for example in Figure 6, which gives contours of constant warmth derived from the psychophysical functions in Figure 3 (0.5-s stimulation of the forehead). The general features of summation are similar in both sets of contours (Figures 5 and 6); the only major difference is that when duration is short, summation disappears only when irradiance is very high.

Reciprocity functions obtained from reaction times measured to radiant heat also resemble the constant-warmth contours. Speed of reaction improves both with increasing stimulus irradiance and areal extent; and again the trade-off between irradiance and size is level-dependent (Banks, 1973).

Inspection of each set of constant-warmth contours suggested that they are dis-

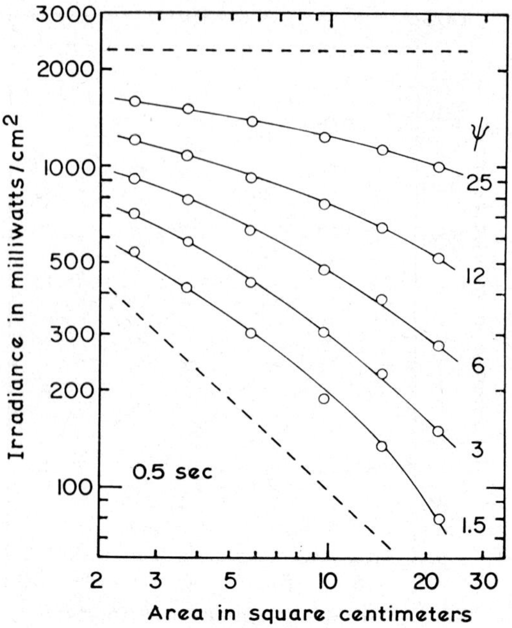

Fig. 6. Equal-warmth contours, showing how irradiance and areal extent of stimulation must convary to maintain constant warmth. The parameter is the level of estimated warmth ψ. The points were determined by uaking horizontal cuts in the psychophysical functions in Figure 3 (0.5-s stimulation).

placed from one another by constant horizontal distances (Marks & J. C. Stevens, 1973). For instance, if all of the contours in Figure 5 (or of Figure 6) are shifted horizontally by appropriate amounts, they will form a single curve. Thus the degree of summation, defined as the rate at which $\log \varphi$ changes with $\log A$ $(\delta \log \varphi / \delta \log A)$ depends solely on stimulus irradiance. Perhaps we have an analogue here to a property of the visual system, where spatial organization, particularly size of receptive field, depends on luminance (Barlow, Fitzhugh, & Kuffler, 1957).

Spatial Discrimination of Warmth

Often there appears to be an inverse relation between a sensory system's capacities to discriminate and to sum spatially. The eye displays fine and precise spatial resolution, and, concomitantly, little spatial summation, except at very low intensities. The warmth sense does the reverse; it displays extensive summation, but poor spatial resolution. Two radiant stimuli that differ in size and irradiance, but feel equally warm, also feel equally large (J. C. Stevens & Marks, 1971). Radiant stimulation of two spots that flank the midline of the forehead produce a single sensation right at the midline (Marks & J. C. Stevens, 1973). No matter how far two radiant stimuli are separated from one another across the back, subjects cannot reliably discriminate the stimulus pair from a unitary field; indeed, subjects often confuse radiant stimulation of the back and the stomach (Cain, 1973). Keen spatial resolution on the skin can only be mediated by the sense of touch. In toto, we see that the warmth sense is highly adapted to say how much heat is applied to the skin, but not where the skin or how much of it is heated.

Biological Significance of Warmth Summation

As was mentioned in the introduction, the thermal senses help to mediate two important biological functions: maintenance of constant internal temperature and prevention of tissue damage from extreme thermal stimulation. Biological regulation can be either automatic and physiological, as when people respond to cold by shivering, or voluntary and behavioral, as when they respond by putting on a sweater. In both cases the thermal senses are an important source of input.

The level-dependence of spatial summation in the warmth sense may be interpreted as a compromise that serves to maintain both a constant internal temperature and the integrity of the skin. At low and moderate levels of stimulus intensity, there is nearly perfect area-irradiance reciprocity (Equation 1). Thus warmth sensation depends not just on irradiance (watts per unit area) but on power (watts), i.e., on total heat input. This latter quantity is obviously of much greater import in the regulation of body temperature. On the other hand, tissue damage due to burning is closely related to perception of pain, and pain is closely tied to the absolute temperature of the skin (Hardy, 1956), but not to how much skin is heated. When irradiance is high or exposure duration is long, the degree of spatial summation diminishes. At high intensity, area is not nearly so significant a determinant of sensation as is intensity itself, and the perception of strong warmth, produced by stimuli of high intensity, serves as a warning of an impending threat to the skin unless either the source of stimulation, or the skin, is removed.

References

Adair, E. R., Stevens, J. C., & Marks, L. E. Thermally induce pain, the dol scale, and the psychophysical power law. *American Journal of Psychology*, 1968, **81**, 147–164.

Banks, W. P. Reaction time as a measure of summation of warmth. *Perception and Psychophysics*, 1973, **13**, 321–327.

Barlow, H. B., Fitzhugh, R., & Kuffler, S. W. Change of organization in the receptive fields of the cat's retina during dark adaptation. *Journal of Physiology*, 1957, **137**, 338–354.

Cain, W. S. Spatial discrimination of cutaneous warmth. *American Journal of Psychology*, 1973, **86**, 169–181.

Craig, J. C. Vibrotactile loudness addition. *Perception and Psychophysics*, 1966, **1**, 185–190.

Greene, L. C., & Hardy, J. D. Spatial summation of pain. *Journal of Applied Physiology*, 1958, **13**, 457–464.

Hardy, J. D. The nature of pain. *Journal of Chronic Diseases*, 1956, **4**, 22–51.

Hardy, J. D., & Oppel, T. W. Studies on temperature sensation. III: The sensitivity of the body to heat and the spatial summation of the end organ responses. *Journal of Clinical Investigation*, 1937, **16**, 533–540.

Kenshalo, D. R., Decker, T., & Hamilton, A. Spatial summation on the forehead, forearm, and back produced by radiant and conducted heat. *Journal of Comparative and Physiological Psychology*, 1967, **63**, 510–515.

Marks, L. E. *Sensory processes: The new psychophysics*. New York: Academic Press, 1974.

Marks, L. E., & Stevens, J. C. Spatial summation of warmth: Influence of duration and configuration of the stimulus. *American Journal of Psychology*, 1973, **86**, 251–267.

Murgatroyd, D. Spatial summation of pain for large body areas. Defense Atomic Support Agency Report, 1964.

Stevens, J. C. Families of converging power functions in psychophysics. In this volume, p. 157–165.

Stevens, J. C., & Marks, L. E. Spatial summation and the dynamics of warmth sensation. *Perception and Psychophysics*, 1971, **9**, 291–298.

Stevens, S. S. The direct estimation of sensory magnitudes – loudness. *American Journal of Psychology*, 1956, **69**, 1–25.

Stevens, S. S. On the psychophysical law. *Psychological Review*, 1957, **54**, 153–181.

MODELS OF ADDITIVITY FOR SUGAR SWEETNESS

HOWARD R. MOSKOWITZ

Pioneering Research Laboratory, U.S. Army Natick Laboratories, Natick, Mass.

Abstract. Observers judged the sweetness of nine different sugars mixed at different concentrations either with glucose or with fructose. Power functions fitted to the sweetness of unmixed sugars were modified to yield two alternate predictors of mixture sweetness: (I) Summation of concentrations or (II) Summation of perceived sweetnesses. Model I and Model II were both appropriate for mixtures with glucose, whereas only Model II appeared appropriate for mixtures with fructose. Both models systematically underpredicted mixture sweetness, suggesting synergistic effects that extend beyond simple additivity. The studies illustrate the use of direct ratio scaling of taste intensity to suggest and to test alternate ways by which the taste system processes mixtures.

Additivity of taste intensities has concerned investigators both for its importance in sensory mechanisms and for its practical use in the food industry. Knowledge of how the taste system integrates complex stimuli having the same taste quality provides clue about whether the mixture is treated as two different stimuli, or as one emergent stimulus of higher effective concentration. Furthermore, most naturally occurring taste stimuli comprise a variety of chemicals, so that the single sugar or acid stimulus presented to the tongue in an experiment provides only an initial probe of the taste experience. In addition, practical implications abound for uncovering the mechanism of taste mixtures. Historically, the increased sweetness that might be obtained via mixtures of artificial sweeteners was of economic interest because of sugar shortages, such as that experienced by Germany during and after World War I. The German chemist Paul (1921) investigated the sweetness of saccharin, dulcin, and their mixtures because they could be potential replacements for sucrose. Invert sugar, a mixture of glucose and fructose, is derived from sucrose, and has received considerable attention as a potentially better sweetener than sucrose (Sale & Skinner, 1922).

Traditionally, sweetness has been assessed through direct matches between an unknown sweetener and a reference sugar (usually sucrose or glucose). Mixtures of sweeteners were evaluated by instructing the observer to find a solution of sucrose equal in sweetness to each component sweetener alone, and to the mixture itself. *Additivity* of sweetness was inferred when the sucrose equivalents of the components added up to the sucrose equivalent of the mixture. When the sum of the equivalents of the components was greater than the mixture's equivalent, then *suppression* was inferred, whereas when the mixture's equivalent was greater than those of the components *synergism* was inferred.

Inferring additivity, suppression, or synergism from equal-sweetness matches poses two major problems. First, the observer balances one stimulus against another, but never provides direct magnitude estimates, thus precluding alternative hypotheses about how the qustatory system might process complex stimuli. Second, as Cameron (1947) and Pfaffmann (1959) have suggested, the success of summing intensity

H. R. Moskowitz et al. (eds.), Sensation and Measurement. 379–388. *All Rights Reserved.*

equivalents in taste depends critically upon the reference chemical. For sweetness, glucose is a better reference than fructose or sucrose, since both these sugars have subjective intensity functions that are curvilinear relative to the functions of most other sugars (Moskowitz, 1971).

Direct estimation of taste intensity by number matching provides a ratio scale of sweetness, on which numerical values can be added, subtracted, and multiplied by a constant. This flexibility permits the construction and testing of a variety of psychophysical models. At least three distinct models have been proposed to account for additivity of taste and smell mixtures:

1. The sensory system adds together the concentrations of the mixture components, treats the sum as a higher concentration of the reference chemical, and then transforms that concentration into subjective magnitude according to an intensity function appropriate for the reference chemical. If sweetness (S) is related to molarity (C) by a power function, $S = kC^p$, then model I can be expressed by three equations:

$$S_a = k_a C_a^m \tag{1}$$

$$S_b = k_b C_b^n \tag{2}$$

$$S_{ab} = k_a (C_a + (k_b/k_a)^{-m} (C_b^n)^{-m})^m . \tag{3}$$

2. The sensory system sums subjective intensities by summing the two sweetnesses

$$S_{ab} = k_a C_a^m + k_b C_b^n \tag{4}$$

3. The sensory system treats the components like vectors in a subjective space, with the angular separation (ϕ) of these vectors corresponding to their subjective dissimilarity in quality. The additivity model is expressed by the equation:

$$S_{ab} = (S_a^2 + S_b^2 + 2S_a S_b \cos(\phi))^{0.5} \tag{5}$$

(S_a = sweetness of a, S_b = sweetness of b), $S_{a\cdot}$: is the sweetness of the mixture.) Equations 3 and 4 were proposed by Moskowitz (1973, 1974) to account for mixtures of sweeteners, and mixtures of acids. Equation 5 was proposed by Berglund, Berglund, Lindvall, & Svensson (1972) to account for the intensity of mixtures of noxious odorants (e.g., methyl monosulfide + methyl disulfide).

The present study assesses the sweetness of a large number of mixtures containing either glucose or fructose as one component. With a broad sample of different sugars it should be possible to evaluate the three models of mixture additivity, and to determine what types of synergism or suppression occur. Because of the wide range of chemicals used, consistent departures from the mixture models also become important as clues to the underlying mechanism by which the gustatory system transforms pairs of chemicals to perceived sweetness.

Method

The study comprised five experiments. In each experiment the observers judged the sweetness of glucose, fructose, and two other sugars, as well as mixtures of the two other sugars with glucose and fructose, respectively. Tables 1 and 2 list the concentrations of each sugar, the mixtures evaluated (schematically, according to the seven to eight pairs tested), and the number of observers participating. The observers were selected from a group of 30 men, and in each experiment two replicate sessions were run with the same observers participating in each session. The *O*s were enlisted military men (ages 18–27), all with previous experience matching numbers to taste intensity.

The *O*s sampled the stimuli from small paper cups filled with 10–15 ml of solution. In each of the five experiments, run on separate days, the stimulus set comprised glucose, fructose, two other sugars, and the mixtures. The *O*s sampled the stimuli in

TABLE 1

Parameters of the power functions for sugars $S = kC^n$

Sugar	(Molarities)	Exponent	St. error	Intercept	Rel. sweetness	R^2	N
I Glucose	(0.125, 0.25, 0.5, 1.2)	1.09	0.08	0.53	3.90	0.94	12
Fructose	(0.12, 0.26, 0.62, 3.5)	0.83	0.07	0.54	4.79	0.95	
Glycerol	(0.43, 0.87, 1.0, 3.2)	1.20	0.18	0.23	1.68	0.65	
Sorbitol	(0.37, 0.80, 1.51, 2.8)	1.15	0.14	0.44	2.76	0.97	
II Glucose		1.18	0.12	0.56	3.90	0.92	10
Fructose		0.82	0.10	0.66	6.37	0.96	
Galactose	(0.26, 0.72, 1.5)	0.93	0.20	0.46	3.40	0.96	
Sorbose	(0.18, 0.45, 1.15, 2.5)	1.04	0.14	0.65	4.96	0.88	
III Glucose		1.20	0.11	0.56	3.90	0.90	10
Fructose		1.15	0.11	0.72	5.91	0.98	
Arabinose	(0.3, 0.65, 1.4, 2.7)	1.49	0.15	0.53	3.35	0.99	
Xylose	(0.32, 0.68, 1.4, 2.5)	1.88	0.15	0.61	3.94	0.99	
IV Glucose		1.36	0.11	0.61	3.90	0.93	12
Fructose		1.03	0.10	0.64	5.22	0.99	
Lactose	(0.16, 0.35, 0.60)	1.27	0.20	0.67	4.84	0.99	
Maltose	(0.25, 0.5, 1, 1.9)	1.74	0.17	0.68	4.09	0.99	
V Glucose		1.19	0.14	0.55	3.90	0.91	10
Fructose		1.15	0.13	0.81	8.43	0.94	
Sucrose	(0.08, 0.20, 0.45, 0.90)	1.39	0.14	1.23	15.09	0.98	

TABLE 2

Schematic for mixtures (Numbers refer to the rank order of concentration, 1 = highest concentration of sugar)

I Glucose + glycerol, glucose + sucrose (4,4; 3,3; 2,2; 1,1; 2,3; 4,2; 2,4; 3,2)

II Glucose or fructose + other sugars (4,4; 3,3; 2,2; 2,3; 4,2; 2,4; 3,2)

(First number refers to glucose or to fructose, second number to the other sugar in the mixture)

irregular order of concentration, compound, and mixture. The first stimulus was selected at random, and *O*s were free to assign to the stimuli numbers that they felt were appropriate. Between samples the *O*s rinsed with 50–100 ml of tap water at room temperature (21 °C ± 2). The responses for all *O*s in each experiment were brought into congruence with each other by the method of *modulus normalization* (Moskowitz, 1970). The responses of each *O* were multiplied by a constant so that the geometric mean of his five judgments of the glucose stimuli came to 10.0.

Results

Figure 1 presents the sweetness functions for the unmixed stimuli. The stimuli had been selected originally to be equally sweet at four concentrations of glucose (0.25, 0.5, 1.0, and 2.0 *M*). In most instances the geometric mean of the magnitude estimates for corresponding levels of different sugars produced approximately the same sweetness rating. The equality of ratings confirms previous findings for the sweetness of these same sugars on the basis of which the concentrations were equated (Moskowitz,1971).

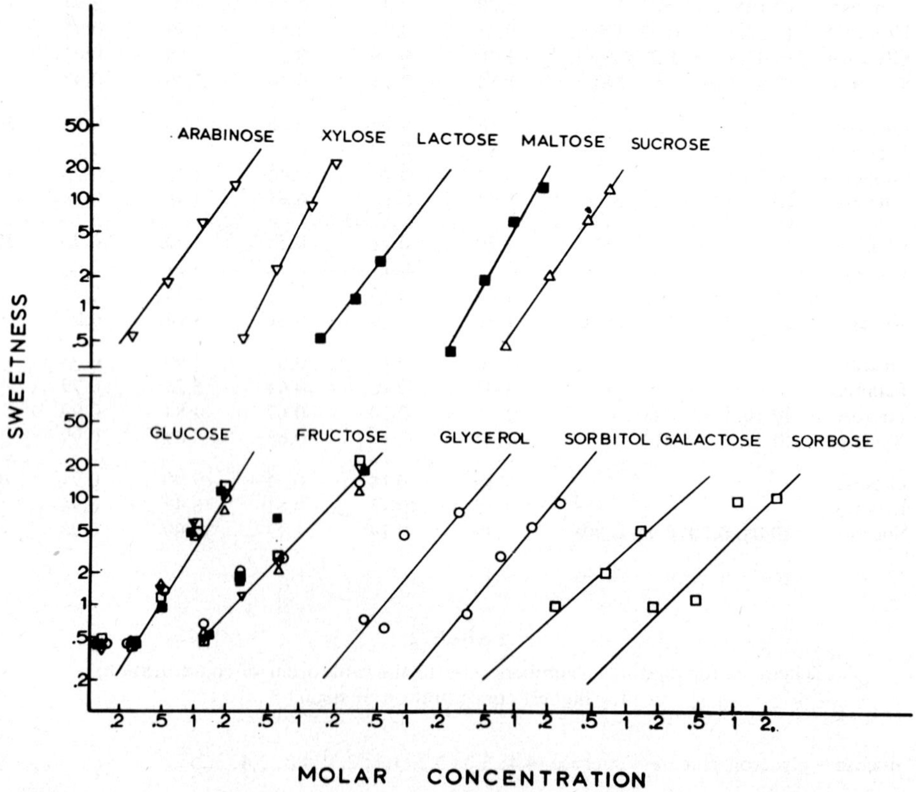

Fig. 1. Sweetness as a function of the molar concentration of sugars. The coordinates are log-log, so that straight lines represent power functions ($S = kC^p$), in which the exponent p is given by the slope of the line. The abscissa values correspond to relative molarities.

Estimates of sweetness obtained from magnitude estimation appear to be robust, and reproducible from one year to the next, and from one group of *O*s to another. Table 1 presents the best-fitting parameters for power functions relating sweetness to concentration. For most sugars (except fructose) the exponent is higher than 1.0, which means that sugar sweetness grows more rapidly than stimulus concentration. The *relative sweetnesses* of sugars (given by the ratio of magnitude estimates) varies somewhat because of exponent differences, so that two sugars equally sweet at one concentration may produce different sweetnesses at higher or lower levels.

SWEETENER MIXTURES

The three models of additivity (Equations 3, 4, and 5) were tested for the mixtures of sweeteners. Since *O*s judged both the components and their mixtures in the same session, the numbers for sweetness are comparable, and the models may be developed directly from the simple sweetness functions. Note that Equations 3 and 4 are formulated in terms of sweetness functions, and thus are expressed in terms of concentrations. Any departure of the simple sweetness function from a strict power function will introduce bias into the mixture equations.

Figure 2 shows the relation between log predicted sweetness (ordinate) and log obtained sweetness (abscissa). The 45° line represents the line of congruity. Points below the line are those in which the obtained mixture sweetness is stronger than the predicted sweetness. Points above the line are those in which the obtained mixture sweetness is less than predicted. Most of the points lie below the line of congruity, so that according to both models sugar mixtures are sweeter than predicted. If synergistic mixtures abound, as they do here, then the vector model of additivity cannot be used to predict additivity. The summation of vectors can lead, at most, to 100% additivity, but never to synergism. For sweetness, therefore, the appropriate models are (*a*) summation of concentrations (expressed in equivalents of either sugar) and (*b*) summation of sweetnesses.

The degree of discrepancy between predicted and obtained mixture sweetness is shown in Table 3. Predicted sweetness ($\log P$) from the models was related to the empirical mixture sweetness ($\log E$) by two equations:

$$\log E = k_1 (\log P) + k_2, \tag{6}$$

$$\log E = 1.0 (\log P) + k_3. \tag{7}$$

In Equation 6, k_1 indexes how rapidly predicted sweetness changes with obtained sweetness. When k_1 exceeds 1.0, then predicted sweetness grows less rapidly than the actual mixture sweetness, whereas when k_1 is less than 1.0, predicted sweetness grows more rapidly. When k_1 equals 1.0 (or is forced to equal 1.0, as in Equation 7), the predicted and obtained mixture sweetnesses grow equally rapidly. The intercept k_3 then represents a constant log difference (or a fixed ratio) between predicted and obtained values. Negative values for k_3 reflect that the models overpredict sweetness of mixtures, whereas positive values of k_3 reflect underpredictions.

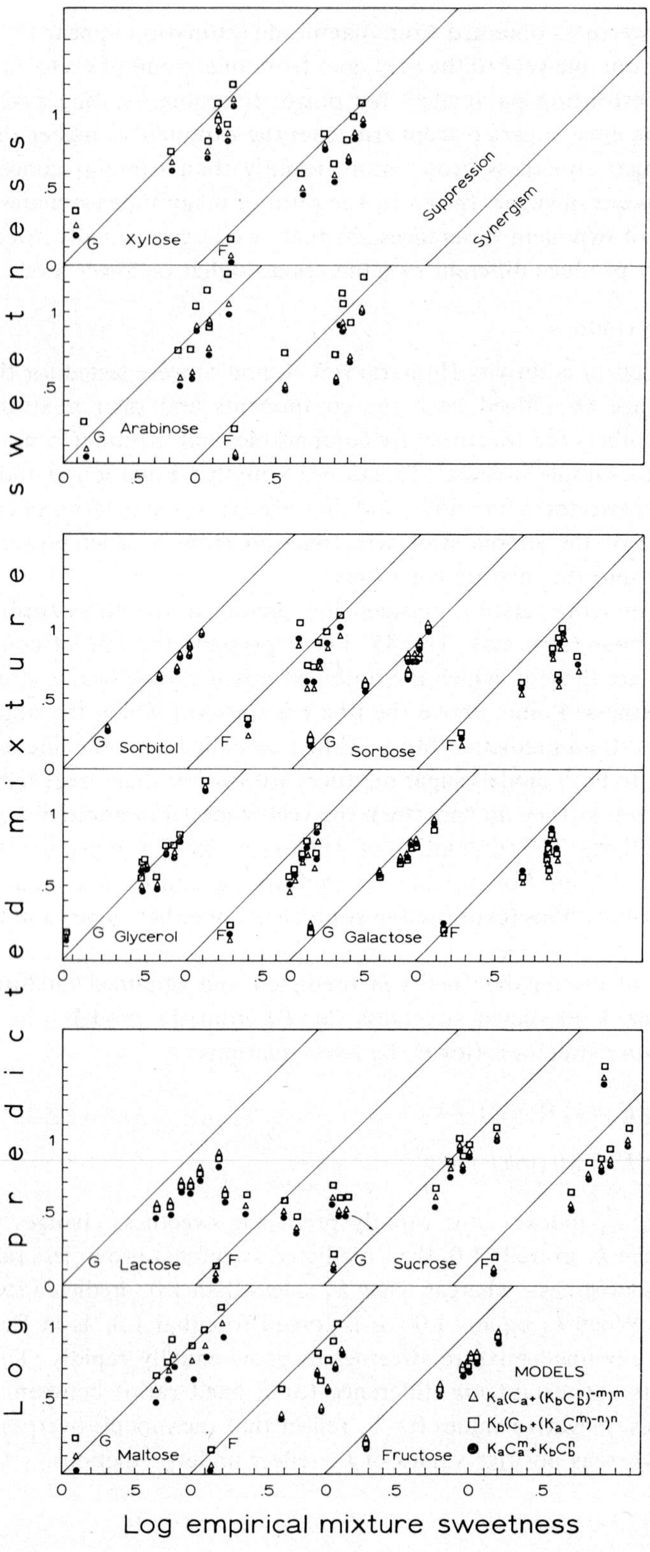
Log predicted mixture sweetness
Log empirical mixture sweetness
Xylose
Arabinose
Suppression
Synergism
Sorbitol
Sorbose
Glycerol
Galactose
Lactose
Sucrose
Maltose
Fructose
G
F
MODELS
$K_a(C_a + (K_b C_b^n)^{-m})^m$
$K_b(C_b + (K_a C^m)^{-n})^n$
$K_a C_a^m + K_b C_b^n$

Sugar mixtures tend to be synergistic, with the degree of synergism between 10% and 50%. Often, k_1 is significantly different from 1.0, so that the degree of synergism varies with sweetness levels of the mixtures (i.e. level-dependency).

Discussion

IMPLICATIONS FOR TASTE MECHANISMS

Additivity of sweetness contrast with partial suppression which occurs when unlike-tasting compounds are mixed and tasted together. Sweet and sour, sweet and salty, and sweet and bitter mixtures each produce an impression of lowered taste intensity, i.e., the numerical sum of the unmixed taste intensities of the components is greater than the intensity of the mixture (Beebe-Center, Atkinson, Rogers, & O'Connell, 1959; Moskowitz, 1972). Mixture laws for gustation differ from those in seeing and hearing – two taste compounds produce a stronger impression only when they are of the same quality.

Since taste qualities are usually divided into four discrete classes, it is possible that taste mixtures may show only a limited range of additivity or suppression. In theory, however, mixtures could range from synergism through 100% additivity, and finally to substantial suppression and even to cancellation. Along this continuum mixtures of substances that taste alike (sugars, acids) may span the upper third (additivity), whereas mixtures of substances that taste different may span the lower third (suppression), leaving the middle range unoccupied. Were sufficient mixture studies to be made, the possibility exists that some mixtures would be found that occupy the middle range of the continuum. The experimental demonstration of the continuum of mixture effects, from synergism to cancellation, rather than only additivity or suppression, argues for a continuum of taste qualities, not for four discrete groups.

According to the parameters in Table 3, when glucose is the reference sugar the summation of concentrations better predicts overall sweetness than summation of component sweetness estimates. Mixtures containing fructose are synergistic, and are sweeter than predicted. Pfaffmann (1959) suggested that fructose and sucrose may not be optimal examples of sugars for use in additivity studies since each produces curvilinear intensity functions. Expressing fructose in terms of equivalents of another sugar improves the fit of Model I, lending credence to Pfaffmann's observation.

Appropriate models of taste additivity also shed light on the relation between the sweetness of disaccharides (e.g., maltose, lactose, sucrose) which comprise pairs of

---

←

Fig. 2. A comparison of three models that predict mixture sweetness. Triangles and squares correspond to a model that adds concentration equivalents, with triangles representing the model that sums glucose or fructose equivalents, and squares the model that sums the equivalents of the second sugar in the mixture. The circles correspond to the model that adds sweetness. All coordinates are log-log, so that relative percentage agreement, rather than absolute agreement, is of interest. *G* represents mixtures with glucose, *F* represents mixtures with fructose. The second sugar is labelled. The ordinate represents predicted mixture sweetness according to the three models, and the abscissa represents the obtained sweetness of the mixture by the method of magnitude estimation.

TABLE 3

Functions relating empirical mixture sweetness (log E) to predicted mixture sweetness (log P)

(*a*) $\log E = k_1(\log P) + k_2$ (*b*) $\log E = 1.0(\log P) + k_3$

		Glucose equiv.	Other equiv.	Summed sweet.	Fructose equiv.	Other equiv.	Summed sweet.
Glycerol	k_1	0.94	0.94	0.94	0.91	0.93	0.92
	k_2	0.02	−0.005	0.04	0.25	0.15	0.21
	r^2	0.88	0.88	0.88	0.91	0.91	0.91
	k_3	−0.02	−0.05	0.00	0.21	0.11	0.17
Sorbitol	k_1	0.98	0.98	0.98	0.73	0.75	0.72
	k_2	0.06	0.04	0.04	0.36	0.22	0.32
	r^2	0.97	0.97	0.97	0.75	0.76	0.76
	k_3	0.04	0.03	0.07	0.20	0.04	0.16
Galactose	k_1	1.23	1.22	1.23	1.30	1.31	1.32
	k_2	−0.14	−0.05	−0.08	0.04	0.00	0.03
	r^2	0.98	0.99	0.99	0.88	0.87	0.87
	k_3	0.02	0.09	0.07	0.22	0.19	0.17
Sorbose	k_1	1.07	1.06	1.07	1.05	1.06	1.06
	k_2	−0.08	−0.04	−0.03	0.25	0.18	0.19
	r_2	0.86	0.87	0.88	0.79	0.79	0.79
	k_3	−0.03	0.01	0.02	0.28	0.22	0.23
Arabinose	k_1	1.32	1.33	1.31	0.97	0.99	0.95
	k_2	−0.19	−0.30	−0.11	0.21	0.10	0.25
	r^2	0.94	0.93	0.94	0.91	0.92	0.91
	k_3	0.04	−0.04	0.09	0.18	0.09	0.22
Xylose	k_1	0.92	0.94	0.91	0.81	0.85	0.81
	k_2	0.13	−0.05	0.19	0.31	0.13	0.34
	r^2	0.90	0.90	0.89	0.86	0.86	0.86
	k_3	0.08	−0.10	0.13	0.19	0.00	0.22
Maltose	k_1	1.09	1.09	1.07	1.00	1.02	1.00
	k_2	−0.04	−0.16	0.07	0.27	0.07	0.28
	r^2	0.97	0.97	0.97	0.90	0.88	0.90
	k_3	0.02	−0.09	0.11	0.27	0.09	0.28
Lactose	k_1	1.32	1.32	1.30	1.56	1.48	1.51
	k_2	−0.14	−0.10	0.00	0.32	0.30	0.31
	r^2	0.98	0.98	0.98	0.49	0.47	0.48
	k_3	0.06	0.09	0.16	0.09	0.05	0.09
Sucrose	k_1	0.98	0.99	0.97	0.50	0.50	0.51
	k_2	0.06	0.00	0.11	0.52	0.48	0.53
	k_3	0.92	0.92	0.92	0.58	0.56	0.58
	k_3	0.05	0.10	0.10	0.12	0.03	0.14
Fructose	k_1	1.26	1.26	1.26			
	k_2	0.03	0.09	0.11			
	r^2	0.98	0.97	0.98			
	k_3	0.20	0.25	0.27			

chemically linked simple sugars (maltose = glucose + glucose, lactose = glucose + galactose, sucrose = glucose + fructose). Is the sweetness of the disaccharide equal to the sum of its component sweetnesses? Table 1 provides a value for relative sweetnesses, corresponding to the expected sweetness of 1 *M* of each sugar. The assumption was made that all sugars are governed by a power function with an exponent of 1.3. A similar convention to obtain relative sweetness was used previously to compare the sweetening capacity of 42 sugars (Moskowitz, 1971).

Both synergism and suppression are evident from Table 1. Sucrose sweetness (15.1) is approximately 25% greater than the sum of glucose and fructose sweetness (3.9 + 8.4). Maltose (4.1) is approximately half as sweet as the sum of its two glucose components (3.9 + 3.9). Finally, lactose, typically considered to be a sugar with low sweetness has a projected value of 4.8, at 1 *M* substantially less than the predicted sum of 7.3. When the component sugars in a disaccharide are different, additivity occurs to a greater extent than when the components are identical (sucrose and lactose vs maltose, respectively). This analysis of disaccharides as sugar mixtures may be a powerful tool for decomposing the response of the gustatory system to a complex molecule of several potentially stimulating moieties that it comprises.

OTHER USES OF ADDITIVITY

A previous study (Moskowitz & Wehrly, 1972) was used to predict the relation between mixture sweetness and the cost of the sweeteners. The solution of the programming problem required both the costs of the components and the appropriate function that transforms pairs of concentrations to a total sweetness level. At that time the mixture equations were obtained empirically only for mixtures of glucose with fructose, sodium cyclamate, sodium saccharin, and saccharin, respectively. The general form of the function (equivalent to Equation 4) was extended to mixtures of sugars not directly tested in experiments (e.g., glucose + sorbitol). The present results extend the data base for economic studies of mixture sweetness, and corroborate the potential applicability of Equation 4 as a simple, but useful model. Studies of mixture sweetness (and of taste mixtures in general) may have as much use in the realm of actual food development and modification as they have potential for uncovering aspects of sensory transduction in taste.

ON THE PROBLEM OF SYNERGISM AND THE PSYCHOPHYSICAL LAW

The most remarkable finding from this series of experiments on sugar mixtures is that 100% additivity and synergism are relatively common, whereas partial additivity is unusual. The opposite occurs in seeing, hearing, and smelling, wherein synergistic mixtures, producing stronger intensities than expected, are rare.

It is quite possible that simple psychophysical functions, such as the power law for magnitude, do not suffice to predict mixtures of taste components. On the other hand, because power functions are very useful for relating sweetness to concentration, our search for mixture models tends to be made with an eye towards the compatibility of the mixture model with the power-function model. This reasoning then raises the possibility that alternative functions besides the power law might be more useful to describe the relation between sweetness and concentration. The alternative functions would be those equations that lend themselves easily to adoption in models of taste mixtures.

The foregoing logic can be extended towards a general rule for psychophysics; namely, that the appropriate functions for simple sensory magnitude are those that are compatible with laws of sensory mixture. This means that one way of validating the psychophysical power law is to see how far it can be extended beyond describing the data. If in the study of mixtures the basic power law must be extensively modified to produce accurate predictions of overall intensity, then it becomes quite important to search either for (*a*) alternative laws of mixtures that are compatible with the simple power function of intensity or (*b*) alternative laws for simple intensity that are compatible with known models of mixtures.

References

Beebe-Center, J. G., Rogers, M. S., Atkinson, W. H., & O'Connell, D. N. Sweetness and saltiness of compound solutions of sucrose and NaCl as a function of concentration of solutes. *Journal of Experimental Psychology*, 1959, **57**, 231–234.

Berglund, B., Berglund, U., Lindvall, T. E., & Svensson, L. T. A quantitative principle of perceived intensity summation in odor mixtures. Report 436, Psychological Laboratories, University of Stockholm, Sweden, 1972.

Cameron, A. T. The taste sense and the relative sweetness of sugars and other sweet substances. Science Report Series No. 9, Sugar Research Foundation, New York, 1947.

Moskowitz, H. R. Ratio scales of sugar sweetness. *Perception and Psychophysics*, 1970, **7**, 315–320.

Moskowitz, H. R. The sweetness and pleasantness of sugars. *American Journal of Psychology*, 1971, **84**, 387–405.

Moskowitz, H. R. Perceptual changes in taste mixtures. *Perception & Psychophysics*, 1972, **11**, 257–262.

Moskowitz, H. R. Models of sweetness additivity. *Journal of Experimental Psychology*, 1973, **99**, 88–98.

Moskowitz, H. R. The sourness of acid mixtures. *Journal of Experimental Psychology*, 1974, in press.

Moskowitz, H. R., & Wehrly, T. Economic applications of sweetness scales. *Journal of Food Science*, 1972, **37**, 411–415.

Paul, T. Der Sussungsgrad von Dulcin und Saccharin. *Chemiker Zeitung*, 1921, **45**, 38.

Pfaffmann, C. M. The sense of taste. In: Handbook of physiology. I: Neurophysiology, 1959 (Ed. by J. Field) pp. 507–533.

Sale, J. W., & Skinner, W. W. Relative sweetness of invert sugar. *Journal of Industrial and Engineering Chemistry*, 1922, **14**, 522–525.

VISUAL PERCEPTUALIZATION OF TETRACHORIC CORRELATIONS

IRWIN POLLACK

Mental Health Research Institute, University of Michigan

Abstract. Random samples drawn from specified distributions were visually presented at high display rates to observers for discrimination. Different levels of tetrachoric correlations were produced by controlling the probability of agreement, PAG, of the signs of the x- and y-coordinates. Differential thresholds are relatively constant, when expressed in terms of the difference in normalized PAG-levels, over a wide range of reference correlations. Although thresholds improve with the number of presented samples, there is a loss of efficiency, relative to the performance of an Idealized Statistical Observer. Sampling from an underlying uniform distribution leads to somewhat lower differential thresholds for tetrachoric correlations than sampling from a normal distribution. Comparisons are drawn with the detection of product-moment correlations.

It is convenient to distinguish between two forms of human operator evaluation of probabilistic information sources. In one, the operator makes successive judgments based upon a developmental scenario of successive samples drawn from the source. In the probability guessing experiment, for example, he may be asked to predict the next item upon successive trials. In the bookbag and pokerchip experiment, he may be asked to update probabilistic estimates as information is aggregated on successive trials. The beauty of this approach is that a developmental history can be obtained as a function of his experience with the source.

However, if we are willing to lose the developmental sequential history, in order to concentrate on the overall source properties, an alternative efficient means of information presentation is available. A large number of the samples of the sources can be presented within a very short time, as a high-speed auditory display or as a visual display. The operator is asked to make a single judgment upon the entire sequence. The essence of the approach is to convert a sequential hypothesis-testing task or problem-solving task into a perceptual discrimination task – hence, the term "perceptualization."

In contrast with the extensive experimental development of the sequential hypothesis-testing approach in psychology (see, for example, the excellent review by Slovic and Lichtenstein, 1967) the "perceptualization" approach has been relatively ignored. Green, White, & Wolf (1959) translated first-order probability distributions into displays differing in brightness. Julesz (1962), Pickett (1964, 1972) and Pollack (1972) have translated second-order probability distributions into displays differing in "texture." When one of two states tends to be repeated, strings of dots and non-dots are perceived as 'coarse' textures; when the two states tend to alternate, strings of dots and non-dots are perceived as 'even' textures. Julesz (1962) and Pollack (1972) have translated third-order probability distributions into displays differing in aggregation. And, most relevant to the present study, correlations based upon continuous

H. R. Moskowitz et al. (eds.), Sensation and Measurement. 389–401.

random noise distributions (Licklider & Dzendolet, 1948) have been presented to the eye (Pollack, 1960) and the ear (Pollack & Trittipoe, 1959) for discrimination.

The present study sought to determine how well the operator can evaluate tetrachoric correlations in the context of a "perceptualized" display. In addition, operator performance will be compared with that of an Idealized Observer in order to obtain measures of relative efficiency.

Method

Apparatus. Samples were randomly selected from defined sources by a PDP-8 computer and were plotted upon a Tektronix 602 display equipped with a fast P-15 phosphor.

TABLE 1

Display parameters for visual correlation detection

g	grid of imaginary matrix upon which points were plotted.
e	linear extent of the display available to x or to y.
d	duration of each dot.
I	off-interval between successive dots.
n	number of dots on the display.
PAG	probability of agreement of the sign of one coordinate, relative to the sign of the other coordinate.
s	number of samples from a uniform distribution contributing to a composite average.

Display parameters. Table 1 lists the display parameters. Points were plotted upon an imaginary matrix grid. The finest grid, g, provided by the display system was 64×64 possible positions extending over an 8×8 cm display surface. The 64×64 grid permitted the 6-bit storage of both x- and y-coordinates within the same 12-bit word of the PDP-8 computer, thus permitting high-speed plotting of the display (Wojnaroski, Bachman, & Pollack, 1972). Restrictions were imposed upon the linear extent, e, available to x- and to y-. In the unrestricted case, x- and y-values ranged from -4 to $+4$ cm, relative to the center of the display. In the most restricted case, each sample was represented by only one of two x-values and of two y-values. Intermediate restrictions employed two display formats: centered and outside-in displays. For example, when $e = \pm 2$ cm in x, the centered display occupied x-coordinates ranging from -2 to $+2$ cm, expressed relative to the center of the display; and the outside-in display occupied x-coordinates of -4 to -2 cm and $+2$ to $+4$ cm, again expressed relative to the center of the display. The centered format concentrated the display area at the risk of confusion of location, relative to the imaginary horizontal and vertical axes. The outside-in format removed ambiguity of location relative to the imaginary axes at the risk of spreading information beyond a central 'focalized' region. The number of possible x- and y-positions was a joint function of the available grid and of the linear extent available to each coordinate. Each two-fold restriction, imposed upon both coordinates, in either g or in e reduced the number of possible plotting positions four-fold. A simultaneous two-fold restriction in both g and e upon both coordinates reduced the number of possible plotting positions 16-fold.

Each sample from the information source was represented by a single dot upon the display. The duration of the dot, d, and the off-interval between successive dots, I, and the number of dots, n, were controlled. Natural binocular viewing was employed. The background illumination was dim. The distance to the display was adjusted for maximum comfort by the observer; the median distance was about 70 cm.

Sampling. Each coordinate was selected from a uniform distribution over the range of available extents. The sign of one coordinate was randomly selected without constraint. The sign of the other coordinate was constrained in terms of the probability of agreement, PAG, with the sign of the first coordinate. When PAG = 1.0, for example, all points were uniformly distributed within the northeast (NE) and southwest (SW) quadrants. When PAG = 0, all points were uniformly distributed within the NW and SE quadrants. When PAG = 0.50, points occurred with equal probability within all quadrants. Manipulation of PAG restricted only the relative frequency balance among the paired quadrants; such manipulation did not restrict positions within a quadrant. The maximum equivalent product-moment correlation when PAG = 1.0 is 0.75 (See Appendix A).

Experimental conditions. Within each block of 25 successive observations, the test parameters were held constant. The display was generated either by a reference PAG (usually, PAG = 0.50) or by another PAG (usually, PAG > 0.50). Each observer, tested individually, was instructed to press one of two buttons to identify each of the two conditions. The task was verbalized in terms of the relative concentration of points within the respective quadrants. Immediate feedback was given. Thirteen paid observers contributed 26 blocks under each of 322 experimental conditions, resulting in a total of 0.21×10^6 observations. The observers previously had extensive experience in perceptual tests of the temporal coherence of auditory and visual displays. Unless specified otherwise, $g = 64 \times 64$, $e = 4$ cm, $d = 0.071$ msec, $I = 0.281$ msec, $n = 1524$, and the reference PAG = 0.50.

Additional tests. Additional tests explored the use of underlying distributions of different shape for the identification of tetrachoric correlations, and for the identification of product-moment correlations.

The transition from uniform to near-normal distributions was achieved by adding together and averaging 1, 2, 4, or 8 successive numbers, s, through a mask of appropriate size. With independent random numbers, a uniform distribution is achieved with only 1 number; a triangular distribution is achieved with 2 numbers; and a near-normal distribution (except for the most extreme cases) is achieved with 8 numbers.

Limitations on the speed and memory of the small PDP-8 computer forced an alternative method. For each sample, a 12-bit number was randomly selected from a uniform distribution. Successive numbers involved a one-bit rotation upon the previous number. With the method of bit-rotation employed, approximations were made to the idealized distributions. Simulations with this procedure indeed show that the normal distribution is closely approximated over most of its range with $s=8$.

Tetrachoric scatterplots were obtained by expressing the selected samples as deviation scores about the mean, randomly assigning a sign for x-, and determining the sign for y- by PAG. The idealized distributions varied from uniform to near-normal by summing $s=1$, 2, 4, or 8 samples from a uniform distribution.

Product-moment correlations were obtained by independent random selection of two samples, x and z. The idealized sampling distributions varied from uniform to near-normal by the method just described. The x-coordinate displayed the x-sample. The y-coordinate displayed:

$$y = cx + (1 - c)\,z, \tag{1}$$

where c is a common factor. With $c=1.0$, x and y are perfectly correlated; with $c=0$, x and y are uncorrelated. Appendix B derives the relation between common factor c and the product-moment correlation, r.

Results

EXAMINATION OF DISPLAY PARAMETERS

Restriction of x- *and* y-. The effect of restricting the range of x- and y- upon the accuracy of identification of the scatterplots is examined in Table 2. The outside-in format was employed with the 64×64 grid. The other experimental parameters are also listed. The percentage of correct observations falls as the extent available (and/or as the number of possible plotting positions) to each coordinate is restricted. The thin diagonal lines connect conditions of equal area extents (the product of $e(x)$ and

TABLE 2

Percentage of correct identifications as a function of the available extent of x- and y-[a]

	$+e(x)$ in cm	Single point	0.5	1	2	4	Aver.
	single point	64	64	71	77	77	71
	0.5	68	76	78	80	82	77
	1	77	82	83	78	80	80
$e(y)$	2	83	80	81	85	76	81
in cm	4	78	79	81	80	88	81
	Aver.	74	76	78	80	82	

[a] Display conditions, $g=64$, $d=0.57$ msec, $I=0.28$ msec, $n=$ $=200$, PAG $=0.5$ vs 0.8, $s=1$, outside-in format.

TABLE 3

Percentage of correct identifications of a function of numbers of grids over entire display area and of the available extents of x- and y- [a]

Number of grids	Single point	$e(x)$, $e(y)$ in cm: 0.5	1	2	4	0.5	1	2	4
2					74				74
4				77	80			79	80
8				83	86			86	86
16			84	85	88		90	94	88
32		77	84	90	92	91	93	93	92
64	73	77	85	85	93	98	97	96	93
(1)	(4)	(16)	(64)	(256)	(1024)	(16)	(64)	(256)	(1024)
	Outside-in format					Centered format			

[a] Experimental conditions, $d = 0.07$ msec, $I = 0.31$ msec, $n = 1524$, PAG $= 0.5$ vs 0.8, $s = 1$.

$e(y)$ constant). Equal area extents yielded roughly equivalent performance levels. Since the total display area subtended by the outside-in format was independent of the available extents, the decrement in performance may be identified either with the higher dot density or with the lower central concentration of points within the restricted display.

An attempt was made to dissociate the contribution of dot density and central concentration. The joint effect of grid density and of the extent available to both x- and y- is examined in Table 3 for outside-in displays (left section) and for centered displays (right section). The entries are the percentage of correct identifications. Entries connected by a thin diagonal line represent a constant number of possible plotting positions per display quadrant. That number is indicated in parentheses. For example, the unrestricted 64×64 grid with available x- and y- extents of ± 4 cm permitted $32 \times 32 = 1024$ positions per quadrant. A two-fold restriction in available extent upon both coordinates with a constant grid, or a two-fold restriction in the number of grids with a constant available extent, reduced the number of possible plotting positions four-fold.

Several points are noted. The previous effect of restricting the available x- and y-extents in the outside-in format with the finest grid, as shown in Table 2, is confirmed under a different set of experimental conditions in Table 3. Performance is substantially better with the centered displays; and the decrement in performance with restricted x- and y- available extents under a fixed grid is markedly reduced with centered displays. For a fixed number of possible plotted positions, shown along the marked diagonals, performance tends to increase as the available extent is increased in the outside-in format, but tends to decrease as the available extent is increased in the centered format. The results suggest that the centered areas of the display can be inspected more efficiently, and within that area, spatial dispersion of the points is effective.

The balance of the tests employed the unrestricted 64×64 grid.

Temporal factors. The rate of plotting successive dots was controlled either by varying the number of successive refreshments of each displayed dot or by varying the interval between successive dots. Aside from brightness differences associated with the number of successive paintings, there was little effect over a 16-to-1 range of the number of successive paintings. Over a range of off-times between successive dots from 0.38 msec to 410 msec, there also was little effect upon performance (a 2% drop). It appears that the correlation detection with the perceptualized display is, within wide limits, relatively insensitive to temporal parameters.

EXAMINATION OF SAMPLING PARAMETERS

Level of reference correlation. Discrimination tests were run with PAG levels below a reference PAG=0.50, and with PAG levels above each of several reference levels from PAG=0.50 to 0.99. The entries in the left section of Table 4 are the PAG thresholds required for 60, 70, 80, and 90% correct identification. (In some cases, the 90% correct level could not be discerned because of the limited range of PAG levels tested.) The entries of the right section are expressed in terms of the difference between the reference and threshold PAG, when each is expressed in z-score, or normalized form. For example, $z(0.80)=0.841$, $z(0.835)=0.974$, $z(\text{difference})=0.133$.

Although somewhat larger normalized differences are required with higher reference PAG levels, the trend is weak. To a first approximation, discrimination is based upon a constant difference, expressed in normalized PAG score units, irrespective of the reference correlation.

TABLE 4

Threshold PAG levels and threshold differences for identification of visual tetrachoric correlations

	Threshold levels					z-differences			
Ref. PAG	60%	70%	80%	90%		60%	70%	80%	90%
0.50−	0.440	0.410	0.360	0.210		0.15	0.23	0.36	0.81
0.50+	0.580	0.640	0.700	0.780		0.20	0.36	0.52	0.77
0.60	0.640	0.680	0.715	0.780		0.10	0.21	0.31	0.52
0.70	0.735	0.770	0.890			0.10	0.21	0.70	
0.80	0.835	0.880	0.925			0.13	0.33	0.60	
0.90	0.929	0.942	0.958			0.19	0.29	0.44	
0.95	0.964	0.972	0.982			0.15	0.27	0.45	
0.97	0.978	0.984	0.989	0.999		0.13	0.26	0.41	
0.98	0.986	0.991	0.995			0.14	0.31	0.52	
0.99	0.994	0.997	0.999			0.18	0.42	0.72	
					Aver.	0.15	0.29	0.52	

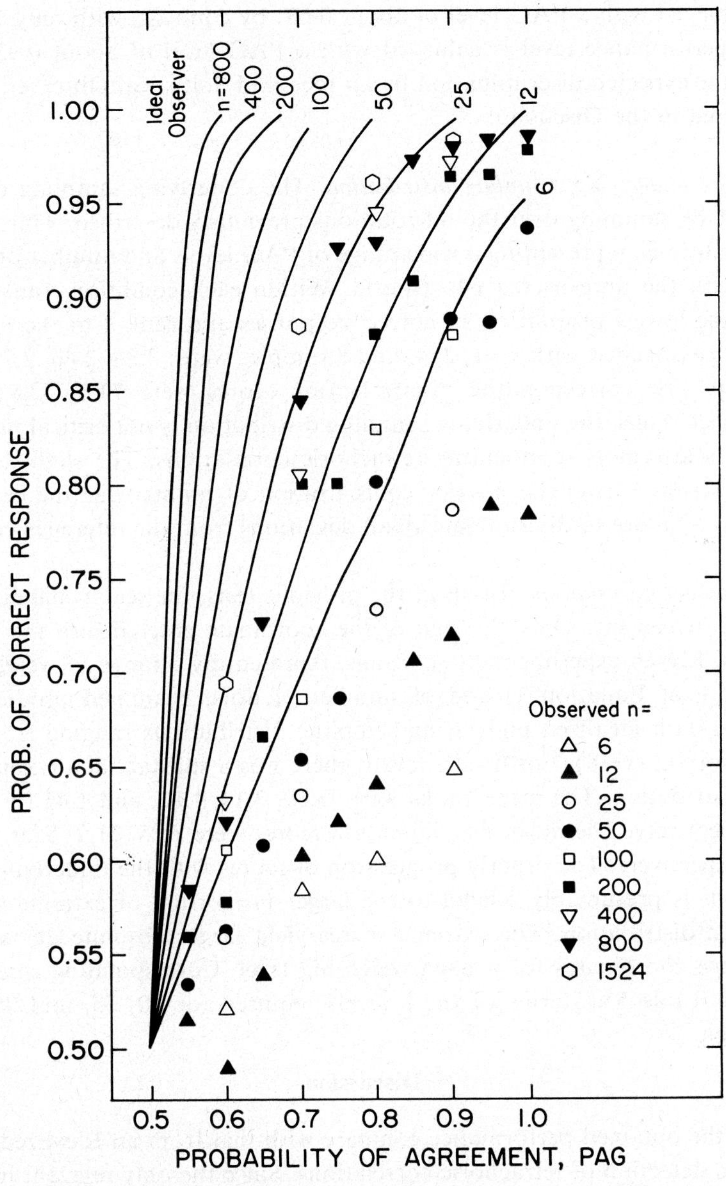

Fig. 1. Accuracy of identification of tetrachoric correlations as a function of the probability of agreement between the signs of the *x*- and *y*-coordinates. The parameter assigned to the points is the number of displayed dots. The thin smooth curves represent the expected discrimination by an Idealized Statistical Observer (see text).

Number of samples. Figure 1 presents the effect of the number of dots within the display upon the identification of tetrachoric correlations. The reference PAG level was 0.50; the other PAG level is plotted on the abscissa. Sensitivity improves with a greater number of observations. With 1524 samples, for example, the 75% correct level is achieved with a PAG level of about 0.63; by contrast, with only 12 samples, the same performance level is achieved with a PAG level of about 0.93. The thin lines plot the expected discrimination by an Idealized Statistical Observer, which will be considered in the Discussion.

Shape of the underlying sampling distribution. The underlying sampling distribution was varied by summing over the bit-rotations previously described. Thirteen experimental conditions, representing a wide range of PAG levels and number of dots, were sampled with the unrestricted 64×64 grid. Within each condition, rank 1 was assigned to the lowest proportion of correct responses and rank 4 to the highest. The mean ranks associated with $s=1$, 2, 4, and 8 samples were: 2.85, 2.46, 2.77, and 1.92 respectively. The corresponding discrimination scores were 73.6, 72.8, 73.0, and 71.5% correct. Thus, the underlying sampling distribution is not critical in the identification of scatterplots representing tetrachoric correlations. The slight loss at $s=8$ may have resulted from the heavier concentration of points near the center of the display and a failure to discriminate small deviations from the reference coordinates.

Product-moment correlations. In all of the previous tests, the scalar magnitude of the sample was irrelevant: Only the sign of the coordinate entered into the tetrachoric correlation. Eleven experimental conditions, representing a range of weighting levels (parameter c of Equation 1) and of number of dots, examined product-moment correlations with idealized underlying sampling distributions ranging from uniform ($s=1$) to normal ($s=8$). For fixed c levels, there was a substantial advantage for the uniform distribution. The mean ranks were: 3.59, 3.14, 1.82, and 1.45 for $s=1$, 2, 4, and 8, respectively. The mean discrimination scores were 75.5, 71.2, 65.9, and 63.1% correct, respectively. The orderly progression of scores with the underlying sampling distributions is presumably related to the larger proportion of extreme scores with the uniform distribution. The extreme scores yield larger absolute deviations from the reference coordinates for a fixed weighting level. Corresponding thresholds are reported in Table 5 in terms of the c levels required for 60, 75, and 90% correct identification.

Discussion

How does the obtained performance compare with that from an Idealized Statistical Observer in detection of tetrachoric correlations. Since the only relevant information is the total number of samples in the NE-SW quadrants relative to the total number of dots, the Idealized Statistical Observer is assumed to make a perfect count of the number of dots in the NE and SW quadrants. With a small number of samples, errors of identification will be made by the Idealized Statistical Observer as a result of probabilistic sampling.

The performance of the Idealized Statistical Observer may be evaluated in several ways. By means of tables of the binomial probability distribution (Harvard University Computational Laboratory, 1955), the exact binomial distribution can be obtained

TABLE 5

Thresholds for detection of product-moment correlations

Level	s	Number of dots, n			
		16	64	256	1024
	1	0.130	0.061	0.033	0.019 [a]
60%	2	0.130	0.078	0.042	0.019
[0.51] [c]	4	0.158	0.094	0.055	0.033
	8	0.209	0.145	0.055	0.044
		(0.233)	(0.141)	(0.300)	(0.120) [b]
	1	0.289	0.123	0.059	0.039
75%	2	–	0.192	0.094	0.045
[1.35]	4	–	0.231	0.100	0.067
	8	–	0.233	0.125	0.097
			(0.316)	(0.349)	(0.154)
	1	–	0.233	0.095	0.059
90%	2	–	–	0.122	0.097
[2.56]	4	–	–	0.172	0.109
	8	–	0.344	0.209	0.177
			(0.372)	(0.367)	(0.138)

[a] Each entry outside of parentheses is magnitude of the common factor, c, common to each of two distributions required to achieve the indicated performance level.

[b] Each item within parentheses is the efficiency of the human operator relative to the Ideal Statistical Observer.

[c] Equivalent d' score.

for each PAG level and number of dots. Assuming symmetrical values and costs, a response criterion can be obtained which will minimize the differences in the areas of the respective tails of the distributions. This method forms the basis for the thin curves of Figure 1.

An approximation to the performance of the Idealized Statistical Observer may also be obtained on the assumption of normality and binomial sampling variance. For the special case where the reference PAG$=0.5$ and the other PAG is abbreviated as p, the performance of the Idealized Observer is:

$$d'_{IO} = \frac{\sqrt{n}(p - 0.5)}{\sqrt{0.25 + p(1 - p)}}.$$

The performance of the human observer in the one-interval test was obtained by converting the percentage correct scores to d'_{HO} scores by means of Elliot's Table I (Swets, 1964). In these calculations, it was assumed that the proportion of misses equalled the false alarm rate.

The *relative efficiency* of the Human Observer, R.E., following Tanner and Birdsall (1958), is defined as:

$$\text{R.E.} = (d'_{HO}/d'_{IO})^2 .$$

TABLE 6

Relative efficiency (R.E.) of the human observer to the Idealized observer

Number samples	R.E.	PAG	R.E.
6[a]	0.208	0.55[b]	0.095
12	0.183	0.60	0.072
25	0.209	0.65	0.078
50	0.190	0.70	0.159
100	0.134	0.75	0.133
200	0.106	0.80	0.158
400	0.082	0.85	0.192
800	0.047	0.90	0.142
1524	0.034	0.95	0.154

[a] R.E. averages for $n=6$, 25, 100, 400, 1524 are based upon PAG levels = 0.60, 0.70, 0.80, 0.90; R.E. averages for $n=12$, 50, 200, 800 are based upon all PAG levels = 0.55 to 0.95.
[b] R.E. averages for PAG = 0.55, 0.65, 0.75, 0.85, 0.95 are based upon n levels = 12, 50, 200, 800; R.E. averages for PAG = 0.60, 0.70, 0.80, 0.90 are based upon all n levels = 6 to 1524.

Relative efficiency scores were computed for the conditions represented in Figure 1. Average efficiency scores as a function of PAG alone and of n alone are presented in Table 6. Over all tests, the average relative efficiency was 0.132. Somewhat higher relative efficiencies are obtained for PAG levels of 0.70 and higher, than for PAG levels below 0.70.

Substantially higher relative efficiencies are obtained for 50 and fewer points than for a larger number of points, where the relative efficiency drops off with the number of points. To this extent, the results suggest that the human operator fails to aggregate information with a large number of samples. Caution must be exercised before the conclusion is accepted uncritically. The normal-curve approximation at $n=6$ and 12, and possibly at $n=25$, is suspect. An exact binomial analysis with $n=6$, employing integer values only, however, suggests that the performance of the Idealized Observer varies from that calculated by, at most, 10%. Moreover, a few 'sloppy' errors, e.g. pushing the wrong button by mistake, have extreme consequences at high d'_{HO} levels. Also, for the very first observation within a one-interval test, the two possible distributions are not available to the human observer. The tentative conclusion is that, while the sharp drop in efficiency with n might be slightly exaggerated by factors peculiar to the testing circumstances, the drop in relative efficiency with larger samples is not artifactual.

It is tempting to ascribe the poor efficiency of the human operator to the non-relevant, but distracting, distribution of points within each quadrant. An argument against this position is the relative insensitivity of the extent of variation, especially in centered displays. Reduction of the extent of available variation, at least in the outside-in displays, is associated with poorer, rather than better performance.

Somewhat different conclusions result when comparing the detection of product-moment correlations to the performance of the Idealized Statistical Observer.

For uniform distributions, it may be shown (Professor W. Ericson, personal communication) that the Idealized Statistical Observer merely determines whether any point is outside of the bounds determined by the lower of two common factors. If so, he responds in favor of the more extreme common factor. If not, he calculates a ratio based upon the magnitude of the two weightings factors and votes accordingly without calculation upon the observations. For Gaussian distributions, it may be shown (Prof. Theodore G. Birdsall, personal communication) that the Idealized Statistical Observer computes for each point the mean squared distance to the positive diagonal and to the negative diagonal, and its predicted performance is

$$d = \text{approximately } (d'_{IO})^2 = \frac{nr^2}{1 - r^2} = \frac{nc^2}{(1 - c)^2}.$$

The efficiency of the human operator, relative to the Idealized Statistical Observer is:

$$\text{R.E.} = \frac{(d'_{HO})^2 \, (1 - c)^2}{nc^2}.$$

The d' scores for the human observer for 60, 75, and 90% correct detection in the one-interval test are listed in square brackets of Table 5 (Elliot, 1964). The relative efficiency scores for $s = 8$ are shown in parentheses.

Up to 256 dots, there is no appreciable loss in efficiency with a greater number of samples. The relative efficiency at the higher performance levels is about 0.35 – a nearly three-fold improvement when compared with tetrachoric correlations.

We are thus left with the following picture:

1. With underlying uniform distributions, the efficiency of the human operator in identifying tetrachoric correlations is relatively poor – about 13% of the Idealized Statistical Observer. Since the Idealized Statistical Observer is insensitive to the underlying distribution, and since the detection by the human observer of tetrachoric correlations is even poorer with underlying normal distributions, the relative efficiency scores would be even lower with normal sampling distributions.

2. With underlying normal distributions, the efficiency of the human operator in identifying product-moment correlations is substantially better – about 30% of the Idealized Observer.

In the identification of product-moment correlations, distance information is relevant; in identification of tetrachoric correlations, only count information is relevant. It would appear, therefore, relative to the performance of an Idealized Statitistical Observer, that the human operator can more effectively extract distance information than counting information.

Appendix A. The Relation between the Product Moment Correlation, *r*, and the Proportion of Agreements of Sign, PAG, for a Uniform Distribution

Without knowledge of x, the mean of y, $M_y = 0$, and the total variance of y is

$$\sigma_y^2 = \int_{-1}^{1} (y - M_y)^2 \, p(y) \, \mathrm{d}y = \left. \frac{y^3}{3} \frac{1}{2} \right]_{-1}^{1} = \tfrac{1}{3}.$$

With knowledge of sign of x, say x is positive, the mean of y,

$$M_{y\,|\,x} = \int_{-1}^{1} y p(y) \, \mathrm{d}y = P \left. \frac{y^2}{2} \right]_0^1 + Q \left. \frac{y^2}{2} \right]_{-1}^{0} = \frac{(P - Q)}{2} = c,$$

where $P = \text{PAG}$ and where $Q = (1 - P)$.

With knowledge of the sign of x, say x is positive, the variance of y

$$\sigma_{y\,|\,x}^2 = \int_{-1}^{1} (y - M_y)^2 \, p(y) \, \mathrm{d}y = P \left[\frac{y^3}{3} - cy^2 + c^2 y \right]_0^1 +$$

$$+ Q \left[y^3 - cy^2 + cy^2 \right]_{-1}^{0} =$$

$$= P\left[\tfrac{1}{3} - c + c^2\right] + Q\left[\tfrac{1}{3} + c + c^2\right] =$$

$$= \tfrac{1}{3} - c^2 .$$

The correlation may be expressed in terms of the ratio between the variance of the test variable accounted by knowledge of one variable, relative to the total variance.

$$r^2 = 1 - \frac{\sigma_{y\,|\,x}^2}{\sigma_y^2} = 1 - \frac{\left(\tfrac{1}{3} - c^2\right)}{\tfrac{1}{3}} = 3c^2 = 0.75\,(2P - 1)^2$$

therefore, when $P = 1.0$ or 0, $r^2 = 0.75$; and when $P = 0.5$, $r^2 = 0$.

Appendix B. Relation between Product-Moment Correlation, *r*, and Common Weighting Factor, *c*, for Two Noise Sources

$$y = cx + (1 - c)\, z \qquad (1)$$

$$\therefore \sum y^2 = c^2 \sum x^2 + 2c\,(1 - c) \sum xz + (1 - c)^2 \sum z^2$$

when x and z are independent distributions,

$$\sum xz = 0, \quad \sum x^2 = \sum z^2$$

$$\therefore \sum y^2 = [c^2 + (1-c)^2] \sum x^2$$

$$r^2 \sum x^2 \sum y^2 = (\sum xy)^2 =$$

$$= [\sum [x_1 (cx_1 + (1-c) z_1] + \cdots [x_n (cx_n + (1-c) z_n]]^2 =$$

$$= [c \sum x^2 + (1-c) \sum xz]^2 =$$

$$= c^2 [\sum x^2]^2$$

$$\therefore r^2 \sum y^2 = c^2 \sum x^2$$

$$r^2 = c^2/[c^2 + (1-c)^2].$$

References

Elliott, P. B. Tables of d'. In Swets, J. A. (Ed.), *Signal detection and recognition by human observers.* Appendix I, 1964, pp. 651–684.

Green, B. F. Jr., Wolf, A. K., & White, B. W. The detection of statistically defined patterns in a matrix of dots. *American Journal of Psychology*, 1959, **72**, 503–520.

Harvard University Computational Laboratory. *Tables of the cumulative binomial probability distribution.* Harvard University Press, 1955.

Julesz, B. Visual pattern discrimination. *Institute of Radio Engineers Transactions on Information Theory*, 1962, **IT-8**, 84–92.

Licklider, J. C. R., & Dzendolet, E. Oscilloscopic scatterplots illustrating various degrees of correlation. *Science*, 1948, **107**, 121–124.

Pickett, R. The perception of a visual texture. *Journal of Experimental Psychology*, 1964, **68**, 13–20.

Pickett, R. Response latency in a pattern perception situation. In Sanders, A. F. (Ed.). *Attention and performance I*. Amsterdam: North-Holland Publishing Company, 1970, pp. 160–169.

Pollack, I. Identification of visual correlational scatterplots. *Journal of Experimental Psychology*, 1960, **59**, 351–360.

Pollack, I. Perception of two-dimensional Markov constraints. *Perception and Psychophysics*, 1971 **9**, 461–464.

Pollack, I., & Trittipoe, W. J. Binaural listening and interaural noise cross-correlation. *Journal of the Acoustical Society of America*, 1959, **31**, 1250–1252. (a)

Pollack, I., & Trittipoe, W. J. Interaural noise correlations: examination of variables. *Journal of the Acoustical Society of America*, 1959, **31**, 1616–1618. (b)

Slovic, P. & Lichtenstein, S. Comparison of Bayesian and regression approaches to study of information processing in judgment. *Organizational Behavior and Human Performance*, 1971, **6**, 649–744.

Tanner, W. P. Jr., & Birdsall, T. G. Definition of d' and η as psychophysical measures. *Journal of the Acoustical Society of America*, 1958, **30**, 922–928.

Wojnarowski, L., Bachman, K., & Pollack, I. High-speed point plotting with computer-controlled displays. *Behavioral Methods and Instrumentation*, 1971, **3**, 210–211.

ROD SIGNALS IN HIGHER COLOR MECHANISMS: THE McCOLLOUGH COLOR AFTEREFFECT OBSERVED IN SCOTOPIC ILLUMINATION

CHARLES F. STROMEYER III[1]

Stanford University

Abstract. The McCollough color aftereffect – a long-lasting color aftereffect specific to both line orientation and spatial frequency – was observed in scotopic illumination well below the rod-cone break. Two color adaptation procedures were used: (*a*) Adaptation to a photopic green vertical grating alternating with a magenta horizontal grating or to an orange vertical grating alternating with a blue horizontal grating; (*b*) Adaptation to vertical green and magenta gratings of different low apatial frequencies. After color adaptation, test patterns were viewed in scotopic illumination. The sftereffects observed were specific to both the orientation and spatial frequency of the test patterns. These results are consistent with physiological observations that rod signals feed into opponent color mechanisms.

The view that rods interact only with rods and that each of the three cones (or Stiles π mechanisms) act independently of each other is a view that is appealing for its simplicity and the wealth of evidence that supports it. The independent action of these mechanisms has been demonstrated in studies on the increment threshold (Stiles, 1949; 1959), the after-flash (Alpern, 1965; Alpern & Ruston, 1965), on sensitization with annular surrounds (Westheimer, 1970; McKee & Westheimer, 1970), and on dark adaptation (Du Croz & Ruston, 1966). These events probably occur quite early in the retina, for the separate channels combine at some level in the retina (Gouras, 1968) and the basic characteristic of later stages of the visual system is an antagonism between different color processes.

An interaction between cone and rod signals has been suggested by studies on brightness contrast (Richards, Luria, & Matteson, 1967) and the conditioning flash (Frumkes, Sekuler, & Reiss, 1972). But the most compelling evidence for interactions comes from studies in which color sensations are elicited via the rods. If the dark-adapted eye is pre-stimulated with a colored light that affects cones, a complementary color afterimage may then be elicited with a scotopic flash (Stabell & Stabell, 1965; 1971b; Stabell, 1967). Rod signals appear to trigger the afterimage, for the color seen does not vary with the wavelength of the scotopic flash, and the level of light required to trigger the afterimage coincides with the dark adaptation curve of the rods (Stabell & Stabell, 1965; 1968a). The scotopic flash may elicit the afterimage even one hour after the colored pre-stimulation (Stabell & Stabell, 1971a). Contrast colors of blue and green can be produced in a bipartite field when one half is illuminated with scotopic light and the other with photopic red, orange, or yellow light (Willmer, 1950; Stabell,

[1] I wish to thank Dr Charles S. Harris for equipment, Mr Richard A. Payne for generously acting as a subject, Mrs Cecilia Bahlman for help on the manuscript, and Professor Karl Pribram for his continued support.

H. R. Moskowitz et al. (eds.), Sensation and Measurement. 403–410. *All Rights Reserved.*

1967; Stabell & Stabell, 1968b). McCann & Benton (1969) obtained similar colors in a Land two-color projection with red and scotopic lights and with red and its photopic blue-green complement. These studies clearly suggest that rod and cone signals converge at some level of the visual system.

The present study shows that McCollough color aftereffects may be seen on test patterns in scotopic light. McCollough (1965) found that after prolonged adaptation to a vertical grating in one color and a perpendicular grating in a complementary color, color aftereffects could be seen for many hours thereafter when the observer viewed a black and white grating whose retinal orientation was similar to the adapting pattern. The color effect was thus orientation-specific and was complementary in hue to the adapting color. The present experiments show that color effects that are specific to both orientation and spatial frequency may be seen at scotopic levels. These aftereffects also appear to induce complementary contrast colors on adjacent gratings, which by themselves appear colorless.

Methods

Three subjects with normal color vision participated in these experiments. One subject, R.A.P., was uninformed about the experiment; the other subjects, who included the author, knew the purpose of the experiment and were very familiar with the McCollough effect.

Dark adaptation curves were first measured on the two experienced subjects. The subject first light adapted 320 s to a very large opal glass field illuminated at 4000 mL by an incandescent bulb. Immediately afterwards the subject fixated a tiny red light in the center of a 10° diameter disk and adjusted a neutral wedge, which controlled the light falling on the disk, so that the disk remained slightly below threshold. The subject also adjusted the intensity of the fixation light so it was just visible. The disk was a piece of white paper on a black ground. These materials had the same reflectance as all test patterns used later. The light came from a regulated projector with accessory lenses, and was filtered through a narrow-band green filter (Wratten 74; under illuminant A, dominant wavelength, 538 nm). The wedges were placed in a narrow part of the beam. Figure 1 shows the dark adaptation curves. The vertical axis represents the luminance of the white disk. The light level at which the break occurs agrees approximately with that found by Chapanis (1947) for a broad-band green spot 3° diameter at 7° from the fovea. It was also noticed that acuity changed very rapidly at the break – especially when the test gratings were viewed in later parts of the experiment.

The color aftereffects in the first experiment were built up with square-wave gratings of 0.75 cycle deg^{-1}, rear-projected on a ground glass screen. The patterns subtended an area about 30° square from the 30-cm viewing distance. All gratings in these experiments were about 95% contrast (Michelson contrast). Gratings were projected in alternate vertical and horizontal orientations and interchanged every second. A tiny fixation light was located in the screen's center. On each presentation the grating was

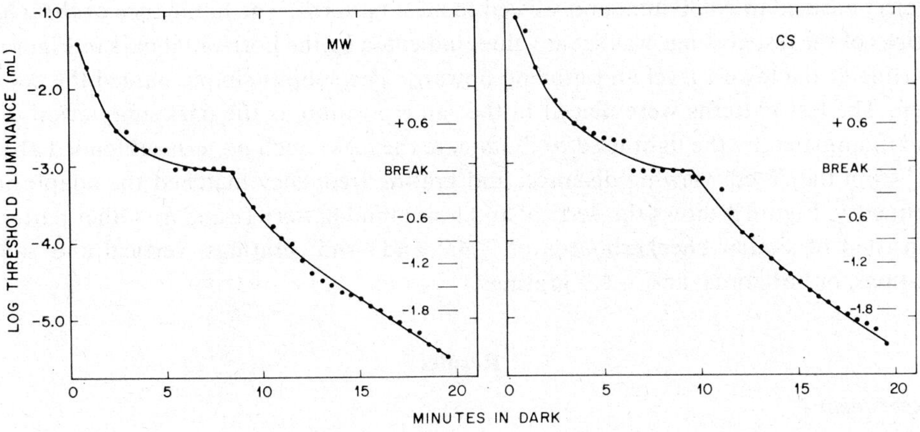

Fig. 1. Dark-adaptation curves measured in narrow-band green light of dom λ538 nm. The luminance of the white stripes of the test gratings is given by bars on right which indicate 0.3 log steps above and below rod-cone break.

projected in the same position or shifted 180° in phase by mirrors. The shift was randomly determined. The subject stared at the fixation light, with head held by a chin and brow rest. This strategy helped to adapt the eyes evenly and prevent a structured afterimage.

In the first session the subject adapted 20 min to a vertical grating projected in green light (Wratten 40; under illuminant A, dominant wavelength, 513 nm and with the luminance of bright bars at 160 mL), and a horizontal grating in magenta light (Wratten 31, 513c nm and 120 mL). In the second session the subject adapted 30 min to a vertical grating in orange light (Wratten 106, 596 nm and 260 mL) and a horizontal grating in blue light (Wratten 47A, 478 nm and 20 mL). After color adaption, the

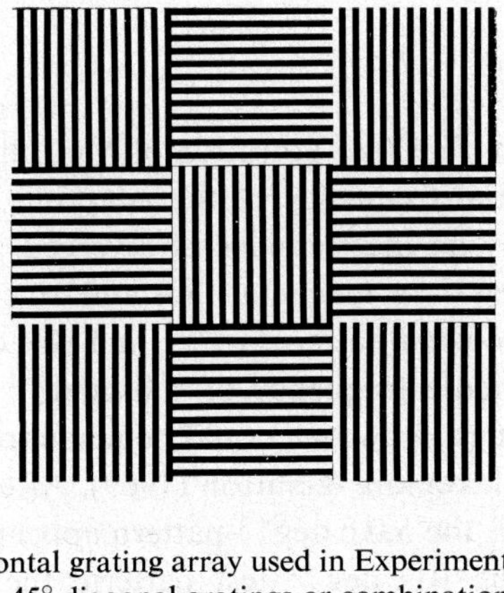

Fig. 2. The vertical and horizontal grating array used in Experiment 1. Other test patterns consisted of similar checkerboards of just 45° diagonal gratings or combinations of vertical and 45° gratings or horizontal and 45° gratings.

subject dark adapted 30 min. and viewed the test patterns. The luminance of the white stripes of the test gratings was set at values indicated by the horizontal bars in Figure 1, starting at the lowest level and moving upward. The subject simply named the colors seen. The test patterns were placed in the same position as the dark adaptation disk and illuminated by the light used to illuminate the disk. Each pattern subtended about 48° from the 50 cm viewing distance, and grating frequency matched the adaptation frequency. Figure 2 shows the vertical and horizontal pattern (v and h). Other patterns consisted of similar checkerboards of +45° and −45° gratings, vertical and +45° gratings, or horizontal and −45° gratings.

Results

Experiment 1

After adapting to vertical green and horizontal magenta gratings, the vertical and horizontal gratings of the v and h pattern (Figure 2) appeared faintly reddish and greenish respectively to all subjects at the lowest scotopic level of −1.8 log units below the rod-cone break. The color became more saturated as the test light was increased. The pattern consisting of just 45° diagonal gratings appeared colorless. However, when diagonal gratings were paired with vertical or horizontal gratings in a checkerboard array, the diagonals then appeared complementary in color to the color seen on the adjacent vertical or horizontal components – green on vertical induced pink on diagonal, for example. All subjects reported this effect when the light was raised to about −0.9 to −0.6 log units.

After adapting to vertical yellow and horizontal blue gratings, the vertical and horizontal components of the v and h pattern appeared respectively blue or blue-green and burnt orange or yellowish for all subjects at levels as low as −1.2 log units.

The inexperienced subject R.A.P. later matched from memory the strongest scotopic colors to Munsell patches viewed in Macbeth daylight. The colors chosen for the first sessions were 10 RP 7/8 and 10 GY 7/8, and for the second session, 2.5 BG 7/4 and 2.5 YR 4/4.5.

Experiment 2

Stromeyer (1972) has shown that the saturation of McCollough aftereffects tended to be strongest when the spatial frequency of the adapting and test patterns matched and decreased progressively as the frequencies diverged. Adaptation to alternating vertical gratings of 2.5 c deg^{-1} in magenta light and 10 c deg^{-1} in green, produced green and pink aftereffects on test patterns of 2.5 and 10 c deg^{-1}, respectively, whereas a test pattern at the middle frequency of 5.0 c deg^{-1} (log scale) appeared colorless. The 5.0 c deg^{-1} pattern, however, could be made to appear colored by the apparent frequency shift of Blakemore & Sutton (1969). After inspecting the 2.5 c deg^{-1} *test pattern* for one minute, the 5.0 c deg^{-1} pattern appeared both finer and pinkish, whereas after inspecting the 10 c deg^{-1} test pattern, the same 5.0 c deg^{-1} pattern appeared both coarser and greenish. The color thus varied with the apparent spatial

Fig. 3. Test patterns used to test whether the McCollough effect is selective to spatial frequency in scotopic illumination.

frequency. When the 5.0 c deg^{-1} pattern was oriented 45° or horizontally, no frequency shift and apparent color was observed. These experiments are now repeated, with the difference that the aftereffects are observed at scotopic levels.

Low frequency, vertical, square-wave gratings of 0.5 and 2.0 c deg^{-1} were used for color adaptation. Shlaer (1937) has shown that below the rod-cone break gratings above 5 c deg^{-1} cannot be resolved. The patterns were about 40° square at the viewing distance of 24 cm. The 0.5 c deg^{-1} pattern alone was projected in the same position or shifted 180° in phase, as before. The subject stared at the central fixation point. Subject M.W. adapted 40 min. to the 0.5 and 2.0 c deg^{-1} patterns projected in the green and magenta lights, respectively. The other two subjects adapted to the opposite condition – C.F.S. for 60 min and R.A.P. for 40 min. For some subjects, the two gratings were shown unequal amounts of time in order to build up good pink *and* green aftereffects. The test patterns are shown in Figure 3. Each grating was 15° by 13° at the viewing distance of 89 cm. After color adaptation the patterns were viewed in Macbeth daylight. The middle frequency pattern of 1.0 c deg^{-1} appeared quite neutral, whereas the other patterns were somewhat pinkish and greenish as predicted. All subjects claimed the colors were more saturated when the patterns were next viewed at high scotopic levels of illumination. (Subjects M.W., C.F.S., and R.A.P. viewed the patterns at the levels -1.0, -0.6, and -0.3 log units respectively – see Figure 1.) The 1.0 c deg^{-1} pattern again appeared quite neutral. However, if the subject first scanned back and forth along the horizontal band separating the 0.5 and 2.0 c deg^{-1} test gratings for 2 min and next fixated the band separating the 1.0 c deg^{-1} gratings, then the two 1.0 c deg^{-1} gratings appeared both different in apparent frequency and colored reddish and greenish accordingly.

Discussion

The color aftereffects observed at scotopic levels are thus both orientation- and frequency-selective, and the hue of the aftereffects is quite similar at both scotopic and photopic levels. However, at the scotopic level, the oranges and yellows effects are weak, yet these same colors are readily seen at photopic levels on patterns viewed in Macbeth daylight (unpublished). The scotopic test patterns appeared to be suffused by a light that was subjectively bluish in tint and this may have partially cancelled any yellow aftereffects. Haig (1941) and Nagel (1924) have noted this blue quality of scotopic light, and Stabell and Stabell (1971a) have shown that negative afterimages triggered by rods are more blue or red than the additive opponent color.

That the aftereffect stays tied to the adapting spatial frequency suggests that the receptive field of the mechanisms underlying these effects does not lose its antagonistic surround in the dark-adapted state. Loss of the surround mechanism would cause test patterns of low spatial frequencies to elicit both the red and green aftereffects, which would cancel each other, and thus frequency-selective colors would disappear. Graham (1972) has shown that adaptation to luminance gratings at low mesopic levels raises the threshold only for gratings of similar spatial frequencies, and the frequency tuning characteristic is identical to that obtained at photopic levels. The present results suggest that adaptation is frequency-selective at even lower, scotopic levels. The existence of the antagonistic surround in the dark-adapted state is further suggested by the occurrence of scotopic brightness contrast (Hollins, 1971), Mach bands (Fiorentini and Maffei, 1973), and sensitization by annular surrounds (Westheimer, 1970). And Gouras (1967) has demonstrated the antagonistic surround in monkey ganglion cells in the dark-adapted state by measuring the areal summation curve for the receptive field.

The present experiment shows that rod signals affect color mechanisms at some level of the visual system. Rod and cone signals converge on single ganglion cells in the monkey retina (Gouras and Link, 1966), and many ganglion cells have receptive fields that receive excitatory signals from a red, green, or blue cone mechanism in the center and inhibitory signals from a different cone mechanism in the periphery (Gouras, 1968). Similar spatial-color units are found in the lateral geniculate nucleus (LGN). Many of these units undergo a Purkinje shift when dark adapted, thus demonstrating a rod input (Wiesel and Hubel, 1966). The color units in the retina and LGN have circularly symmetric receptive fields. The McCollough effect is orientation-selective and it does not transfer from eye to eye. Dow and Gouras (1973) have found in monkey cortex many orientation-selective color cells. Many of these color-opponent cortical cells have receptive fields whose excitatory and inhibitory areas receive inputs from the same cone type (Gouras, 1974), and thus they are highly sensitive to the spatial properties of, say, a red or green pattern – unlike the pre-cortical cells. And most of these cells respond to one eye only (Gouras, 1974). Adaptation to a colored grating might thus depress sensitivity in a subset of units tuned to the adapting color, spatial frequency, and orientation. A test pattern similar to the adapting pattern will then produce less activity in these units, and this imbalance of response may thus signal the complementary color. Rod signal may also feed into these units, and thus the color aftereffects might also be seen in scotopic illumination. (Stabell and Stabell, 1973, present a somewhat similar theory for rod triggered afterimages.)

Simultaneous color contrast was observed in the present experiments. Thus a grating that appeared colorless when viewed alone, could be made to appear colored by pairing it with an adjacent grating that did appear colored. A single grating could be made reddish or greenish by this contrast effect. Color contrast elicited via the rods cannot be explained by the classical theories which postulate lateral inhibitory interactions between only receptor mechanisms of the same type (Rollett, 1867; McDougall, 1901; Alpern, 1964). Nor can it be explained by the Hering opponent theory (Jameson and Hurvich, 1964) which postulates a black-white luminance system independent from the red-green and blue-yellow systems. Both Wiesel and Hubel (1966) and De Valois and Pease (1971) have not found units at pre-cortical levels that might plausibly serve as a mechanism of color contrast. They both suggest that color contrast may be a cortical affair. The mechanism thus remains elusive.

References

Alpern, M. Relation between brightness and color contrast. *Journal of the Optical Society of America*, 1964, **54**, 1491–1492.

Alpern, M. Rod-cone independence in the after-flash effect. *Journal of Physiology*, 1965, **176**, 462–472.

Alpern, M., & Rushton, W. A. H. The specificity of the cone interaction in the after-flash effect. *Journal of Physiology*, 1965, **176**, 473–482.

Blakemore, C., & Sutton, P. Size adaptation: A new aftereffect. *Science*, 1969, **166**, 245–247.

Chapanis, A. The dark adaptation of the color anomalous measured with lights of different hues. *Journal of General Physiology*, 1947, **30**, 423–437.

Dow, B. M., & Gouras, P. Color and spatial specificity of single units in Rhesus monkey foveal striate cortex. *Journal of Neurophysiology*, 1973, **36**, 79–100.

De Valois, R. L., & Pease, P. L. Contours and contrast: Responses of monkey lateral geniculate nucleus cells to luminance and color figures. *Science*, 1971, **171**, 694–696.

Du Croz, J. J., & Rushton, W. A. H. The separation of cone mechanisms in dark adaptation. *Journal of Physiology*, 1966, **183**, 481–496.

Fiorentini, A., & Maffei, L. Contrast in night vision. *Vision Research*, 1973, **13**, 73–80.

Frumkes, T. E., Sekuler, M. D., & Reiss, E. H. Rod-cone interaction in human scotopic vision. *Science*, 1972, **175**, 913–914.

Graham, N. Spatial frequency channels in the human visual system: Effects of luminance and pattern drift rate. *Vision Research*, 1972, **12**, 53–68.

Gouras, P. The effects of light-adaptation on rod and cone receptive field organization of monkey ganglion cells. *Journal of Physiology*, 1967, **192**, 747–760.

Gouras, P. Identification of cone mechanisms in monkey ganglion cells. *Journal of Physiology*, 1968, **199**, 533–547.

Gouras, P. Opponent-colour cells in different layers of foreal striate catex. *Journal of Physiology*, 1974, **238**, 583–602.

Gouras, P., & Link, K. Rod and cone interaction in dark-adapted monkey ganglion cells. *Journal of Physiology*, 1966, **184**, 499–510.

Haig, C. The course or rod dark adaptation as influenced by the intensity and duration of preadaptation to light. *Journal of General Physiology*, 1941, **24**, 735–751.

Hollins, M. Brightness contrast at low luminances. *Vision Research*, 1971, **11**, 1459–1472.

Jameson, D., & Hurvich, L. M. Theory of brightness and color contrast in Human vision. *Vision Research*, 1964, **4**, 135–154.

McCann, J. J., & Benton, J. L. Interaction of long-wave cones and rods to produce color sensations. *Journal of the Optical Society of America*, 1969, **59**, 103–107.

McCollough, C. Color adaptation of edge-detectors in the human visual system. *Science*, 1965, **149**, 1115–1116.

McDougall, W. IV – Some new observations in support of Thomas Young's Theory of light – and colour-vision (III. Conclusion.) *Mind*, 1901, **10**, *N.S.*, 347–382.

McKee, S. P., & Westheimer, G. Specificity of cone mechanisms in lateral interaction. *Journal of Physiology*, 1970, **206**, 117–128.

Nagel, W. Adaptation, twilight vision, and the duplicity theory, an appendix in H. Helmholtz, *Treatise on Physiological Optics*, Vol. II, 1924 (translated from the third German Edition by J. P. C. Southall) Optical Society of America.

Richards, W., Luria, S. M., & Matteson, H. H. Interacting spectral sensitivity functions obtained in a contrast situation. *Vision Research*, 1967, **7**, 629–644.

Rollett, A. Zur Physiologie der Contrastfarben. *Sitzungsberichte Akademie der Wissenschaften, Wien, Mathematisch-naturwissenschaftliche Klasse*, 1867, **55**, *Abth. 2*, 741–766.

Shlaer, S. The relation between visual acuity and illumination. *Journal of General Physiology*, 1937, **21**, 165–188.

Stabell, B. Rods as color receptors in scotopic vision. *Scandinavian Journal of Psychology*, 1967, **8**, 132–144.

Stabell, U., & Stabell, B. Rods as color receptors. *Scandinavian Journal of Psychology*, 1965, **6**, 195–200.

Stabell, B., & Stabell, U. Color threshold measurements in scotopic vision. II. Test-stimulation varied. *Scandinavian Journal of Psychology*, 1968a, **9**, 129–132.

Stabell, U., & Stabell, B. Color threshold measurements in scotopic vision. III: Simultaneous color contrast. *Scandinavian Journal of Phychology*, 1968b, **9**, 133–137.

Stabell, U., & Stabell, B. Duration of scotopic contrast colors. *Scandinavian Journal of Psychology*, 1971, **12**, 106–112. (a)

Stabell, U., & Stabell, B. Chromatic rod vision. II: Wavelength of pre-stimulation varied. *Scandinavian Journal of Psychology*, 1971, **12**, 282–288. (b)

Stabell, B., & Stabell, U. Chromatic rod vision. IX: A theoretical survey. *Vision Research*, 1973, **13**, 449–455.

Stiles, W. S. Increment thresholds and the mechanisms of colour vision. *Documenta Ophthalmologica*, 1949, **3**, 138–163.

Stiles, W. S. Color vision: The approach through increment-threshold sensitivity. *Proceedings of the National Academy of Science*, Washington, 1959, **45**, 100–114.

Stromeyer, C. F. III. Edge-contingent color after-effects: Spatial frequency specificity. *Vision Research*, 1972, **12**, 717–733.

Westheimer, G. Rod-cone independence for sensitizing interaction in the human retina. *Journal of Physiology*, 1970, **206**, 109–116.

Wiesel, T. N., & Hubel, D. H. Spatial and chromatic interactions in the lateral geniculate body of the Rhesus monkey. *Journal of Neurophysiology*, 1966, **29**, 1115–1156.

Willmer, E. N. Low threshold rods and the perception of blue. *Journal of Physiology*, 1950, **111**, 17P.

THE DOUBTFUL PHENOMENON OF OVER-CONSTANCY

MARTHA TEGHTSOONIAN[1,2]
Smith College

Abstract. Originally "over-constancy" meant the growth of matched size with distance, in contrast to invariance (constancy) or decrease (under-constancy). There are logical reasons for restoring this definition and distinguishing over-constancy from over-estimation, where matched size exceeds the physical size of the standard at one or several distances. Some studies cited as demonstrating over-constancy fail to show the functional relation between matched size and distance. Of eight studies that do show this relation, two demonstrate constancy without measuring it and an additional one presents a clear picture of growth in matched size with distance, whereas the other five either obtained constancy or found over-constancy only for some standards or over a limited range of distance. Still lacking are systematic studies of size-matching for a wide range of size over a wide range of distance. Meanwhile, on the evidence currently available, the existence of over-constancy remains in doubt.

It is a widely-held belief among students of size perception that, when an observer is asked to match the physical size of an object, his matches increase in size as the distance of the object increases; see, for example, reviews by Epstein, Park, & Casey (1961), Wohlwill (1963), and Baird (1970, pp. 77–89). The phenomenon is called over-constancy, in contrast to size constancy – an invariance of matched size with increased distance – and under-constancy – a decrease in matched size with increased distance. Over-constancy is a peculiarly puzzling phenomenon for several reasons. First, it is a laboratory finding unconfirmed by everyday observation: phenomenally, an object seems to remain the same size or to get smaller as it moves further away (Leibowitz & Harvey, 1967). Second, from an evolutionary point of view, over-constancy seems at best non-functional, at worst maladaptive (Gilinsky, 1955). Third, the experimental evidence reveals little agreement about the ranges of size and distance over which over-constancy occurs, much less a general quantitative specification of the effect.

In previous papers (e.g., M. Teghtsoonian, 1965, 1972; R. Teghtsoonian & M. Teghtsoonian, 1970a, 1970b) R. Teghtsoonian and I have applied the techniques of scaling developed by S. S. Stevens to the general field of size perception, and it seems an especially useful perspective from which to review the problem of over-constancy. Such a perspective emphasizes the determination of a functional relation between dependent and independent variables, thus suggesting that over-constancy be regarded as a *growth* in matched size with the increase in distance of a given target, rather than as simple over-estimation of a target at a single distance. A review of the

[1] I dedicate this paper to S. S. Stevens. I remember him as a wrestler-scientist, stubbornly intent on wrenching truth from a disorderly and recalcitrant universe. I am grateful to him for many lessons, perhaps most of all for showing me the power of simplicity.

[2] This paper was prepared with support from grant GB 38292 from the National Science Foundation while I was a visitor in the Psychological Laboratories of the University of Stockholm, and I thank the Laboratories for the facilities they provided. I am also thankful to Robert Teghtsoonian for his careful reading of, and critical comments on, this paper, which have substantially improved it.

H. R. Moskowitz et al. (eds.), Sensation and Measurement. 411–420.

experimental literature in the light of this more restrictive definition shows that the evidence for over-constancy is neither as extensive nor as compelling as has generally been thought.

Two Criteria for Including Studies

One condition for obtaining over-constancy about which there is no disagreement is that the observer attempt to make his matches equal to the physical size of the standard, usually under explicit instructions to do so. Both Gilinsky (1955) and Leibowitz & Harvey (1967, 1969) have demonstrated a clear difference in the functions obtained under "retinal" and "objective" instructions; the former produce a decrease in matched size with distance, whereas the latter may produce an increase. In the studies reviewed here, observers either were instructed to make "objective" matches, or adopted an "objective" attitude.

A second criterion imposed on studies to be included in this review is that they occurred in natural settings and permitted unrestricted viewing – that is, free head movement and binocular regard. Experimental manipulation of setting and viewing conditions can, by the appropriate selection of parameters, produce nearly any functional relation between perceived size and distance: Vogel & M. Teghtsoonian (1972), for example, showed that the apparent size of a target object of fixed physical size may either increase (over-constancy) or decrease (under-constancy) as distance increases, depending on the perspective context in which the object is viewed. Without denying the interest and importance of such studies, this review is concerned *only* with studies of the relationship between perceived size and distance as it occurs in the natural environment. It is this relationship, after all, that laboratory analysis is intended to explain, and it seems desirable to have in hand a complete and accurate description of it. Two experiments that have been cited as showing over-constancy are eliminated by this criterion: Chalmers (1952) used a severely-reduced viewing situation; Sonoda (1961) used photographic stimuli. A study by Holway & Boring (1941), strictly speaking, does not meet the criterion, since there was no illumination in the setting save for that provided by the standard and comparison stimuli. However, it is so often cited as the first demonstration of over-constancy that a detailed consideration seems necessary.

Over-Estimation vs Over-Constancy

Holway & Boring (1941) reported a growth of matched size with distance. In their procedure, the comparison stimulus, adjustable by the observer, was always at the same distance. The series of standard stimuli, which were, like the comparison, circles of light projected on a screen, varied in distance from the observer; the size of the standard varied with distance in such a way that it always subtended the same visual angle. The results were that matched size increased faster than physical size of the standard as its distance (and physical size) increased. Holway and Boring say, "... the apparent size ... of a standard stimulus varies directly with the distance from *O* to the standard. ... At first thought, it seems as if we had here to do with a case in which apparent size is 'more than constant' [p. 26, 27]." It is clear that they meant to specify by "more than constant" a relation in which the apparent size of a standard of fixed size *increases* with distance, and to contrast it with the alternative hypotheses of constancy, in which apparent size will be unchanged with distance, and under-constancy, in which it will decrease as distance increases (a hypothesis based on consideration of the decreasing visual angle subtended by the standard). This meaning – of a monotonic increasing function relating matched size and distance for an object of fixed size – was maintained by Smith (1953), by Gilinsky (1955), and by Jenkin (1959).

However, Carlson (1960, 1962) used "over-constancy" to refer to the over-estimation of the standard at a single separation from the comparison, and Wohlwill (1963), among others, has equated over-estimation with over-constancy; moreover, this change in definition was not accompanied by an explicit recognition that it *was* a change. Consequently, "over-constancy" is now used indiscriminately to refer either to a particular functional relation between matched size and distance or to simple over-estimation of size when standard and comparison are separated in distance. Logically, however, over-estimation can occur *without* any growth in matched size with distance; there are factors that may influence the matched size of the standard at several separations of standard and comparison without producing an increasing relation between matched size and distance.

One such factor is the regression effect described by Stevens & Greenbaum (1963): observers tend to restrict the range of their responses in cross-modal matching tasks, with the result that a linear matching function (on log coordinates) will have a flatter slope than the theoretical ideal function. I have reported a regression effect even when the target continuum, line length, was the same as the matching continuum (M. Teghtsoonian, 1972). If this result is general for intramodal matching tasks, i.e., that observers produce a set of matches that cover a shorter range than the set of targets, then matched size may exceed target size over some portion of the target range. (More generally, matched size and target size will interact.)

It is also possible that differences between the standard and comparison objects, in nature or location, could produce an "illusory" size difference that would be consistently reflected in the observer's size matches at *every* distance. Such results were obtained by Leibowitz & Harvey (1967, 1969). Using a person as target object, they found no *increase* in matched size with distance, although matched size was 2–6% greater than physical size at *every* distance. With vertical boards as targets, objective-size matches again proved independent of distance, although there was an over-estimation of target objects by 10–20%. With a horizontally-placed tube as target, matched size again showed no effect of distance; when the tube was laid on an athletic field, its size was over-estimated by 20–40%, at all distances, whereas when it was laid on railroad tracks, there was no over-estimation at any distance. Finally, with a vertical board or a human as target, size matches under objective size instructions showed no change with distance; the board was overestimated by about 10% at all distances, but there was no over-estimation for the human. These studies are remarkably consistent in failing to show any effect of distance on matched size under "objective" instructions over distances from 33 to 560 yd, although their generality is limited by a narrow range of size – 60–72 in. They also demonstrate that characteristics of the target object and its setting, in conjunction with an "objective" set, can produce a considerable over-estimation of size, but to the same degree over a five-fold range of distance.

It is the argument of this paper that the two effects – over-constancy and over-estimation – ought to be discriminated from each other. Over-estimation can occur without over-constancy, and therefore variables producing one phenomenon need not produce the other. To talk about the two as if they were equivalent may lead to false conclusions about the existence and controlling variables of over-constancy.

If the term "over-constancy" is reserved for the functional relation between apparent size and distance in which the former increases with the latter, then any experiment that uses a single distance cannot establish the existence of over-constancy. Carlson (1960, 1962) showed that, under objective-size instructions, the near comparison was set to a greater value than the far standard. But only one separation between standard and comparison was used, and, since distance was not varied, Carlson did not discover the functional relation between matched size and distance in his viewing situation. His results are *consonant* with the existence of over-constancy, but they may as well have resulted from characteristics of the viewing situation other than distance, or from constraints exerted by the matching task, that would have led the observer to set the comparison larger than the standard. For example, he used an unfamiliar target object, a condition shown by Leibowitz & Harvey (1969) to be conducive to over-estimation independently of distance.

The Holway and Boring Design Does not Demonstrate Over-Constancy

The same criticism that was made of Carlson's design as a means of demonstrating over-constancy can also be made of the Holway & Boring (1941) design, since, as in Carlson's studies, only one distance was used for any given target size. The comparison was at a fixed distance; a different size of the standard occurred at each of several distances (in order to maintain a constant visual angle). Thus, there was (and could be) no direct evidence that the matched size of a single standard increased with distance. The result that led the authors to conclude that matched size did increase with distance was that the matched size was always larger than the physical size of the standard; this was true at every distance, and the absolute size of the error increased with the physical size of the standard (and its distance). Holway and Boring *assumed* that, if standard and comparison had been presented at the same distance, then the comparison would have been set to physical equality with the standard; if this assumption was correct, then the larger matched size of the standard when it was further away indicated a growth in matched size with distance, and so over-constancy.

But there are reasons for doubting the correctness of this assumption. First, one standard (a circle of 2-in. diameter) was presented at the same distance as the comparison, with the result that the comparison was set, on the average, about 20% greater than the standard! Second, an examination of the data for individual observers suggests that the judgmental ranges are shorter than the stimulus ranges, and hence that the regression effect was at work. (Since distance and standard size are linearly related, Holway and Boring's matched size vs distance plots can be redrawn as matched size vs standard size.) Power functions for individual observers are excellent fits, with coefficients of determination all near 0.99, but the exponents are all less than 1.00, ranging from 0.88 to 0.99. The slight downward concavity implied by an exponent less than 1.00 is obvious to visual inspection. We may speculate that the observers restricted the range over which they produced matched sizes, with the result that their matches to small standards were markedly greater than the physical sizes of those standards, the error (relative to the size of the standard) decreasing as the standards grew larger (and further away); we might anticipate that, had Holway and Boring used even larger stimuli, the error would have reversed its direction and the observers would have made matches smaller than the physical size of the standard. Indeed, one observer, EGB, who had the smallest exponent, did make matches smaller than the larger standards.

Since Holway and Boring confounded size and distance of standard, it is not possible to tell from their data whether constancy or over-constancy was manifested; the control observations – of each size at the same distance as the comparison – are missing. A similar criticism may be made of a study by Leibowitz, Pollard, & Dickson (1967), which used the same design as Holway & Boring (1941). They found that the size of the comparison chosen to match the standard increased linearly with distance for adults viewing binocularly, but matched size increased at a faster rate than the physical size of the standard. Making the same assumption as Holway and Boring, that the matched size would be the same as the physical size of the standard when comparison and standard were at the same distance, they concluded that their adult observers "exhibited a tendency toward 'over-constancy.' [p. 266]" They used a method of limits, so that the regression effect evident in Holway and Boring's data does not appear in theirs: matched size appears to be a linear function of distance – and physical size – of standard. But their test objects were unfamiliar, and the setting was out-of-doors, conditions that Leibowitz & Harvey (1969) have demonstrated are conducive to an over-estimation of the standard that does not depend on distance: the near comparison is set to a larger value than the far standard regardless of the distance of the standard, by an amount that varies between about 5 and 20% when the method of limits is used. If, in the Leibowitz *et al.* (1967) study, one assumes that the observer would have selected a comparison about 7% larger than the standard regardless of relative distance, then one can account for their results as readily as by an assumption of over-constancy. Again, as in the Holway and Boring study, the control observations – of the match between comparison and each standard at the same distance – are not available, and thus it is not possible to decide between the two hypotheses.

In brief, these two experiments – one the first to be cited as demonstrating over-constancy, the second apparently extending the results to an outdoor situation – are in fact ambiguous in the meaning of the outcome. Whereas the results obtained may have resulted from a growth in matched size with distance, and so indicated over-constancy, they may also have resulted from response biases or illusory effects associated with the methods, settings, or stimuli used, and so indicated only a tendency for the observer to manifest those biases or effects at all distances. The ambiguity results from the design, which by increasing the physical size of the standard as distance is increased, makes it impossible to directly inspect the functional relation between apparent size and distance for a standard of fixed physical size.

Designs Varying Distance for a Fixed Standard Size

Experiments that have varied the distance of a fixed standard size, or of a series of standard sizes, include: in outdoor settings, Gibson (1947), Smith (1953), Gilinsky (1955), Joynson, Newson, & May (1965), and Leibowitz & Harvey (1969); in indoor settings, Joynson, Newson, & May (1965), and R. Teghtsoonian & M. Teghtsoonian (1970a). The outcomes of these studies defy concise summary. Although all had similar designs and all used unfamiliar test objects, natural settings with free binocular regard, and objective-size instructions (explicit or implicit), they resulted variously in increasing, constant, and decreasing functions relating matched size to distance of the standard.

OUTDOOR SETTINGS

A brief recapitulation of outcomes of studies in an outdoor setting includes the following. (*a*) Gibson (1947) demonstrated constancy for standards 63–75 in. up to 784 yd; averaged over standard heights, matched size rose only slightly and irregularly, by about 4%. (*b*) Gilinsky (1955) demonstrated over-constancy for standards 42–66 in., constancy for a 78-in. standard, up to 1333 yd; averaged over heights, matched size increased by 18%. There was a clear interaction of size with distance, however: matched size for the two smallest standards showed a 26% increase; for the 66-in. standard, 11%; for the largest, 1%. (*c*) Joynson, Newson, & May (1965) demonstrated marked over-constancy for a 12-in. standard, and over-constancy, constancy, or under-constancy for other standards up to 168 in., for distances up to 440 yd. In one experiment, estimated size increased by about 20% up to 440 yd for all standards, except by 250% for the 12-in. standard; in another experiment, estimated size increased up to 250 yd for 12- and 42.5-in. standards, but remained constant or decreased for 87- and 168-in. standards. (*d*) Smith (1953) demonstrated over-constancy for standards 2 and 4 in. high up to 107 yd; matched size increased by 25% for the 2-in. standard, 14% for the 4-in. standard. (*e*) Leibowitz & Harvey (1969) demonstrated constancy for 60- and 72-in. standards up to either 167 or 560 yd; matched size showed no change with distance, although there was consistent overestimation in some conditions.

Reliability of increases in matched size. In none of the first four experiments reviewed was the reliability of the trend to increasing matched size with distance evaluated statistically. In Gibson's (1947), Gilinsky's (1955), and Joynson, Newson, & May's (1965) data, the standard deviations are often large relative to the differences between means at different distances; Smith (1953) did not provide standard deviations. The trends may be reliable, but in the absence of statistical tests, it is difficult to know how seriously to take them. This problem becomes more critical as the number of distances decreases (to as few as three in Smith's 1953 study). Leibowitz & Harvey (1969), who did perform tests of the effect of distance, consistently found it not reliable.

Conflicting outcomes for same-sized standard. Three studies included at least some standards between 60 and 78 in.; Gibson (1947) reported constancy for four standards 63-75 in.; Gilinsky (1955) reported over-constancy for 66 in. and constancy for 78 in.; Leibowitz & Harvey (1969) reported constancy for standards 60 and 72 in. Gilinsky concluded that the results for smaller stimuli were typical and that over-constancy was the best general description of her results; she omitted data from the 78-in. standard in reaching this conclusion, because she believed those results to be artifacts of the upper size limit of the comparison (whose greatest value was only 10% taller than the largest standard). Gibson's tallest comparison was only 11% greater than his tallest standard, and, by inference, his results may have been artifactual. Leibowitz and Harvey do not specify the limiting value of the comparison for two experiments; however, in a third experiment, it was 8 ft for a 5-ft standard, and can scarcely have accounted for their finding of constancy. When different studies, basically similar in design, suggest such different conclusions, it seems wise to be cautious in choosing one conclusion rather than the other. But for this small but homogeneous set of studies, over-constancy is an exceptional result.

Psychophysical method. Psychophysical method *per se* does not seem to be a factor in determining the occurrence of over-constancy. Leibowitz & Harvey (1969) used both a method of limits and a method of adjustment, and measured invariance of matched size with distance in both cases. Joynson, Newson, & May (1965) used a method of magnitude estimation and found estimated size to be increasing, constant, and (perhaps) decreasing functions of distance, depending on size of standard.

Limited range of standard size. These studies have restricted themselves to a rather limited range of size: excluding the Joynson, Newson, & May (1965) study, nine of 12 standard heights used in four studies have fallen in the interval from 60 to 78 in. In view of the marked interaction of physical height with distance in determining estimated height (or perhaps the dependence of estimated height on visual angle) demonstrated by Joynson, Newson, & May (1965) – who spanned a range from 12-168 in. – it seems unwise to generalize about size constancy or departures from it on such a limited sampling of sizes.

INDOOR SETTINGS

A series of experiments by Jenkin (1957, 1959) varied the distance of the comparison but not of the standard.[3] Studies that varied distance for fixed standard sizes include Joynson, Newson, & May (1965) and R. Teghtsoonian & M. Teghtsoonian (1970a).[4]

Jenkin (1957, 1959) had observers select a comparison at various distances to match a 4-in. standard at a single fixed distance, and measured the change in size of the comparison necessary to compensate for changes in its distance. The results provide equal – matched-size contours: in Experiment I (1959), for instance, to match a 4-in. square at 8.9 yd, observers required a 4.56-in. square at 0.6 yd, a 4.47-in. square at 1.1 yd, and a 4.28-in. square at 4.4 yd. In three experiments with the 4-in. standard at 8.9 yd, the comparison selected to match it decreased by about 0.4 in. as the comparison increased in distance from 0.6 to 4.4 yd, a small but reliable change. It seems justified to infer from this, as Jenkin did, that the matched size of an object of fixed size increases with distance, but his data do not demonstrate this directly nor provide a measure of the effect of distance on matched size, since any single size appeared only at one distance. (For a discussion of the relation between equal-attribute contours – e.g., equal-volume or equal-size contours – and the psychophysical functions relating that attribute to physical variables, see Terrace & Stevens, 1962.)

Joynson, Newson, & May (1965) presented standard heights 3 to 96 in. high, at distances of 2 and 6.7 yd. Only for the 3-in. standard was there an increase in estimated size with distance; estimated size showed no increase for standards 15-96 in. high. This outcome suggests strongly that Jenkin's conclusions ought not be generalized to other sizes without experimental verification. Again, as in Gilinsky's (1955) and Joynson, Newson, & May's (1965) outdoor studies, size of standard is implicated as a critical variable.

R. Teghtsoonian & M. Teghtsoonian (1970a) presented irregular polygons, ranging in average height from about 3 to about 25 in., at distances from 1.7 to 15 yd. In Experiment I magnitude estimations of apparent area increased by about 30% from 1.7 to 8.3 yd and remained constant from 8.3 to 15 yd; this was true for all sizes, and both the linear and quadratic trends of the function relating size estimations to distance were reliable. In Experiment II, a replication of Experiment I, there was no increase in magnitude estimations with distance for any size. Teghtsoonian and

[3] There is some question whether Jenkin's studies meet the criterion of a natural setting: the viewing situation was not reduced but special homogeneous backgrounds were provided for standard and comparisons.

[4] Both Joynson, Newson, & May (1965) and R. Teghtsoonian & M. Teghtsoonian (1970a) used a method of magnitude estimation. The other studies reviewed used variously a method of adjustment, of limits, or of constant stimuli, so that the size of the comparison was matched by the observer to the size of the standard. In magnitude estimation, the observer matches numbers to the size of the standard, an operation that does not differ in principle from matching size (Stevens, 1966). Over-constancy is demonstrated when the observer matches successively larger sizes or numbers to the same standard as its distance increases.

Teghtsoonian could only speculate about the reasons for this difference in outcome; the fact is that the over-constancy manifested over a segment of the distance range in the first experiment was not obtained at all in the second.

It appears that, in experiments with indoor settings, over-constancy is by no means the rule, and, when it does occur, it is associated with small stimulus figures.

Summary and Conclusions

Of those studies, both indoors and out, whose designs are adequate to demonstrate over-constancy or its absence, three demonstrate over-constancy for all values of the standard and all distances used (Smith, 1953; Jenkin, 1957, 1959), three demonstrate over-constancy under some conditions and constancy under others (Gilinsky, 1955; Joynson, Newson, & May, 1965; R. Teghtsoonian & M. Teghtsoonian, 1970a), and two demonstrate constancy for all values of the standard and all distances used (Gibson, 1947; Leibowitz & Harvey, 1969). These studies differed in the number and size of standards, in the number and value of distances, in physical setting, and in psychophysical method: it is not surprising that there should be some lack of agreement in outcome. On the other hand, they were alike in basic design, in using unfamiliar test objects, in allowing free binocular regard and head movement, in providing natural or non-reduction settings, and in inducing an objective-size attitude: if over-constancy is a robust and sizeable phenomenon, it could be expected to manifest itself more consistently. Of the eight studies, only two used a range of size as great as ten to one; the others confined themselves to one, or a few similar, sizes. And of the eight studies, none used a range of distance as great as one hundred to one, whereas four had ranges less than ten to one. Still lacking are the systematic studies of size-matching for a wide range of size over a wide range of distance that are needed to confirm the existence of over-constancy.

References

Baird, J. C. *Psychophysical analysis of visual space.* Oxford: Pergamon Press, 1970.

Carlson, V. R. Overestimation in size-constancy judgments. *American Journal of Psychology*, 1960, **73**, 199–213.

Carlson, V. R. Size-constancy judgments and perceptual compromise. *Journal of Experimental Psychology*, 1962, **63**, 68–73.

Chalmers, E. L. Monocular and binocular cues in the perception of size and distance. *American Journal of Psychology*, 1952, **65**, 415–423.

Epstein, W., Park, J., & Casey, A. The current status of the size-distance hypotheses. *Psychological Bulletin*, 1961, **58**, 491–514.

Gibson, J. J. *Motion picture testing and research.* AAF Aviation Psychology Program Research Report No. 7. Washington, D.C.: U.S. Gov't. Printing Office, 1947.

Gilinsky, A. S. The effect of attitude upon the perception of size. *American Journal of Psychology*, 1955, **68**, 173–192.

Holway, A. H., & Boring, E. G. Determinants of apparent visual size with distance variant. *American Journal of Psychology*, 1941, **54**, 21–37.

Jenkin, N. Effects of varied distance on short-range size judgments. *Journal of Experimental Psychology*, 1957, **54**, 327–331.

Jenkin, N. A relationship between increments of distance and estimates of objective size. *American Journal of Psychology*. 1959, **72**, 345–363.

Joynson, R. B., Newson, L. J., & May, D. S. The limits of overconstancy. *Quarterly Journal of Experimental Psychology*, 1965, **17**, 209–216.

Leibowitz, H. W., & Harvey, L. O., Jr. Size matching as a function of instructions in a naturalistic environment. *Journal of Experimental Psychology*, 1967, **74**, 378–382.

Leibowitz, H. W., & Harvey, L. O., Jr. Effect of instructions, environment, and type of test object on matched size. *Journal of Experimental Psychology*, 1969, **81**, 36–43.

Leibowitz, H. W., Pollard, S. W., & Dickson, D. Monocular and binocular size-matching as a function of distance at various age levels. *American Journal of Psychology*, 1967, **80**, 263–268.

Smith, W. M. A methodological study of size-distance perception. *Journal of Psychology*, 1953, **35**, 143–153.

Sonoda, G. Perceptual constancies observed in plane pictures. In Y. Akishige (Ed.), *Experimental researches on the structure of the perceptual space*, Vol. 4. Fukuoka, Japan: Fac. Lit., Kyushu Univ., 1961.

Stevens, S. S. On the operation known as judgment. *American Scientist*, 1966, **54**, 385–401.

Stevens, S. S., & Greenbaum, H. Regression effect in psychophysical judgment. *Perception and Psychophysics*, 1966, **1**, 439–446.

Stevens, S. S., & Guirao, M. Subjective scaling of length and area and the matching of length to loudness and brightness. *Journal of Experimental Psychology*, 1963, **66**, 177–186.

Teghtsoonian, M. The judgment of size. *American Journal of Psychology*, 1965, **78**, 392–402.

Teghtsoonian, M. Apparent length as a function of tilt does not depend on orientation of the standard. *Journal of Experimental Psychology*, 1972, **94**, 191–197.

Teghtsoonian, R., & Teghtsoonian, M. The effects of size and distance on magnitude estimations of apparent size. *American Journal of Psychology*, 1970, **83**, 601–612. (a)

Teghtsoonian, R., & Teghtsoonian, M. Two varieties of perceived length. *Perception and Psychophysics*, 1970, **8**, 389–392. (b)

Terrace, H. S., & Stevens, S. S. The quantification of tonal volume. *American Journal of Psychology*, 1962, **75**, 596–604.

Vogel, J. M., & Teghtsoonian, M. The effects of perspective alterations on apparent size and distance scales. *Perception and Psychophysics*, 1972, **11**, 294–298.

Wohlwill, J. F. The development of "overconstancy" in space perception. In L. P. Lipsitt and C. C. Spiker (Eds.), *Advances in child development and behavior*, Vol. I. New York: Academic Press, 1963.

PART IV

A BRIEF AUTOBIOGRAPHY

NOTES FOR A LIFE STORY[1]

Being recollections assembled in no particular order for a volume *History of Psychology in Autobiography*, December 1970

S. S. STEVENS

November 4, 1906–January 18, 1973

In 1929 my uncle sent me off to Stanford to study law, or so he thought. I wanted to be a writer or an artist, or so I thought. A writer writes and a painter paints, and if you have passed 23 with neither pen nor brush constantly in hand, you are neither writer nor artist. So what did I want to do? A romantic answer had popped out on a soft spring night when the moon lit the snowfields on the Wasatch peaks above the campus of the University of Utah. Two students were projecting their yearnings into the future, and I shocked the girl, my sweetheart since childhood, by opting for the role of spectator on the comedy of life. The girl, Phyllis, glowed with purpose, though. She knew what she wanted, and she went on to win accolades in the world of the theater and to have a New York playhouse named for her. Why, she asked, had I no ambitions?

So I was shipped off to Stanford for the junior year, only to indulge anew my predilection for courses that promised wide-roaming talk and conceptual excitement. Nothing in science, nothing in mathematics, nothing elementary. Only the windy subjects. The philosopher image seemed most congenial. But mainly, that first year at Stanford, I suffered the shock of severance. I knew no one, whereas the year before at Utah I had known almost everyone. Joining the debating team helped, but not much. We lost to some wits from Oxford, but we triumphed over St. Mary's in the hills behind Berkeley. The then-famous St. Mary's football team made up most of the audience.

Another transfer student, shipped west for some of the same reasons that may have motivated my own family, happened to land next door to me in a Palo Alto rooming house at 257 Byron Street. We were both intensely people-shy and succeeded in avoiding conversation until one day when we bobbed up at the same time on the edge of the swimming pool. That set off an intellectual sparring that grew into friendship. Dane Wilsey was wild, brilliant, and wealthy. His red convertible, and sometimes my green roadster, took him to San Francisco for most of his adventures, but the intellectual life of Stanford absorbed a share of his breathless energy. He bounded in one day and said, "I've got it, we can't waste our time on these philosophy courses. We should study medicine. The world needs us." So in our senior year we both registered for freshman physics, chemistry, and biology. In addition I registered

[1] From *History of Psychology in Autobiography*, Vol. 6, Appleton-Century-Crofts (in press), by permission of Prentice-Hall.

H. R. Moskowitz et al. (eds.), Sensation and Measurement. 423–446. *All Rights Reserved.*

for golf, because happiness, I was beginning to think, was an endless fairway. Fortunately, I got higher grades in science than in golf.

Wilsey could not spare the time for the laboratory toils. His adventures in San Francisco produced a wife (his second) and a job with a broker. But the market was tumbling, and one morning he got up from breakfast, walked into the bedroom, and took the exit by bullet, the exit that he and I had many times argued for and against as we bulled through the night at the rooming house.

The laboratory work was a bore, but I liked some parts of the exercises. Perhaps I was setling down now, because the rooming house days were past. During the spring vacation I had taken the train back to Salt Lake City and had returned, much to my own surprise, with a beautiful young wife named Maxine. No one was home at the rooming house, so we first had to scale the walnut tree to the roof of the back porch to find an open window. The landlady and her sloe-eyed daughter took a sour view of the marital proceedings and we soon moved to a duplex at 228 Kipling Street.

Adjustment to life at Stanford was impeded partly by age. I was three years older than most of my classmates. After finishing high school at 17 I had been sent on a 3-year mission for the Mormon Church. Both parents had died that same year, 1924, and I was carrying on my father's electrical equipment business, Stevens Sales Company, where I had always worked after school. The business was prospering and life was blithe and gay. My friends, Richard L. Evans chief among them, would assemble at closing time, and we would take off in my new 1924 Overland with its huge balloon tires that could ride high in the loose gravel on the dusty roads of the unpaved West. Gaiety subsided, however, on a seasick voyage from Montreal to Liverpool, and then from Harwich to Antwerp on the night boat. I reported in at the mission office in Liège, Belgium, knowing not a word of French, and was assigned a companion who was "counting the days" till his release. He was a musician and he tried to elevate my taste by a weekly exposure to opera, but I always slept through the second act.

Sometime near the end of the third month, that chattering, machine-gun language called French, which had been going by in a staccato blur, began to break up into words. A cloud was lifting. Soon I was taking my turn at the pulpit and taxing the ears of the faithful with fractured French in diphthonged accent. Two years later, though, my thinking and daydreaming had shifted over to French and I found myself translating back into English.

Every four months or so a missionary got a new companion, often accompanied by a change of scene. With a young Brother Nelson I was sent to open a branch in Charleroi, a sooty town noted for its mines and glassblowing factories. We rented a small upstairs room with a gas heater and a water pitcher. You carried water up from ground level. The house was owned by two maiden sisters, angular and spare, somewhat on the design of gargoyles. They served us breakfast and cackled at our protests about its insufficiency. And when we discovered a back room with a bathtub, they refused to empty out the cans and bottles stored therein. You could buy a bath at the local hotel, they said, if you couldn't keep clean with rag and basin.

For a few weeks we knocked on doors, passing out brochures and a handbill announcing a coming *Conférence* in a hotel ballroom we had rented. The day of the *Conférence* dawned in a howling Belgian deluge, and all we had to preach to were the two landladies, a waiter, and a few missionaries from nearby towns. A miserable start, but I am told that many people have since joined the Mormon Church in Charleroi.

There was already a flourishing branch in Liège where earlier missionaries had leased a former beer hall complete with gas lights, stage, and balcony. Backstage there was a pistol target range and a boxing ring. Both saw action.

When two close friends were released early in 1927 I received a 3-month furlough to accompany them on a trip to Egypt and Palestine. The style and extent of the journey were dictated by the minimum fund of $362 saved up by one of them. Missionaries paid their own way, helped, of course, by family and friends; the Church paid only the passage home. By eating one meal a day, supplemented by bread, oranges, and chocolate, and by riding third class on the railroads and "deck" (without bed) on the ships, we got as far south as a day's camel ride to the Step Pyramid, and as far east as the Dead Sea. Swimming there was much like that in our own Great Salt Lake, where you float about like an empty bottle. Then from Tel Aviv by boat to Rumania on the Black Sea and back to Turkey, and then by train through the Balkans and on to Switzerland, where I reported in again and was placed in charge of the Swiss Conference of the French Mission. I was stationed in Lausanne, but my travel beat ranged from Besançon, France, to La Chaud de Fonds in the Jura Mountains, and my chief duty was to buck up the resident missionaries and visit the church members.

My own release came in time to enter the University of Utah in 1927 and begin a hind-end-to education, starting with advanced courses in philosophy, political science, Japanese sociology, history, and the like. It was rich fare, but it should have included some mathematics. As a matter of fact, I had registered for college algebra, but initiation into the πKA fraternity had set me so far behind in the exercises that I had to drop the course. Disaster! But how is a student to know what only a playback can reveal?

Money for mission and college came mainly from my father's insurance, about $15000, supplemented by such jobs as teaching in the French phonetics laboratory. Summers I worked for the Idaho Power Company, starting as a grunt (hole digger and lineman's helper), living in a tent in a construction camp beside a mountain stream where you almost froze to death at night. I later worked up to summer utility man. That meant that I had a new job almost every two weeks as I replaced the man on vacation, whether meter reader, waterheater installer, or night troubleshooter. Forty years later, it becomes clear that my education for science took place more in the summers than in the winters.

Summer was for education in boyhood too. Released from the tyranny of inkwell and desk, I was transported by cinderbelching train from Salt Lake City to the paradise of Logan, Utah, where barn and corral and garden and river and irrigation ditches became the playground for three glorious months among cousins of all ages. My grandfather, Orson Smith, and his two remaining wives occupied houses on a major part of a town block, and some of his two dozen children had homes nearby. A polygamous household was a wonderful institution under a patriarchal mesomorph who had been born in a covered wagon and who had subdued his land by brains and energy. He educated himself and rose to the highest position in Cache Valley, but his vision often raced ahead of reality. Since markets sometimes plummet, it was almost inevitable that his elevator would be full of the valley's wheat crop when the panic of 1897 broke the price. Off he went to the Klondike to recoup in the gold rush, but again he overreached by trying to move in machinery while most others were panning the bright metal.

So there stood the great grain elevator tower for boys to climb and explore, forbidden and tightly locked, of course, but a boy could squeeze through a foundation vent if someone helped by pushing or pulling. And next door stood the "new house," waiting through the years, half finished, for lathe and plaster. We could climb up the studs from floor to floor and catch bats among the rafters. But all those boyhood castles held second place to the barn. We were not supposed to play in the hay, but no one kept watch as we burrowed and tunneled and contrived a slick chute down which we could plunge from ridge to stable – and frighten the chickens as we landed.

Best of all, though, was the running water. Whenever I was missing they knew exactly where to look: the wooden culvert that carried the irrigation stream across the road to plunge into a pool where toads sat fat on the bank and horses stretched their necks to drink. The clear swirling water was my first love, and the pool was my first point of call after the train ride from Salt Lake City. Other things could wait. The contriving of dams and water wheels delighted me and led the family to predict the career of hydraulic engineer.

Twice a week there were "water rights." During certain hours you could dam up the ditch and open the sluice gate to your own garden. Then barefoot with hoe you guided the precious water down the rows until the dusty earth would make mud curls through your toes. And you opened another weir and flooded the lawn, and the little kids ran splashing and rolling in four inches of sparkling water.

Then summer would end, as all things must, and my mother and I would take the branch line from Logan to Cache Junction to connect with the Oregon Short Line for Salt Lake City, and school would start and Phyllis would be there to stoke the tormenting fires of puppy love, as unfeeling adults presumed to call it. School was O.K., I guess, but they thought I would never learn to read. They had to give me a second try at conquering the first grade, but thereafter I seemed somehow to stand a little higher in class during each successive year. I was considered listless, as they phrased it, low in energy, and my round-shouldered posture had not responded to various braces and harnesses, except to provide a handle by which larger cousins could lift me to hang helpless off the ground.

My mother, who suffered a heart-valve leakage from girlhood rheumatic fever, worried much about me and about the gangs of boys that played and warred throughout the 8th East neighborhood, where the houses ranged from shacks to mansions. Some of us showed up now and then in juvenile court, but I can see now that even as boys we knew which of us were the bad guys and which went along for the fun. Three of the true delinquents later made it to the state penitentiary, one of them for a capital offense.

One day, when I was beginning the fourth grade, Mother asked me if I would like to go to live in Logan. What a question! My father's asthma was kicking up and his business was touch and go. We would be able to eat better in Logan, where we would stay with Aunt Maggie, my mother's oldest sister. Her husband, Will, was the genial chief clerk in the general store, a large endomorph, but a vigorous man, who pedaled a bicycle back and forth and brought home each night a big leather pouch full of coins to be counted. That Christmas two young cousins developed a theory, based on someone's offhand remark about a "windbag," that a pin would deflate Uncle Will. As he bent his great bulk over the coal scuttle they tested the hypothesis, and everyone thought Uncle Will had lost his wits as he cried out in shaking rage and grabbed one of the fleeing experimenters.

But the hardships of the adults were mostly lost on us children, even though the talk of the grownups in the evening circle about the potbellied stove told of trials – and of comedy. Whatever the childhood game in progress, you kept an ear cocked for a salty tale – and you appeared not to be listening. And when finally sent to bed you could undress by the warm stove in the kitchen where the bread was rising in its big pan under the dish towel, and you could poke in a finger and pull out a tangy swatch of dough to comfort your stomach and help ease the shock of the cold leap into bed.

Asthma, I was later to learn, was not the only thing troubling my father. There was another woman. My semi-invalid mother was walking out. Later on came a divorce, but it did not take. On many occasions Dad would be sitting by her bed when I came home at night and then one evening they told me they had married again. God, it made me happy. Mother's circulation grew worse and a couple of years later she suffered a stroke and died. Thereafter, Dad and I shared the cooking while I finished my last year at high school. We had always pulled well together, both at work and in our travels, and we continued to do so, always with very few words, for neither of us was a talker. Our silences never clamored to be broken.

One afternoon I returned to the school after a hard but exhilarating day at the finals of the state debating competition only to be told that they were looking for me. There had been an auto accident and Dad was dying. He was only 42, and everyone said "so young to die." I was 17 and I wondered that a parent could be anything but old.

Dad had been 18 when he lost his father, and he too had been sent on a mission – to Holland. He returned to start an electrical business in Ogden, Utah, the town where I was born in 1906 in a small wooden house on Stewart Lane, now called Ogden Avenue. The business failed and we moved to Salt Lake City, where Dad worked for Fairbanks-Morse until he could once again start his own business. His technical training came through correspondence schools, because the death of his father precluded college and ended his hope to study medicine.

Dad's father, Thomas J. Stevens, was born in Bristol, England, on the day gold was discovered in California. Soon thereafter his parents joined the Mormon Church, and at 16 he drove two yoke of oxen across the plains from the Missouri River to the mountains of Utah. Coming from a family of mechanics he had apprenticed the blacksmith trade, and he worked for the Union Pacific Railroad before he and his brothers started their own foundry and machine shop in Ogden. He later made a mark as treasurer of several institutions, and as Commissary General of the National Guard. And for 13 years he served the Mormon Church as Bishop of the Fifth Ward. A bishop is a kind of works manager, a chief of chores, the link pin in the chain between spiritual dispensation and temporal care. The bishop tithes, builds, counsels, buries, blesses, arbitrates, marries, christens, visits the sick, and carries food and fuel to the poor. My grandfather's journal records those daily acts of service.

For a time he filled in as head of the local Academy – now Weber State College. Like so many of those self-educated pioneers, he showed an exaggerated faith in formal education, despite being surrounded by examples of men whose achievements owed nothing to classroom or curriculum. Perhaps the generations produce little change, for here am I at Harvard teaching formal courses in subjects I was never taught, and seeming thereby to imply that the course is the only door to mastery.

I never knew Grandfather Stevens, but I remember his wife and the big house in Ogden, with its carriage barn behind. The house stood at 2575 Jefferson Avenue, across the street from the Eccles mansion – one of the grander places in the town. Grandma Stevens was one of 27 children fathered by Briant Stringham, pioneer and rancher, who built a house for each of his four wives, three of them Ashby sisters from Salem, Massachusetts. I was 6 when Grandma Stevens died, and her funeral was my first view of death, with Grandma lying serene and still in the parlor under the heavy overcast of odor from banks of flowers.

One of the questions we debated my senior year in high school was the mandate for compulsory education to age 16. We had to stand ready to debate either side of the question, and the background research led me to the new excitement concerning the intelligence test and the remarkable invariance of the IQ. That kind of library searching and reading struck a responsive resonance, I now think, but in those days I had no idea where I was going. "What do you want to be?" everybody kept asking. How could I tell them something I had never heard of? How could I answer, "I would like to become the world's first Professor of Psychophysics"?

It was in March 1929 in a philosophy class that I first became curious enough to ask Professor Ericksen what was meant by psychology. He said I could find out on the top floor. (Psychology was always relegated to the attic or the basement.) I climbed to the top floor and asked Dorothy Nyswander. She said I ought to take a course and find out. She was teaching comparative psychology and she challenged me to try to catch up with the reading and join the course. I accepted. Mostly I learned about the phyla, which is useful, and about rats running mazes, which is not. Dr

Nyswander despaired of making me appreciate animal training, as I called it. The text was a ponderous tome by J. B. Watson, but I gathered that he had written a more lively volume on *Behaviorism*, a volume that was supposed to have shaken psychology.

The next summer in Pocatello, Idaho, I discovered that Watson could also shake the parents' class in Sunday School, where I was conducting the lessons. Watson's blatant environmentalism went down hard with those anxious parents, some of whom had done everything they could to steer a wayward boy. Give him a dozen infants at birth, boasted Watson, and he could make each of them anything you named. Such rot made for a good sermon, and I believed it then, though the evidence leads me to wager that biology would have shattered Watson's myth if someone had supplied the infants he asked for. So much of our behavior style seems to be wired in at the start. Those parents, many from ranch and farm, had a sense of biology sounder than mine.

Teaching the parents' class seemed somehow to be my specialty, even after leaving the West for Harvard. In Boston in 1931 we met on Sunday mornings in an upstairs night club that featured green walls and a bilious odor. The group later moved to Cantabrigia Hall near Harvard Square, and now there are Mormon churches in many towns around. I finally gave up the parents' class after another upsetting issue had been aired: whether there is a conflict between science and religion. Mormon doctrine says no, and the lives of many distinguished scientists have demonstrated that churchgoing does not preclude first-rate research. But on method, I tried to argue, science and religion must stand opposed. Belief is what the ideal scientist, if there were such, would be totally free of. Only evidence would count for him, evidence viewed with dispassionate objectivity. But the suspension of intense belief comes hard. Few manage it at all. The young almost never do.

The parents' class churned with argument as I tried by Socratic induction to force the members to set the prophet's injunction to believe against the scientist's injunction to question. In that confrontation the teacher may have learned more than the students, for I was then trying to sort out from among my tangled intellectual inputs an explicit philosophy that I could live with. Many years later I would call it the schemapiric view, but in the early 1930's the quest for a congenial approach was leading me toward operationism, a topic on which I later wrote a series of articles.

But the problem of belief persisted, for believing, it seems, holds many attractions. Believing is easy – and lazy. And it fills people with a warm glow, so that when two or more believers are gathered together in common conviction about philosophy, politics, or divinity, they sense the cozy, comforting contagion of zeal. The zealot detects virtue in blind belief. The uncommitted mind regards such allegations of virtue with high skepticism. I was beginning to aspire to the suspension of belief.

My graduation from Stanford had been threatened by a failure to major in anything. I had never read the catalogue, except to shop for courses, and beginning a premedical course in the senior year did not appear to fit the rules. It was then that my chemistry professor, who was also the registrar, dredged out of his memory a long-forgotten bit of legislation that prescribed a major for anyone who could offer at least one course in a half dozen different areas of social science. I could do that with no trouble at all. But there was one penalty. Despite election to $\Phi\beta$K at the end of junior year, graduation with honors was ruled out because I was taking freshman courses in the senior year. Curricular rules take funny twists. I warn students not to let the curriculum interfere with their education.

Those freshman science courses in the senior year persuaded me that my previous studies were fitting me to talk about anything, but to do nothing. No skills acquired, no procedures mastered, no craft apprenticed. To be sure, I was by then getting my hands on something concrete in the laboratories, but in your 25th year you should be finishing, not starting. I was cheered a bit by comparative anatomy under Professor Stark, who liked to claim that his main mission in life was to keep the wrong people out of medical school. I hit one of his exams for 100, which he told the class had never before been done, and so I found myself admitted to Harvard Medical School, with two provisos: (1) that I send fifty dollars and (2) that I take organic chemistry during the summer. Neither condition seemed attractive. When I vacillated, a student who had been turned down offered me $5000 to go in my place.

Decision never comes easy to me, and trying to decide to do something often tears me apart more than doing it. So I dallied and the deadline passed and I still had my $50 and there was no need for a 4-year grind through medical school. What to do? Someone recommended the vocational interest test that E. K. Strong was developing. It told about interests, not abilities, and it told me that my interests correlated highly with those of the mathematician, the psychologist, and a few other academic types, and very poorly with the YMCA secretary. Mathematics was out, of course, so I talked to C. P. Stone, who was known as a rat man, but who also taught abnormal psychology and who took the class on hospital excursions where we had exhibited to us dramatic examples of the classic psychotic syndromes. Stone advised me against psychiatry, which in those days meant tending a hospital, and he remarked that people trained in solid experimental psychology seemed best able to find jobs, which were then becoming scarce in the deepening depression. Stone scorned my thought of going to Harvard, because Yale and its new Institute of Human Relations heralded the hope of the future. I promised to limit myself to one year at Harvard, which seemed to mollify the professor, and he then gave me some choice advice: "Wherever you go," he said, "ask the professor first off if there isn't some small problem you can work on for him."

The road to Harvard led first to Los Angeles for a combined summer school and marital vacation. I drove out to the new campus at UCLA, where gawky buildings rose lonely and comical from a treeless waste of hills and eroded gullies. Nothing much seemed to be stirring except rabbits. I wandered about and found the office of Knight Dunlap, a name I had heard of, but no one was home. So I drove back into town and signed up at USC, where things turned out to be bouncing. I found an old friend from Utah named Van Tanner, another college wanderer and bon vivant, who was in charge of student activities and who combatted boredom as a movie extra and stunt man. He led me through many novel exploits, a good supplement to courses in philosophy and psychology. I took statistics from H. E. Garrett and history from J. F. Dashiell, a pair of distinguished summer imports. For diversion one could sit in the old wooden house where Milton Metfessel had his laboratory and watch comedian Joe E. Brown making a movie with the USC football team.

Then back to Salt Lake City, where Maxine had been visiting her parents, and thence down the long dusty road "back east." Pavement began around Chicago and had become fairly continuous by Cleveland. There we visited some Stanford friends and were startled to find them a "first family" in a fabulous estate. We saw for the first time what great wealth and gracious living could be like.

We drove into Cambridge in a September drizzle, bought a newspaper, and telephoned a want-ad number that advertised rooms at 9 Sumner Road. It cost $10 per week for two small rooms separated by a curtain. One room served as bath and kitchen. Mrs Clark, a Victorian-style Cambridge widow, was quite alarmed when we said we would move right in. Who were we, she wondered. Maybe we should come back tomorrow, she suggested. I pointed out that we would still be the same people tomorrow. Did we know someone she could call? No one in Cambridge. Gradually as the talk continued, the alarm subsided, and we unloaded. The location turned out to be so wonderfully convenient to Harvard and Radcliffe that we were able to sell the faithful Hupmobile.

Having eschewed medical school I began to cast about for some other option. Always, it seems, I was looking for the easiest. While hunting around in the catalogue, which I had now decided was for reading, I turned up the interesting fact that tuition in the School of Education was only $300. We were borrowing money for Maxine's tuition at Radcliffe ($400), and so any bargain was appreciated. When I appeared at the office in old Lawrence Hall – the same building where in 1876 William James had set up a "laboratory for psychophysics" – the secretary assured me that I could not register because I had not applied for admission. "You don't just walk in," she admonished. My offer to go back and crawl in did not seem to amuse her. But officialdom finally bent and I was admitted.

There was only one course in Education that looked interesting – advanced statistics under T. L. Kelley who, like me, had just arrived from Stanford. About twenty of us registered for the course, but only two of us took the final exam. I had nothing to lose, and the other fellow was a Negro principal on leave who was required by his school board to take all exams. Kelley could not bring himself to flunk even half the class, but the questions made no more sense to either of us than the lectures had. Kelley was a bad teacher. Or was he? He pioneered in his field and he turned out distinguished students. Is there some surer mark of good teaching?

The $300 tuition purchased four courses, so for the other three I scanned the listings under Arts and Sciences. I wanted physiology, I thought, and I found W. J. Crozier in a vast new building that was then less than half full. Crozier gave me a room overlooking a pleasant quadrangle guarded by two great bronze rhinos, newly cast, whose cost seemed scandalous to him. "Think how much research that money would support!" Each time I pass those handsome bronze beasts I wonder whether they feel guilty.

The course started out with Crozier's blast at mentalism, followed by his display of the evidence that the tropism exhibited by young rats climbing a slope obeys the Mendelian laws. The rats inherit a climbing angle. Then Crozier disappeared and various other people showed up to tell about their research. Again a bad job of teaching. Or was it?

As the year ground on I found that Crozier had attracted an interesting array of talent into the south wing of the Biological Laboratories. On the first floor one day I walked in on a man who was busily plotting data. He said they were "eating curves" for rats and could be described by power functions. I told him I didn't know much math, and what was a power function? For the first time he turned and looked at me; then he waggled his head and dismissed me by saying, "The only way to get over an inferiority complex about mathematics is to learn some." That was my first and possibly my most profitable encounter with B. F. Skinner. Both his diagnosis and his prescription were just right, as it turned out.

Up in Emerson Hall I located E. G. Boring, Harvard's lone Professor of Psychology, the de facto chairman of a nonexistent department, for psychology was part of philosophy. Boring admitted me to the "systematic" course on perception, although he doubted its suitability for a student in the School of Education. Then I startled Boring by asking if I could work on some problem of his. Well, yes, perhaps. He had heard that when you mix red and green on a color wheel it looks gray only if you stand at the right distance. That seemed interesting, and up in the attic under the rafters I found a place where I could try it out. It worked all right, but so what? I tried various arrangements and noted that if I looked slightly away from the color wheel the gray turned greenish. Finally I got around to mixing a black and white to provide a gray that could be compared with the gray produced by red and green.

Then late one afternoon my scientific career began. There occurred that surge of elation, the *eureka*! that drives the investigator. I suddenly sensed that there was a law to be worked out. You could mix some green with the black and white and you could vary the amount in a way that would just cancel the effect of a change in distance. A function could be measured! Bursting with elation, I bounded down from the attic that evening and ran all the way back to Sumner Road.

Boring was right about students in the School of Education and their deficient background. During most of his lectures on perception that first semester I felt submerged under a strange, unstructured flow of esoteric words and concepts. Perception had no back, front, or sides. The final examination over, Boring wrote me one of his famous scrap-paper missives announcing my failure, but according me the courtesy of a passing grade because I was not a graduate student in psychology.

What do you do when the blast of your first failure shatters your prospects and your newly formed hope for a scientific career? I crawled up to my improvised desk in the attic and sat staring. The emotion of dismay was shot through from time to time by a surge of diffuse anger. Finally I went home and told Maxine that I had blown it.

Not long thereafter I asked one of the instructors in Crozier's physiology course how to go about getting a degree in biology. He said there were a lot of required courses, but that he had taken his degree in experimental psychology. There, he explained, you had only to pass the "prelims" and write a thesis. Why didn't I try that? Well, why not, even though I had already visited Yale and arranged to transfer there. It was then February, and exactly 100 days later the four 3-hour written examinations would begin. If I read and mastered 100 pages per day for 100 days, making 10000 pages, that ought to tell whether experimental psychology was for me.

So the grind began. Boring agreed that I might be allowed to take the prelims, although he saw little prospect of success. Maxine, fortunately, had walked in on Radcliffe and been admitted despite initial assurances from everyone except the president that the college was full and that transferring from the University of Utah was out of the question. She later earned $\Phi\beta$K and was graduated with high honors in philosophy, so during the 100 days she was too busy herself to object to my 16-hour daily stint. Tension built up with the growing exhaustion, and spirits drooped as my conviction grew firmer that a Ph.D. lay far beyond reach. After all, I told myself, I was the first of either of my families to go to college, why should I aim so high? And then, when the examinations had been written and the cruel wait for the verdict began, I felt sure by the way Boring and Beebe-Center and the other arbiters of my fate looked at me in the hallway – or didn't look at me – that I had blown it again.

Not at all! In fact, when the grades came out Boring seemed so pleased at my performance that one would have thought it was he who had passed. Now, said Boring, if I would transfer from the School of Education they would offer me the half-time Emerson Hall assistantship which paid $900. Imagine! You could earn money and go to school, too. No more thought of Yale, cancel the application to transfer. No more wondering whether we could make it through. Instead, we packed up and sailed on the Bremen to Europe, for the round trip fare was then at the all-time low of $120, third class, with all the food you could eat.

The International Congress of Psychology convened in Copenhagen that summer of 1932, so I had my first look at some of the people I had been reading about. I listened in on an animated discussion with Pavlov, his son serving as translator. The elder Cattell avoided the meetings but held court on the steps, smoking a big cigar. Warren had spent the summer in a German nudist camp and testified regarding the artificiality of clothes. Köhler sat handsome and serenely superior as chairman of one of the sessions. In the eyes of a graduate student it made a tremendous show.

Before leaving for Europe I had sent to a journal the manuscript describing the visual experiments with the color mixing wheel. It would have seemed sensible to continue the visual studies, but there occurred one of those minor accidents that deflect careers. P. M. Zoll got himself admitted to Medical School. Zoll was the man using the oscillator – that wonderful new instrument out of which you could get an assortment of pure tones – and Boring suggested that I might take over Zoll's experiments on tonal volume. The field of audition, as it turned out, was then the scene of great ferment, generated by a new tool, the vacuum-tube amplifier. Audition was indeed the place to be. It was easy to make a thesis out of tonal volume, but my real excitement stemmed from other discoveries – that pure tones have the attribute of density, as well as pitch, loudness, and volume, and that intensity by itself can change the pitch of a tone. Those were new things.

By May of 1933 I had three papers in press and a thesis defended before the full assemblage of all the philosophers and all the psychologists. I therefore applied for the Ph.D. No, said the administrative board, the year in Education plus the year at half-time in Arts and Sciences do not add up to the two-year residence requirement. But, I pointed out, the catalogue says the Ph.D. is not predicated on the accumulation of courses. Besides, didn't I have a summer session at USC in 1931, and didn't I finish the A.B. requirements at Stanford one full quarter early? Should not that last quarter count as graduate work? Back and forth went the argument both written and oral. I can still see the Graduate Dean, staring ruefully at my record and muttering, "Graduate credit for freshman physics, freshman chemistry, freshman biology and golf." He came down hard on the word *golf.*

They finally let me have the degree, though, because administrators would rather change their rules than look silly. No great advantage accrued, except relief from tuition, because there were no jobs to be had. I pleaded for another year as Emerson Hall assistant, because $900 would keep us eating. Boring said I had been the worst assistant they had ever had, and if they let me stay on would I do something besides my own research? I promised to clean up the laboratory.

One day I tackled the mess in the so-called battery room, where the upper reaches were ringed with shelves holding great crocks, each containing a human brain. The collection was said to date back to William James. Anyhow, the James brains had to go, and so did the shelves of reagents and chemicals that no one ever used, among them a two-gallon bottle of ammonia.

Whenever you started a job like that, E. B. Newman was sure to poke his head in to see what was going on, and then start helping. We thought it would scare the janitor if he found brains in his barrels, so we decided to cut them up and flush them down the lone toilet in the laboratory. We set the crocks and the chemicals in the hallway and then arranged a fast system for chopping and flushing the brains. Toward the end, however, the chopping grew careless, and a thick slice of somebody's frontal lobe got stuck. No standard remedy by plunger seemed to work so we unwound the fire hose and Newman jammed the nozzle tightly into the toilet. When I gave the signal, another helpful student, J. G. Needham, turned the valve. The water shot up out of the toilet like a geyser and the fire hose thrashed about like a stricken snake. The hose tipped over the ammonia bottle and the ammonia ran flooding down the hallway, and when Needham picked up the bottle and sniffed it, the fumes almost did him in.

Brute pressure was getting us nowhere, it seemed, so we decided to try chemical warfare. Sulfuric acid ought to dissolve a few brain cells. But pouring H_2SO_4 into water, as we knew, generates a lot of heat. "Pour slowly," I said. Newman dribbled it in, but not slowly enough. The water bubbled and steamed, and long before the brain gave way there was a loud bang and the bowl cracked open. We mopped up the mess, called the college plumber, and reported a toilet out of order.

One of the diversions that attenuated my effectiveness as a laboratory assistant was the brokerage business. From 10:00 A.M. to 3:00 P.M. the market tape in a Harvard Square office would go clacking by, displaying the rise and fall of prices. Dane Wilsey at Stanford had introduced me to the world of stocks and bonds, and in 1930 I had bought 10 shares of General Motors which promptly rose to a profit. Making a living from the market looked like the easy way to support a would-be scientist. But action found itself stifled by scholarship, market scholarship, I mean. I subscribed to a course on stock chart reading, and I devoured all the broker's advisory manuals. Then I combed the library at the Harvard Business School and brought back a great stack of books. Since my growing erudition was occasionally consulted in the back room of the broker's office, I toyed for a time with the possibility of becoming a professional security analyst. My temperament ruled out stock trading, because in order to be successful you have to average two correct decisions on each trade. I am congenitally unsuited to the making of even one decision – correct or not.

Another demand on my time was electrophysiology at the Medical School. I had dropped in at Building C one day and asked Hallowell Davis if I could help with an experiment. Yes, I could keep protocol, meaning, write down everything that Davis or Derbyshire called out. It was a deadly job, but a first-rate apprenticeship, and after a time they allowed me to operate on the animals and run some of the experiments. The following year an NRC Fellowship enabled me to spend full time at the Medical School mapping the frequency response of the guinea pig's cochlea by damaging the hair cells at various positions along the organ of Corti and noting the change in the electrical response. The Medical School activities culminated in the book *Hearing* that Davis and I published in 1938.

Not long after I began work at the Medical School, Davis allowed me to give one of the colloquium lectures attended by the medical students. So there I was, a medical drop-out, lecturing to some of the students whose class I would have joined had I sent along the $50. Davis also arranged for me to join the Neurological Supper Club, a lively, articulate group devoted to shop talk and new ideas. Lashley later joined the club, as did Norbert Wiener, and it was there that cybernetics was born – in arguments about the control of body movements through information and feedback. Years later, in 1948, Wiener recounted those origins in his book, *Cybernetics.*

When the NRC found itself out of funds, my request for the renewal of the Fellowship came to the attention of a part of the Rockefeller Foundation that wanted to foster interdisciplinary research by sponsoring training in a second science. They discussed my going back to school for a three-year retreading, this time in physics and chemistry. It sounded wonderful, despite their insistence that research was to be out for the duration (except perhaps during vacation), and also despite the offer of a job in psychology as instructor at $2500. So I turned down the job and became a Research Fellow in Physics with an office in Lyman Laboratory, where I had already been auditing courses in physics and mathematics. But a man can absorb only so much schooling. There comes a stage of saturation when he drops it off at one end as fast as he takes it on at the other. Consequently, the following year, 1936, when the offer was raised to $2750 I gave up physics to become a psychologist – until psychology later changed its central concern. I taught the laboratory course and four sections in Psychology 1. Later on I worked up an offering in mathematics for psychologists.

Psychology had the virtue of providing a haven for one who could never decide which star to steer by. Where else could a man be considered properly on the job even though he carried on research at the Medical School and dabbled in activities that ranged from electronic circuit design to philosophy? For extra money I sold various electronic devices to other laboratories and made hearing aids for a few customers who were willing to carry around an amplifer in a box.

But philosophy and the theory of measurement occupied many of my non-experimental hours. The philosophers inhabited the first floor of Emerson Hall, and it was convenient to take a seat at their lectures. A. N. Whitehead was the chief luminary in the early 1930's, but toward the end of the decade there was an influx from Europe, particularly from the Vienna Circle, which produced an enormous ferment. Rudolf Carnap climbed up to my laboratory one day and proposed that we should form a shop club to discuss the Science of Science. I sent out the invitations, and on Halloween 1940 we inaugurated monthly meetings by listening to P. W. Bridgman defend his solipsistic brand of operationism. Many notables followed. G. D. Birkhoff, called by one historian America's greatest mathematician, discoursed on the importance of invariance. The central problem in science, he insisted, is to locate the invariances.

My own central problem throughout the 1930's was measurement, because the quantification of the sensory attributes seemed impossible unless the nature of measurement could be properly understood. At a Congress for the Unity of Science in 1939, I had tried to describe the nature of measurement and to illustrate the different kinds of scales by examples from sensory psychophysics. It was a botch. Something was still missing, but I felt that I was groping in the right direction. In addition to the ordinal scale, I had distinguished between intensive and extensive scales and had tried to relate them to the determination of differences and ratios. In the aftermath of the debates that followed, most of them over semantic issues, I began to tabulate the various kinds of scales and the kinds of operations needed to create them. Then it became clear that each kind of scale permitted a different mathematical transformation, and suddenly one evening in Emerson Hall the picture snapped into focus – there exists a hierarchy of scales defined by the mathematical transformations that leave the scale form invariant.

The discovery of a simple principle generates two conflicting emotions: elation because of the new insight, and embarrassment because of the failure to see it sooner.

It remained to fix up the terminology by inventing new names, interval scale and ratio scale, names that I did not care for at first, but which have now become standard. When I called at Birkhoff's study in Widener Library to invite him to talk to us, I tried to interest him in the scale problem. My empirical orientation probably impeded communication, but he brightened up at the transformation feature, and spoke of the group structure of the scales. That was enough to send me to the mathematics library to learn more about mathematical groups.

At the next Congress for the Unity of Science in 1941, I was ready with a paper that outlined the theory of scales in a form that has since become rather widely accepted, so widely, in fact, that many authors feel no need to cite the origin.

Actually, my first presentation of the schema that defines measurement scales in terms of group invariance occurred in a symposium at the 1940 meeting of the Psychological Round Table, the PRT, a youth-fired rebellion organized in 1936. Five others – Graham, Hunt, Jacobsen, Marquis, and Newman – joined me in sponsoring the invitations. We called it initially the Society of Experimenting Psychologists, which was enough to incur the angry displeasure of my senior professor, and to draw blackballs against my name when I was later nominated for membership in the august Society of Experimental Psychologists. The PRT had no membership, but was run by a self-perpetuating band of six who issued invitations to an annual and thoroughly uninhibited meeting. One key rule was enforced: ejection at the age of 40. I am told that the PRT still carries on, and that its noisy good fellowship is still climaxed by a banquet that features the William A. Hunt Memorial Address, and that the Address is till unprintable. But I wonder, does the spirit run as fierce and free as it did in the early years? Some of those who attended the first meeting will doubt it.

As it happened, I missed a part of that first meeting. In a tense face-off a few days earlier, Boring had insisted that no permission had been granted for me to be absent from my four Saturday sections in Psychology 1. I would either teach the sections or be cited for insubordination. I taught the sections. That retreat proved fortunate both for me and for the PRT. While I taught sophomores in Cambridge, the brethren gathered at a business meeting in New London, Connecticut, where they considered and rejected the set of rules that were supposed to govern the fraternal sodality. The business meeting dissolved after someone remarked that if six of us could organize such a splendid muster, who needed rules? So the PRT, like Harvard University, came to be governed by a small autocratic and self-perpetuating minority.

In 1936, shortly after our son Peter was born, a postpartum psychosis overwhelmed Maxine and devastated our lives. Maxine moved in and out of various hospitals as therapy by shock or insulin made dramatic tub temporary changes in her state. During one of the brighter periods she returned to Utah to live with her parents, where she died some two decades later. My own reaction to the anguish of those wretched days was to plunge furiously into the job at hand. Work seemed the only road to relief. While Peter was small enough to be carried in a basket, I could take him with me to the laboratory, but he soon outgrew my ability to care for him alone. He then went to board with a warm-hearted, motherly woman in a nearby town. Peter is now an architect and father of three, and is here at Harvard this year on a Guggenheim Fellowship.

With nothing to do but work, it was easy to be productive. I could work all day and far into the night. Boring noted one year that my papers had produced more entries in the *Abstracts* than those of any other psychologist, and he cautioned that a reputation for superficiality might result. But research and writing could not be slowed, especially when they were going well. In one of my spurts, a 65-page manuscript called "Psychology and the Science of Science" got itself written between the APA meetings in early September and the 25th of October. The editor never quite believed it.

And when not writing my own papers, I was sometimes writing for others. W. H. Sheldon showed up at Harvard with a staggering pile of photographs, data, and tables concerned with somatotypes and temperaments. The challenge appeared to me to lie in the measurement problem: can you really identify and scale the principal components of human physique?

I ran a test to see how well a person, given only brief instructions, could use 7-point scales to rate the three components of physique as exhibited in photographs of 50 men. Twenty people cooperated, and the correlations for all three components were high, 0.9, which was good enough to convince me.

Sheldon is by nature an observer, a naturalist, a systematizer of phenomena. He was once an ornithologist, and as a numismatist he is the author of a charming and definitive book on the early American cent – the large coppers – for which he devised a system that put an end to classificational chaos for the 327 known die varieties. I am by nature quite the opposite: more interested in abstract principle than in concrete fact. Together, however, we effected a fruitful collaboration, producing a pair of books, one on physique, the other on temperament. Sheldon taught me to look and to observe, or at least he tried. It has often impressed me that a principal difference between the psychologist and the medical man lies in the unwillingness of the psychologist to scrutinize the object of his study. Rather, he keeps his distance and permits no closer contact than a pencil-and-paper test, or a button to be pressed. Watching people the way a naturalist watches terns or foxes might instruct the psychologist concerning the limitations that nature has imposed on sociogenesis, the seductive myth that experience writes on an empty slate.

In 1937 Davis and I were making progress on our book on hearing. As I combed the literature in psychophysics it became clear that the experiments of a Hungarian physicist named Georg von Békésy would command much space in the book, provided we could trust his claims. His descriptions of procedure left much unsaid. Helped by funds from the American Otological Society, I went to Budapest in 1937 to see whether Békésy was a reality. Fortunately, E. B. Newman, who went with me, was fluent in German. At the end of the streetcar line we tramped down a dusty road and found Békésy in a large building belonging to the Hungarian post-telephone-telegraph. Békésy, who appeared to be the Bell Telephone Laboratories of Hungary, harbored a lively suspicion of time-wasting visitors, and it was not easy to convince him that we were serious. He showed us nothing, but he did not refuse our request to visit him the next day. On the second day we got to see some of Békésy's experiments and learned of his frustration at not having easy access to the superior amplifying devices made in America. As we warmed to one another, Békésy invited us to return the following morning, a Saturday, so that he could take us on a tour of the city. At dinner, in a great vaulted hall, Newman and I said we would like to try real goulash. Which one? We didn't know. So the waiter brought half a dozen different dishes on a Lazy Susan and we sampled them all. Then Békésy recommended a local specialty for dessert, which turned out to be corn on the cob.

Some 25 years later, after Békésy had become a member of our Psycho-Acoustic Laboratory, he won a Nobel Prize for his early work on the ear. Békésy was indeed a reality.

Although it did not get named until several months later, the Psycho-Acoustic Laboratory began its operation in 1940, more than a year before the Japanese attack on Pearl Harbor. My research has been supported by public funds continuously ever since, which probably makes me the oldest non-stop scientific dole in existence.

The process started when a Captain Dent of the Air Force called a meeting of some experts in acoustics to ask what could be done to quiet the intense noise in military aircraft, which was thought by some to cause pilot error in landings after long flights. The captain wanted some research done. A young physics instructor, L. L. Beranek, had prepared an estimate of the equipment he would need to study airplane quieting. He could borrow most of the instruments, but if he were to employ a part-time assistant, he would need at least a couple of thousand dollars. The captain asked how much faster it could be done with ten times that much money. Beranek gulped and said, a lot faster. "Speed is what we need," said the captain. He then turned to me and asked whether a project to determine the effects of noise would need to be at least as large. I allowed that it would. Two young scientists reeled out of that meeting, dazed and incredulous, for we had never conceived of so much money for research.

Next began a frantic hunt for a place to make a noise. Led by the chief of buildings and grounds, R. B. Johnson, I searched through attics and basements in every Harvard building that appeared at all likely to yield a laboratory, and even considered walling off a section under the stadium. We were growing thoroughly discouraged when Johnson hit upon it. "Let's look in Memorial Hall," he said. Harvard's flamboyant Gothic edifice had been built in 1875 in order, as William James said, to dispense honor to the dead and food to the living. Down among the reaches of abandoned kitchens we found a huge furnace room, unused since 1915 and black with soot. I said no, but Johnson argued that he could tear out the pipes, pave the floor, and produce a first-rate laboratory. He was right.

We put subjects in the furnace room and pummeled them with 7-hour noise exposures at 115 dB. The subjects went from test to test through a battery of tasks designed to measure everything we could think of. We proved that the noise did nothing to performance, but it produced a temporary hearing loss. More important, when we tried to use the standard aircraft intercoms to communicate in the noise, the results were so bad that the design and testing of communication gear became the focus of our research. By the time Germany surrendered, all components of the intercoms had been redesigned. The tail gunner could now understand what the pilot was hollering about, even at high altitude. He was aided by an earphone cushion that was patented in my name and produced in vast quantity. For the patent rights, I was supposed to receive $1.00 from the government. I am still waiting.

As the Psycho-Acoustic Laboratory expanded to include some 50 people, more and more of the subterranean space under Memorial Hall – "inter-cellar space," it was called by Licklider – found itself partitioned and made usable. I hired a carpenter and we did much of the work with our own hands.

Then after the war the Provost, Paul Buck, allotted us $150000 to finish the rest of the basement, plus the upstairs serving kitchens, in order to create room for the Psychological Laboratories, which could thereupon relinquish Emerson Hall to the new Department of Social Relations. The Provost exacted a promise that I would never ask for any more space. Two decades later a new president, Nathan Pusey, forced me to move out of that wonderful basement laboratory and into an office tower named for William James. Administrations, I have learned, have no memory.

Why did they create a new Department of Social Relations, or why, as a sociologist grumbled, did they move the disaffected professors into Sociology? There are many theories, but whatever the potential causes, the critical incident turned, I think, on the vote of the Psychology Department to require mathematics as well as statistics in the examinations for the Ph.D. The chairman, G. W. Allport, our most eminent social psychologist, opposed the motion, but it carried. Allport had never lost before, and shortly thereafter we began to hear talk of secession.

Earlier in my career, one of the instructors had taken delight in issuing periodic warnings that I should move out of Harvard because the chairman would never promote me. The instructor was correct, in a sense. Allport opposed my promotion in a long letter that detailed my shortcomings, a chief one of which was my open disparagement of teaching. Another was the aversion shown me by some of the students.

Since President Conant thought that insight might mend the defects, he discussed the letter with me. Allport was right, of course, for in neither temperament nor appearance am I the outgoing teacher. A constraining shyness, a longish face, and a low tolerance for prattle have too often defeated my efforts at affability. "Qu'il est sévère!" the Belgians used to say. A treasured need for solitude frequently overrides my need for people, and I have often sensed the bitter sweetness of melancholy. I told Conant, as I had already told Allport, that I would teach my courses faithfully, but to enjoy standing before classes was beyond my power.

Actually, two forms of teaching give me great joy: the joint endeavor of laboratory apprenticeship, and editorial give and take. In those two ways I seem always to be teaching. But deans count you at work only when you stand before a group with your mouth moving.

The promotion to a tenured position was made in 1944, without benefit of Conant's famous procedure of first convening an extradepartmental *ad hoc* committee to consider all potential candidates. "Sometimes," said Conant, "we feel competent to make the judgment ourselves." That was good to hear, for Conant had assured me four years earlier that there was no opening and no possibility of my remaining at Harvard, despite Boring's exertions in my behalf. My assistant professorship was to be considered terminal. Pearl Harbor changed all that.

The war finally over, I got around to publishing the prewar work on the theory of scales of measurement, but then began seven lean years.

Other people saw those seven years as rich and full of achievement. They could not sense the gnawing fear that the fire was spent, that science, the jealous mistress I had abandoned for war research, had now abandoned me, so that no new fruit would fall. There were honors, to be sure, and the Psycho-Acoustic Laboratory grew renowned for the eminence of its roster. Three different agencies vied to give us financial support, and since I served as chief mentor, I was later awarded a plaque and $1000 by the Beltone Institute to signal my accomplishments as an educator! There was election to the National Academy of Sciences while still in my thirties, to be followed by the chairmanship of a division of the National Research Council. That meant commuting to Washington and sitting on numerous Boards, Committees, Study Sections, and Panels. I was becoming a wheel in the bureaucratic busy work – the overhead of science. And when President Eisenhower invited a score of scientists to a State Dinner at the White House, I was among them, in white tie and tails. But somehow the road to Washington glittered less and less.

In my 42nd year I took up skiing – on a pair of elderly boards that someone had left in the laboratory. That imprudence led to Silver Lake, New Hampshire, and the purchase of an old farmhouse abandoned by a 75-year-old lady because nothing worked. Friends, students, and colleagues pitched in to renovate the place and turn it into a ski lodge with 18 beds, a pool table, and a practice ski slope out behind the barn. If happiness had once seemed an endless fairway, it now seemed an endless snowfield. But skis, I found, left much to be desired, and I began to experiment with them and to write articles for ski magazines. Since ski length was a principal variable, I cut some 18 pairs to various sizes, ranging from 2 feet upward, and determined that my standard skis had been twice too long. My new 40-inch skis have made the wonders of the high Alps into an alluring playground for a sexagenarian who skis in spite of the exercise.

I am really not a mesomorph, managing only a 4-4-4 in somatotype, an almost equal distribution among the three components of physique: fat, muscle, and lean. Sheldon says I am lucky, because with only a 4 in mesomorphy I have been spared the monkey trap of serious athletic competition. I could never quite make the team. But it sometimes seems as though a balance among the three components puts you on a horse that tries to gallop off in three directions at once.

Three of the seven lean years were squandered on the *Handbook of Experimental Psychology*. The writing, editing, and rewriting of that million-word tome was a consuming chore – enlivened and lightened by the excellence of the contributors, 17 of whom have won election to the National Academy of Sciences. Most of the editing really fell to Geraldine Stone, who has ministered to the laboratory since its inception in 1940, and who became my wife in 1963. To celebrate that event our friends held a champagne reception on the snowfield near the summit of Mount Washington, and we then skied down Tuckerman's Ravine.

How do you break into research of your own when you have passed middle age and have grown rusty from directing others? In 1953 the barriers seemed firm. If I started to pick up a piece of apparatus, my shop assistants wanted to do it for me. How could I grasp my own soldering iron to fix a loose connection when my desk bloomed with important papers pressing for attention? Could I risk looking foolish on a piece of research that might flop, while at the same time my presence was wanted at the riskless tables of high council? If you insist on doing your own research, you have to perform the trivial and forsake the grand.

Actually, it was a former student who rescued me. W. R. Garner had conducted some very thorough experiments on the equisection and fractionation of loudness, two problems that had concerned me off and on for two decades. Could it be that equisection and fractionation gave results that differed as much as Garner seemed to find? What good is a scale of subjective loudness if intervals disagree with ratios? The problem troubled me so much that in the spring of 1953 I took over a small room, assembled some apparatus, and began to run subjects. Everyone who passed the door was hauled in and asked to make loudness judgments. Once again I was doing my own research!

One day during a coffee break Richard Held accused me of acting as though a person has a built-in loudness scale from which values can be read. That was an interesting idea. Why not try it? I presented a series of sound intensities in irregular order, and Held assigned numbers to them, apparently with no trouble at all. That method, magnitude estimation, which calls for the matching of numbers to perceived intensity, was soon to transform psychophysics. The procedure of matching subjective impressions is so simple, and yet so powerful. Why are the simplest things the hardest to discover?

R. J. Herrnstein hired on as assistant that decisive summer of 1953, and together we found ourselves working all day and half the night. To me it was like living again, thinking up new experiments and rushing to complete them. A curious effect (hysteresis) occurred in loudness bisections, and we wondered whether the effect would occur in visual brightness. We found a box – a rat shipping cage – cut a hole in one end, inserted some lamps, and before the day was done we had satisfied ourselves that hysteresis occurs also in vision. We rigged the laboratory projector so that subjects could make magnitude estimations of brightness, and we carried equipment upstairs to the lecture hall where a summer school class matched numbers to the brightness of a spot projected on a screen.

The summer over, Herrnstein went back to his pigeons, and I was left with sheets of data that seemed somehow to be trying to tell me something. There was contradiction and confusion in the evidence, but the main trend emerged strong enough to push the message through: in both vision and hearing the subjective magnitude of the sensation grows as a power function of the stimulus intensity. Not only that, but the two modalities, vision and hearing, seem to have the same exponent, namely, $\frac{1}{3}$. I ventured to put that finding on record in *Science* (November 13, 1953) and to tell about it at the autumn meeting of the National Academy of Sciences.

No one seemed much impressed, as I recall, nor did it appear to me that anything especially startling had been discovered. Perhaps my power law would merely join the long parade of claims that psychophysicists had made since that day when Fechner lay abed on October 22, 1850, and conjectured a logarithmic law for the growth of sensation. Anyhow, it was good to be back at work.

So good, in fact, that I canceled a sabbatical leave for which arrangements had been made to spend a year at the Institute for Advanced Study at Princeton. When I explained the dilemma to the director, Robert Oppenheimer, he agreed that I should stay with the research. "You must lick that pot clean," he said. But he promised a rain check.

I finally got around to a sabbatical leave in 1966, thirty years after I first became an instructor. Even then, my wife and I left the laboratory only for a 3-week tour of nine Alpine ski resorts in France, Italy, and Switzerland. Didi and I have introduced short skis to skeptical Europeans by skiing the slopes arm in arm.

By 1958 the measurement of sensation was going so well that the seven lean years had become only a cankered memory, but I still clung to some of the protective baggage of boards and committees, despite a growing distaste for paper shuffling. You can tell whether you are a scientist by noting what you do first each day: tend the experiment or read the mail. When my letters began to threaten a hopeless disarray, I wrote a batch of letters and resigned from all but one distraction. That distraction was the Space Science Board, which was trying to hold the space program together until Congress could set up NASA. Early in 1960 I resigned from the Space Science Board too. That cleaned the slate, and by August of that year a nine-chapter monograph on visual brightness had been completed, with J. C. Stevens (no relation) as co-author.

Research must feed on itself if it is to hold its excitement. One discovery must lead to another, with serendipity calling the turns. Over and over for 30 years I have had to stop and write a project proposal for the next year's funds – they ask you to predict what research will get done. Save for the first few years during World War II, I have chalked up a near perfect score: unless already half completed, the research fancied in the project proposal has never been performed. Something more exciting has always turned up when the time came to set to work – something no project proposal could have foreseen.

How could I have foreseen that every sense modality would respond according to a power law – what some of the textbooks now call Stevens' law? (It would of course delight any scientist to see his name become an eponym, if history so decided.) How could it have been foretold that a simple quantitative invariance would describe the operation of every sensory system that we have been able to stimulate? That basic invariance can be stated very simply: equal stimulus ratios produce equal subjective ratios. And the procedures that have served to confirm the invariance have also been used to scale many nonsensory variables, ranging from the prestige of occupations to the seriousness of crimes. That too lay beyond the reach of project-proposal prophecy.

In the 17 years since 1953, research in psychophysics has disclosed important but unsuspected human capacities. The normal sentient observer turns out to be a marvelous matching instrument. With surprising consistency he can assign numbers to any aspect of nature that appears to him to vary in degree, and he can make the numbers proportional to the strength of his subjective impressions. Already more than 40 perceptual continua have been scaled by simple number matching – magnitude estimation, as it is called. Equally important, the human subject can match any variable to any other variable, such as apparent loudness to apparent brightness, or force of handgrip to warmth on the skin, or apparent duration to apparent area, and so on. The demonstrated success of such cross-modality matching means that the interrelations among all subjective variables can be quantified. Definitive descriptions of the operating characteristics of all the sensory systems are placed within reach. Much remains to be done. The prospect excites me.

Epilogue

I break off here, just as I begin my 65th year, in order to comment on the design of the foregoing career and to inquire what residues, if any, give promise of survival.

The career itself exhibits no plan or purpose, no overreaching strategy, only tactical maneuvers brought on when circumstance has confronted desire. A series of accidents, in fact. Any man's life builds on a succession of accidents. That explains only part of it, however, for among the chance encounters there are some that take effect, whereas against other exposures a person stands as though inoculated with some natural antibody, as though his ingrained nature has created immunity to alien rhetoric. One man's great teacher scores as another man's humbug.

Accidents of time and juncture seem to have determined the content of my career, including, of course, the languages spoken and the principles learned. You cannot study discoveries yet to be made. But a replay of all the circumstances with a different man on scene would probably not have produced a professor of psychophysics. The students who fail to warm to the virtues of that subject are legion, which is good, for it averts the disaster of everybody's crowding in to toil at the same bench.

As an undergraduate I wallowed joyfully in the verbal compost of philosophy and the social sciences. Why did that exposure not produce a sociologist, or something similar? Why am I now put off by the chanting of a hypersyllabic idiom in which social scientists make nouns into modifiers, and correlation into causation? A man is a hunter, not for the food that our ancestors had to seek, but for the consonant path of life. Some men can sniff the agreeable trail first off, but others must keep on hunting decade after decade to locate the congenial calling.

As I write these lines on floor 9 in a tower named for William James, I look down on his house on Irving Street, where his grandson once presented me with a New Hampshire scene painted by William James, Jr., artist son of William. Think how

William James struggled to locate his proper pursuit. He went through medical school, became instructor in physiology, and set up a laboratory of psychophysics. But then he drifted slowly into philosophy. His nature was coded by a template vastly different from mine, for my drift has been in the opposite direction. I started where James finished and finish where James began. Floor 9 is now called the Laboratory of Psychophysics. Had we been contemporaries at Harvard, our concerns might have coincided momentarily – perhaps where James shifted his interest from the physiology of emotion to the psychology of will.

Despite excursions here and there, my career has centered on the psychophysics of sensory function, which was once central to experimental psychology, but which may now stand so distant as to form a separate discipline. Students ask, why desert psychology? It is quite the other way: psychology has deserted psychophysics. There are now more than 30000 psychologists who probably care nothing about sensory measurement, nor about how the sense-organ transducers operate to bring about the miracle of sensation. Psychology has moved so far toward social relevance, and has spilled so widely into media and market place, that those who man the old-fashioned experimental workshop must find a new label for their métier. My own choice was to become Professor of Psychophysics, a title exacted from the University in 1962 as the price for my resignation as Director of the Psychological Laboratories. I was being fired for trying to obstruct what was then called progress – the transplanting of the laboratory.

We moved. I have stuck it out. Békésy tried for a couple of years to sustain his research activites, spread vertically over four floors served by reluctant elevators, but he finally tendered his resignation.

Is there any residue from my career that will interest the future? Who knows? On an airplane flight from Washington, following the State Dinner at which Eisenhower honored the scientists, the wife of the President's Science Advisor said, "What's the matter with you scientists, why do you think you have to leave something permanent?" That is a good question. Especially when our great historian of science, George Sarton, observed that science is progressive and therefore ephemeral, whereas art is nonprogressive and therefore eternal. Unlike the artist, the scientist engages in the business of putting both himself and his colleagues out of business. New discoveries negate old notions, fashions in thought stir new enthusiasms, and only a few principles pass on to become gospel for future generations.

Many of my intellectual products of the past four decades promise to give way to better formulation and thereby demonstrate their ephemeral character. Some of them may ebb, perhaps to return on another tide. The operational outlook, which seeks to equate the meaning of a term with the concrete operations that underly it, seems currently to have lost its vogue. Its day will probably come again, however, even if under a different banner, for the issue remains too basic to disappear.

The outcome of experimental work can always be improved. My loudness scale has been standardized by an international body, but already I am proposing to change it slightly. And the standard procedure for calculating the loudness of noise, a procedure employed to assess noise pollution, has been renovated in a paper I am now preparing. Such matters undergo continual change, although a few sturdy principles may stay put. One such principle seems to me to concern the direct relation between the subjective scale of pitch, measured in mels, and the location in the inner ear where the different sound frequencies produce their excitation. But here again, the measurements of both pitch and place can be improved.

Then what about permanent residue? History likes to make comedy out of predictions, but predictions tell at least how it seemed at the time. With that in mind, in this year 1970 I venture to suggest that the remainders of long-term interest may prove to be the two principles of invariance that I have tried to formulate: one that applies to scales of measurement, and one that governs the ratio relation between stimulus and sensation – the so-called power law. Other than that, what has there been except the joy of search and solution in the contest to decipher nature's ways, and the great good fun of carrying on?

S. S. STEVENS' BIBLIOGRAPHY

Major Articles

1934

The attributes of tones. *Proceedings of the National Academy of Science*, **20**, 457–459.

The localization of pure tones. *Proceedings of the National Academy of Science*, **20**, 593–596 (with E. B. Newman).

The relation of saturation to the size of the retinal image. *American Journal of Psychology*, **46**, 70–79.

Tonal density. *Journal of Experimental Psychology*, **17**, 585–592.

The volume and intensity of tones. *American Journal of Psychology*, **46**, 397–408.

1935

The localization of pitch perception on the basilar membrane. *Journal of General Psychology*, **13**, 297–315 (with H. Davis & M. H. Lurie).

The operational basis of psychology. *American Journal of Psychology*, **47**, 323–330.

The operational definition of psychological concepts. *Psychological Review*, **42**, 517–527.

The relation of pitch to intensity. *Journal of the Acoustical Society of America*, **6**, 150–154.

1936

The localization of actual sources of sound. *American Journal of Psychology*, **48**, 297–306 (with E. B. Newman).

On the nature of aural harmonics. *Proceedings of the National Academy of Science*, **22**, 668–672 (with E. B. Newman).

The nature of tonal brightness. *Proceedings of the National Academy of Science*, **22**, 514–521 (with E. G. Boring).

Psychology: The propaedeutic science. *Philosophy of Science*, **3**, 90–103.

Psychophysiological acoustics: Pitch and loudness. *Journal of the Acoustical Society of America*, **8**, 1–13 (with H. Davis).

The psychophysiology of hearing. *Proceedings of the American Society of the Hard of Hearing*, **17**, 30–35.

A scale for the measurement of a psychological magnitude: Loudness. *Psychological Review*, **43**, 405–416.

1937

Cardiac acceleration in emotional situations. *Journal of Experimental Psychology*, **21**, 72–87 (with J. G. Beebe-Center).

H. R. Moskowitz et al. (eds.), Sensation and Measurement. 447–455.

1937

Factors in the production of aural harmonics and combination tones. *Journal of the Acoustical Society of America*, **9**, 107–118 (with E. B. Newman & H. Davis).

On hearing by electrical stimulation. *Journal of the Acoustical Society of America*, **8**, 191–195.

On the method of bisection and its relation to a loudness scale. *American Journal of Psychology*, **49**, 134–137 (with J. Volkmann & E. B. Newman).

A scale for the measurement of psychological magnitude: Pitch. *Journal of the Acoustical Society of America*, **8**, 185–190 (with J. Volkmann & E. B. Newman).

1938

The emotional responses: Changes of heart rate in a gun-shy dog. *Journal of Experimental Psychology*, **23**, 239–257 (with J. G. Beebe-Center).

On the pitch of frequency-modulated tones. *American Journal of Psychology*, **51**, 521–526 (with R. E. P. Youtz).

1939

The mechanism of hearing by electrical stimulation. *Journal of the Acoustical Society of America*, **10**, 261–269 (with R. C. Jones).

Psychology and the science of science. *Psychological Bulletin*, **36**, 221–263.

1940

The quantum of sensory discrimination. *Science*, **92**, 583–585 (with J. Volkmann).

The relation of pitch to frequency: A revised scale. *American Journal of Psychology*, **53**, 329–353 (with J. Volkmann).

Three mechanisms of hearing by electrical stimulation. *Journal of the Acoustical Society of America*, **12**, 281–290 (with R. C. Jones and M. H. Lurie).

1941

Theory of the neural quantum in the discrimination of loudness and pitch. *American Journal of Psychology*, **54**, 315–335 (with C. T. Morgan & J. Volkmann).

1942

Rectilinear rectification applied to voltage integration. *Electronics* (Jan.), **15**, 40–41.

1943

Vision, hearing and aeronautical design. *Journal of Aeronautical Science*, **10**, 127–130 (with L. D. Carson & W. R. Miles).

1946

Machines cannot fight alone. *American Scientist*, **34**, 389–400.

The masking of speech by sine waves, square waves, and regular and modulated pulses. *Journal of the Acoustical Society of America*, **18**, 418–424 (with J. Miller & I. Truscott).

The science of noise. *Atlantic Monthly*, **178** (1), 96.

The selection of hearing aids. *Laryngoscope*, **56**, 85–115, 135–163 (with H. Davis *et al.*).

On the theory of scales of measurement. *Science*, **103**, 677–680.

1947

Methods of measuring speech spectra. *Journal of the Acoustical Society of America*, **19**, 771–780 (with J. P. Egan & G. A. Miller).

The new Harvard Psychological Laboratories. *American Psychologist*, **2**, 239–243 (with E. G. Boring).

Premodulation clipping in AM voice communication. *Journal of the Acoustical Society of America*, **19**, 125–131 (with K. D. Kryter & J. C. R. Licklider).

Psychological writing, easy and hard. *American Psychologist*, **2**, 230–235 (with G. Stone).

1948

A psychological scale of weight and a formula for its derivation. *American Journal of Psychology*, **61**, 343–351 (with R. S. Harper).

1950

The masking of pure tones and of speech by white noise. *Journal of the Acoustical Society of America*, **22**, 6–13 (with J. E. Hawkins, Jr.).

1951

Mathematics, measurement, and psychophysics. In S. S. Stevens (Ed.), *Handbook of experimental psychology*. New York: Wiley, pp. 1–49.

1952

The NAS-NRC and psychology. *American Psychologist*, **7**, 119–124.

1954

Biological transducers. *Convention Records of the Institute of Radio Engineers*, Pt. 9, 27–33.
The ear and the eye (El oido y la vista). *Acta Prima Congresso Extraordinario Sociedad Internationale Audiolojico*, Buenos Aires, pp. 408–416.
Pitch discrimination, mels, and Kock's contention. *Journal of the Acoustical Society of America*, **26**, 1075–1077.

1955

Apparent reduction of loudness: a repeat experiment. *Journal of the Acoustical Society of America*, **27**, 326–328 (with M. S. Rogers and R. J. Herrnstein).
On the averaging of data. *Science*, **121**, 113–116.
Decibels of light and sound. *Physics Today*, **8** (10), 12–17.
On the halving and doubling of the loudness of white noise. *Journal of the Acoustical Society of America*, **27**, 329–331 (with E. C. Poulton).
The measurement of loudness. *Journal of the Acoustical Society of America*, 27, 815–829

1956

Calculation of the loudness of complex noise. *Journal of the Acoustical Society of America*, **28**, 807–832.
The direct estimation of sensory magnitudes – loudness. *American Journal of Psychology*, **69**, 1–25.
The estimation of loudness by unpracticed observers. *Journal of Experimental Psychology*, **51**, 71–78 (with E. C. Poulton).

1957

Calculating loudness. *Noise Control*, **3** (5), 11–22.
Concerning the form of the loudness function. *Journal of the Acoustical Society of America*, **29**, 603–606.
Critical bandwidth in loudness summation. *Journal of the Acoustical Society of America*, **29**, 548–557 (with E. Zwicker & G. Flottorp).
On the psychophysical law. *Psychological Review*, **64**, 153–181.
Ratio scales and category scales for a dozen perceptual continua. *Journal of Experimental Psychology*, **54**, 377–411 (with E. H. Galanter).

1958

Adaptation level vs. the relativity of judgment. *American Journal of Psychology*, **71**, 633–646.

Measurement and man. *Science*, **127**, 383–389.

Problems and methods of psychophysics. *Psychological Bulletin*, **55**, 177–196.

A scale of apparent intensity of electric shock. *Journal of Experimental Psychology*, **56**, 328–335 (with A. S. Carton & G. M. Shickman).

Some similarities between hearing and seeing. *Laryngoscope*, **68** (3), 508–527.

1959

Cross-modality validation of subjective scales for loudness, vibration, and electric shock. *Journal of Experimental Psychology*, **57**, 201–209.

Finger span: Ratio scale, category scale and jnd scale. *Journal of Experimental Psychology*, **57**, 91–95 (with G. Stone).

Measurement, psychophysics and utility. In C. W. Churchman & P. Ratoosh (Eds.), *Measurement: Definitions and theories*. New York: Wiley, pp. 18–64.

The quantification of sensation. *Daedalus*, Fall, **88** (4), 606–621.

Tactile vibration: Dynamics of sensory intensity. *Journal of Experimental Psychology*, **57**, 210–218.

On the validity of the loudness scale. *Journal of the Acoustical Society of America*, **31**, 995–1004.

1960

Binaural summation of loudness. *Journal of the Acoustical Society of America*, **32**, 1337–1344 (with G. S. Reynolds).

The dynamics of visual brightness. Harvard University: Psycho-Acoustic Laboratory, August (with J. C. Stevens).

Growth of sensation on seven continua as measured by force of handgrip. *Journal of Experimental Psychology*, **59**, 60–67 (with J. C. Stevens & J. D. Mack).

On the new psychophysics. *Scandinavian Journal of Psychology*, **1**, 27–35.

Ratio scales, partition scales and confusion scales. In H. Gulliksen & S. Messick (Eds.), *Psychological scaling: Theory and applications*. New York: Wiley, pp. 49–66.

Subjective intensity of coffee odor. *American Journal of Psychology*, **73**, 424–428 (with T. S. Reese).

Warmth and cold: Dynamics of sensory intensity. *Journal of Experimental Psychology*, **60**, 183–192 (with J. C. Stevens).

1961

The auditory input-output function. *Proceedings of the Third International Congress of Acoustics*. Amsterdam: Elsevier, pp. 78–80.

To honor Fechner and repeal his law. *Science*, **133**, 80–86.

Procedure for calculating loudness, Mark VI. *Journal of the Acoustical Society of America*, **33**, 1577–1585.

Psychophysics of sensory function. In W. A. Rosenblith (Ed.), *Sensory communication.* M.I.T. Press, Cambridge, Mass., pp. 1–33; *American Scientist*, 1960, **48**, 226–253.

Toward a resolution of the Fechner-Thurstone legacy. *Psychometrika*, **26**, 35–47.

Voice level: Autophonic scale, perceived loudness and the effects of sidetone. *Journal of the Acoustical Society of America*, **33**, 160–167 (with H. L. Lane & A. C. Catania).

1962

Loudness, reciprocality, and partition scales. *Journal of the Acoustical Society of America*, **34**, 1466–1471 (with M. Guirao).

In pursuit of the sensory law. Northwestern University: 2nd Klopsteg Lecture, November.

The quantification of tonal volume. *American Journal of Psychology*, **75**, 596–604 (with H. Terrace).

The scaling of subjective roughness and smoothness. *Journal of Experimental Psychology*, **64**, 489–494 (with J. R. Harris).

The surprising simplicity of sensory metrics. *American Psychologist*, **17**, 29–39.

1963

The basis of psychophysical judgments. *Journal of the Acoustical Society of America*, **35**, 611–612.

Brightness function: Effects of adaptation. *Journal of the Optical Society of America*, **53**, 375–385 (with J. C. Stevens).

The dynamics of subjective warmth and cold. In C. M. Herzfeld (Ed.), *Temperature – Its measurement and control in science and industry*. New York: Reinhold, Vol. 3, Part 3, pp. 239–243 (with J. C. Stevens).

Subjective scaling of length and area and the matching of length to loudness and brightness. *Journal of Experimental Psychology*, **66**, 177–186 (with M. Guirao).

1964

Concerning the psychophysical power law. *Quarterly Journal of Experimental Psychology*, **16**, 383–385.

Measurement of auditory density. *Journal of the Acoustical Society of America*, **36**, 1176–1182 (with M. Guirao).

Relation of brightness to duration and luminance under light- and dark-adaptation. *Vision Research*, **4**, 391–401 (with T. S. Aiba) .

Scaling of apparent viscosity. *Science*, **144**, 1157–1158 (with M. Guirao).

Sensory transform functions. In R. W. Gerard & J. W. Duyff (Eds.), *Information processing in the nervous system*. Excerpta Medica, pp. 53–60.

Subjective hardness of compliant materials. *Quarterly Journal of Experimental Psychology*, **16**, 204–215 (with R. Harper).

1965

Effect of glare angle on the brightness function for a small target. *Vision Research*, **5**, 649–659 (with A. L. Diamond).

Loudness, a product of volume times density. *Journal of Experimental Psychology*, **69**, 503–510 (with M. Guirao & A. W. Slawson).

On the uses of poikilitic functions. In D. I. Mostofsky (Ed.), *Stimulus generalization*. Stanford University Press, pp. 24–29.

1966

Duration, luminance, and the brightness exponent. *Perception and Psychophysics*, **1**, 96–100.

Matching functions between loudness and ten other continua. *Perception and Psychophyscis*, **1**, 5–8.

A metric for the social consensus. *Science*, **151**, 530–541.

On the operation known as judgment. *American Scientist*, **54**, 385–401.

Operations or words? *Psychological Monographs*, **80**, No. 627, 33–38.

Power-group transformations under glare, masking, and recruitment. *Journal of the Acoustical Society of America*, **39**, 725–735.

Quantifying the sensory experience. In P. Feyerabend & G. Maxwell (Eds.), *Mind, matter, and method*. University of Minnesota Press, pp. 215–233.

Regression effect in psychophysical judgment. *Perception and Psychophysics*, **1**, 439–446 (with H. B. Greenbaum).

Saturation of red: A prothetic continuum. *Perception and Psychophysics*, **1**, 59–66 (with D. Panek).

Scaling of saturation and hue. *Perception and Psychophysics*, **1**, 253–272 (with T. Indow).

Transfer functions of the skin and muscle senses. Ciba Foundation Symposium on *Touch, heat and pain*. London: J. & A. Churchill, pp. 3–17.

1967

Intensity functions in sensory systems. *International Journal of Neurology*, **6**, 202–209.

Loudness functions under inhibition. *Perception and Psychophysics*, **2**, 459–465 (with M. Guirao).

Masking and sensory dynamics. In *Acoustic noise and its control*, Institute of Electrical Engineers Conference, Publication 26, January, pp. 1–3.

1968

Edwin Garrigues Boring: 1886–1968. *American Journal of Psychology*, **81**, 589–606.

Measurement, statistics, and the schemapiric view. *Science*, **161**, 849–856.

Psychophysics and the measurement of loudness. *Sixth International Congress of Acoustics*, Tokyo, Japan.

Le quantitatif et la perception. *Bulletin de Psychologie*, 1968–69, **22**, 696–715.

Ratio scales of opinion. In D. K. Whitla (Ed.), *Handbook of measurement and assessment in behavioral sciences*. Reading, Mass.: Addison-Wesley, pp. 171–199.

Tactile vibration: Change of exponent with frequency. *Perception and Psychophysics*, **3**, 223–228.

1969

Cross-modality matching of brightness to loudness by 5-year-olds. *Perception and Psychophysics*, **6**, 337–339 (with B. Bond).

Measurement and social science. *et al.* [sic], **2** (1), 5–6.

On predicting exponents for cross-modality matches. *Perception and Psychophysics*, **6**, 251–256.

Sensory scales of taste intensity. *Perception and Psychophysics*, **6**, 302–308.

1970

Neural events and the psychophysical law. *Science*, **170**, 1043–1050.

On the quantitative evaluation of noise. In J. D. Chalupnik (Ed.), *Transportation noises: A symposium on acceptability criteria*. Seattle: University of Washington Press, pp. 114–128.

1971

Issues in psychophysical measurement. *Psychological Review*, **78**, 426–450.

Sensory power functions and neural events. In W. R. Loewenstein (Ed.), *Handbook of sensory physiology, Vol. 1*. Berlin: Springer-Verlag, pp. 226–242.

1972

Calculating the perceived level of light and sound. *Journal of Sound and Vibration*, **23**, 297–306.

A neural quantum in sensory discrimination. *Science*, **177**, 749–762.

Perceived level of noise by Mark VII and decibels (E). *Journal of the Acoustical Society of America*, **51**, 575–601.

Psychophysics and social scaling. General Learning Press, Morristown, New Jersey, 27 pp.

Stability of human performance under intense noise. *Journal of Sound and Vibration*, **21**, 35–56.

In Press

Notes for a life story. In *History of Psychology in Autobiography*, Vol. 6. Appleton-Century-Crofts.

Perceptual magnitude and its measurement. In E. C. Carterette & M. P. Friedman (Eds.), *Handbook of perception*, Vol. 2. New York: Academic Press.

Books

Hearing, its psychology and physiology. New York: Wiley, 1938 (with H. Davis).

The varieties of human physique. New York: Harper, 1940 (with W. H. Sheldon & W. B. Tucker).

The varieties of temperament. New York: Harper, 1942 (with W. H. Sheldon).

Transmission and reception of sounds under combat conditions. (Summary Technical Report of NDRC Div. 17, Vol. 17-3). Washington, 1946 (with G. A. Miller & F. M. Wiener).

Hearing aids. An experimental study of design objectives. Cambridge: Harvard University Press, 1947 (with H. Davis *et al.*).

Handbook of experimental psychology (Ed.). New York: Wiley, 1951.

Bibliography on hearing. Cambridge: Harvard University Press, 1955 (with J. C. G. Loring & D. Cohen).

Sound and hearing. New York: Time, Inc., 1965 (with F. Warshofsky and the Editors of *Life*).

Psychophysics (in preparation, being prepared for posthumous publication by G. Stevens).

INDEX OF NAMES

INDEX OF SUBJECTS